Optometry A–Z

To Suzanne, Zoe and Bruce

For Elsevier Butterworth-Heinemann:

Commissioning Editor: Robert Edwards
Development Editor: Kim Benson
Project Managers: David Fleming, Christine Johnston
Design: Stewart Larking
Grading scale artwork: Terry R. Tarrant
Schematic artwork: Kathy Underwood and Lisa Dixon of J&L Composition Ltd
Illustrator: Ian Ramsden
Illustration Manager: Gillian Murray

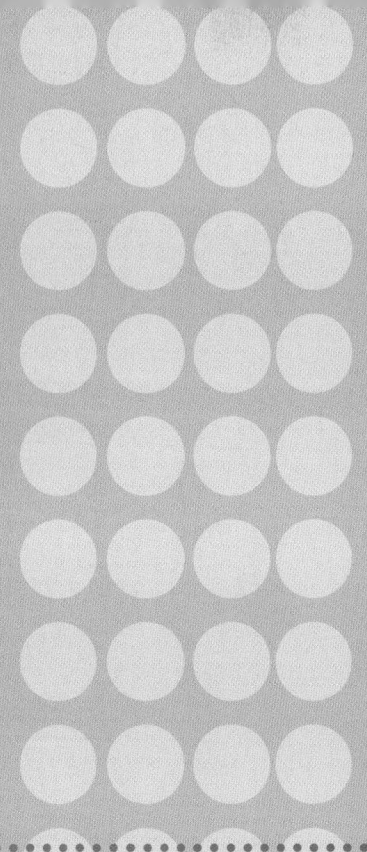

Optometry A–Z

Edited by

NATHAN EFRON

BScOptom PhD DSc
FAAO (Dip CL) FIACLE FCLSA FBCLA ILTM

Research Professor
School of Optometry
and
Institute of Health and Biomedical Innovation
Queensland University of Technology
Brisbane, Australia

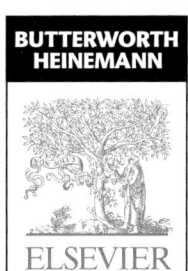

EDINBURGH   LONDON   NEW YORK   OXFORD   PHILADELPHIA   ST LOUIS   SYDNEY   TORONTO   2007

BUTTERWORTH
HEINEMANN
ELSEVIER

© 2007, Elsevier Limited. All rights reserved.
First published 2007

The right of Nathan Efron to be identified as author of this work has been asserted by him in accordance with the Copyright, Designs and Patents Act 1988

No part of this publication may be reproduced, stored in a retrieval system, or transmitted in any form or by any means, electronic, mechanical, photocopying, recording or otherwise, without the prior permission of the Publishers. Permissions may be sought directly from Elsevier's Health Sciences Rights Department, 1600 John F. Kennedy Boulevard, Suite 1800, Philadelphia, PA 19103-2899, USA: phone: (+1) 215 239 3804; fax: (+1) 215 239 3805; or, e-mail: healthpermissions@elsevier.com. You may also complete your request on-line via the Elsevier homepage (http://www.elsevier.com), by selecting 'Support and contact' and then 'Copyright and Permission'.

ISBN-13: 978-0-7506-4913-1
ISBN-10: 0-7506-4913-5

British Library Cataloguing in Publication Data
A catalogue record for this book is available from the British Library.

Library of Congress Cataloging in Publication Data
A catalog record for this book is available from the Library of Congress.

Note
Neither the Publisher nor the Editor assume any responsibility for any loss or injury and/or damage to persons or property arising out of or related to any use of the material contained in this book. It is the responsibility of the treating practitioner, relying on independent expertise and knowledge of the patient, to determine the best treatment and method of application for the patient.

The Publisher

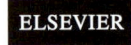

ELSEVIER your source for books, journals and multimedia in the health sciences

www.elsevierhealth.com

Working together to grow
libraries in developing countries

www.elsevier.com | www.bookaid.org | www.sabre.org

ELSEVIER   BOOK AID International   Sabre Foundation

The publisher's policy is to use paper manufactured from sustainable forests

Printed in Spain

Contents

Dedication   *ii*
Preface   *vi*
Acknowledgements   *vii*
Associate Editors   *viii*
Contributors   *ix*

A–Z   1

APPENDICES

A Reported ocular side effects of selected systemically administered drugs   395

B Optometric grading scales   399

C Efron grading scales for contact lens complications   401

D Vertex distance correction   406

E Extended keratometer range conversion   408

F Corneal curvature – corneal power conversion   410

G Contact lens manufacturing tolerances   412

H Contact lens terms, symbols and abbreviations   414

Preface

The practices and procedures that define optometry are constantly evolving. This evolution can be attributed to a number of factors, such as emerging technologies, advances in our understanding of the normal and abnormal eye, changes in the eye care needs of our patients, modifications to the regulatory framework of the health professions and continual redefining of the way in which governments choose to organize the provision of health care generally.

New textbooks of optometry need to reflect this constant state of flux, and indeed that is the aim of this book. The classic textbook approach is to provide a thorough account of the field, organized into chapters, and offering a discursive overview of different topics and themes, supplemented by numerous illustrations, pictures, tables and reference sources. This work is designed to supplement conventional books by providing an easily accessible ready-reference source for information about all aspects of optometric practice. Entries are set out alphabetically in what is more of an encyclopedic than a dictionary approach. Thus, in comparison to a dictionary of the same size and covering the same material, Optometry A–Z contains fewer entries, but each entry is of greater length. Therefore, there are few narrow 'technical definitions' in this book; rather, the entries tend to cover more general themes. It is hoped that this book will be a useful aid to students who need a quick explanation of a key term during a lecture or period of study, and to practitioners who require rapid access to material in the course of their clinical work.

Thus, this is a true reference text that is not really designed to be read from cover to cover.

As with any reference book of this kind, decisions have had to be made concerning which entries to include and which to leave out, how extensive the various entries should be, and what terminology should be used to describe a given concept, idea or technique. I have tried to give appropriate weighting to entries to reflect their current importance in the field, and to adopt the terminology that is most widely used. Thus, while this book covers all aspects of optometry, it can not cover every topic within the various aspects. For example, it is not possible in a book such as this to describe every known eye disease; instead, the most common eye problems – and especially those of more immediate interest to optometric practice – are covered. Extensive cross-referencing and the incorporation of alternative terminology (cited alphabetically with cross-references to the primary entry) will hopefully allow readers to quickly find the information they are seeking.

The layout of the book is straightforward. Each term is set in blue type, and the descriptive text follows in plain black type. Useful cross-references are sometimes given at the conclusion of an entry, and occasionally key synonyms and antonyms are provided.

I hope that students and practitioners of optometry will find this to be a valuable reference source.

Nathan Efron

Acknowledgements

I am grateful for the continuing support provided by Butterworth-Heinemann – especially Caroline Makepeace, Robert Edwards and Kim Benson. Book production really is a team effort, and the help and advice I receive from the Butterworth-Heinemann team are very much appreciated.

Over many years, my family – Suzanne, Zoe and Bruce – have allowed me to indulge in my passion for textbook writing, and I shall be forever grateful. I am especially thankful to Suzanne for all her efforts in assisting at the proof-reading stage.

Special thanks must go to my team of Associate Editors, who are listed on page viii. All of these colleagues have written authoritative textbooks in their chosen areas of expertise, and I am honoured that they have agreed to share their knowledge by way of preparing entries relating to these specialist areas. My Associate Editors and I have been assisted by numerous other colleagues (see list of 'Contributors' listed on page ix), whose indirect contributions are also greatly appreciated.

Photographs and illustrations are an integral part of an academic textbook, and in this regard I wish to pay tribute to the extraordinary clinical insights and technical skills of my many colleagues who have supplied photographs and illustrations of outstanding quality. The clinical photographers and illustrators I refer to are:

Joe Barr, Figures H.5 and H.6; Biocompatibles-Hydron, Figure S.19; Adrian Bruce, Figures I.4–7, K.5 and V.5; Hilmar Bussaker, Figures P.21, I.6 and I.7; Leo Carney, Figure R.9; Patrick Caroline, Figures D.4*, L.6*, N.1* and O.2*; W. Neil Charman, Figures A.1, D.5, E.4, F.3, H.2, O.5 and S.10; Suzanne Fleiszig, Figures O.1 and P.22; Des Fonn, Figures F.7*, P.23* and S.16*; Andrew Gasson, Figure K.4*; Tim Grant, Figure S.5*; Nizar Hirji, Figure F.1; Brien Holden, Figure W.3*; Sarah Hosking, Debbie Jones, Figures B.2* and C.9*; Lyndon Jones, Figures I.1–3, M.1*, N.2, N.3, O.3, O.4, P.1, P.2, P.8, S.7, S.8, S.12 and S.19*; Jan Kok, Figure P.16*; John Lawrenson, Figures C.6, C.11, C.13, E.13, G.1, L.2, L.5 and O.6; Richard Lindsay, Figures S.14 and S.15; Ron Loveridge, Figure D.3; Philip B. Morgan, Figures B.4, E.5, F.8, H.3, H.7, M.7, R.10, S.2, S.11, T.2 and T.7; Sarah Morgan, Figure P.9; John Mountford, Figure O.7; Eric Papas, Figure L.7; RD Parashar, Figure P.12*; Sudi Patel, Figures I.9, K.6, R.3 and S.1; Richard Pearson, Figure M.6; Frank Pettigrew, Figure E.12*; Ken Pullum, Figures T.4 and T.5; Trevor Rowley, Figure P.17; Ralph Salazar, Figure R.1*; Maki Shiobara, Figure P.7*; Sarita Soni, Figure R.4*; Luigina Sorbara, Figure K.3*; Joe Tanner, Figures L.4 and P.13; Rob Terry, Figure V.2*; Brian Tighe, Figures P.14 and S.4; Brian Tompkins, Figures M.5, V.1 and NE-1; Cindy Tromans, Figures P.3–5; C Vervaet, Figure P.10*; Rients Visser, Figure S.3*; Barry Weissman, Figures K.2 and P.15; Craig Woods, Figure M.2*; Graeme Young, Figures D.8, E.1, E.2, F.4, F.7, F.9 and F.10; and Steve Zantos, Figures E.6 and E.7.

(*Courtesy of the Bausch & Lomb Contact Lens Slide Collection)

Associate Editors

Jennifer Birch, MPhil
Senior Lecturer
Department of Optometry and
Visual Science
The City University
London, UK

Adrian S Bruce, PhD
Chief Optometrist
Victorian College of Optometry
and
Department of Optometry and
Vision Sciences
University of Melbourne
Melbourne, Australia

Christine Dickinson, PhD
Professor of Clinical Optometry
Faculty of Life Sciences
The University of Manchester
Manchester, UK

Sandip Doshi, PhD
Optometrist
Surrey, UK

Colin Fowler, PhD
Senior Lecturer
School of Life and Health Sciences
Aston University
Birmingham, UK

William Harvey, BSc(Hons)
Director of Visual Impairment
Clinic
Department of Optometry and
Visual Science
The City University
London, UK

David Henson, PhD
Professor
Department of Ophthalmology
The University of Manchester
Manchester, UK

John Lawrenson, PhD
Professor
Department of Optometry and
Visual Science
The City University
London, UK

Rachel V North, PhD
Professor
School of Optometry and Vision
Sciences
Cardiff University
Cardiff, UK

Richard Pearson, MPhil
Optometrist
Kent, UK

Stephen Taylor, PhD
Optometrist
Dorset, UK

Contributors

Paul Adler
Alec Ansons
Joe Barr
Angela Bishop
Noel Brennan
Dick Bruenech
Adrian Bruce
Roger Buckley
Leo Carney
Pat Caroline
Neil Charman
Chantal Coles
Keith Edwards
Frank Eperjesi
Bruce Evans
Nizar Hirji
Sharon Ho
Milton Hom
Graham Hopkins
Sarah Hosking
Tony Hough
Adrian Jennings

Lyndon Jones
John Lawrenson
Richard Lindsay
Michael Loughnan
John Meyler
Philip Morgan
Sarah Morgan
Clare O'Donnell
Sudi Patel
Keziah Latham Petre
Ken Pullum
John Siderov
Alison Spencer
Loretta Szczotka
Joe Tanner
Brian Tighe
Cindy Tromans
Barry Weissman
Craig Woods
Graeme Young
Karla Zadnik

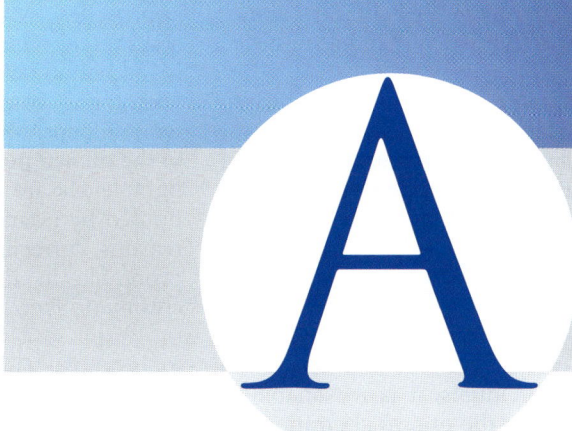

Aberration, chromatic

Since the refractive indices of all the ocular media vary with wavelength, the eye suffers a defect due to the unequal refraction of light of different wavelengths; this may manifest as longitudinal and transverse chromatic aberration. At the fovea, the former is more important – the amount of aberration approximating to that which would occur if the eye media were all water. Unlike the monochromatic aberrations, longitudinal chromatic aberration varies very little between individuals and equals about 2.00D across the visible spectrum. Since the visual axis is usually displaced from the nominal optical axis of the eye by about 5°, some transverse chromatic aberration is found at the fovea, amounting to about 36 sec arc; this further degrades foveal image quality.

Aberration control, rigid contact lens

The steep surface curvature of rigid lenses means that their major aberration in relation to foveal imagery ought to be spherical aberration. Although a well-centred aspheric contact lens might reduce the overall spherical aberration with respect to a lens with spherical surfaces, this advantage could break down if the lens decentred by more than about 1mm, when substantial amounts of coma and defocus could be introduced (depending upon the exact lens parameters involved). Image quality with a spherical lens is generally more robust against decentration. Although the effects of rigid lens spherical aberration on visual performance at photopic levels are generally small, there is some evidence that asphericities that optimize vision for the individual are appreciated by the wearer.

Aberration control, soft contact lens

For foveal vision and well-centred contact lenses having steeply curved surfaces, the classical aberration of greatest potential importance is spherical aberration, in which the power of the contact lens varies with distance from its axis. This is in contrast to spectacle lenses where, since the eye moves with respect to the lens, oblique astigmatism, distortion, field curvature and transverse chromatic aberration are all introduced whenever the visual axis moves away from the optical centre of the lens. Indeed, spherical aberration is of little importance in spectacle lenses, whereas control of the off-axis aberrations is a major design aim. With the exception of diffractive lenses for presbyopia, longitudinal chromatic aberration is normally of negligible importance in either spectacle or contact lens design, since any contribution from the correcting lens is much smaller than that of the eye itself.

The benefits of aspheric lens surfaces need to be considered in terms of the combined aberration of the lens-eye system; a contact lens with minimal spherical aberration does not necessarily lead to the best visual performance.

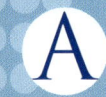

In principle, the aberration of the lens should balance that of the eye so that the combined system has minimal aberration.

With soft lenses, the draping of the lens to conform to the conicoidal corneal surface results in the anterior surface of the flexed lens retaining the natural benefit of peripheral corneal flattening in reducing spherical aberration. It is only if lenses are of high power (outside the range –6.00D – +3.00D) and pupils are large that amounts of spherical aberration will have a detectable impact on visual performance.

In the light of developments in our understanding of the wide variations in corneal contour and aberration found among different individuals, it is reasonable to suggest that the interaction of the optical aberrations of any particular design of soft lens with those of the eye is likely to vary with the individual, rather than being the same across all the population.

Although the concept of neutralizing the spherical aberration of the eye by that of the contact lens is attractive, the realities of the situation should be borne in mind. Most eyes do not suffer only from primary spherical aberration but have a complex mixture of regular and irregular aberrations. Movement and flexure of the soft lenses on the eyes may introduce additional asymmetric aberrations. Thus, correction of the spherical aberration component will still leave substantial uncorrected monochromatic aberration, together with chromatic aberration. It may be that the ocular aberration of a minority of eyes is amenable to correction; such patients may be identifiable in the future if simple routine measurement of individual ocular aberration becomes possible.

Aberration, correction of ocular

Until recently, the irregular nature of the monochromatic wavefront aberration of the eye has made it impossible to correct fully, although some reduction can be achieved with appropriately aspheric contact lenses. Longitudinal chromatic aberration can be corrected by a suitable achromatizing doublet lens, but the improvement in retinal image quality in white light is small and occurs mainly at intermediate spatial frequencies; no improvement in conventional high contrast white-light visual acuity is normally detectable. More recently, however, real progress has been made in correcting monochromatic aberration using either adaptive optics or liquid crystal phase plates. While all these corrections are at present only feasible in the laboratory, they do show that marked improvements in spatial vision can be achieved over the uncorrected eye, particularly if both monochromatic and chromatic aberrations are corrected. If only monochromatic aberrations are corrected, performance in white light only improves modestly.

In theory, having measured the wave aberrations of the individual eye, the form of the cornea could be appropriately shaped (e.g. by a computer-controlled scanning-spot excimer laser) to compensate for the aberrations – although currently our limited knowledge of regression effects would make this difficult to achieve exactly. Alternatively, a tight-fitting contact lens with minimal transverse and rotational movement might be engineered to play the same role. At best, however, such approaches would only reduce the monochromatic aberrations, which in any case may change with the level of accommodation. The blur effects due to chromatic aberrations would remain uncorrected. Moreover, the worst monochromatic aberration occurs in the periphery of the dilated pupil, and pupil dilation only occurs when light levels are low and visual performance is largely limited by neural, rather than optical, factors. For these reasons, correction of aberration only seems likely to be profitable in the case of individuals whose monochromatic aberration is particularly high.

Aberration, monochromatic

Aberration acts to introduce additional blur into both in-focus and out-of-focus images. Monochromatic aberration can arise from a variety of causes. The eye would be expected to display the classical Seidel aberrations (spherical aberrations, coma, oblique astigmatism, field curvature and distortion) inherent in any system of spherical centred surfaces but, due to the various asphericities, tilts, decentrations and irregularities that may occur in its optical surfaces, its aberrational behaviour is much more complex than that which would be expected on the basis of simple schematic eye models.

Aberration is most commonly expressed in terms of the wavefront aberration. The behaviour of a 'perfect' optical system, according to geometrical optics, can either be visualized as involving rays radiating from an object point to be converged to a unique image point, or as spherical wavefronts diverging from the object point to converge at the image point, so that the object point is the centre of curvature of the object wavefronts and the image point that of the image wavefronts (Figure A.1A). The rays and wavefronts are everywhere perpendicular to one another. If we have aberration, the image rays fail to intersect at a single image point. Similarly, the wavefronts, which are still everywhere perpendicular to the rays, are no longer spherical (Figure A.1B). It is usual to express the wavefront aberration at any point in the pupil as the distance between the ideal spherical wavefront, centred on the Gaussian image point, and the actual wavefront, where both are selected to coincide at the centre of the exit pupil (Figure A.1C).

Abrasion

- See *Relief of pain, therapeutic contact lenses for*.

AC/A ratio

The accommodative convergence to accommodation ratio, or AC/A ratio, is significant because of the influence it has on the type of phoria (or tropia). It also has an influence on the choice of treatment. There is an inborn link between accommodation and convergence. For every dioptre of accommodation, a certain amount of accommodative-convergence occurs. The linear relationship between accommodative-convergence and accommodation is expressed as the AC/A ratio. In simple terms, a patient who has a 60mm inter-pupillary distance and who is fixating a target at 1m will accommodate 1.00D and his convergence will be 6^Δ. The AC/A ratio would therefore be 6:1 but a pre-existing phoria (or tropia) would modify this figure.

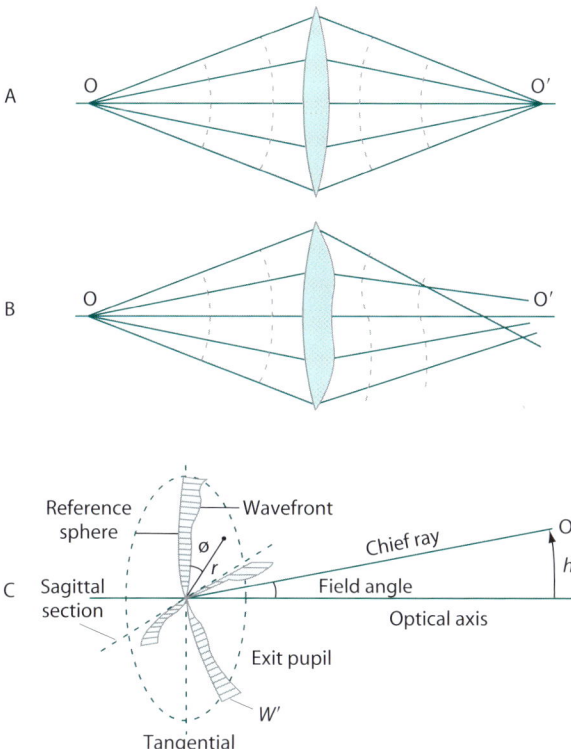

Figure A.1 • (A) With a perfect lens, rays from the object converge to a single image point. Alternatively, we can visualize divergent spherical wavefronts (shown dashed) from the object point converging as spherical wavefronts to the image point. (B) If the lens suffers from aberration, the imaging rays fail to converge to a single point and the corresponding wavefronts are not spherical. (C) The wavefront aberration, W′, is specified as the distance between the ideal wavefront, or reference sphere, centred on the gaussian image point, O′, and the actual wavefront in the exit pupil. It is usually adjusted to be zero at the centre of this pupil.

There are several methods of calculating the AC/A ratio. In each method, convergent (esophoric) values are taken as positive values and divergent (exophoric) as negative values.

The *heterophoria/tropia* method of calculating the AC/A ratio is given by the formula:

$$AC/A = \frac{\text{interpupillary distance in centimetres} + (\text{near phoria/tropia} - \text{distance phoria/tropia})}{\text{near distance in dioptres}}$$

Near and distance phorias (or tropias) should be measured using prism and the cover test. Using this method, the normal values range from 4:1 to 7:1.

The *gradient method* of calculating the AC/A ratio requires determination of the effect of spherical lenses on convergence. It can be measured either at distance or near. If measured at distance only minus lenses can be used; at near, plus or minus lenses can be used. The phoria (or tropia) is measured by prism and the cover test or by Maddox rod first without any additional lenses and then again with additional minus or plus lenses. The AC/A ratio is derived by:

$$AC/A = \frac{\text{phoria/tropia with lenses} - \text{phoria/tropia without lenses}}{\text{dioptric power of lens used}}$$

This method gives a lower result than the heterophoria/tropia method because it excludes proximal convergence; however, it is regarded as the most accurate method of determining the AC/A ratio.

The *fixation disparity* method of calculating the AC/A ratio in heterophoria is undertaken as follows. A graph is constructed with prism base-in as negative values and prism base-out as positive values on the x-axis and with convergent (esophoric) disparity and divergent (exophoric) disparity on the y-axis. The amount of disparity induced by base-in or base-out prism while maintaining binocular single vision at a constant near distance is plotted. The amount of convergent (esophoric) or divergent (exophoric) disparity induced by plus or minus lenses is plotted. The results are compounded to give the amount of prism base-in or base-out associated with changes in plus or minus lenses.

Clinically it is important to be able to designate the AC/A ratio as high or low. If it is low, the convergence response for accommodation at near will be less than normal, resulting in exophoria of the convergence-weakness type or a convergence insufficiency. Treatment for convergence insufficiency will improve the fusional convergence so that the patient becomes symptom-free, but it will not alter the basic AC/A ratio. If the AC/A ratio is too high, it will produce over convergence at near resulting in a convergence-excess esophoria (or esotropia). Occasionally, a high AC/A ratio will produce pseudo-divergence excess where the near divergence appears to be less than at distance. However, if fusional convergence is suspended by occlusion and the angle re-measured, it will be seen to be the same at distance and near.

Acanthamoeba keratitis

Acanthamoeba is a protozoa that has chameleon-like tendencies in that it is able to transform from a chemotherapeutically susceptible trophozoite to a resistant cystic form. The trophozoites are polygonal and can be up to 45μm in diameter, and the cysts are double-walled and up to 16μm in length. Acanthamoeba species are widely distributed in the natural environment, and have been isolated from swimming pools, hot tubs, soil, dust, reservoirs, under ice, the nasopharyngeal mucosa in healthy humans, and even the air we breathe.

A fully developed corneal ulcer may take weeks to form. Typical signs include:

- corneal staining
- pseudodendrites
- epithelial and anterior stromal infiltrates, which may be focal or diffuse
- radial keratoneuritis – a characteristic circular formation of opacification that becomes apparent relatively early in the disease process (Figure A.2).

Acanthamoeba keratitis has a slow time course of recovery. The condition may progress over many months with periods of apparent improvement followed by regression. Patients are inevitably left with superficial nebulae corresponding to the site of infection. See *Antimicrobial efficacy.*

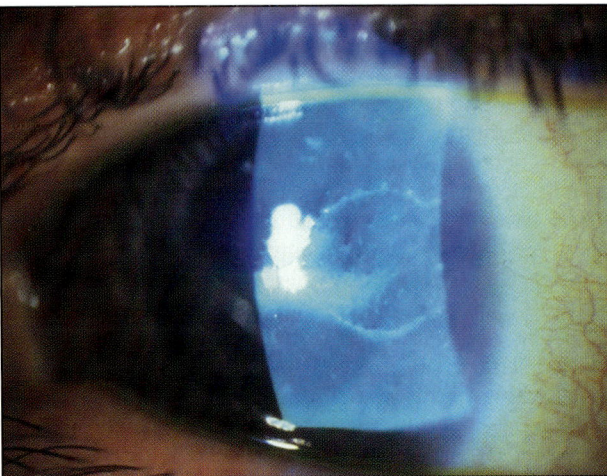

Figure A.2 • Characteristic pattern of radial keratoneuritis in a soft lens wearer with Acanthamoeba keratitis.

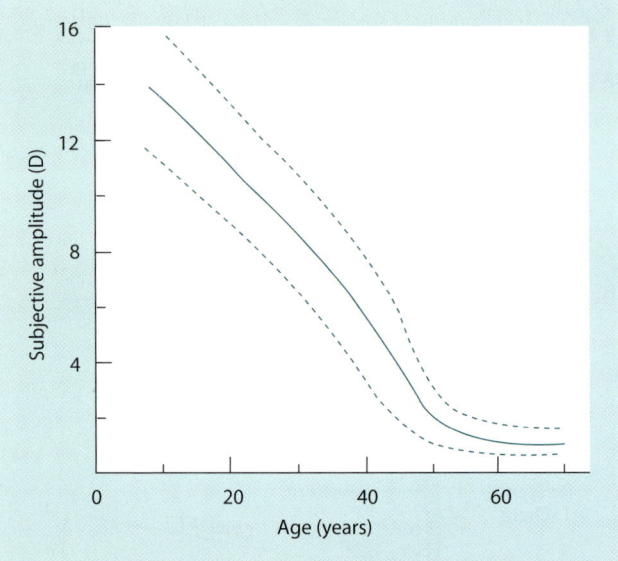

Figure A.3 • The decline in monocular amplitude of accommodation, referenced to the spectacle plane, with age. After A. Duane (1922) Studies in monocular and binocular accommodation with their clinical implications. Am. J. Ophthalmol., 5, 865–877.

Accessory lacrimal glands

Numerous small accessory lacrimal glands, which include the eponymous glands of Wolfring and Krause, are found within the conjunctival stroma. They have a particular predilection for the upper fornix and above the tarsal plate, and on the basis of proportion of total lacrimal tissue, it has been estimated that they contribute 5–10% of aqueous tear volume. Structurally, they have a similar appearance to the lacrimal gland proper. However, true acini are absent, and glands consist of elongated tubules that connect with ducts that open onto the conjunctival surface.

Accommodation

Accommodation is the process of causing the crystalline lens of the eye to change shape so that it has greater plus power, thus allowing near objects to become clear. The amplitude of accommodation declines with age (Figure A.3). Few everyday tasks require accommodation in excess of about 4.00D, so it is normally only as individuals approach 40 years of age that marked problems with near vision start to appear. It is, however, important to recognize that, even for objects lying within the available range of accommodation, accommodation is rarely precise. 'Lags' of accommodation usually occur in near vision, and 'leads' for distance vision. Since the accommodation system is driven via the retinal cones, these lags increase if the environmental illumination is reduced to mesopic levels and the accommodation system is inoperative at scotopic light levels. See *Presbyopia*.

Accommodation demand

Just as the position of the correcting lens affects the correcting power required and the spectacle magnification, so it also influences the accommodation required to view a near object. The accommodation necessary with any particular correction can easily be calculated for any given object distance, lens position and correcting power by determining the difference between the vergence of the light striking the cornea when viewing a near object and that for a distant object. However, an adequate approximation for most purposes is that the accommodation demand in dioptres is given by:

$$A \approx -L(1 + 2aK)$$

where L is the object vergence (negative for real objects), a is the vertex distance and K is the ocular refraction. In this approximation, a is zero for a contact lens, so that it can be seen that for a myope (negative K) the accommodation demand is higher with contact lenses than with spectacles lenses, whereas the reverse is true for hypermetropes. For an object at 33cm (L= –3.00D) and a spectacle vertex distance a = 14mm, the difference in demand with the two types of correction becomes significant (>0.25D) when the magnitude of the refractive error, K, is larger than about 3.00D. Thus, higher myopes approaching presbyopia might slightly delay the need for a reading addition by wearing spectacles, whereas hypermetropes would find near vision easier with a contact lens correction.

ACLM

- See *Association of Contact Lens Manufacturers*.

Achromatopsia

Achromatopsia refers to absence of colour vision. Those with this condition ('achromats') cannot distinguish wavelengths in the visible spectrum or pigmented surfaces which have the same perceived lightness. Achromatopsia is often used to describe acquired absence of colour vision due to intracranial pathology. See *Monochromatism*.

Acne rosacea

- See *Systemic disease, contact lens wear in*.

Table A.1 • Classification and characteristics of acquired colour deficiency.

Classification	Characteristics	Association
Type 1 Red-Green	Similar to protan deficiency. Maximum relative luminous efficiency displaced to shorter wavelengths. Reduced sensitivity to long wavelengths. Reduced visual acuity.	Cone dystrophies and disease affecting the cone receptors (e.g. Stargardt's disease, chloroquine toxicity)
Type 2 Red-Green	Similar to deutan deficiency. Reduced sensitivity to short wavelengths. Reduced visual acuity	Optic neuropathy (e.g. retrobulbar neuritis, ethambutal toxicity, digoxin toxicity)
Type 3 Tritan	a) Similar to tritan deficiency. Reduced sensitivity to both long and short wavelengths. Abnormal visual fields. b) Similar to tritan deficiency. Maximum relative luminous efficiency displaced to shorter wavelengths (pseudo-protanomaly). Reduced visual acuity.	Rod dystrophies (e.g. retinitis pigmentosa) Retinal vascular lesions (e.g. diabetic retinopathy) Peripheral retinal lesions (e.g. glaucoma, retinal detachment) Macular oedema (e.g. diabetic maculopathy, central serous chorioretinopathy, exudative age-related macular degeneration)

Acoustic neuroma
- See *Eyelid pathology, therapeutic contact lenses for*.

Acquired colour vision deficiency
Abnormal colour vision can be acquired as a result of ocular or general pathology, intracranial injury or toxicity caused by the prolonged use of some therapeutic drugs. 'Dyschromatopsia', meaning abnormal colour vision, is most frequently used to describe acquired colour deficiency but can also be used in the context of congenital colour deficiency.

Acquired colour deficiency is not easy to classify using the same terms as those used to describe types of congenital colour deficiency (Table A.1). The severity of hue discrimination loss changes with time and may either recover or progress in stages equivalent to anomalous trichromatism and dichromatism and eventually monochromatism. Monocular differences in severity are common and monocular colour vision examination is needed.

Acquired red-green colour deficiency (Type 1 and Type 2) is always associated with reduced visual acuity which limits the use of some tests designed to assess congenital colour deficiency. Short wavelength sensitivity is also abnormal. Acquired Type 3 ('Tritan') colour deficiency is the most common type of acquired abnormality and is usually associated with visual field defects. Measurement of wavelength detection thresholds (Wald-Marré mechanisms) show that both red and green colour vision mechanisms are reduced in severe Type 3 colour deficiency and there is an enlarged neutral zone in the yellow-green region of the spectrum which justifies the term 'blue-yellow' colour deficiency. In the early stages a tritan axis of confusion is obtained with the Farnsworth Munsell 100 hue test. Overall loss of hue discrimination is found with this test when colour deficiency is severe and red-green mechanisms are involved. A series of saturated and desaturated D15 tests are also useful for assessing hue discrimination losses in acquired colour deficiency. A Farnsworth D15 test with enlarged caps can be used when visual acuity is reduced, for example in age-related macular degeneration. A clinical test battery is recommended for the assessment of acquired colour deficiency. This should include pseudoisochromatic plates for tritan deficiency and hue discrimination tests which examine neutral zones. See *Pseudoisochromatic plates; Lanthony colour vision tests*.

A simple handheld colour target may be reported to change hue or saturation when moved into an area of the visual field associated with abnormal colour vision. The Red Dot test can also be used (see *Confrontation tests*). Psychophysical methods such as short wavelength automated perimetry (SWAP) have been developed for examining acquired colour vision changes in the peripheral retina. Electrodiagnostic tests, such as the 'blue' cone electroretinogram, computerized measurements of discrimination ellipses and colour contrast sensitivity have also been used to study acquired colour deficiency. See *Kollner's rule*.

Acute red eye reaction
- See *Contact lens induced acute red eye (CLARE)*.

Aerosol saline
- See *Saline solutions for contact lens care*

Aesthesiometry, contact
- See *Cochet-Bonnet aesthesiometer*.

Aesthesiometry, non-contact
- See *Non-contact aesthesiometry*.

Table A.2 • Suggested aftercare schedules

soft lens daily wear	soft lens extended wear	rigid lens daily wear	rigid lens extended wear	therapeutic use
1–2 weeks	1 day (a.m. visit)	1–2 weeks	1 day (a.m. visit)	1 week
1 month	1 week	1 month	1 week	3–4 weeks
3 months	1 month	2 months	2 weeks	2 months
6 months	3 months	3 months	1 month	3 months
every 6–12 months thereafter	every 3 months thereafter	6 months	3 months	6 months
		every 6–12 months thereafter	every 3 months thereafter	every 6 months thereafter

Aftercare, contact lens

Contact lenses are generally very well tolerated by the majority of patients; however, appropriate aftercare of the contact lens patient is essential to ensure that long-term success is maintained. Aftercare procedures are as important as the original lens fitting, because the lenses that were fitted initially may develop unanticipated complications that require correction at any time during post-fitting patient care. In fact, it is commonly held that contact lens aftercare represents a continuum and as such can never be considered to be complete.

Aftercare schedules will vary based on lens type, mode of wear, and underlying corneal physiology (Table A.2). For example, patients wearing rigid lenses should be examined more frequently during the first few months of lens wear. Patients using lenses for extended wear must be monitored more frequently, with the initial visits in the early morning hours to assess lens adherence or excessive overnight corneal swelling. Additionally, the following groups of patients generally require more frequent aftercare as part of their management compared with uncomplicated cosmetic lens wearers: those with corneal pathology such as keratoconus or corneal dystrophy; those post-keratoplasty or post-refractive surgery; those using contact lenses for other therapeutic applications such as aphakia or high ametropia; and also paediatric patients.

The general strategy adopted for aftercare visits is to consider the procedures in two phases: those conducted with the patient wearing lenses (assuming that the patient presented wearing lenses), and those conducted following lens removal. Certainly, patients should present to all aftercare visits while wearing lenses, unless a complication warrants lens discontinuation. It is rarely necessary to conduct all possible aftercare procedures at every follow-up visit. Essential procedures (such as those outlined below) should generally be performed; these can be supplemented with ancillary testing to solve specific problems. The aftercare visit may on occasions be very brief; for example, if a patient presents with a minor problem soon after having been given a full aftercare examination, and the solution is straightforward, it may only be necessary to see the patient for a few minutes. The only caveat here is that, for medico-legal reasons, vision should always be measured if the patient enters the consulting room, no matter how brief the visit. The procedures conducted during the two phases of an aftercare examination are as follows.

1. Procedures conducted with the patient wearing lenses:
- history taking
- visual acuity
- over-refraction
- over-keratometry
- external examination
- slit-lamp biomicroscopy
- lens surface assessment
- lens fitting characteristics
- lens-eye interactions.

2. Procedures conducted following lens removal:
- uncorrected vision
- refraction
- keratometry and corneal topography
- slit-lamp biomicroscopy
- lens inspection and verification
- additional procedures, which may not be readily available to all contact lens clinicians, include corneal thickness measurements (pachometry) and endothelial specular microscopy; digital slit-lamp imaging is a valuable method of recording clinical information
- other procedures as required, including visual fields, ophthalmoscopy, tonometry, gonioscopy, binocular vision assessment, corneal sensitivity, tearscope evaluation, colour vision assessment etc.
- concluding discussion with patient.

Ageing, contact lens

The pre-insertion water content of all soft lenses decreases significantly over time. This ageing process is different from the well-known phenomenon of lens dehydration over the course of a number of hours throughout a day. The extent of ageing must be considered in the context of the intended life of the lens; thus, adverse ageing-related effects of a lens that occur at a constant rate over a 1-month period can be minimized or avoided if the lens is replaced weekly instead of monthly.

It is clear that a combination of physical and/or physiological factors cause this irreversible reduction in water content of the hydrogel lenses over time. It follows that some change to the lens appears to have caused a progressive reduction in water uptake by the lens each night during storage, in what amounts to a 'lens ageing'

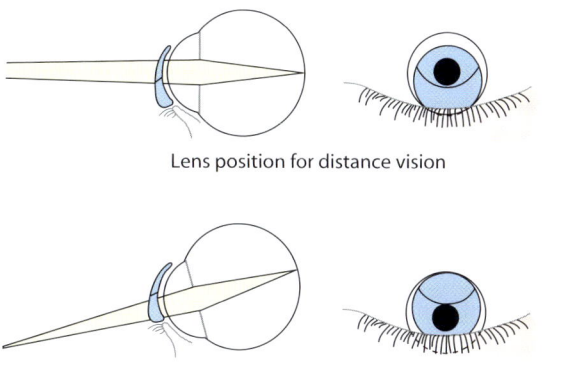

Figure A.4 • Rigid bifocal lens positions for distance and near vision.

effect. The most likely explanation for this ageing effect is that lens spoilation acts either to displace water from the lens, or it alters the nature of the lens material in such a way that less water is absorbed by it. This phenomenon occurs more in some patients than in others. A negative clinical ramification of this phenomenon is that there is an associated loss of oxygen performance with dehydration. Thus, the corneas of patients wearing lenses that display significant cyclic ageing will be generally more prone to chronic hypoxic complications, as well as specific acute hypoxic complications in the period immediately preceding lens replacement.

Alignment rigid bitoric contact lenses
- See *Cylindrical power equivalent rigid toric contact lenses*.

Alkali burns
- See *Chemical injuries, therapeutic contact lenses for*.

Alternating vision contact lenses for presbyopia

These contact lenses have distance and near powered portions, set out in a similar way to that observed in a bifocal spectacle lens. Although soft alternating bifocals have been available in the form of concentric and crescent segment designs, they have not generally proved successful due to ineffective translation. Translating designs are therefore almost exclusively available as rigid lenses. During primary gaze, the distance portion of the contact lens is positioned over the pupil. When gaze is directed downwards during reading, the near portion translates upwards to allow near vision correction (Figure A.4). Segment position and lens translation are the keys to success, and the lower lid has an important role in positioning and stabilizing the lens against the globe. The position of the lower lid should be no lower than the inferior limbus, otherwise translation is less effective and often inadequate. Upper lid movement also plays an important role in lens translation, as the upward movement of the lower lid is restricted to about 0.8mm. It may be more challenging to fit patients with ambient pupil sizes greater than 3mm, as the segment has to be positioned lower to avoid the pupil margin and consequently requires greater translation to achieve adequate pupil coverage by the near portion.

The two distinct portions that make up an alternating lens may be either fused or solid and a range of alternative segment shapes are available. Lens stability, position and translation can be controlled by introducing prism onto the lens, truncating the lens, or both. Regardless of lens design, the success of alternating vision contact lenses is made possible by adequate lower lid tone, which facilitates upward translation of the lens during downgaze. This positions the near portion of the lens over the pupil and allows near vision. The truncated edge should be finished in such a way to encourage comfortable effective translation and minimize the risk of the lens slipping beneath the lower lid.

Solid designs can be cut from a single piece of material, and the segment shape and design can vary. If the optical centres of the distance and near portion do not coincide, image jump will occur with down gaze, and lenses of 3.00D or greater frequently result in intolerable diplopia for the wearer. For this reason, it is better to avoid solid construction lenses in these powers unless using a monocentric design. In these designs optical centres of both distance and near portions of the lens are coincident, which produces a straight top segment bifocal contact lens with the same properties as an 'executive' bifocal spectacle lens.

Fused-segment rigid lenses use a fused insert of higher refractive index than the rest of the lens to generate the add power, whilst the front surface curvature remains continuous. There is minimal image jump and blanks are supplied to laboratories, allowing individual lens specifications to be made to order, including more complex front and back surface geometries. Care must be taken not to fit these lenses with the segment position too high as this increases the risk of reflections being noticed from the top of the segment. The fused segment is fluorescent, allowing easy observation using a Burton lamp.

Alternating lenses are generally fitted on alignment or with minimal apical corneal touch. The truncation should rest on the lower lid. The lens should have a vertical diameter at least 2mm smaller than the horizontal visible iris diameter; this encourages the required inferior centration and rapid recovery of lens position following blink as well as upward movement during depressed gaze. Translation over the corneal surface is more likely if there is unimpeded vertical movement, so a steep fitting approach should be avoided. In general, a lens fitted too steeply will tend to swing nasally and show poor translation, unlike a flat lens fit, which decentres temporally.

Most alternating bifocal contact lenses are fitted so that the segment is positioned in line with the inferior pupil margin during primary gaze in ambient illumination. Alternatively, some solid designs are such that the segment should be fitted higher to occupy approximately 20% of the pupil area. More importantly, the near segment should occupy at least 75% of the pupil diameter during depressed gaze to allow adequate near vision. An exception is when fitting fused rigid lens designs, as the segment position should be positioned approximately 0.4–0.7mm below the pupil margin when observed under slit-lamp illumination. This minimizes light reflections from the segment line interfering with distance vision performance. As a general rule, it is best to err on setting the segment top a little high, as this can subsequently be lowered by increasing truncation. A near horizontal segment line position is preferred; however, a small amount of nasal rotation is acceptable because the natural convergence of the eyes at near helps offset this rotation.

Observing segment positions under slit-lamp illumination can be deceptive due to the resultant pupil miosis. A better assessment can be made using an ophthalmoscope focused on the lens surface. If an optimal alignment fit shows significant rotation away from the desired position, the lens can be re-ordered with prism offset by the angle through which the lens mislocates to compensate for the rotation. For example, if the lens persists in rotating by 15° nasally in the right eye, ordering the prism base at 285° rather than 270° orientates the lens correctly. Increasing the amount of prism can also be useful in reducing superior centration.

Amblyopia

Amblyopia is characterized by reduced acuity in one eye. It is typically caused by abnormal or insufficient stimulation of the binocular system in the early years of life. Anomalies such as congenital cataract and ptosis cause gross visual deprivation, and result in a deep amblyopia characterized by greatly reduced acuity. Strabismus and anisometropia exert their influence a little later in life and typically cause less severe amblyopia. Some strabismics avoid amblyopia by alternating. For example the larger esotropes often cross-fixate. If the refractive error allows, anisometropes may use one eye for near and the other for distance, thus avoiding amblyopia.

In strabismic amblyopia the loss of acuity is restricted to the foveal region, whereas in anisometropia the reduction in sensitivity is proportionally the same centrally and peripherally. Amblyopes with both strabismus and anisometropia follow strabismic characteristics. The distinction between anisometropes and strabismics has to be made with care because many anisometropes may also have a small strabismus. It was originally suggested that the 2.0 log unit neutral density filter test distinguished between the reduced acuity caused by pathology (organic amblyopia) and the amblyopia of anisometropia and strabismus (functional amblyopia). However, it has been demonstrated that the response of an anisometropic amblyope is similar to that of organic amblyopia. That is, organic and anisometropic amblyopias both show a reduction in acuity after adapting for a few minutes through the filter, whereas the acuity in strabismic amblyopia is unaffected. This test is difficult to perform and a goggle arrangement is necessary to ensure that light only enters the eye through the filter. If a trial frame is used the eye may never actually adapt.

Prediction of amblyopia based on risk factors makes prevention a possibility. Heredity seems to be relevant, principally in the inheritance of abnormal refractive error. Abnormal refractive error in the first year of life has been shown to be a good predictor of later amblyopia and strabismus. Studies show the 5% of the population with > +3.50DS hypermetropia at 9 months are significantly more likely to have strabismus or amblyopia by the age of 4 years than infants with normal refractive errors. A lesser but also valid alternative to prediction and prevention is early detection. In some parts of Scandinavia there has been screening at the age of 4 years for about 20 years. Retrospective studies have shown that the prevalence of amblyopia and strabismus have been reduced by a half in these regions.

The initial measure of acuity establishes the presence and the extent of the amblyopia. A perfunctory measure can give a low value and therefore a false sense of 'improvement' on later reassessment. It is advisable to use the same test and examination distance at each appointment, preferably with charts with crowding contours such as the Cambridge Crowding cards or the Glasgow Acuity cards. LogMAR charts give a more precise measure of acuity and facilitate more robust statistical analysis. If available, contrast sensitivity charts add a further dimension by revealing performance across the whole spatial frequency spectrum.

In treating amblyopia promising results have been reported with drugs related to L-dopa, that cause an increase in visual plasticity. Acuity has been shown to improve in children and to a lesser extent in adults. However, at present the improvement would seem only temporary. Atropine in the eye with better acuity and an extra +3.00DS spectacle prescription in the amblyopic eye forces the better eye to be used for distance and the amblyopic eye for near. Such an approach has cosmetic advantages over occlusion and does not totally disrupt binocular vision. However, careful monitoring is necessary to be sure that the desired alternation actually occurs.

Occlusion using adhesive patches remains the favoured treatment (preferably reinforced with pencil and paper exercises to encourage hand–eye co-ordination). The best occlusion regimen for amblyopia, total occlusion, is controversial because of fears of promoting intractable diplopia in older patients and of destroying binocularity in the young. The risk of causing diplopia is difficult to quantify. However, the speed and complexity of visual development in the first few years certainly makes too early intervention potentially hazardous.

Optometrists are usually involved with managing amblyopic children of six or seven years or older, an age when visual plasticity is declining. Constant occlusion usually proves necessary at this age and though careful monitoring is prudent, occlusion amblyopia is unlikely. Constant occlusion is best arranged during school holidays and it is essential to ensure that the child is adequately supervised while occluded. Occlusion is generally found to be more effective the younger the child, although success continues until mid-teens. Several years after treatment the acuity often deteriorates. More than half of patients show regression of at least a line of acuity; anisometropes usually more. This problem is seldom quantitatively addressed and it is critical in any assessment of the effectiveness of amblyopia treatment.

American Optical Company (Hardy, Rand and Rittler) pseudoisochromatic plates

- See *Pseudoisochromatic plates*.

Ametropia

An emmetropic eye is defined as one in which the fovea lies at the posterior principal focus of the system. All departures from emmetropia, where the refractive components of the eye focus light away from the fovea and are therefore said to have a refractive error, can be defined as ametropia. However, a range of variations from emmetropia can be considered as within normal limits. More than 80% of all children 1 to 7 years of age have a cycloplegic spherical equivalent refractive error of between +0.50D and +3.00D of hypermetropia (where the point focus is behind the plane of the fovea). Less than 5% of all 5 to 7 year olds are more than +5.00D hypermetropic and less than 3% are myopic (where the focus is in front of the plane of the fovea). These high refractive errors are almost exclusively congenital. Only 8% of 5 to 7 year olds have more than 0.75D of astigmatism, more commonly 'with the rule' (the vertical meridian has maximum refractive power and the cylinder axis is horizontal).

Juvenile myopia is the most common form of myopia. It can be defined as myopia with onset at any age between 6 and 15 years. Of all children in this age group, 15 to 30% are myopic, though large increases in this percentage have been measured, particularly in far eastern countries. Those 5 to 7 year olds with refraction close to emmetropia (especially those with 'against the rule' astigmatism) are at the greatest risk of developing juvenile myopia. This is because from the age of 8 years there is a myopic shift and mean refractive error drops by an average of +0.25D per year. The earlier the onset of juvenile myopia, the higher the ultimate refractive error. There is a slight increase in incidence of 'against the rule' astigmatism with onset and progression of juvenile myopia.

Higher levels of hypermetropia are likely to result in amblyopia and possibly a convergent strabismus related to the accommodative effort exerted in overcoming the refractive error. Lower amounts of hypermetropia may cause little problem as they can be easily overcome by accommodation, only coming to light as the accommodation reserve reduces with age (latent hypermetropia becoming manifest).

Changes in the adult refractive error may be related to disease processes; for example, a myopic shift with nucleosclerotic cataract, hypermetropic shift with macular oedema, or a variable refraction due to crystalline lens dehydration and rehydration in a poorly controlled diabetic.

Understanding the expected reduction in vision related to an uncorrected refractive error is essential for an accurate refractive assessment of a patient. The uncorrected vision allows an estimate of the refractive error, the change in acuity with trial lenses gives information about the subjective response, and the use of plus-powered 'fogging lenses' and their subsequent impact on acuity, give information about the accommodative state of the eye. As a general rule, 0.25D represents one line of acuity such that an uncorrected 1.00D myope (or presbyopic myope) of 6/5 corrected acuity will have vision of around 6/12. For astigmatic errors, the mean sphere should be considered, such that the visual ability in this example would also apply to a 2.00D astigmat. See *Refraction, subjective*.

Table A.3 • Expected amplitude of accommodation and reading addition for age.

Age	Expected amplitude (D)	Near add (D)
20	10	0.00
30	8	0.00
40	5–6	0.00 – 0.50
45	3–4	0.00 – 1.00
50	2	1.00 – 1.75
55	1	1.50 – 2.25
60	0	1.75 – 2.50

Amplitude of accommodation, measurement

Measurement of the amplitude of accommodation is useful, not only in deciding upon a near addition requirement for the early presbyope, but also to ascertain information about ocular and physical or emotional general health. The RAF rule is usually used, though a 'budgie stick' and measuring tape is just as good. The target is moved slowly towards the patient along the ruler held slightly below the straight-ahead position until it becomes blurred. The patient is then asked if they can bring the target back into focus. If so, it is moved towards the patient until the target can no longer be focused. This distance is noted in centimetres from the spectacle plane ('push-up' value). The target is then moved back until the patient can see it clearly, and this distance also noted ('pull-back' value). The amplitude of accommodation is the average of the 'push-up' and 'pull-back' values. The target should be the smallest print that can be seen clearly when the target is at the remote end of the ruler or at arms length if using a budgie stick or separate card. Accommodation should be measured both monocularly (to screen for third nerve anomalies), and binocularly.

The normal amplitude of accommodation declines with age until around 55 years (Table A.3). Inter-patient variation in amplitudes is expected. However, reduced accommodation may be associated with latent or inadequately corrected hypermetropia, poor health (e.g. Graves disease, alcoholism) or drug treatment (e.g. for asthma, antidepressants) or abuse, hysteria and stress, over-stimulation of the sympathetic nervous system, ocular disease (e.g. glaucoma, anterior uveitis), myopia, or a history of sunny or tropical environment. Girls around the age of 12 to 14 may experience a temporary accommodative palsy which usually resolves spontaneously after a short time. Help with reading may be necessary for a while. Higher than expected amplitudes of accommodation may be recorded in older patients or those with small pupils due to enhanced depth of focus and hence this is artefactual. Patients on pilocarpine will have small pupils and ciliary spasm and some adults (more often females) will develop spasm of the near reflex as a response to excessive demands on accommodation or convergence.

Amsler charts

Many perimetric instruments have relatively few stimuli within the central 10° and it is, therefore, often difficult, if not impossible, to accurately map central defects. One solution to this problem is to use Amsler charts. The charts consist of a series of cards, each with a central fixation point and a regular pattern of markings. The most widely used chart has a regular 1° square matrix of white lines on a black background.

The patient's task is to fixate the centre of the chart, which is held 30cm from the eye, and to describe, or draw – on a separate recording chart that mimics the Amsler chart – where the lines are missing or distorted. Research has shown that these areas coincide with regions of retinal disturbance.

The attractions of this test are its simplicity, and high sensitivity. The vast majority of patients with central serous retinopathy and optic neuropathy report changes in the appearance of the Amsler charts. Amsler testing is both considerably faster and more sensitive than either conventional tangent screen examination or full-threshold perimetry.

Anaesthetics, local

Local or topical anaesthetics can temporarily block conduction of nerve impulses along sensory fibres. They enhance the corneal penetration of any drugs or stains subsequently instilled. As a result of interaction with a specific binding site associated with the sodium channel, these drugs block the transient boost in cell membrane permeability to sodium ions which increases the threshold value for cell firing and decreases the excitability of the cell.

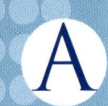

The principal uses of local anaesthetics in optometric practice include:

- Applanation tonometry
- Ocular first aid when removing a foreign body on the cornea or conjunctiva
- Gonioscopy
- The Schirmer II tear test
- Lacrimal procedures such as dilation, irrigation and insertion of punctual plug
- Eye impressions for the construction of scleral lenses
- Fitting of rigid corneal lenses. This is rarely necessary but may be justified when only a rigid lens can provide satisfactory visual acuity for a very apprehensive patient.
- Reduction of reflex lacrimation prior to the instillation of a cycloplegic to enable it to have a quicker and deeper effect.

Local anaesthetics should *never* be used solely for the alleviation of ocular symptoms including those caused by contact lens wear.

Examples of local anaesthetics listed in *increasing* order of the discomfort that they cause are:

- Proxymetacaine – also known as Proparacine, Ophthaine, Alcaine and Ophthetic. Initial stinging is least with this drug making it the most appropriate choice for use with children. It causes very little epithelial disturbance. Proxymetacaine is also available in combination with fluorescein (see *Fluorescein sodium*) for use in applanation tonometry. Hypersensitivity reactions to this drug are rare. The duration of its anaesthetic effect is about 15min.
- Oxybuprocaine or benoxinate – also known as Novesine and Dorsacaine. It causes less epithelial staining than amethocaine. Toxic effects are unlikely with this drug. The duration of its anaesthetic effect is about 15min.
- Lidocaine or lignocaine – is available in combination with fluorescein for use in applanation tonometry. The duration of its anaesthetic effect is about 30min. Lidocaine, with or without adrenaline (epinephrine), can be injected into the eyelids for minor surgery, while retrobulbar or peribulbar injections are used for surgery involving the globe.
- Tetracaine – also known as Amethocaine, Anethaine, Decicain and Pontocaine. The initial smarting sensation that it commonly produces subsides within 30s. Following instillation, patients should close their eyes for a few moments in order to reduce discomfort. Since a more profound anaesthesia is produced by tetracaine it is suitable for use prior to minor procedures such as the removal of corneal sutures. Tetracaine does have a temporary disruptive effect on the corneal epithelium and dermatitis is a possible adverse reaction. The duration of its anaesthetic effect is about 20min.

Each of the above anaesthetics exerts its effect within a few seconds and clinical procedures necessitating their use can generally be undertaken 30s after their instillation. There is a significant inter-subject variation in the time required to return to baseline sensitivity following corneal anaesthesia. Allergic responses to local anaesthetics are more likely to occur with the older ester-linked compounds – proxymetacaine, oxybuprocaine and tetracaine – than with lidocaine, which is an amide. The esters are less stable and more readily metabolized than the amides.

Single dose preparations of local anaesthetics are shown in Table A.4.

Precautions for the use of local anaesthetics include the following:

- Explain to the patient the reason for using a local anaesthetic.
- As with any other drug, it is wise to ask patients whether they have previously had corneal anaesthesia and whether there was any adverse reaction to the drug used. For example, if an ester-linked compound caused a hypersensitive or allergic response, it is appropriate that an amide be used in future.
- On most occasions a *single* drop produces adequate anaesthesia.
- Ideally, patients should not leave the practice until corneal sensitivity has largely returned to normal which is usually 15 to 20min following instillation of the drops. Within this period of time, patient should be discouraged from rubbing their eyes.
- Following use of a local anaesthetic, re-examine the state of the cornea.
- Issue a note which states the local anaesthetic used and provides advice on what action the patient should take in the event of an adverse reaction.
- If contact lenses are worn, they should not be inserted until 30min after the instillation of the local anaesthetic.

Table A.4 • Local anaesthetics: unpreserved single dose preparations.

Non-proprietary name	Proprietary name	Formulation
Lidocaine hydrochloride	Minims® Lignocaine and Fluorescein	Drops 4% with fluorescein sodium 0.25%
Oxybuprocaine hydrochloride	Minims® Benoxinate (Oxybuprocaine) Hydrochloride	Drops 0.4%
Proxymetacaine hydrochloride	Minims® Proxymetacaine	Drops 0.5%
	Minims® Proxymetacaine and Fluorescein	Drops 0.5% with fluorescein sodium 0.25%
Tetracaine hydrochloride	Minims® Amethocaine hydrochloride	Drops 0.5 and 1%

Angioscotoma
- See *Visual field artefacts*.

Aniseikonia
Aniseikonia is a binocular perceptual distortion of space that is induced when corresponding retinal images of the two eyes are unequal. This occurs when anisometropia is corrected by spectacle lenses, causing marked differences in spectacle magnification between the two eyes. This condition can be disturbing and disorientating to the patient. A small amount of aniseikonia can also be induced when the magnitude and/or axis of cylinder correction is changed. The effect is usually transient, and patients adapt within hours of receiving a new or changed optical correction. These distortions are much reduced in the case of contact lenses, which therefore minimize the possibility of aniseikonic symptoms. See *Spectacle magnification*.

Anisocoria
This refers to the pupils of the two eyes being of unequal size. Anisocoria may be physiological, whereby the extent of the difference is small and constant irrespective of the level of illumination. The most common conditions where anisocoria is a feature are Adie's pupil and Horner's syndrome. Anisocoria can manifest as a result of direct injury to the iris, inflammation or disease of the iris, paralysis of the third nerve, angle closure glaucoma, systemic disease or drug instillation into one eye (e.g. a miotic or mydriatic).

Anisometropia
Anisometropia refers to a difference in refractive status between the two eyes whereby a different optical correction is required for each eye. Correction of anisometropia can result in aneisekonia. Anisometropia can be classified in a variety of ways, as follows:

- Refractive error. Isoanisometropia means that both eyes are either hyperopic (anisohyperopia) or myopic (anisomyopia). Antimetropia means that one eye is hyperopic and one eye is myopic.
- Magnitude. Anisometropia can be classified as low (a difference in best sphere refraction between the two eyes of 0.00 to 2.00D), high (a difference of 2.00D to 6.00D) and very high (a difference of > 6.00D). A patient with low anisometropia can usually tolerate a full correction, and a patient with high anisometropia will usually have binocular vision problems. A patient with very high anisometropia will typically be asymptomatic because of the presence of central suppression.
- Aetiology. Anisometropia can be classified as being hereditary or acquired. Hereditary anisometropes are those due to congenital glaucoma, congenital cataract, and conditions causing eyelid closure such as congenital third nerve palsy, ptosis and obstetric trauma. Acquired anisometropia includes those caused by trauma or space-occupying lesions, or iatrogenic causes such as unilateral aphakia, refractive surgery and penetrating keratoplasty.
- Contributing ocular components. Differences in axial length account for almost all cases of anisometropia greater than 5.00D. Lenticular anisometropia is observed in patients who have an inter-ocular difference of between 3.00D and 5.00D. Inter-ocular differences in corneal power are rarely the cause of anisometropia.

Anomaloquotient
An anomaloquotient is useful for comparing results obtained with different anomaloscopes, which obtain a spectral Rayleigh match, or redefining the mid point of the normal matching range after the light source of a particular instrument has been changed. An anomaloquotient is calculated by dividing the numerical value of an individual mean match on the red/green mixture scale by the numerical value of the normal mean match obtained for 100 people with normal colour vision. Population studies with the Nagel anomaloscope have estimated that 95% of normal trichromats have anomaloquotients between 1.42 and 0.76 and a matching range of less than 6 scale units on the red-green mixture scale. Anomaloquotients are of limited value in defining the severity of anomalous trichromacy because the calculation is based on the midpoint of a matching range which can vary enormously in size. A single abnormal colour match followed by calculation of an anomaloquotient is completely inadequate for determining the type and severity of red-green colour deficiency. In general, deuteranomalous trichromats have an anomaloquotient greater than unity and protanomalous trichromats have an anomaloquotient less than unity.

Anomaloscope
An anomaloscope is a colour matching instrument. Psychophysical methods of examination are employed.

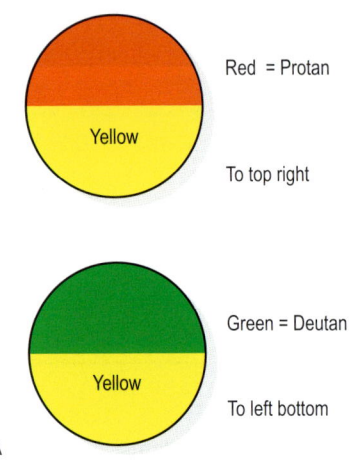
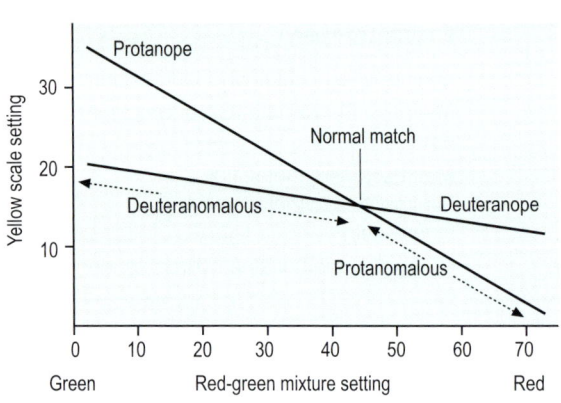

Figure A.5 • Graphic representation of diagnostic results obtained with a Nagel anomaloscope showing different matching ranges and yellow luminance values in protan and deutan colour deficiency.

A spectral anomaloscope is the "gold standard" reference test for red-green colour deficiency. Spectral anomaloscopes present a Rayleigh match which measures the proportions of monochromatic long wavelength (red) and middle wavelength (green) needed to match an intermediate monochromatic yellow wavelength. Anomaloscopes are less useful for identifying tritan colour deficiency because there is no appropriate spectral wavelength match which results in a fully saturated intermediate wavelength. Variations in normal short wavelength sensitivity produce large individual differences in blue-green colour matches in the population. (See *Macular pigment; Ocular lens light absorption*.) A simple Engelking–Trendelenburg match (blue added to green to produce blue-green) is inadequate and some anomaloscopes offer a Moreland match. However, wavelength detection thresholds, either on a white or yellow background adapting field, are the 'gold standard' reference test for tritan colour deficiency. See *Wavelength detection thresholds*.

The Nagel anomaloscope is the gold standard reference test for identifying and diagnosing congenital red-green colour deficiency. The anomalosope consists of a Maxwellian view spectroscope in which the two halves of a 2 to 3 degree bipartite field are illuminated respectively by monochromatic yellow (589nm) and a mixture of monochromatic red and green wavelengths (670nm and 546nm). A system of reciprocating slits keeps the luminance of the mixture field constant for any red-green mixture ratio. Accurate diagnosis of red-green colour deficiency begins by determining the normal red-green matching range for the instrument. Subjects are required to make several exact colour matches by adjusting the red-green mixture ratio and the luminance of the yellow test field. These matches are used as a guide to the more important second stage of the examination in which the examiner determines the limits of the matching range by setting red-green mixture ratios and ascertaining whether an exact match can be obtained by the subject altering the luminance of the yellow test field (Figure A.5). Normal trichromats make precise matches within a small range of red-green mixture ratios. The matching ranges of protanomalous and deuteranomalous trichromats are outside this range and form two separate distributions which vary in magnitude and show the severity of the discrimination deficit produced by the abnormal photopigment. Pigment density and neural post-receptoral gain mechanisms also contribute to the size of the matching range. Protanomalous trichromats require significantly more red light and deuteranomalous trichromats require significantly more green light compared with normal. Protanopes and deuteranopes have only one photopigment within the spectral range of the instrument and are able to match all red-green mixture ratios with yellow, including pure red and pure green. Protanopes are distinguished from deuteranopes by the very low yellow luminance needed to match pure red. Deuteranopes match pure red and pure green with approximately the same yellow luminance value.

The Neitz anomaloscope is similar to the Nagel anomaloscope except that interference filters are used to provide the test and mixture wavelengths. The test field is darker than that of the Nagel anomaloscope but comparable results have been reported. The Neitz anomaloscope is therefore considered to be a reliable substitute for the Nagel anomaloscope.

The Spectrum Colour Vision Meter was developed from the Besancon anomaloscope and is a 4 channel instrument intended to examine acquired colour deficiency. Two colour matches are obtained with interference filters – a Rayleigh match and a Moreland match. The Moreland match is intended for identifying tritan deficiency. The test field consists of a mixture of blue-green (480nm) and a desaturating yellow wavelength (580nm). The matching wavelengths are green (490nm) and blue (436nm) which are selected in order to minimize the effect of variations in macular pigment density. The instrument is interfaced with a computer and the examination routine is fully automated.

The HMC (Oculus) anomaloscope was developed from the Heidelberg anomaloscope and this instrument also presents a Rayleigh match and a Moreland match. The examination routine is automated and the viewing time for making a match is very short. After each brief match presentation the test field is replaced by an intense white adapting field which people find very disturbing.

The Pickord–Nicolson anomaloscope is a direct vision instrument constructed with broad band filters. Filter anomaloscopes cannot be used as reference tests for colour vision deficiency because desaturated colour matches neither identify the type of colour deficiency precisely nor classify dichromats. Expertise is needed to administer the test since there is no fixed examination protocol. The Pickford–Nicolson anomaloscope was

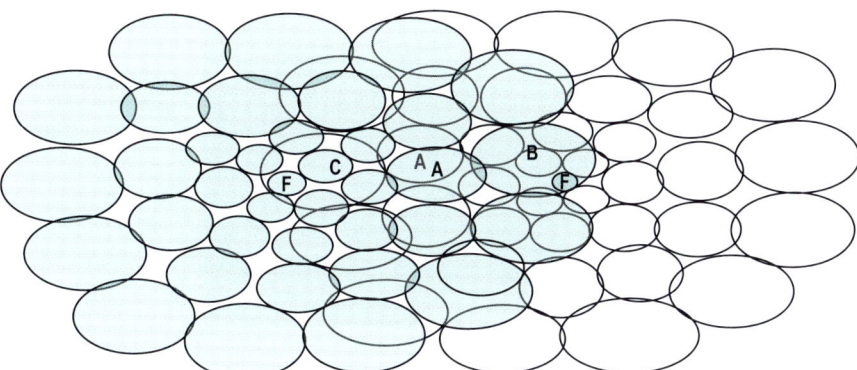

Figure A.6 • Schematic illustration of re-mapping. Adapted from B. Evans, S. Doshi (2001) Binocular Vision and Orthoptics. Butterworth-Heinemann-Optician, Oxford.

mainly utilized to study acquired colour deficiency. Three colour matches are available. These are red added to green to match yellow, blue added to green to match blue-green and blue added to yellow to match white. The luminance of the mixture field varies and the results are therefore only comparative.

Anomalous retinal correspondence

Binocular alignment in normal (non-strabismic) observers can shift by about 2° without losing fusion and stereopsis. During everyday vision the eyes and head are constantly moving hence small errors in vergence occur: the visual axis of one eye may become misaligned with the object of fixation. This is particularly likely to happen after a large saccade and represents a small breakdown in Hering's law. These vergence errors are typically of the order of 20min arc but can be as much as 1 to 3° for a 30° horizontal saccade. This is significantly larger than the size of Panum's areas. Yet, in everyday vision, we do not experience momentary periods of absence of stereopsis. Thus, the flexibility in the system which allows fusion and stereopsis during a vergence error of about 2° has probably evolved to help us overcome mechanical limitations in the ability to maintain precise motor fusion as the eyes move. In other words, sensory fusion has evolved with the plasticity required to compensate for inherent errors in motor fusion.

This cortical processing is far surpassed by the ability of children, who are young enough to possess considerable neural plasticity, to exhibit large shifts in retinal correspondence to compensate for strabismus. The purpose of this anomalous retinal correspondence (ARC) is for a point on the retina of the good eye to correspond with a new point on the retina of the strabismic eye (not its natural, innate, corresponding retinal point). The newly corresponding points are set at the angle of strabismus. This is nearly always the case in ARC and there is said to be *harmonious anomalous retinal correspondence* (HARC). The angle through which the retinal correspondence has been shifted from the normal is called the *angle of anomaly*. It should be noted that the term anomalous *retinal* correspondence has been criticized because the abnormal correspondence occurs cortically, not on the retinae. Despite this semantic objection, it is often easier to conceptualize the effect of the HARC by considering retinae.

The precise mechanism of HARC remains unclear. One view is that re-mapping of Panum's areas occurs. Another view is that Panum's areas become enlarged. The latter view may be supported by the observation that HARC is uncommon in vertical strabismus as Panum's areas are horizontally oval. A third hypothesis is that in HARC the bi-foveal assumption is abandoned and the position of each eye is registered separately, probably on the basis of muscle activity. This form of HARC would be most likely to facilitate the perception of direction, not depth and distance. It might account for HARC in large angle strabismus, with the "cortical re-mapping hypothesis" accounting for HARC in cases of small-angle strabismus.

Although the precise neurophysiological basis of HARC is not known, it has certain limitations. One of these relates to the requirement for the visual system to be plastic for HARC to develop. It is therefore not surprising that a younger age of onset of strabismus is associated with a greater likelihood of HARC being present. In cases of intermittent strabismus the visual axes will sometimes be straight and the patient will have normal retinal correspondence (NRC), yet at other times there will be a strabismus and the patient might have HARC. The change from NRC to HARC can be sudden (abrupt switching) or gradual (smoothly varying HARC). The term co-variation has been used to describe the situation when the angle of anomaly co-varies with the objective angle of strabismus. Co-variation is likely to place additional neural demands on the visual system and hence constant strabismus will be more likely to develop HARC than intermittent or variable strabismus. For similar reasons, unilateral strabismus is more likely to develop HARC than alternating strabismus.

Photoreceptor types, receptive field sizes, and ganglion cell types vary across the retina. One degree of retina near the fovea has a much greater cortical representation than one degree in the periphery. The cortical processing required to re-adjust retinal correspondence in HARC is likely to be easier if neo-corresponding points are at similar eccentricities from the fovea. Hence a small angle strabismus is more likely to develop HARC than a large angle strabismus (Figure A.6).

The obvious alternative to HARC is NRC with diplopia or global suppression. A third option, *unharmonious anomalous retinal correspondence* (UARC), is very rare and is best understood by the following example – imagine a young child who develops a small stable strabismus and associated HARC. Now, assume that after many years in this adapted state the patient suffers, for example, trauma and an extra-ocular muscle paresis resulting in a

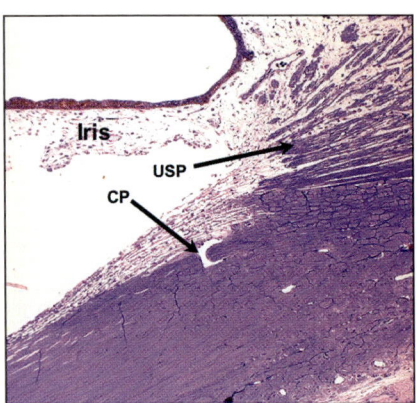

Figure A.7 • Histological section through the anterior angle showing aqueous outflow pathways. CP = conventional pathway through the canal of Schlemm. USP = uveoscleral pathway.

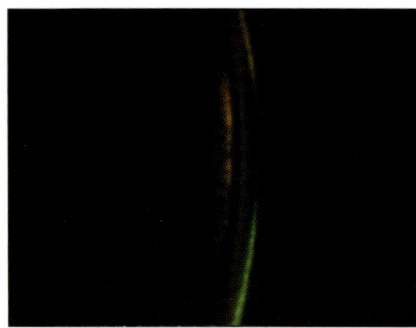

Figure A.8 • Estimating anterior chamber depth using the Van Herrick's technique.

change in the angle of strabismus, with consequent diplopia. If the HARC was not deep then the patient would revert to NRC. However, if the HARC associated with the old strabismus was very deep then the patient may continue with this HARC in the presence of the new strabismus. It is unlikely that a long-standing stable HARC could co-vary with a new change in the angle of the strabismus. Instead, the patient has developed a 'strabismus on top of a strabismus'. The objective angle will be the angle of the new strabismus and the subjective angle will be the difference between the angle of the old strabismus and the new strabismus. The angle of anomaly will be neither zero nor equal to either of the subjective angles.

This sequence of events is extremely unlikely to occur (although UARC can also occur secondary to any surgery), so the question arises as to why UARC is given such prominence in some textbooks. The reason is that many early methods of investigating retinal correspondence created very artificial conditions, which tended to cause HARC to break down. It was sometimes concluded that these techniques were detecting UARC. If the patients really had UARC then they would complain of diplopia.

Anoxia
- *Absence of oxygen. adj: anoxic*

Anterior angle of the eye

The external features of the drainage angle can be visualized gonioscopically. Schwalbe's line is the most anterior structure, and represents the termination of Descemet's membrane and the transition from corneal endothelium to trabecular cells. In the absence of pigment, the trabecular meshwork appears as a featureless band, approximately 750 microns in width. The posterior border of the trabecular meshwork is marked by a pale translucent ridge that corresponds to the location of the scleral spur.

In meridional histological section, the trabecular meshwork and canal of Schlemm can be seen to lie within a scleral sulcus that encircles the anterior chamber angle (Figure A.7). The trabecular meshwork is triangular in profile, with its base opposite the scleral spur and its apex adjacent to Schwalbe's line. Anatomically, the meshwork can be resolved into three distinct regions:

- Uveal meshwork
- Corneoscleral meshwork
- Juxta-canalicular tissue (cribiform layer)

The trabecular meshwork provides a resistance to aqueous outflow to generate an intra-ocular pressure. It also acts as a filter, and trabecular cells have a selective phagocytic capacity.

The canal of Schlemm is a circular venous channel approximately 36mm in circumference that lies deep within the scleral sulcus adjacent to the trabecular meshwork. Collector channels deliver aqueous from the canal of Schlemm into the intra-scleral venous plexus that in turn connects with episcleral veins (Aqueous veins represent a special case where mixing of aqueous with blood occurs at the ocular surface). The pressure within the drainage system decreases from the anterior chamber through to the ocular surface. Consequently aqueous flows down a pressure gradient.

Aqueous can also leave the anterior chamber via the uveoscleral pathway. Since there is no epithelial barrier between the anterior chamber and the ciliary body, aqueous is able to enter the loose connective tissue in front of the ciliary muscle and pass between the muscle fibres into the supraciliary and supra-choroidal spaces. From here, it can potentially be absorbed by vessels draining the uvea. The pressure-lowering action of prostaglandin analogues is thought to be the result of an increase in uveo-scleral outflow.

Anterior chamber depth assessment, Van Herrick's technique of

Anterior chamber depth can be estimated with a slit-lamp biomicroscope using Van Herrick's technique. A typical procedure is as follows:

- magnification of the slit-lamp biomicroscope should be set at 10x to 16x to allow an adequate depth of focus.
- With the patient positioned comfortably and staring straight ahead towards the microscope, the illumination system is set at 60° temporal to the patient's eye. This angle is chosen so that the illuminating beam is approximately perpendicular to the limbus. The routine employment of a 60° angle ensures consistency of interpretation every time the patient is assessed.
- A section of the cornea as close to the limbus as possible is viewed (Figure A.8).
- A comparison is made between the thickness of the cornea and the gap between the back of the cornea

Table A.5 • Van Herrick's grading system		
Cornea:gap ratio	Grade	Angle
1:1 or greater	4	Open
1:0.5–1.0	3	Open
1:0.25–0.5	2	Narrow, angle closure possible
1:less than 0.25	1	Narrower angle, closure likely
Closed	0	Angle-closure glaucoma

and the front of the iris where the beam first touches.
- The ratio of these two measurements can be graded and interpreted, as outlined in Table A.5.
- A measurement can also be made at the nasal limbus, and that if a large difference is found between nasal and temporal angles, the narrower angle should be considered. (See Appendix B.)

Anterior chamber depth assessment, Smith's method of

First described by Smith in 1979, this technique of assessing anterior chamber depth provides the practitioner with a measurement (in millimetres) of anterior chamber depth. The procedure is carried out as follows:

- The microscope is placed in the straight-ahead position in front of the patient, with the illumination placed at 60° temporally. To examine the patient's right eye, the practitioner views through the right eyepiece, and for the left eye through the left eyepiece.
- A beam of moderate thickness (1 to 2mm) is orientated horizontally and focused on the cornea. In this position, two horizontal streaks of light are seen, one on the anterior corneal surface and the other on the front surface of the crystalline lens.
- Altering the slit-height adjustment on the instrument is seen as a lengthening or shortening of the two horizontal reflexes.
- Beginning with a short slit, the length is slowly increased to a point at which the ends of the corneal and lenticular reflections appear to meet.
- The slit length at this point is then measured (it is assumed that the slit lamp is calibrated for slit length).
- This length may be multiplied by a constant to yield a figure for the anterior chamber depth.

From a clinical point of view, a chamber depth of 2mm should be treated with caution when considering pupil dilation. An adapted version of the above method has been proposed for use in those situations in which variable slit height is not possible. In this case, the slit length is noted prior to measurement at a point where it corresponds to 2mm. The instrument is then set up exactly as in the Smith method (above), but with the initial angle of incidence at 80°. By gradually closing the angle, the two reflected images on the cornea and lens appear to move closer and the angle at which they first touch is noted. A corresponding value for the anterior chamber depth for differing angles is then calculated. Verification of the accuracy of this result with pachymetry and ultrasonography results shows a good correlation between the methods.

Anterior limiting lamina of the cornea

This second layer of the cornea is also known as Bowman's layer. It varies in thickness between 8 and 14μm. With the light microscope, it appears as an acellular homogeneous zone. Ultrastructurally, it is composed of a randomly orientated array of fine collagen fibrils, which merge with the fibrils of the anterior stroma. Fibrils are composed primarily of collagen types I, III and V. Collagen type VII associated with anchoring fibrils is also present. There is evidence that the anterior limiting lamina is formed and maintained primarily by the epithelium, although its function is unclear. The absence of this lamina from the cornea of most mammals, and the fact that corneas devoid of this lamina over the central cornea following photorefractive keratectomy apparently function normally, suggest that it is not critical to corneal integrity.

Antibacterial drugs

Bacterial eye infections are usually treated topically with eye drops and eye ointments. However, in some conditions, such as posterior blepharitis, systemic administration of a broad-spectrum antibiotic may be appropriate. Systemic, intracorneal or intravitreal routes of administration of antibacterials are necessary in the treatment of intra-ocular infection.

The following topical antibiotics are in common use:

Chloramphenicol is a bacteriostatic antibiotic that inhibits protein synthesis in the bacterial cell and has a broad spectrum of activity against Gram-positive and Gram-negative organisms, particularly *Staphylococcus aureus*. It is considered to be the drug of choice for the treatment of superficial eye infections such as bacterial conjunctivitis and blepharitis and is the most commonly prescribed ophthalmic antibiotic in the UK. Chloramphenicol can also be used prophylactically in the management of a corneal abrasion or following removal of a foreign body. Concern that the use of this well-tolerated antibiotic was associated with aplastic anaemia is no longer considered to be justified.

Fluorinated quinolones are broad-spectrum bactericidal antibacterials that interfere with the production of DNA by inhibiting the enzyme, gyrase, which is responsible for producing the coils of the nucleic acid in the bacterial cell. Ciprofloxacin and ofloxacin are topical fluoroquinolones that are held in reserve for use when other drugs have failed and for the treatment of more serious infections. Ciprofloxacin is effective against *Pseudomonas aeruginosa* and is licensed for the treatment of corneal ulcers. Its use has been associated with the occurrence of fine white corneal deposits in some patients. Ofloxacin is licensed for the treatment of conjunctivitis and keratoconjunctivitis and was thought to be less toxic to the cornea. However, it may be associated with a greater incidence of corneal perforation than fortified antibiotics. Although resistance to fluoroquinolones has been found in some countries such as the USA and India, it has not yet been encountered in the UK.

Levoflaxin and norflaxin, together with the fourth generation fluoroquinolones, moxifloxacin and gatifloxacin, are used in the USA for the treatment of bacterial conjunctivitis, but they are not currently available in the UK. The newer fluoroquinolones are claimed to have better penetration of the cornea, conjunctiva and anterior chamber together with less tissue toxicity.

The aminoglycoside antibiotics, framycetin, gentamicin and neomycin inhibit protein synthesis and have rapid bactericidal action. Framycetin sulphate, otherwise known as neomycin B, has a broad spectrum of activity against Gram-positive and Gram-negative bacteria and is effective against a wider range of bacteria than penicillin or streptomycin. Gentamicin is effective against many strains of *Pseudomonas aeruginosa* and is the treatment of choice for this organism. Gentamicin resistant strains of *Pseudomonas* have been found and may be the consequence of its use in the treatment of minor infections such as conjunctivitis. Neomycin sulphate has a broad spectrum of activity but is not effective against *Pseudomonas aeruginosa*. It is combined with polymixin B and gramicidin in order to achieve a broader spectrum of activity.

Fusidic acid inhibits protein synthesis and has potent bacteriostatic or bactericidal activity against Gram-positive bacteria, which is achieved by the inhibition of protein synthesis. It is commonly used as a front line treatment of bacterial conjunctivitis and is useful in recurrent blepharitis associated with rosacea. Although it has a narrow spectrum of activity, fusidic acid is very effective in staphylococcal infections.

Polymixin B sulphate interferes with cell wall synthesis and is effective against Gram-negative organisms and many strains of Pseudomonas aeruginosa. In order to achieve a broader spectrum of activity, it is combined with bacitracin, which has similar properties to penicillin and is mainly effective against Gram-positive bacteria such as staphylococci and streptococci. This combination is supplied as an ointment. Polymixin B can also be combined with trimethoprim as ointment or eye drops.

Propamidine isethionate is an aromatic diamidine that interferes with DNA synthesis and has a broad-spectrum of activity being staphylococcicidal and amoebistatic. It is available over-the-counter from a pharmacy as eye drops for treatment of minor ocular infections such as blepharitis and conjunctivitis. It is of some value in the treatment of *Acanthamoeba* keratitis and is effective against the active trophozoite form of *Acanthamoeba* but not against the dormant cyst form. Unfortunately, propamidine can induce encystment making this condition refractory to treatment.

Dibromopropamidine isethionate, the dibromo derivative of propamidine, is also available over-the-counter from a pharmacy as an ointment for treatment of minor ocular infections such as blepharitis and conjunctivitis and can be used prophylactically following a procedure such as removal of a foreign body.

Topical antibiotics in multidose, single dose and ointment forms are listed in Tables A.6, A.7 and A.8, respectively.

Antifungal drugs

Although fungal ocular infections, or mycoses, are rare in temperate climates compared to those caused by bacteria, they can be very serious and require prompt, effective treatment, ideally at a specialist centre. Ocular mycosis generally occurs in patients who have undergone trauma (especially if of agricultural origin) or surgery, or may result from the spread of infection from the paranasal sinuses. Those at greater risk of infection are the elderly, debilitated or immunocompromised, and those living in the tropics.

Since host cells and fungal cells are eukaryotic, both have the potential to be affected by antifungal agents. For this reason, evidence that an ocular disease has a fungal involvement, together with mycological identification, is usually required before treatment is undertaken. The essential challenge is to use drugs that are effective against the invading fungal cells without having a toxic effect upon the host cells.

A range of antifungal agents is available that can be administered topically, usually as drops, or by subconjunctival injection. Systemic administration, which is required for deep corneal infections, can be taken orally (as tablets) or by intravenous injection. The choice of drug and its means of administration are determined by the causative fungus, the ocular structures that are affected and the severity of the infection.

Antifungal drugs fall into two principal categories – polyene antibiotics and imadiazoles – both of which disrupt membrane function. The hydrophobic groups of a polyene, such as amphotericin-B, become inserted into the plasma membrane of the fungus creating small pores through which cellular components leak. Amphotericin toxicity may be the consequence of a similar effect upon the host cells. As a generalization, the polyenes are more effective against superficial infections since they exhibit poor penetration if the corneal epithelium is intact. However, if there is an epithelial defect, high levels can reach the stroma.

Since amphotericin is not absorbed orally, it is administered topically or by injection. Irritation may occur as a side effect and punctuate epithelial erosions may result from its use at higher doses. Although natamycin is less toxic than amphotericin, it may cause conjunctival hyperaemia and corneal epithelial defects.

The imadiazoles disrupt the synthesis of sterols and their reduced numbers make the fungal membrane unstable. As most imadiazoles achieve good penetration of ocular tissues, they can be used topically and are well tolerated. Oral administration of ketoconazole, itraconazole and fluconazole results in significant absorption by

Table A.6 • Topical antibacterials: preserved multidose preparations.

Non-proprietary name	Proprietary name	Formulation	Preservative
Chloramphenicol	Chloromycetin®	Drops 0.5%	Phenylmercuric nitrate 0.002%
Ciprofloxin hydrochloride	Ciloxan®	Drops 0.3%	Benzalkonium chloride 0.006%
Framycetin sulphate	Soframycin®	Drops 0.5%	Benzalkonium chloride 0.024%
Fusidic acid	Fucithalmic®	Gel 1% that liquefies	Benzalkonium chloride 0.01%*
Gentamicin sulphate	Garamycin®	Drops 0.3%	Benzalkonium chloride 0.01%
	Genticin®	Drops 0.3%	Benzalkonium chloride 0.02%
Neomycin sulphate	Neosporin®	Drops neomycin sulphate 1700 units, gramicidin 25 units, polymyxin B sulphate 5000 units/mL	Benzalkonium chloride 0.005%
Ofloxacin	Exocin®	Drops 0.3%	Benzalkonium chloride 0.005%
Polymixin B sulphate	Polytrim®	Drops trimethoprim 0.1%, polymyxin B sulphate 10 000 units/mL	Benzalkonium chloride 0.005%
Propamidine isethionate	Brolene® and as Golden Eye® Drops	Drops 0.1% Drops 0.1%	Benzalkonium chloride Benzalkonium chloride 0.01%

* with disodium edetate

Table A.7 • Topical antibacterials: unpreserved single dose preparations.

Non-proprietary name	Proprietary name	Formulation
Chloramphenicol	Minims® Chloramphenicol	Drops 0.5%
Gentamicin sulphate	Minims® Gentamicin Sulphate	Drops 0.3%

Table A.8 • Topical antibacterials: ointments.

Non-proprietary name	Proprietary name	Formulation
Chloramphenicol	Chloromycetin®	Ointment 1%
Polymixin B sulphate	Polyfax®	Ointment polymyxin B sulphate 10 000 units, bacitracin zinc 500 units/g
	Polytrim®	Ointment trimethoprim 0.1%, polymyxin B sulphate 10 000 units/g*
Dibromopropamidine isethionate	Brolene® and as Golden Eye® Ointment	Ointment 0.15%

* preserved with thiomersal

ocular tissues. Although itraconazole is particularly effective, it is hepatotoxic.

Flucytosine (5-fluorocytosine) represents a third category of antifungal agent that, in susceptible organisms, is converted to fluorouracil, which inhibits RNA function and DNA synthesis.

Since no ocular antifungal drugs are generally available in Europe due to the low prevalence of ocular

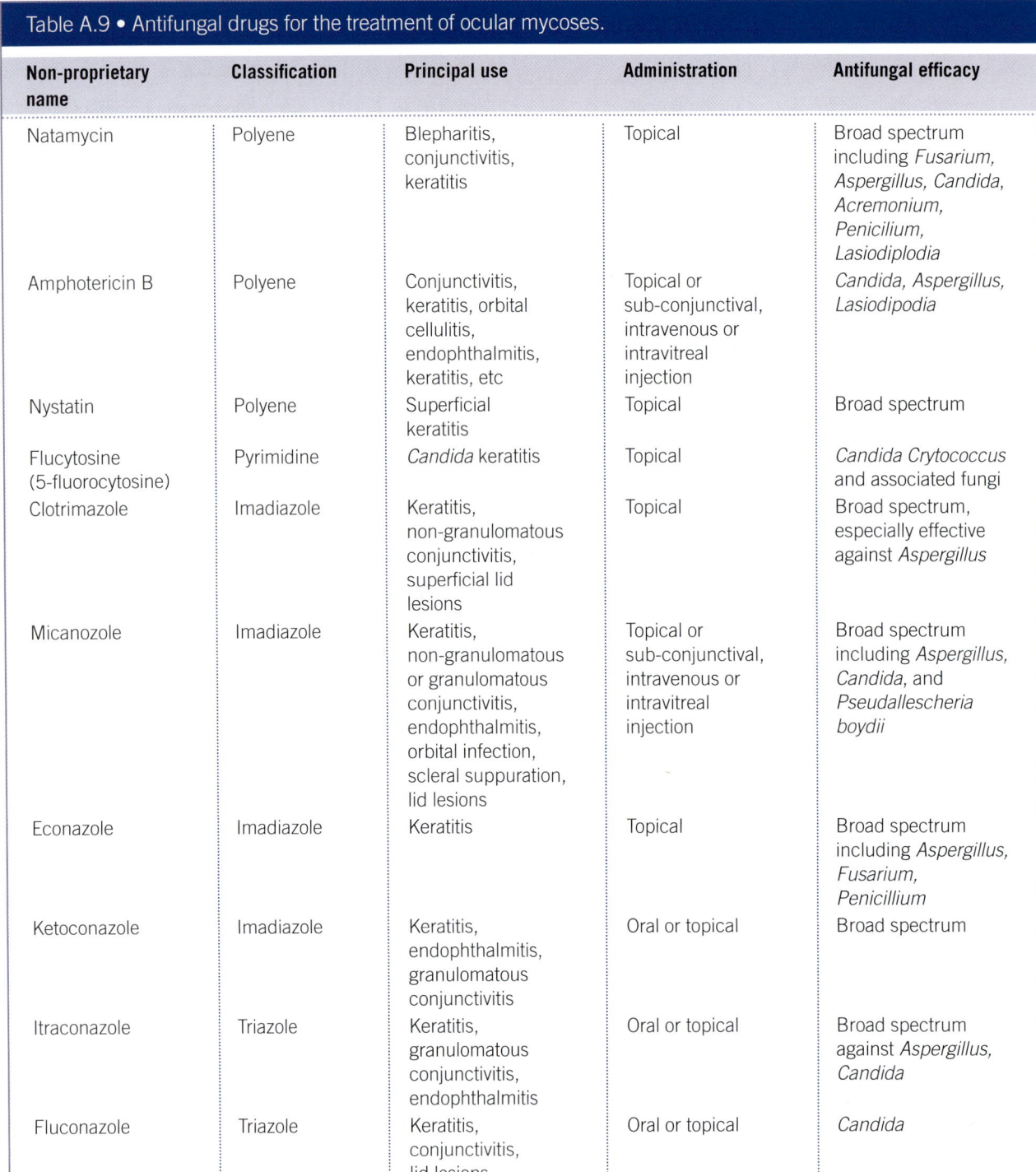

Table A.9 • Antifungal drugs for the treatment of ocular mycoses.

Non-proprietary name	Classification	Principal use	Administration	Antifungal efficacy
Natamycin	Polyene	Blepharitis, conjunctivitis, keratitis	Topical	Broad spectrum including *Fusarium, Aspergillus, Candida, Acremonium, Penicilium, Lasiodiplodia*
Amphotericin B	Polyene	Conjunctivitis, keratitis, orbital cellulitis, endophthalmitis, keratitis, etc	Topical or sub-conjunctival, intravenous or intravitreal injection	*Candida, Aspergillus, Lasiodipodia*
Nystatin	Polyene	Superficial keratitis	Topical	Broad spectrum
Flucytosine (5-fluorocytosine)	Pyrimidine	*Candida* keratitis	Topical	*Candida Crytococcus* and associated fungi
Clotrimazole	Imadiazole	Keratitis, non-granulomatous conjunctivitis, superficial lid lesions	Topical	Broad spectrum, especially effective against *Aspergillus*
Micanozole	Imadiazole	Keratitis, non-granulomatous or granulomatous conjunctivitis, endophthalmitis, orbital infection, scleral suppuration, lid lesions	Topical or sub-conjunctival, intravenous or intravitreal injection	Broad spectrum including *Aspergillus, Candida*, and *Pseudallescheria boydii*
Econazole	Imadiazole	Keratitis	Topical	Broad spectrum including *Aspergillus, Fusarium, Penicillium*
Ketoconazole	Imadiazole	Keratitis, endophthalmitis, granulomatous conjunctivitis	Oral or topical	Broad spectrum
Itraconazole	Triazole	Keratitis, granulomatous conjunctivitis, endophthalmitis	Oral or topical	Broad spectrum against *Aspergillus, Candida*
Fluconazole	Triazole	Keratitis, conjunctivitis, lid lesions	Oral or topical	*Candida*

mycosis, they have to be specially prepared by the hospital pharmacy.

Table A.9 illustrates the uses and effectiveness of several antifungal drugs in the treatment of various conditions in which a mycotic involvement has been established.

Antihistamine drugs

An antihistamine drug blocks the effect upon small blood vessels of histamine that, following its release from mast cells, is the primary mediator of the acute or early phase of an allergic response. In a condition such as allergic conjunctivitis, which affects approximately 25 per cent of the US population, the allergen-antigen reaction results in an increased influx of calcium ions into the mast cells and histamine is released from them stimulating nerve endings and causing symptoms of pain and itching. The permeability of capillaries increases causing loss of cells and proteins. In turn, the loss of protein raises the osmotic pressure of the fluid and oedema ensues from the increased loss of water into tissues. Redness results from a diffuse vasodilation. Accordingly, the characteristic symptoms of ocular allergy are itching, redness, tearing and chemosis.

Two types of histamine receptors, H_1 and H_2, have been found in the human conjunctiva. Stimulation of the H_1 receptors gives rise to itching while stimulation of H_2 receptors elicits dilation of conjunctival blood vessels without itching. The essential function of an antihistamine such as antazoline is to act as an H_1-receptor antagonist. Accordingly, such drugs prove to be more effective in relieving itching (the hallmark symptom of allergic conjunctivitis) than redness.

Topical administration of antihistamines has the advantage that the drug is delivered directly to the affected site to provide faster relief with reduced risk of adverse systemic effects and drug interactions. However, oral administration may be preferred in cases of severe or chronic allergy and a number of non-sedating antihistamines are available. While these are effective and well tolerated, several hours must elapse before the maximum therapeutic effect is achieved. A range of side effects from the use of topical antihistamines has been reported and those most frequently mentioned are transient irritation, blurred vision and headache.

Examples of topical antihistamines are:

- Antazoline, which is combined with the sympathomimetic or α-adrenergic agonist, xylometazoline hydrochloride, which constricts conjunctival vessels (see *Decongestants*) to provide a dual mode of action. Although the symapthomimetic causes very little mydriasis, it is considered that the use of these drops in patients with narrow angle glaucoma should be avoided. This product can be obtained from a pharmacy as an over-the-counter preparation.
- Azelastine inhibits histamine release and interferes with activation of other mediators of allergic inflammation. It has been shown to be at least as effective as levocabastine in improving itching and conjunctival redness in patients with moderate to severe perennial allergic conjunctivitis.
- Emedastine decreases the extent of itching of the eye and conjunctival hyperaemia in children with acute allergic conjunctivitis, its effects being exerted within minutes. Various studies suggest that emedastine is superior to nedocromil, loratadine and levocabastine in relieving the symptoms of this condition.
- Ketotifen, a benzocycloheptathiopane derivative, has been used for many years in the treatment of asthma. In addition to its potent non-competitive H_1 antagonist activity, it stabilizes conjunctival mast cells and decreases chemotaxis, activation and degranulation of eosinophils. The late phase of an allergic response occurs from 2 to 24 hours after exposure to an antigen and results from the infiltration and activation of inflammatory eosinophils and macrophages. Ketotifen has been shown to provide a faster onset of action and better relief of symptoms than emedastine.
- Levocabastine is more potent than antazoline and has a rapid onset of action, relieving symptoms within 10 minutes of instillation. It also has a long duration of action and is well tolerated in the treatment of vernal conjunctivitis, seasonal allergic rhinoconjunctivitis and allergic conjunctivitis caused by dust mites. A levocabastine preparation licensed only for the treatment of seasonal allergic conjunctivitis is available from a pharmacy as an over-the-counter preparation.
- Olopatadine is a topical ocular dibenzoxepin derivative that has selective H_1 receptor blocking activity and a mast cell stabilizing effect. One investigation showed that ketotifen is more effective than olopatadine in inhibiting degranulation of mast cells and the release of histamine. However, the results of another study found that olopatadine was more effective than ketotifen in the treatment of allergic conjunctivitis and that it caused less ocular discomfort.

Although it is unlikely that patients would wish to wear hydrogel contact lenses while suffering from vernal conjunctivitis, seasonal allergic rhinoconjunctivitis or allergic conjunctivitis, they should be cautioned that antihistamine eye drops are preserved with benzalkonium chloride. If contact lens wear is essential, the lenses could be inserted after at least 15 minutes following each instillation of the drops.

Mast cell stabilizers are also used in the treatment of allergic conjunctivitis.

Table A.10 shows some preserved multidose antihistamine preparations.

Anti-inflammatory drugs

- See *Corticosteroids*; *Non-steroidal anti-inflammatory drugs*

Antimicrobial efficacy of contact lens solutions

This is the capacity of a lens care product to eradicate or minimize microbial organisms. An important consideration for the contact lens practitioner when dispensing a care product is its performance in terms of cleaning and – perhaps more importantly in terms of wearer safety – antimicrobial efficacy.

The first safeguard for the practitioner is that, in many parts of the world, contact lens disinfectants are required to meet a number of criteria before they can be labelled and sold. For example, in the European Union all such products are required to display the 'CE mark', which indicates that the product has displayed a minimum level of disinfecting performance and that a number of other criteria such as satisfactory manufacturing conditions have been met. The CE mark requires a contact lens disinfectant to meet the performance requirements of the international standard EN ISO 14729:3 (Microbiological requirements for products and regimens for hygienic management of contact lenses). To achieve this, the product must show activity against three bacteria (*Pseudomonas aeruginosa*, *Staphylococcus aureus* and *Serratia marcescens*) and two forms of yeast (*Candida albicans* and *Fusarium solani*).

Products are first tested on a 'stand-alone' basis. Here, the disinfectant must be able to reduce the population of each of the bacteria by 99.9% (or a three log reduction) and the yeasts by 90% (a one log reduction). This testing is performed in laboratory conditions without the use of contact lenses – that is, there is a mixing of the test organisms with a fixed quantity of the solution under test.

Table A.10 • Topical antihistamines: preserved multidose preparations.

Non-proprietary name	Proprietary name	Formulation	Preservatives (% w/v)
Antazoline sulphate	Otrivine-Antistin®	Drops 0.5% with xylometazoline hydrochloride 0.05%	Benzalkonium chloride 0.01%*
Azelastine hydrochoride	Optilast®	Drops 0.05%	Benzalkonium chloride 0.0125%*
Emedastine difumarate	Emadine®	Drops 0.05%	Benzalkonium chloride 0.01%
Ketotifen hydrogen fumarate	Zaditen®	Drops 0.025%	Benzalkonium chloride 0.01%
Levocabastine chloride	Livostin®	Drops 0.05%	Benzalkonium chloride 0.015*
Olopatadine hydrochloride	Opatanol®	Drops 0.1%	Benzalkonium chloride 0.01%

* with disodium edetate

If the product fails to meet the stand-alone criteria the 'regimen procedure' can be invoked, whereby the performance of the product in a more 'real world' situation is analyzed. However, to proceed to this stage, solutions must at least have demonstrated that they are able to achieve stasis for yeast in the stand-alone test, and an overall combined five log reduction for the three bacteria, with at least one log reduction for each of the bacteria. In the regimen procedure, contact lenses are inoculated with the panel of test organisms, and then treated according to the instructions provided by the manufacturer for cleaning, rinsing and soaking. To satisfy the criteria, there must be at least a four log reduction for all the test organisms.

In order to reach the marketplace, therefore, contact lens solutions are required to achieve a set standard of performance. However, of further interest is the relative performance of the various products that are available. Although this might seem to require simply generating comparative data for a range of care products, this area is fraught with problems. For example, an approach that has been used in the past to demonstrate the disinfection capabilities of disinfectant systems is the 'D-value'. This parameter denotes the time taken for a disinfectant product to reduce the population of an organism to 10% of its original level (a one log reduction).

Although this appears to be a useful indication of solution performance, there are a number of problems with its use. The D-value assumes a linear relationship between the logarithm of the number of survivors and time. However, the action of contact lens disinfectants tends to be non-linear, which suggests that the use of D-values is inappropriate and can lead to misleading representations of product performance. Another drawback to the D-value approach is that no account is made of the minimum recommended disinfection time (MRDT) recommended by the manufacturer. For example, a product may offer a one log reduction in 20 minutes and a three log reduction in 1 hour; the clinical success of this product, however, must depend to some extent on the MRDT, which could be 10 minutes or 6 hours. A new measure of solution potency – solution 'power' – overcomes this problem. This parameter is defined as the MRDT divided by the D-value.

A difficulty with this sort of approach is that no account is made of any cleaning or rinsing (as distinct from disinfecting) that may be employed as part of the overall care system. Some wearers might tend to omit these steps with some systems and not with others; this must impact on the overall disinfecting capabilities of the regimen.

Another significant problem when assessing differences between products is that different laboratory conditions and techniques can be employed. A relevant example here is the effectivity of disinfectants against Acanthamoeba. A number of variables exist when analyzing the performance of products against Acanthamoeba, including the strain of Acanthamoeba used, growth conditions, and contact time of the disinfectant. Indeed the results in this area are highly dependent on methodology, which has led, in part, to the efficacy of contact lens disinfectants against Acanthamoeba being omitted from ISO 14729:3.

Despite this, the effectiveness of contact lens disinfectants against Acanthamoeba is of considerable interest to contact lens practitioners. On a stand-alone basis, hydrogen peroxide is effective at killing both Acanthamoeba trophozoites and cysts, with overnight storage in 3% hydrogen peroxide providing better performance in this regard than the shorter contact time with a one-step system. Multipurpose solutions have poor anti-Acanthamoebal efficacy, although the combination of MAPD and polyquad may improve this. In a clinical setting, cleaning and rinsing is likely to remove some Acanthamoebae. Furthermore, Acanthamoeba is thought to require the presence of bacteria to survive and grow, so the antibacterial efficacy of a contact lens disinfectant will have an effect on Acanthamoebal contamination.

Anti-reflection coatings

In order to reduce surface reflections from a lens and maximize transmittance of light through the lens, a thin film coating is applied in a vacuum chamber. The

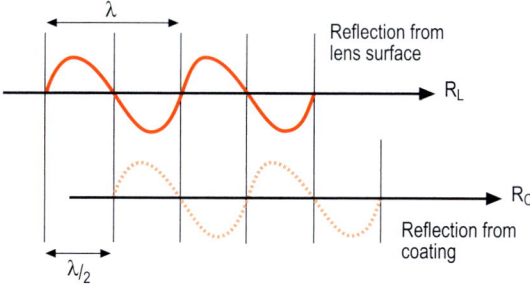

Figure A.9 • Use of destructive interference.

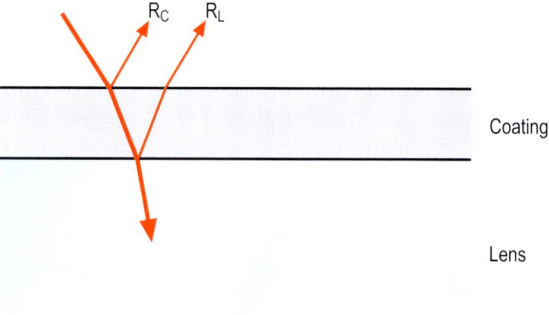

Figure A.10 • Anti-reflection surface.

properties of this film must be very carefully controlled in order that it reduces reflections in the desired manner.

The theory of anti-reflection coatings depends on light acting as a wave (Figure A.9). Assume the reflected light from the lens has a wavelength λ; if it is combined with light which is half a wavelength out of phase ($\lambda/2$ path difference), then the two waves will destructively interfere, reducing the reflection to zero. Light not reflected is then transmitted. Thus, in Figure A.10, if a thin film is coated on the lens such that the extra path length of the light passing through the coating is half a wavelength, then interference will take place. As the light passes twice through the coating, the thickness should be half of $\lambda/2 = \lambda/4$. Hence the required thickness of an anti-reflection coating is one quarter of the wavelength of light.

The other optical property that needs to be considered in constructing an anti-reflection coating is the refractive index. For a lens of refractive index n' in a surrounding medium of index n, the reflection from a surface (σ) is given by:

$$\sigma = [(n'-n)/(n'+n)]^2 \qquad \text{Equation 1}$$

Equation 1 gives a value for σ of between 0 and 1, where 0 indicates that no light is reflected at the surface, and 1 indicates that the entire incident light is reflected at the surface. The equation shows that reflectance increases with higher index lens materials. It also shows that reflectance is greater at the blue end of the spectrum, since any lens material has a higher refractive index for short wavelengths than for longer wavelength light. If the amount of reflection from the coating/lens surface (σ_L) is made the same as the amount of reflection from the coating/air surface (σ_C), then the reflections will destructively interfere if the thickness condition discussed above is met. Thus, for a lens material of refractive index n' with a coating of index n_c, in air:

If:

$$\sigma_L = [(n'-n_c)/(n'+n_c)]^2$$
$$\sigma_C = [(n_c-1)/(n_c+1)]^2$$
and $\sigma_L = \sigma_C$
then $[(n'-n_c)/(n'+n_c)]^2 = [(n_c-1)/(n_c+1)]^2$

taking square roots of both sides and expanding

$$(n'-n_c)(n_c+1) = (n_c-1)(n'+n_c)$$
$$n'n_c + n' - n_c^2 - n_c = n'n_c + n_c^2 - n' - n_c$$
$$2n_c^2 = 2n'$$
$$n_c = \sqrt{n'} \qquad \text{Equation 2}$$

Thus, the refractive index of the coating must be the square root of the refractive index of the lens material. For ophthalmic crown glass of index 1.523, this requires a coating of index 1.234. For a practical coating, there are two fundamental problems here. First, the theory shows that this coating is only effective at one wavelength of light, but spectacle lenses are used in conditions of broad band lighting across the full visible spectrum. Second, there is the problem of obtaining a coating material which is not only the correct wavelength, but is also durable enough to withstand the rough treatment given to spectacle lenses. Unfortunately, there is no material that satisfies these criteria fully. Magnesium fluoride ($n = 1.38$) is the most practical coating, despite having a less than ideal refractive index for many lens materials. However, for high refractive index materials, for example $n=1.80$, it is much closer to the ideal value which in this case would be 1.34. The majority of coatings used for ophthalmic lenses now consist of several layers. This enables a lens to have reduced reflections over a wider range of wavelengths.

Antiviral drugs

Viruses are intracellular parasites that can only replicate within a host cell, making viral infections more difficult to treat than those caused by bacteria. Antiviral drugs interfere with the enzymes responsible for viral replication and can be used to treat *Herpes simplex* and *Herpes zoster* infections. However, there is no specific antiviral treatment for several other ocular viral conditions such as adenovirus infection.

Idoxuridine, vidarabine and trifluorothymidine (F_3T) are examples of first generation non-specific antiviral agents that suffered from the disadvantage of damaging host cells. Aciclovir, ganciclovir and valaciclovir are specific antivirals that have a minimal effect upon uninfected host cells.

Idoxuridine, a derivative of thymidine, is the oldest antiviral compound. Viral metabolism incorporates idoxuridine into the DNA inhibiting further synthesis or leading to mutations. When used topically, idoxuridine is very selective and does not impair epithelial growth but it cannot be used following keratoplasty because it inhibits stromal healing.

Vidarabine, also known as adenine arabinoside, is a purine analogue that inhibits DNA polymerase arresting the growth of the nuclear chain. It is effective against

Table A.11 • Antiviral drugs for ocular administration.			
Non-proprietary name	Proprietary name	Formulation	Preservatives (% w/v)
Aciclovir	Zovirax®	Ointment 3%	None
Ganciclovir	Virgan®	Drops/gel 0.15%	Benzalkonium chloride 0.075%

both strains 1 and 2 of *Herpes simplex* which cause infections above and below the waist, respectively. Since its mode of action differs from idoxuridine, it can be used in patients who are allergic to that agent or to treat idoxuridine resistant cases. While vidarabine does not diminish epithelial growth, it does slow the repair of stromal defects.

Trifluorothymidine (F_3T or trifluridine) is a thymidine derivative that becomes incorporated into the viral DNA creating defective new virus particles. It has better ocular penetration than idoxuridine or vidarabine and appears to provide somewhat swifter healing providing early treatment is given.

There are strains of virus that are resistant to idoxuridine, vidarabine and trifluorothymidine and although each of these agents is very potent in terminating viral replication, they exhibit toxicity with extended use. Due to such limitations, they are no longer used in the UK and have been superseded by a second generation of antivirals such as aciclovir that are selectively active in virus-infected cells and less toxic.

Aciclovir (acycloguanosine) becomes phosphorylated into a triphosphate by the viral enzyme in infected cells, thymidine kinase. Replication is then prevented because the triphosphate form of this drug strongly inhibits viral DNA polymerase enzymes resulting in chain termination.

Aciclovir is effective against infections with strains of *Herpes simplex* that are resistant to idoxuridine and its selective mode of action ensures that it is less toxic and does not impede epithelial or stromal wound healing. Aciclovir is widely employed, both orally and topically in the treatment of *Herpes zoster* infections. The ointment form achieves excellent corneal penetration. Although resistance to aciclovir is uncommon, it can occur in immunocompromised patients.

Ganciclovir is another DNA polymerase inhibitor which has similar efficacy to aciclovir in the treatment of corneal ulceration in *Herpes simplex* dendritic keratitis. It is a broad-spectrum virustatic agent which is effective against both strains of *Herpes simplex, cytomegalovirus,* Epstein-Barr virus and *Herpes Zoster* virus. Topical ganciclovir gel achieves good corneal penetration.

Cytomegalovirus (CMV) retinitis ultimately affects about 40% of patients with AIDS and slow-release ocular implants containing ganciclovir are available for surgical insertion in its immediate treatment. Ganciclovir, which is also given intravenously or intravitreally for this condition, is far more toxic than aciclovir.

Treatment with aciclovir necessitates high dosage and frequent administration and valaciclovir, a prodrug of aciclovir, was introduced to address this problem. It provides high oral bioavailability being rapidly and almost completely converted to aciclovir and valine.

Famciclovir, a nucleoside analogue, is the oral prodrug of penciclovir which is well absorbed and rapidly converted to the active compound and is effective against herpes viruses. It has similar efficacy to aciclovir but requires less frequent dosing. The pharmacological mode of action is similar to that of aciclovir, virus-induced thymidine kinase rapidly and efficiently converting penciclovir into the triphosphate which results in inhibition of replication of viral DNA. However, in uninfected cells the concentrations of penciclovir-triphosphate are barely detectable. Penciclovir has been shown to be active against a recently isolated aciclovir-resistant herpes simplex virus strain that has an altered DNA polymerase.

Aciclovir tablets have been used in the systemic treatment of Herpes zoster ophthalmicus but due to its low bioavailability and short plasma half-life, high doses and frequent administration are required. The two prodrugs, valaciclovir or famciclovir, overcome these limitations.

Antiviral drugs for ocular administration are shown in Table A.11.

Aphakia, contact lens correction of

Aphakia – the absence of the crystalline lens – is now rare in adults due to the high success rate of intra-ocular lenses. However, in cases where intra-ocular lens implantation is impossible – for example when the patient has ancilliary pathology such as aniridia, chronic uveitis or glaucoma – contact lenses may be indicated. Such lenses typically have high plus power (i.e. >10.00D). Hydrogel lenses may be used with close monitoring, but silicone elastomer, silicone hydrogel or high-Dk rigid lenses are preferred to ensure adequate corneal oxygenation. Extended wear is desired to minimize frequent lens handling. Patients wearing lenses on an extended wear basis may, with proper monitoring, wear their lenses for a month at a time. High water content hydrogel lenses may be preferred for comfort, and should be selected to maximize oxygen transmissibility for extended wear. Low water content lenses may be preferred due to durability for daily wear, but the risk of hypoxic problems is high. Interestingly, the aphakic eye may swell less than an unoperated eye.

Handling will typically be difficult in bilateral aphakic patients due to poor uncorrected vision and reduced manual dexterity in the elderly. Some aphakes may prefer to handle soft lenses due to their large size, and some may prefer rigid lenses because of their stiffness. Corrections for residual astigmatism and near work can be placed in spectacles to be worn over the contact lenses. Patients with conjunctival filtering blebs should be monitored closely, and contact lenses should not impinge on these blebs excessively. Preferably, topical

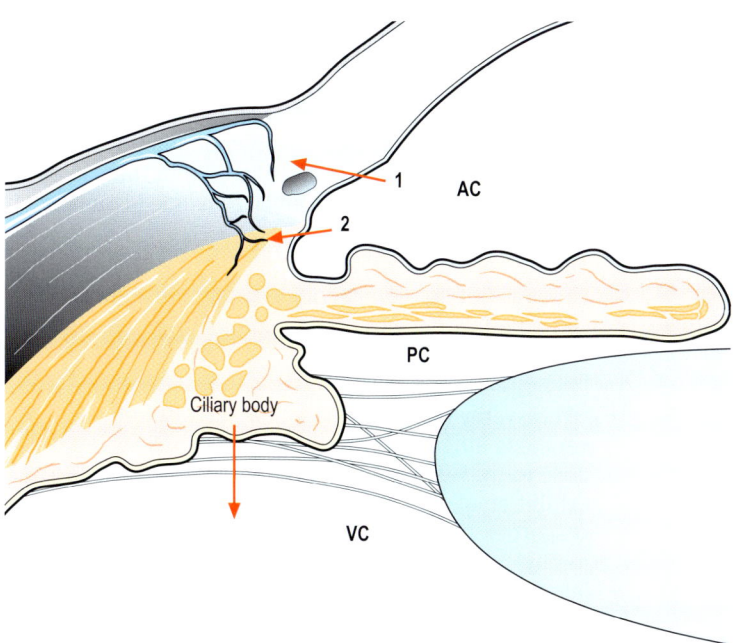

Figure A.11 • Schematic representation of aqueous dynamics. Arrows indicate the direction of aqueous flow. There are two routes for aqueous outflow:
1 = conventional route via the canal of Schlemm
2 = uveoscleral outflow.

ocular medication is instilled before and after lens wear and only under close supervision during contact lens wear. See *High plus power contact lens design*.

Apparent eye size

A cosmetic disadvantage of spectacle lenses is that they alter the apparent size of the eyes of the wearer as seen by other people; the eyes appear larger with positive spectacle corrections and smaller with negative ones. Using a thin lens approximation, where the power of the correcting lens is F_c and the eye is at a distance l from the lens, it is easy to show that the paraxial magnification, M, of the anterior eye is given by:

$$M = 1/(1 + F_c l)$$

Since l is small (0.02m), this can be approximated by:

$$M = 1 - F_c l$$

Thus, if l is –20mm and F_c is –10.00D, the eyes nominally appear only 80% of their true size. In fact, for the viewer, the apparent size will vary depending upon the viewing direction, since conditions will not necessarily be paraxial. Clearly, with contact lenses this cosmetic disadvantage is absent.

Aqueous humour

Aqueous humour is a transparent colourless fluid that is essential for the nutrition of the avascular cornea and lens and the removal of metabolic waste products. It also generates an intra-ocular pressure that is determined by the balance between aqueous production and drainage. Flow rates vary between 2 to 3 microlitres per minute. Much higher flow rates have been recorded during waking hours than during sleep, possibly as a result of circadian variation in endogenous hormones. The composition of the aqueous reflects the secretory activity of the ciliary epithelium and the metabolic processes within the eye. The electrolyte concentration is broadly similar to plasma, although the two fluids differ in the concentration of particular electrolytes e.g. Cl^-, Ca^{2+}, Mg^{2+} and HCO_3^-. Aqueous also differs in the concentration of certain organic solutes, e.g. the levels of ascorbate and lactate are much higher than in plasma. In the interests of optical clarity, the aqueous contains a very low concentration of protein, and is generally <1% of the level in plasma. This situation is maintained by the blood-aqueous barrier, which acts as an exclusion filter. Inflammation of the anterior uvea can lead to a breakdown of this barrier and the presence of protein in the aqueous. The resulting light scatter by protein molecules is manifest clinically as 'flare'.

Aqueous is secreted into the posterior chamber by the ciliary processes. It passes around the equator of the lens, and then flows through the pupil into the anterior chamber (Figure A.11). Aqueous circulates within the anterior chamber due to convection currents, which derive from temperature differences between the cornea and iris. Aqueous then leaves the eye via two alternative routes:

- Conventional pathway: through the trabecular meshwork into the canal of Schlemm from where it drains into episcleral veins
- Uveo-scleral pathway: through the ciliary muscle into the supraciliary and suprachoroidal spaces.

Aqueous leak

- See *Post-trauma or post-surgery, therapeutic lenses for*.

Artificial tears and ocular lubricants

Artificial tears are used to alleviate mild to moderate signs and symptoms of reduced or abnormal tear secretion. In severe cases of dry eye, treatment to conserve tears may include occlusion of the puncta and lateral tarsorrhaphy. The most widely used tests for the diagnosis of dry eye are the Schirmer I test, assessment of tear meniscus height, tear film break-up time and staining with rose bengal. While dryness is a frequent complaint in wearers of hydrogel contact lenses, it is usually managed with comfort drops (also known as conditioning or cushioning drops) rather than with artificial tears, many of which are preserved with benzalkonium chloride.

Artificial tears do not contain an active pharmacological agent but do employ a water soluble polymer that acts as a viscoliser which mimics the actions of mucin in making the hydrophobic surface of the corneal epithelium more hydrophilic and serves as a lubricant between the eyelids and the cornea. The polymer first used for this purpose was the synthetic colloid, methylcellulose which has a high viscosity that caused blurring of vision, sticking and uncomfortable crusting of the eyelids.

The osmolarity of newly produced tears is about 300mOsm/L and in the region of 305 to 310mOsm/L in the tear film. Most artificial tear preparations are iso-osmolar. However, some patients with aqueous deficiency have a higher tears osmolarity than normal. In such cases, artificial tears with an osmolarity of 210 to 230mOsm/L (e.g. Hypotears) are intended to dilute the hyperosmolar tear film and lower the osmolarity to that of normal tears. Although a hypo-osmolarity value of 150mOsm/L is well tolerated, at 75mOsm/L ocular irritation occurs. Distilled water represents the limit of hypo-osmolarity (0mOsm/L) and causes itching and epithelial oedema. It has been shown that in keratoconjunctivitis sicca, hypo-osmolarity alone does not guarantee relief from symptoms and that factors including viscosity and colloid osmotic pressure may be more significant.

At a temperature of 32 to 33°C, the viscosity of normal tears is 9mP and most artificial tears have a value within the range of 10 to 44mP. Highly viscous solutions remain in contact with the eye for a longer time but they make blinking more difficult and disturb vision more. Solutions with a viscosity above 1000mP fail to mix with natural tears. Artificial tears generally have a pH value on the alkaline side of neutral to achieve optimal comfort.

The most widely used preservative in artificial tears is benzalkonium chloride 0.01%, a concentration at which the tear film can destabilize. In some formulations, the concentration of preservative is halved in order to avoid this problem. It has, nevertheless, been suggested that patients with keratoconjunctivitis sicca should use *unpreserved* eye drops.

Due to significant variation in the formulation and viscosity of the various products, it may be necessary for the patient to try several of them in order to find one that is acceptable. Immediately following the instillation of artificial tears, patients may experience transient irritation, blurring or a sticky sensation and should not drive unless certain that their vision is clear.

Artificial tears and ocular lubricants available in eye drop form include the following:

- Hypromellose (hydroxyproplymethylcellulose), a substituted cellulose ether, is the long-standing choice of treatment for aqueous tear deficiency and is available in both preserved multi-dose and unpreserved single dose forms. It has been in ophthalmic use since the 1940s. In one product, hypromellose is combined with phenylephrine hydrochloride which constricts conjunctival vessels, but its prolonged use is not recommended. Although the weak concentration of sympathomimetic causes very little mydriasis, it is considered that the use of these drops in patients with narrow angle glaucoma should be avoided.
- The mucolytic agent, acetylcysteine (the N-acetyl derivative of the amino acid L-cysteine) has been combined with hypromellose and is beneficial when mucous strands or filaments are present as in filamentary keratopathy.
- Hydroxyethylcellulose is another substituted cellulose ether which is available in unpreserved single dose form. Hydroxyethylcellulose and hypromellose exhibit emollient and film-forming (cohesive) properties that are at least equal to those of methylcellulose but they are less viscous and cause less blurring of vision.
- Carmellose sodium (sodium carboxymethyl cellulose) is widely used as an agent in which to suspend active ingredients as an emulsifying and thickening agent. It is also used to make artificial saliva solutions for patients suffering from a dry mouth caused by radiotherapy or antimuscarinic drugs.
- Polyvinyl alcohol acts not only as a viscoliser but as a nonionic surfactant which is helpful in patients with mucin deficiency and at a concentration of 1.4% it has almost the same surface tension as normal tears. Polyvinyl alcohol has been used in artificial tears since the 1960s.
- A mucomimetic agent, hydroxypropylguarpolysaccharide (HP-guar) is employed in a novel product together with two demulcants, polyethylene glycol 400 and propylene glycol and is preserved with polidronium chloride (Polyquad). This agent has been shown to be more effective than carboxymethylcellulose in reducing the signs and symptoms of dry eye.
- Povidone (polyvinyl pyrrolidone) is a mixture of essentially linear synthetic polymers of 1-vinylpyrolidin-2-1 of different chain lengths and molecular weights that functions as a non-ionic surfactant and in a concentration of 3 to 5% it increases the viscosity of solutions.

Artificial tears and ocular lubricants are also available in gel form. Carbomers are synthetic, high molecular weight polymers of acrylic acid cross-linked with either allyl ethers of sucrose or allyl ethers of pentaerithrityl. Carbomer 980 (polyacrylic acid) is supplied as a gel that has thixotropic (i.e. reversible) properties. During blinking, liquefaction of the gel occurs followed by reformation of the gel to reduce elimination from the tear film. The significantly greater retention time has the advantage that fewer instillations are required in order to achieve relief from symptoms and there is a further advantage of a correspondingly lower corneal exposure to preservatives such as bezalkonium chloride.

Liquid paraffin is an ocular lubricant that is supplied as preservative-free ointment and has a much longer retention time than eye drops. Since ointment is likely to

Table A.12 • Artifical tears: preserved multidose preparations.

Non-proprietary name	Proprietary name	Formulation	Preservatives (% w/v)
Hypromellose	Isopto Alkaline®	Drops 1%	Benzalkonium chloride 0.01%
	Isopto Plain®	Drops 0.5%	Benzalkonium chloride 0.01%
	Tears Naturale®	Drops 0.3% with dextran 70 0.1%	Benzalkonium chloride 0.01%*
	Isopto Frin®	Drops 0.5% with phenylephrine hydrochloride 0.12%	Benzethonium chloride 0.01%
	Ilube®	Drops 0.35% with acetylcysteine 5%	Benzalkonium chloride 0.01%*
Carbomer 980	GelTears®	Liquid gel drops 0.2%	Benzalkonium chloride 0.01%
	Liposic®	Liquid gel drops 0.2%	Cetrimide 0.01%
	Viscotears®	Liquid gel drops 0.2%	Cetrimide 0.01%*
Polyvinyl alcohol	Hypotears®	Drops 1% with macrogol '8000' 2%	Benzalkonium chloride 0.01%*
	Liquifilm Tears®	Drops 1.4%	Benzalkonium chloride 0.005%*
	Sno Tears®	Drops 1.4%	Benzalkonium chloride 0.004%*
HP-guar with PEG and PG	Systane™	Drops (concentration not disclosed by manufacturer)	Polidronium chloride 0.001%

*with disodium edetate

Table A.13 • Artificial tears: unpreserved single dose preparations.

Non-proprietary name	Proprietary name	Formulation
Hypromellose	Artelac®	Drops 0.32%
Hydroxyethylcellulose	Minims® Artificial Tears	Drops 0.44%
Carmellose sodium	Celluvisc®	Drops 1%
Carbomer 980	Viscotears®	Liquid gel drops 0.2%
Polyvinyl alcohol	Liquifilm® Tears Preservative Free or REFRESH OPHTHALMIC™	Drops 1.4% with povidone
Povidone K25	Oculotect®	Drops 5%
HP-guar with PEG and PG	Systane™	Drops (concentration not disclosed by manufacturer)

blur vision, it is best used before sleep as an adjunct to drops that are used during the daytime. Ointments are also of value in the treatment of recurrent epithelial erosion.

The recommended dose for most artificial tears is in the region of one or two drops, applied three to four times a day. Examples of artificial tear products in multi dose and single dose forms are listed in Tables A.12 and A.13, and examples of lubricant ointments are shown in Table A.14.

Aspheric ophthalmic lenses

Aspheric ophthalmic lenses are lenses where at least one of the surfaces is made aspherical. Literally speaking an aspherical surface could be any surface which is non-spherical in form, so could include cylindrical or toroidal surfaces. Equally, progressive power lens surfaces are aspherical in nature, but vary in their characteristics in different parts of the lens. A more appropriate definition for an aspheric lens is therefore a lens that has one surface which is of rotationally symmetrical aspherical form. These lens forms were originally used exclusively for single vision lenses, but are now used for all types of spectacle lens.

The most straightforward aspheric surface is the conic section, shown in Figure A.12. With the origin of an x,y coordinate system at the vertex of a surface, the curve is defined as:

$$y^2 = 2r_0x - px^2$$

Table A.14 • Ocular lubricants: ointments.

Non-proprietary name	Proprietary name	Formulation
Liquid paraffin	Lacri-Lube®	White soft paraffin 57.3%, liquid paraffin 42.5%, wool alcohols 0.2%.
	Lubri-Tears®	White soft paraffin 60%, liquid paraffin 30%, wool fat 10%.
Paraffin Yellow soft (Simple Eye Ointment)	None	liquid paraffin 10%, wool fat 10%, in yellow soft paraffin 80%

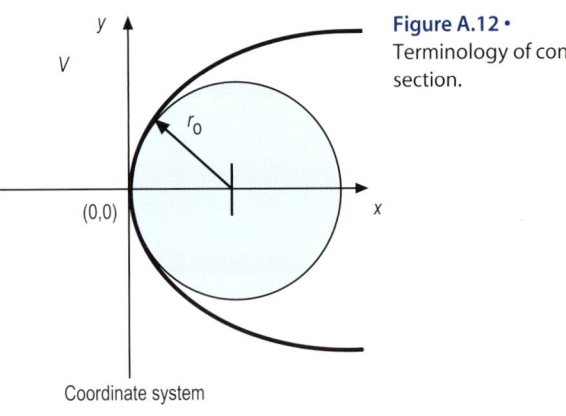

Figure A.12 • Terminology of conic section.

Coordinate system

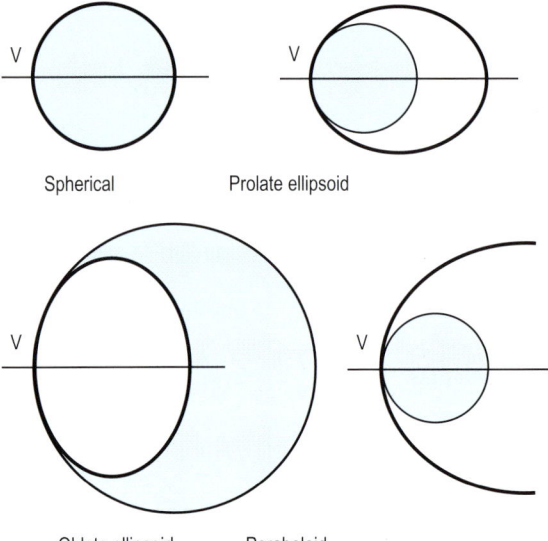

Spherical   Prolate ellipsoid

Oblate ellipsoid   Paraboloid

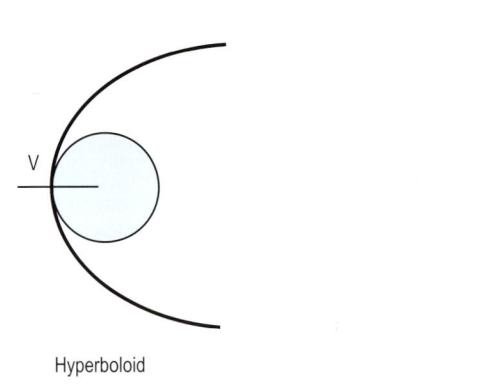

Hyperboloid

Figure A.13 • Conic surfaces.

where r_o is the paraxial radius of curvature, and p is the conic coefficient of the surface. The relationship of conic coefficients to various types of conic surface is given below:

$p < 0$ Hyperboloid
$p = 0$ Paraboloid
$1 > p > 0$ Prolate ellipsoid
$p = 1$ Spherical
$p > 1$ Oblate ellipsoid

The types of curve yielded by these various forms are shown in Figure A.13. The peripheral flattening of the lens is the amount by which a curve departs from the spherical, as shown in Figure A.13, towards the edge of the lens. Note that in terms of peripheral flattening, the order is in relation to the value of p. Thus a hyperboloid will have the flattest aspheric form for a given value of r_o.

Aspheric surfaces are useful in ophthalmic optics as they neutralize the oblique astigmatism caused by off axis viewing, by means of the astigmatism inherent in the surface. Thus any point, apart from the optical centre, will have surface astigmatism. This can be calculated for the tangential and sagittal meridians of the surface in terms of the localized radius in each meridian. The sagittal radius (r_s) is given by:

$$r = v\,[r_o^2 + (1-p)y^2]$$

And from this the tangential radius (r_t) is given by:

$$r_t = r_s^3 / 1 r_o^2$$

Using these expressions, ray tracing programs can be written to derive the oblique astigmatism and curvature error. For steeply curved surfaces, a small change in p has a significant effect upon the optical performance of a lens. Table A.15 illustrates the optical effects of changing the front surface of a +14.00DS lens from spherical to various aspherical forms, while the rear surface remains spherical and of constant power.

It will be apparent that all three major aberrations cannot be reduced to zero at the same time. Astigmatism reaches a minimum with a p_1 of 0.5, curvature error or mean oblique error is at a minimum with a p_1 of 0.7, and distortion is minimized with a p_1 of −0.3.

With the widespread use of intraocular implants after cataract surgery, there are far fewer high positive power lenses supplied than was once the case. Hence the majority of aspheric form lenses are now supplied in low and medium (up to +6.00D) powers. Typically, the front surface is made aspheric, with the rear surface spherical or toroidal depending on the demands of the prescription. A few lenses are supplied in bi-aspheric form, and aspheric toroidal (atoroidal) surfaces are sometimes used to give the optimum correction in both astigmatic meridians.

Although aspherical minus lenses have the benefit of a small reduction in edge thickness compared with their spherical equivalent, the greatest benefits are undoubtedly in plus power lenses where a substantial improvement in appearance can be achieved because of the flatter front surface in aspherical form. Thus, the majority of lenses currently used in aspherical low powers are positive. It must be emphasized that the aspherical surface is used primarily to improve appearance and reduce weight, and does not give improved optics over what is possible with the optimum spherical meniscus form.

Aspheric rigid contact lens designs

A surface that is not spherical (i.e. progressively flattening or steepening) is said to be aspheric. Aspheric rigid lenses have two important disadvantages compared with spherical lenses: firstly, they are more difficult to manufacture, particularly using conventional lathes; and, secondly, they cannot easily be checked using a radiuscope or keratometer. Nevertheless, they offer a number of advantages that arguably outweigh their disadvantages. The main advantages of aspheric designs relate to comfort. Aspheric designs tend to show less edge clearance and therefore induce less edge sensation from contact with the palpebral conjunctiva. Poor blending of back surface junctions in spherical lenses can cause irritation on version when the lens moves off-centre and the peripheral zones come into contact with the cornea. This is generally avoided with aspheric lenses unless the periphery is poorly blended.

The gradual flattening of aspheric lens surfaces results in a thinner periphery, which may also help reduce edge sensation.

Optically, aspheric designs can both improve and degrade image quality. When not aligned with the visual axis, aspheric lenses will induce astigmatism. On the other hand, with higher power lenses, aspheric optics can reduce spherical aberration. In myopic early presbyopes, the reduced minus power in the periphery of aspheric lenses can help with near vision and delay the need for a presbyopic correction.

Aspheric designs take different forms, but these differences are usually so subtle as to be evident only from the manufacturer's product literature. The simplest aspheric design is an elliptical shape selected to be close to, or slightly flatter than, the average cornea. More complex aspheric designs change their degree of flattening, or eccentricity, from centre to edge. Some designs are spherical in the centre and change to an aspheric geometry towards the periphery. Most aspheric designs incorporate a much flatter, often spherical, peripheral zone about 0.2mm wide. This peripheral zone helps to avoid mechanical irritation when the lens decentres to the peripheral cornea.

Association of Contact Lens Manufacturers (ACLM)

UK-based association of companies involved in the contact lens field. Its mission statement is: 'Promoting and growing contact lens wear'. Website: www.aclm.org.uk

Association of Optometrists

Formed over 60 years ago, the Association of Optometrists represents individual independent optometrists and those working with corporate bodies, and undertakes a number of activities designed to support its members.

The organization promotes the professional and clinical independence of its members and encourages the development and promotion of high standards of practice. It also represents members in negotiations on

Table A.15 • Aberration values for +14.00D lens made with various front surface conic asphericities.					
Lens aberrations					
$F'v$	14.00				
F_2	−2.00				
t (mm)	10.00				
n	1.50				
z (mm)	27.00				
Angle (°)	35.00				
p_2	1.00				

Front surface asphericity (p_1)	Oblique astigmatism	Mean oblique power (D)	Mean oblique error (D)	Distortion (%)	
1.00	3.69	16.26	2.26	20.05	
0.70	1.03	13.89	−0.11	13.45	Minimum curvature error
0.50	−0.27	12.65	−1.35	9.91	Minimum oblique astigmatism
0.00	−2.50	10.31	−3.70	3.05	
−0.30	−3.39	9.26	−4.75	−0.13	Minimum distortion
−0.40	−3.36	8.95	−5.05	−1.07	

fees, conditions and terms of service and in disputes, and uses its position to promote the interests of its members to Parliament, Government departments and other Institutions.

The Association has approximately 9000 members and is administered by a Board of Directors of 11 appointed from an elected council of 45 members.

Asthenopia

Asthenopia is a term used to denote a non-specific set of adverse symptoms thought to be attributed to the use of the eyes. Asthenopic symptoms are often vague and the patient may experience difficulty in communicating the apparent type of ocular discomfort they are experiencing. Symptoms that come under the general classification of asthenopia include headache, ocular tiredness, 'pulling' or 'drawing' of the eyes, diffuse ocular pain or discomfort, photophobia and general visual disturbance. Asthenopia can be attributed to any form of ocular dysfunction, such as:

- optical, e.g. ametropia, presbyopia
- visual, e.g. field loss, glare sensitivity
- binocular, e.g. phoria, tropia
- oculomotor, e.g. A-V problem, convergence insufficiency
- pathological, e.g. glaucoma, conjunctivitis
- ophthalmic prostheses related, e.g. uncomfortable spectacles, contact lens discomfort

Practitioners should always be prepared to investigate whether asthenopia symptoms are related to problems that are unrelated to the eyes, such as general stress, fatigue, systemic disease, pathology of the head and neck etc.

Asthenopia is also sometimes referred to as 'eyestrain', although this term relates more to problems with near vision.

Astigmatism

Astigmatism is a refractive defect of the eye in which light from a distant object is focused as two orthogonal focal lines rather than a single focal point. Astigmatism is corrected with toric lens forms.

Astigmatism can be classified in a variety of ways, as follows:

- Regular or irregular astigmatism. In regular astigmatism, the two axes are separated by an angle of 90°. In irregular astigmatism, the two axes are separated by an angle other than 90°. The latter may occur in cases of irregular corneal shape, such as following trauma or surgery, or as a result of keratoconus.
- Contributing ocular component. Astigmatism can arise due to toricity of one of the major refracting optical components of the eye, such as the anterior or posterior cornea or anterior or posterior lenticular surfaces. Tilting of the crystalline lens can also cause astigmatism. Other anatomical causes of astigmatism include the fovea being displaced from the optic axis and the retina being tilted with respect to the other optical components of the eye.
- Orientation. If the corneal meridian that has the least refractive power is horizontal, this is described as 'with-the-rule astigmatism'. If the corneal meridian that has the least refractive power is vertical, this is described as 'against-the-rule astigmatism'. If the corneal meridian that has the least refractive power is neither horizontal nor vertical, this is described as 'oblique astigmatism'.
- Refractive error. Astigmatism may be classified with respect to the relative positions of the retinal images of a distant object under conditions of minimal accommodation. These are: simple astigmatism – one image is located on the retina; simple myopic astigmatism – one image is located on the retina and the other is in front of the retina; simple hyperopic astigmatism – one image is located on the retina and the other is behind the retina; compound astigmatism – both images are located either in front of, or behind, the retina; compound myopic astigmatism – both images are located in front of the retina; compound hyperopic astigmatism – both images are located behind the retina; mixed astigmatism – one image is located in front of the retina and the other is located behind the retina.

Astringents

An astringent is an agent that causes cells to shrink by precipitating proteins from their surfaces. Topical application of these agents therefore usually produces a local contraction of tissue.

Zinc sulphate, a heavy metal, is a good example of a traditional astringent that has had a long history of use in the treatment of angular conjunctivitis, which is usually caused by the Gram negative Morax-Axenfeld bacillius (*Moraxella*). Although zinc salts were considered to be specific in their effect on this type of conjunctivitis, they have been superseded by topical antibiotics. Since zinc sulphate precipitates protein and clears mucous from the ocular surface, it has also been used in the treatment of epiphora.

A number of collyria (eyewashes) and non-specific over-the-counter eye preparations continue to incorporate zinc sulphate because of its astringent action. A non-proprietary formulation of zinc sulphate (0.25%) eye drops can still be supplied by a pharmacy.

Witch hazel, the extract of the shrub *Hamamelis virginiana*, is another example of a mild astringent that forms the basis of a commonly used eye lotion (Optrex). Witch hazel is also used in lotions to soothe and cool sprains and in other preparations to alleviate the discomfort caused by haemorrhoids.

Atopic eczema

- See *Systemic disease, contact lens wear in.*

Atopic keratoconjunctivitis

- See *Degenerations of the corneal epithelium, therapeutic lenses for.*

Autorefraction

The use of a machine to measure refractive error has a long history. The original optometers could use either subjective methods, the forerunners of modern phoropters, or objective methods, and it is the automated objective refraction instruments that are now described as autorefractors. Autorefractors use an infra-red light source (around 800 to 900nm), which allows good ocular transmission, but requires a –0.50D adjustment to the final refraction due to error introduced by reflection from the choroid and sclera. The source projects light via a beam splitter and a Badal lens system to form a slit image within the eye, the reflection of which passes out via the beam splitter to reach a light sensor. Throughout, the patient is encouraged to relax accommodation (a major source of error for autorefractor measurement) by use of a fixation target or, in some cases, an open view to allow fixation on a distant target. The calculation of refractive error is based upon analysis of how the eye of the patient influences the infra-red radiation.

There is a variation in the way refractive error is analyzed by different autorefractors. Most of the original instruments used some form of image quality analysis, relying on positioning of the Badal lens system to achieve a maximum signal to the light sensor. The majority of modern autorefractors, of which there are many, rely on an adapted Scheiner disc principle. The original Scheiner disc consisted of two holes in a card placed before the eye. A myopic eye will see the two images from the holes swapped over or crossed, while the hypermetrope sees them uncrossed. This may be done in various meridians to give information about the nature of astigmatism. Autorefractors simulate this using light emitting diodes (LEDs), the image of which are detected by a light sensor or photodetector and the position of the LED needed to achieve a single image over the photodetector is related to the patient's refractive error. A further method employed by a few machines is an adaptation of retinoscopy, where the instrument analyses the speed of movement of a reflex of infra-red light to measure the refractive error.

Most studies suggest that autorefractors are quick, simple, repeatable and accurate (with some qualification). With cycloplegia or good accommodative control, the results are very accurate. Indeed, the spherical aberration introduced by the dilation of pupils with a cycloplegic makes the method preferable to retinoscopy in many cases. The ease of use of an autorefractor makes it suitable to be carried out by ancillary staff, so reducing the workload of the optometrist. The machines may directly link to an automated phoropter head, again making the routine refraction more fluid. It is useful to remember that

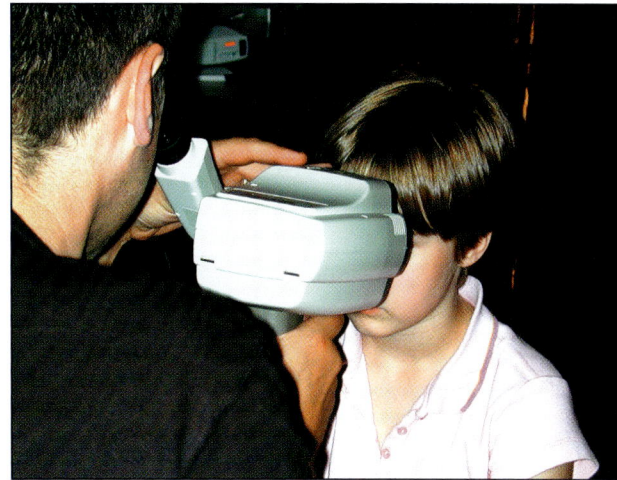

Figure A.14 • Portable autorefractor in use.

even the most accurate objective measurement may not be that preferred by the patient so a subjective approach is always preferable to ensure a tolerable refractive correction, even though this is sometimes modified away from the actual refractive error present.

The main error with autorefractors is due to poor fixation (dependent very much on the target of the instrument), accommodative fluctuation (proximal accommodation in the young invariably leads to excess minus power being recorded) and media difficulties (which are also likely to reduce the effectiveness of retinoscopy). Portable models are available, some of which have found use in child screening programmes where the main outcome is not precise error measurement but detection of large amounts of ametropia or anisometropia (Figure A.14). Other new models incorporate some subjective assessment also, with the patient responding to prompts to clarify a presented image.

Average thickness of a lens
- See *Lens thickness*.

Axial edge lift
- See *Edge lift*.

Babies, contact lenses for
- See *Paediatric contact lenses; Paediatric contact lens examination; Paediatric contact lens fitting.*

Back optic zone diameter (BOZD) of a contact lens
The diameter of the optic zone on the back of the lens as measured through the lens centre (Figure B.1). The back optic zone diameter (BOZD) of a rigid lens is generally fixed for a given design in a given total diameter (TD), and is generally 1–1.5mm smaller than the TD. The BOZD should be large enough to cover the pupil in most conditions, including low illumination.

With toroidal corneas, using a smaller BOZD can increase the area of alignment and therefore improve the fit. However, if the BOZD is reduced while maintaining the same TD, this will result in a wider periphery, and flatter peripheral curves are required in order to maintain edge clearance.

If the BOZD is changed, it is usually necessary to change the BOZR in order to maintain a clinically equivalent fit. Reducing the BOZD, without reducing the BOZR, results in a sagittal depth that is shallower and therefore a flatter fit. As a rule of thumb, an increase in BOZD of 0.5mm requires an increase in BOZR of 0.05mm.

Back optic zone radius (BOZR)
The back optic zone radius (BOZR, or 'base curve') is the radius of curvature of the back surface of a contact lens (Figure B.1). It is the main parameter to be modified when attempting to optimize the fit of a soft lens, a steepening of BOZR being required to tighten a soft lens fit and *vice versa*. However, even with lenses that are relatively inflexible, such as thick, low water content lenses, large changes in BOZR are required in order to have a significant effect on lens movement. With more flexible, thinner, high water content lenses, changes in BOZR have even less effect. The labelled BOZR is therefore of little help in soft lens fitting.

Knowledge of soft lens BOZR is not necessarily helpful when comparing different brands of lens. Lenses of similar BOZR can show widely differing sagittal depths because of differences in back surface design. This phenomenon, and differences in material mechanical properties, means that widely differing fitting characteristics can be observed on a given cornea with different brands of lenses of the same nominal BOZR.

Back surface rigid toric contact lenses
- See *Cylindrical power equivalent rigid toric contact lenses.*

Back vertex power (BVP) of a contact lens
This is the optical power of the lens measured in dioptres. Modifications are often made to the design of soft lenses at the extremes of the power range. At

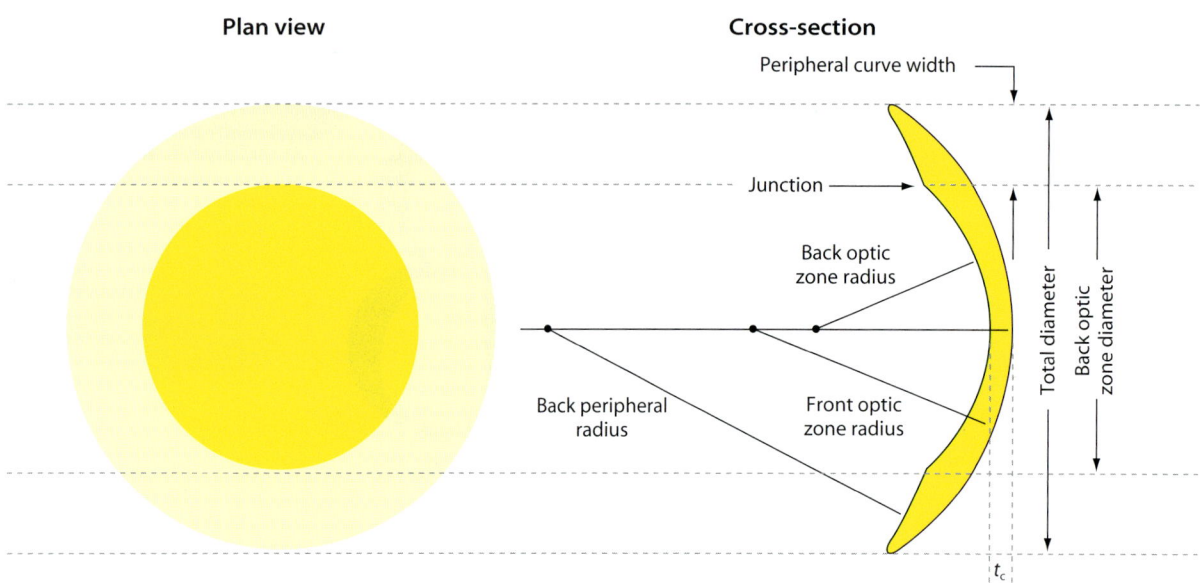

Figure B.1 • Plan and cross-sectional view of a minus-powered contact lens with a single curve front surface and bicurve back surface.

the lower end of the minus power range (<–1.50D), lens centre thickness is usually increased to improve lens handling. At the higher end of the power range, lens centre thickness is often reduced and the optic zone diameter kept to a minimum in order to reduce lens bulk and maximize oxygen transmission.

The thickness of high minus lenses can be further reduced, and the optical performance improved, by incorporating aspheric optics in order to overcome lens spherical aberration. With plus power lenses, the optic zone diameter is again minimized in order to minimize centre thickness. Some manufacturers have utilized a larger diameter in order to counterbalance the anticipated greater movement of plus-power lenses; however, hyperopic eyes tend to be smaller in diameter and therefore this is of doubtful benefit.

There tends to be little difference in lens fit between low minus and higher minus lenses of similar design. However, plus power lenses tend to show significantly more post-blink movement than minus power lenses of the same dioptric power, probably due to their greater thickness, leading to increased interaction with the upper lid. (See Appendix D.)

Back vertex power
- See *Lens power*

Bacterial keratitis

Bacterial infections of the cornea are acutely sight threatening and if left untreated can rapidly progress to marked stromal loss and even perforation. Bacterial keratitis almost always occurs in the presence of a significant risk factor such as contact lens usage, especially with poor lens care or extended wear. The most common bacteria in contact lens-related bacterial keratitis is *Pseudomonas aeruginosa*, a bacteria that is notable due to its ability to spread rapidly and lead to severe inflammation and tissue damage. For overnight wear, high oxygen transmission silicone hydrogel lenses carry a 5× lower risk of causing bacterial keratitis compared with hydro-

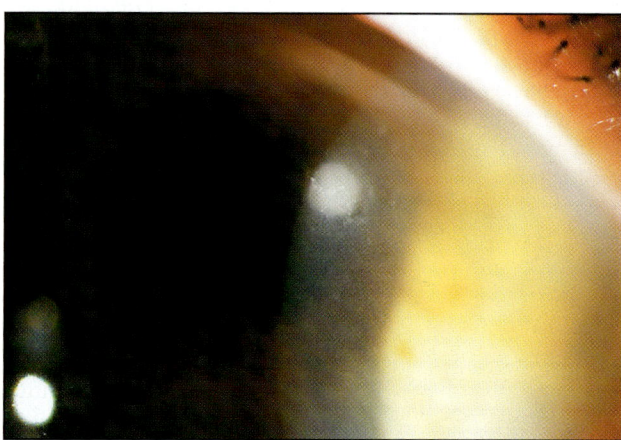

Figure B.2 • Small focal corneal infiltrate in early bacterial keratitis.

gel lenses. Other risk factors include a poor ocular surface, lid disease, prolonged topical steroid usage, lacrimal drainage system dysfunction, corneal abrasion and recurrent corneal erosion syndrome.

Patients usually present with increasing photophobia, lid swelling, blur and a watery discharge. They also frequently experience a foreign body sensation and increasing pain, although wearing a contact lens may mask symptoms. Occasionally there may be a mucopurulent discharge from an associated bacterial conjunctivitis. There are several acute inflammatory signs within the cornea itself with an inflammatory infiltrate (Figure B.2), stromal oedema, stromal loss and keratic precipitates. The anterior chamber also displays signs of inflammation with cells and flare and frequently a hypopyon and synechiae. These are not usually due to infection within the anterior chamber but rather signs of sterile inflammation secondary to the inflammatory mediators and bacterial toxins released within the cornea. This condition is potentially sight threatening.

Whether all cases of microbial keratitis need to be thoroughly investigated for the causative organism is debatable. Certainly, investigation is essential if the

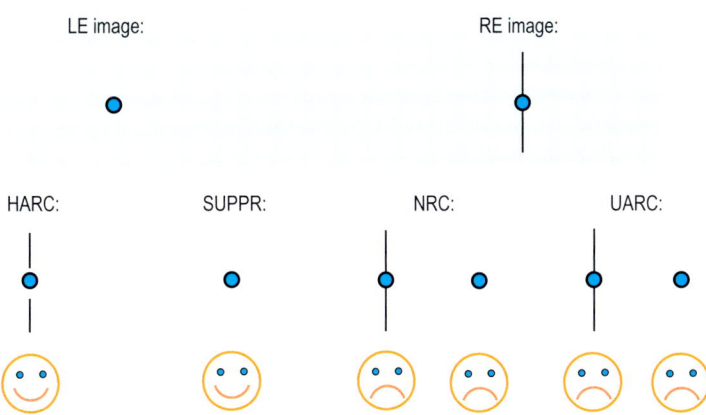

Figure B.3 • The likely results of the Bagolini test.

infection is not responding appropriately to treatment to ensure other causative organisms such as herpes simplex virus, *Acanthamoeba*, fungi and atypical mycobacteria are not missed. Routine investigation includes inoculation of slides for Gram and Blankaphor stains, and bacterial culture plates and broth. Special stains for viruses and cultures for viruses, fungi, protozoa and mycobacteria may also be added if thought appropriate.

Prior to bacterial stains and culture results, treatment with broad-spectrum antibiotics is commenced. Current practice is with either monotherapy with a fluoroquinolone (either ciprofloxacin or ofloxacin), or with dual therapy with both a fortified cephalosporin (cephalothin 5%) and aminoglycoside (tobramycin 1.3%). Drops are commenced hourly and the patient may be admitted to hospital if compliance is thought to be an issue. After considering the stain results antibiotics should not be withdrawn because of the risk of polymicrobial infection, but they may be added. The usage of topical steroids in the treatment of bacterial keratitis is controversial. They are not used initially but may be added after an appropriate clinical response is noted to reduce inflammation and thereby the degree of scarring and epithelial defects.

Bagolini striated lens

The Bagolini striated lens is a plano trial-case lens which has a fine grating of lines ruled on it. This allows the patient to see through the lens with very little disturbance of normal vision, but when looking at a spot of light the lens produces a faint streak crossing the light. In unilateral horizontal strabismus, one lens can be used before the deviated eye to produce a vertical streak rather like a 'see-through' Maddox rod, while the patient looks at a spot of light with both eyes open. If the streak appears to pass through the spot of light, harmonious anomalous retinal correspondence (HARC) is demonstrated. A local suppression area may result in a gap in the central part of the streak, but the patient may be able to report that the ends of it can be seen in line with the spot. If the streak and the spotlight are not perfectly aligned, this does not necessarily mean that there is unharmonious anomalous retinal correspondence (UARC), but can result from an imperfection in the new anomalous sensory relationship. The diagnosis of UARC (which is very rare) or normal retinal correspondence (NRC) is confirmed by the presence of diplopia and confusion (Figure B.3).

Occasionally, patients may change fixation to the deviating eye and hence see the streak passing through the light. Close observation of any eye movements during the test and a confirmatory cover test should be used to verify that the eye behind the Bagolini lens is still deviating. Unnecessary repeated covering should be avoided because this could cause HARC to break down to UARC or suppression.

If the streak is misaligned and the patient is diplopic, then either normal retinal correspondence (NRC) or UARC is revealed, depending on whether the angular separation of the spot and the streak is the same as the angle of the deviation. If the patient reports diplopia during the Bagolini lens test, but not during everyday viewing, then the patient has HARC which has 'broken down' under the very slightly abnormal viewing conditions. Such cases are rare and careful questioning may reveal that the HARC also breaks down when the patient is fatigued, or in dim illumination. In these cases, the 'pseudo-binocular vision' breaks down in an analogous way to the breaking down of binocularity in a decompensated heterophoria. If the patient reports an unstable perception of the streak in the Bagolini test, then this can be indicative of an instability in the HARC. Again, this can be associated with symptoms and such cases may require treatment.

In alternating deviations, it is usually necessary to use a striated lens before both eyes so that they produce streaks at 45° in one eye and 135° in the other. When the two streaks appear to pass through the light spot, HARC is demonstrated.

The depth of ARC can be quantified by introducing filters in front of the strabismic eye. The filters are usually in the form of a filter bar or ladder: this is a series of filters of increasing absorption mounted in a continuous strip. The depth of the filter is gradually increased (usually in 0.3 neutral density steps) until suppression of the streak occurs or the patient reports diplopia (less common). If a deep filter is needed then this suggests that the ARC is deep, which is associated with a worse prognosis for treatment. If global suppression is present then the streak will not be seen. The depth of the suppression can be measured by using a filter bar placed in front of the non-deviated eye.

Two kinds of Bagolini striated lenses are available: the No. 2 and the No. 4, with the No. 4 giving a slightly brighter streak. An approximation to a Bagolini lens can be made by using a plano (or –0.12D) trial lens with a spot of grease (e.g., from the skin) lightly smeared across it. The more faint the streak produced, the more likely it is that HARC and suppression will be detected, as there is very little disturbance of the patient's habitual vision.

Bandage contact lens
- See *Relief of pain*, therapeutic contact lenses for; *Therapeutic contact lenses*.

Bar and flat field magnifiers
Bar and flat field magnifiers are single solid lenses of hemicylindrical (bar; magnifying only in the vertical meridian) or hemispherical form (flat-field; magnifying the image overall), designed to be placed directly onto the object. They are therefore only suitable for reading on a firm, flat surface: a newspaper, for example, would need to be placed on a board. To avoid scratching the lens it may be made from glass (although this increases the weight), or the lower lens surface may be held about 1mm away from the task by a flange around the lens. They are also known as 'paperweight' or 'Visolett' magnifiers. Despite the fact that these magnifiers are obviously plus lenses, their magnifying properties are derived from lateral magnification of the object, 'real-image magnification,' rather than from the change in viewing distance which other plus lens magnifiers allow. That is, the image size can be measured with a millimetre scale and compared to the size of the original object. The real image is formed by the magnifier at approximately the same distance from the eye as the original object. This means that the user can adopt their habitual reading posture, use binocular viewing, and that any reading addition already prescribed will still be appropriate.

Magnification, M, of the device is given by

$$M = \frac{nr}{t(1 - n) + nr}$$

where t is the thickness of the magnifier, n is the refractive index of plastic/glass of the magnifier, and r is the radius of curvature of the bar magnifier. When the magnifier is exactly hemispherical with the thickness equal to the radius of curvature (t = r), then

$$M = n$$

The thicker the magnifier in relation to its radius of curvature, the higher will be its magnification, but this is unlikely to exceed 3× in practice. Decreasing the eye-to-magnifier distance will not increase the field-of-view: the number of words seen through the magnifier will only be affected by the lens diameter (which ranges from about 20 to 90mm). The periphery of the lens suffers none of the aberrations usually associated with optical systems, the image having equal clarity across its full width. A useful additional feature of these magnifiers is their light-gathering property, whereby the illumination of the working plane viewed through the magnifier is increased relative to the surrounding area in the presence of diffuse background illumination.

Basal cells of the epithelium
- See *Corneal epithelium*.

Basal lamina of the corneal epithelium
This is the basement membrane of the corneal epithelium, and is synthesized by basal epithelial cells. It varies in thickness between 0.5 and 1.0μm, and under the electron microscope can be differentiated into an anterior clear zone (lamina lucida) and a posterior darker zone (lamina densa). The basal lamina is part of a complex adhesion system which mediates the attachment of the epithelium to the underlying stroma. Hemidesmosomes link the cytoskeleton, via a series of anchoring fibrils, to anchoring plaques in the anterior stroma. The molecular components of this adhesion complex include type VII collagen, integrins, laminin and bullous phemphigoid antigen.

Base curve of a contact lens
- See *Back optic zone radius (BOZR) of a contact lens*.

Basement membrane dystrophy
- See *Recurrent erosion syndrome*, therapeutic contact lenses for.

BCLA
- See *British Contact Lens Association*.

Bebie curve
The Bebie curve is an alternative form of graphically representing the data from a threshold visual field examination that has certain advantages for interpreting results. The ability to produce a Bebie curve is built into the software of the Octopus perimeters (1–2–3 and 101). With a Bebie-curve the individual defect values (difference between the measured threshold and the age-matched normal value) are ranked according to depth and then plotted, in rank order, along the x-axis, the y-axis being the defect level (Figure B.4). A patient with only diffuse loss will have a curve that shows a relatively constant deviation from the norm. A patient with local loss will have a curve that follows the normal range until it gets to the right hand side where the large individual defects are plotted. It then shows large deviations from the norm. Changes in overall loss and localized loss will have different effects upon the Bebie curve. Changes in overall loss will result in a lowering of the curve, while increases in the size of a scotoma will produce a shift to the left of the sharp line demarcating between normal and defective test points.

Bedewing
- See *Endothelial bedewing*.

Best form ophthalmic lens
An ophthalmic lens which is designed to have some control of aberration is sometimes known as 'best form'. As this description is often used somewhat indiscriminately, it is worth considering the British Standard definition (BS 3521: Part 1: 1991) of 'best form lens': "a lens whose curvatures are computed to eliminate or minimize a stated

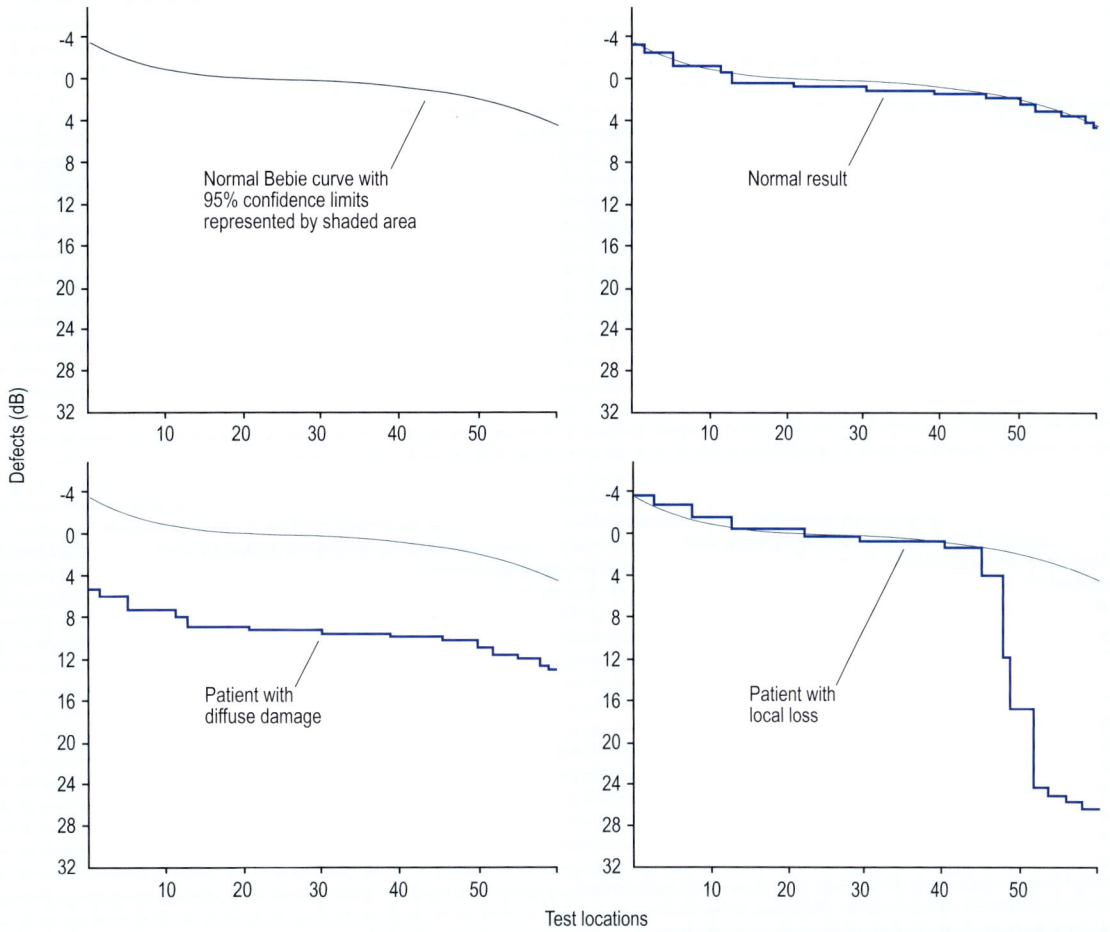

Figure B.4 • Bebie curves.

image defect or defects under defined conditions." Thus a best form lens may only attempt to reduce a single aberration for a given fixation distance. It is not guaranteed to be the best optical or cosmetic solution for a given prescription. In the USA, best form lenses are known as 'corrected curve lenses'.

The aberrations which can most readily be controlled by changing lens form are oblique astigmatism, curvature and distortion. These aberrations are normally computed by trigonometric ray tracing. However, if some approximations are applied, a simpler, graphical representation can be used, known as Tscherning's ellipse. An example is shown in Figure B.5, computed to illustrate lens forms which are free from oblique astigmatism. This is the solution of a quadratic equation and makes various assumptions as follows:

- The lens is thin
- A small oblique angle of gaze such that 'third order' approximations can be made
- Specific refractive index for the lens
- Specific centre of rotation distance (z)
- Specific fixation distance, in this case infinity.

Thus, in the range of powers with a real solution for the quadratic, there are two forms for zero oblique astigmatism for any given back vertex power. The steep form (Wollaston), with a highly powered rear surface (F_2), is shown by the lower portion of the curve. The shallower form (Ostwalt) is shown by the upper portion. In fact, even the shallow forms have a much steeper shape than curves commonly used today for spectacle lenses. One reason for this is that single vision lenses are commonly used for a wide variety of fixation distances, and that a different ellipse would be computed for near vision which would have flatter forms. Also, it should be realized that the ellipses for other aberrations would give different lens forms for their elimination. To make a lens free from distortion, for example, requires a very steep lens form. Thus, a general purpose lens series must be a compromise between the requirements of distance and near vision, as well as being cosmetically acceptable to the wearer.

Note that the range of lenses which can be made free from oblique astigmatism using spherical curves is very heavily biased towards minus powers. Lenses with a power of greater than +7.00D would require the use of an aspheric form to control this aberration.

Best vision sphere, determination of

Changing the sphere in front of the patient until they can see clearly will leave the circle of least confusion upon the retina and is an integral part of subjective refraction. This may be done using a sequence of lenses or by using

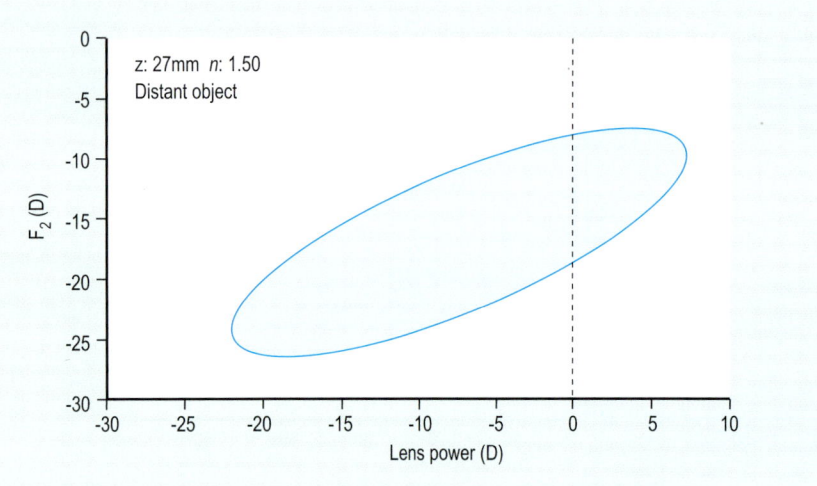

Figure B.5 • Tscherning's ellipse for a distant object viewed through a lens of refractive index (n) 1.50 by an eye whose centre of rotation (z) is 27 mm from the lens. The ellipse gives the rear surface power(s) (F_2) that a lens of any given back vertex power (F'_v) should have in order to eliminate oblique astigmatism.

the duochrome target. The key factor is to avoid any accommodative effort by the pre-presbyopic patient, as it may result in too much minus power being placed in front of the eye prior to determination of the cylindrical component of the refraction, and lead to error. Two approaches are commonly employed to avoid such problems. The first relies on a fogging lens being placed before the eye immediately after objective results have been found (usually by retinoscopy). This lens should be of sufficient plus power to fog the patient's eyes by around four lines on the acuity chart from the line they see with the objective result. This 'fog' should then be reduced in 0.25D steps until the best acuity is reported and where the next 0.25D reduction fails to result in any improvement.

A second and perhaps more commonly used method is to hold a positive lens in front of the objective refraction. Assuming reasonable acuity, say 6/9 or better, this should be a +0.25D lens, although for poorer objective results or where objective refraction has not been possible, the lens power should be chosen to allow some possibility of appreciation of change by the patient. So, for example, at 6/60 a +1.00D lens should be presented. If this lens improves the acuity or, importantly for the pre-presbyope, fails to blur the acuity, it should be included and the step repeated until the plus power lens actually causes noticeable blur at which stage the best mean sphere has been achieved. If a patient with reduced acuity shows an improvement as lenses are presented, the power of subsequent lenses needs to be reduced, as appropriate, to the new acuity. A negative power lens should only be presented if the initial positive power lens causes blur. This power should then only be included, and a further negative lens presented, if the first results show an actual improvement in the acuity in that the patient actually reads more letters on the target, rather than the target appearing smaller and darker, which would indicate accommodation having been stimulated.

The response to the presentation of spheres may occasionally not be as expected, for example in older patients with small pupils it is important to remember unaided vision and objective results when deciding upon the magnitude of the mean sphere.

Before attempting to measure the cylindrical part of the refractive error, a small allowance for depth of focus may be made by reducing the final power of the sphere by 0.25D. This slight technique is most useful for younger patients with a small depth of focus and active accommodation to ensure the circle of least confusion is close to the retinal plane.

Bifocal and multifocal contact lenses

Bifocal and multifocal contact lenses can be simultaneous or alternating vision designs. Simultaneous designs generally require the lens to be relatively stable on the eye and will be associated with some form of visual compromise because objects at both distance and near are imaged simultaneously on the retina. Alternating vision bifocal lenses require significant lens movement so that the distance and near portions of the lens can be positioned over the pupil by interaction with the lids. See *Alternating vision lenses for presbyopia; Monovision correction for presbyopia; Simultaneous vision lenses for presbyopia*.

Bifocal ophthalmic lenses

As their name implies, bifocal lenses have two discreet focal powers. They are principally used for the alleviation of presbyopia, and are sometimes used to help control binocular vision disorders in the young. Most bifocal lenses have a large area for distance, with a small area of higher positive power for near vision. Bifocal lenses can be classified by their method of construction as split, fused (or cemented) or solid bifocals.

Split bifocals were first described by Benjamin Franklin in 1784. These are made by the relatively crude method of splitting a distance and a near lens, then mounting the top half of the distance onto the bottom half of the near to form a single lens. This approach is still in use for prescriptions which cannot be manufactured using mass-produced lenses, an example being where a large amount of prism is required at near but not at distance.

Fused bifocals are glass lenses where the extra positive addition for near is produced by fusing (or cementing) in a higher refractive index piece of material into the major portion. This design has the advantage of good cosmetic appearance. The required addition depends on:

- The refractive indices of the two glass materials
- The contact radius between the components (the depression curve)
- The curve worked on the segment side of the lens.

A variety of different segment shapes is possible. Shapes of segment currently available include:
- D segment
- Semi-circular segment
- B segment, sometimes known as a ribbon segment
- Curved top D segment.

Solid bifocals can be considered as a one piece solid version of the cement bifocal. There are two basic types. A bifocal can be produced by grinding a negative power curve into a single vision lens, thus giving a negative addition. This type of lens is used currently as the upcurve bifocal, and is extremely rare. The segment contains the highest minus power and is therefore the distance portion. This is the most straightforward type of lens to produce as a 'one off' item, but unfortunately suffers from the fact that the near vision area is normally required to be smaller than the distance.

An alternative and more popular type of solid bifocal is one where the segment stands proud of the main lens, and has a positive power addition in the segment. This is more complex to manufacture as the lens is thicker in the near portion rather than the distance, and hence cannot be made from a single vision lens as with the upcurve. Solid bifocals of this type are known as downcurve bifocals. In glass material, the segment is positioned conventionally on the rear surface, but in plastic materials it is generally incorporated into the front surface.

Solid bifocals with the appearance of one piece Franklin split bifocals are also popular, these are called 'Executive' bifocals, a trade mark of American Optical, or sometimes 'E style'. The advantage of this type of lens is the wide field of view at near, as well as improvement in optical quality. However, care must be exercised when using the E style in hypermetropic prescriptions as the lens can be excessively thick in the distance, particularly in high additions. This excessive thickness can be reduced to some extent by the careful use of prism thinning.

Solid shaped segments are also manufactured in plastic materials. The only problem with these designs is that there must be a ledge along any straight surface which can accumulate dirt and is also prone to damage. At one time, round segment blended bifocals (generally known as seamless bifocals) were popular in the USA. These lenses have the least conspicuous segment of any bifocal, but are seriously compromised optically in the blending zone around the segment. They have been largely superseded by progressive addition ophthalmic lenses, that have an excellent cosmetic appearance, and much improved optical quality.

Binocular balancing

This technique is necessary to ensure equal accommodative demand in each eye when the final binocular prescription is presented. If one eye is over-minussed by –0.25D in a young patient, the eyes may have equally good acuity but the extra 0.25D that this eye will need to accommodate may cause asthenopic symptoms in the binocular state. It is not necessary to balance if a binocular refraction has been carried out, or if the patient has no significant accommodation (e.g. the over sixties or pseudophakes). There are many methods of balancing but the most commonly used techniques require one eye to be fogged by several lines of acuity, but not by so much that any further fogging by accommodation will not be appreciated. Lenses are then presented to the non-fogged eye to determine how much power, if any, is needed to fog this eye or change preference on the duochrome test. The same is then done for the other eye and, if balanced, the result will be the same; if not, the difference needs to be incorporated into the final correction. So, if the unfogged right eye accepts +0.50DS before clarity is lost, and the other +0.25DS, then there is an imbalance of +0.25D which may be removed by adding +0.25D to the first eye, or +0.50 to the first and +0.25 to the second. In each case the balance is achieved as the accommodative difference is addressed.

Binoculars

Binoculars are two telescopes – one for each eye – mounted side-by-side so that both can be used simultaneously to give magnified binocular vision of a distant object. The images are erected using a negative powered eyepiece, prisms, or compound lens systems. The optical configuration of a set of binoculars is given as M × D, whereby M is the magnification and D is the diameter of the objective or entrance pupil.

Biomicroscope
- See *Slit-lamp biomicroscope*.

Blebs
- See *Endothelial blebs*.

Blepharitis

Blepharitis is an infection and/or inflammation of the eyelid margins. The condition is usually bilateral, symmetrical and chronic in nature. Anterior blepharitis affects the margins anterior to and including the lash line, whereas posterior blepharitis affects the Meibomian glands. Anterior blepharitis affects the glands of Moll which are modified sweat glands at the base of the lashes, and the glands of Zeis which are oil secreting glands on the anterior lid margin. Staphylococcal overgrowth and seborrhoea are thought to be intimately involved in the development of anterior blepharitis. Staphylococci are known to produce markedly inflammatory exotoxins and it is likely that sensitivity to these toxins plays a major role. Staphylococci overgrowth is probably encouraged by the excess production of lipid associated with seborrhoea.

Posterior blepharitis affects the 30 to 35 meibomian glands opening onto both the upper and lower eyelid margins, posterior to the lash line. As such, dysfunction of the secretion of lipid (meibome) from these glands can lead to both local inflammation and dry eye symptoms. Blockage of the glands can lead to sterile (chalazia) or infected cysts (internal hordeolum).

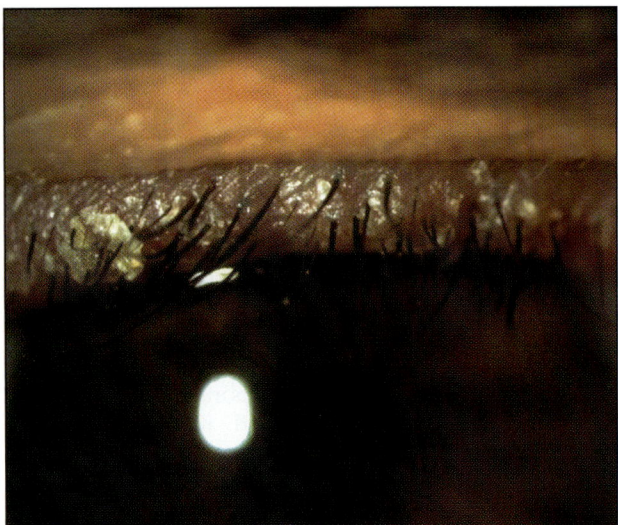

Figure B.6 • Staphylococcal anterior blepharitis.

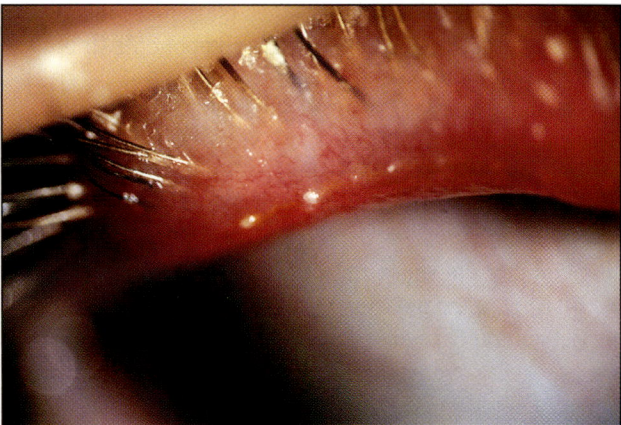

Figure B.7 • Blocked meibomian gland orifices associated with lid thickening, telangiectasias, and lid scarring in chronic posterior blepharitis.

Anterior and posterior blepharitis tend to be associated with similar symptoms, and a disparity between the degree of signs and symptoms is a common feature of this disease. Symptoms result from disruption to normal ocular surface function and reduction in tear stability as reflected in a decrease in the tear break-up time (BUT). Typical symptoms include burning, grittiness, a foreign body sensation and mild photophobia as well as crusting and redness of the lid margins. Symptoms typically fluctuate and are usually fairly symmetric. There may be exacerbations during winter especially in cold climates. As with most forms of dry eye, symptoms are also often made worse in drying environments such as with air travel and air conditioned offices.

Anterior blepharitis shows changes to the lashes, which may be reduced in number (madarosis) and non-pigmented (poliosis) (Figure B.6). They may be matted together and encrusted with scales, staphylococcal scales are typically hard and brittle and form collarettes around the base of the lashes, while seborrhoeic scales are soft and greasy (scurf). Scarring within the lid margin from chronic blepharitis can lead to individual lashes becoming misdirected and touching the ocular surface (trichiasis).

The key sign in posterior blepharitis is an abnormality of the meibomian gland secretions. In Meibomian seborrhoea excess secretions manifest as oil globules capping the meibomian gland orifices and an oily or foaming tear film. In Meibomianitis there is inflammation or obstruction of the glands which may be manifest as little pustules at the orifice. Expression of the contents of the glands demonstrates many to be blocked, those that do express release yellowy, viscous, even toothpaste like secretions.

Both anterior and posterior blepharitis show variable lid margin inflammation and thickening; also vascular dilatation and telangiectasia. Chronic posterior blepharitis can lead to scalloping of the lid posterior margin secondary to scarring (Figure B.7). There are frequently associated ocular surface signs with punctate fluorescein and rose Bengal staining adjacent to the lower lid margin. Marginal keratitis may occur during acute exacerbations. An external hordeolum (stye) may develop if the glands of Moll or Zeiss become infected. Both forms of blepharitis are usually associated with low-grade symptoms and a cosmetic problem. They can also cause tear film instability, and secondary changes in the conjunctiva and cornea. When associated with marginal keratitis and rosacea keratitis, posterior blepharitis can be sight threatening.

The chronic recurrent nature of the disease should be explained to the patient. Lid hygiene is the mainstay of long-term treatment for anterior blepharitis and is aimed at decreasing seborrhoea and staphylococcal antigen load. Scrubbing of the lashes and lid margin is performed with a mild detergent to remove built up scale and oils. This can be done with either a commercially available product or diluted baby shampoo. In posterior blepharitis, lid hygiene is also an important component of long-term treatment, but cleaning should be supplemented with warm compresses to melt solidified sebum and with lid massage to promote expression of meibomian gland secretions. In anterior blepharitis, topical weak corticosteroids such as fluorometholone and antibiotics such as chloramphenicol may be useful in acute exacerbations to reduce inflammation and staphylococcal load. They are used 4 times a day for 1–2 weeks. They are very much a short-term measure until other treatment modalities begin working.

Systemic tetracyclines are the mainstay of the treatment of posterior blepharitis. They are broad-spectrum antibiotics and are also thought to have a primary action in altering the nature of the lipid produced by the meibomian glands. Systemic tetracyclines are also useful in the management of any associated facial rosacea. They are usually used initially at a high dose and then reduced to a lower dose for maintenance. A typical regime is Doxycycline 100mg oral daily for 1 month followed by 50mg orally for 2 months. Instability of the tear film due to chronic inflammation and dysfunction of the lipid component of tears leads to many of the symptoms seen in these conditions. Comfort can be improved with the sparing use of tear supplements.

Blindness

- See *Registered visual impairment; Low vision*

Blinking with contact lenses

Contact lenses elicit reflex blinking during lens insertion and removal and other instances of manual manipulation.

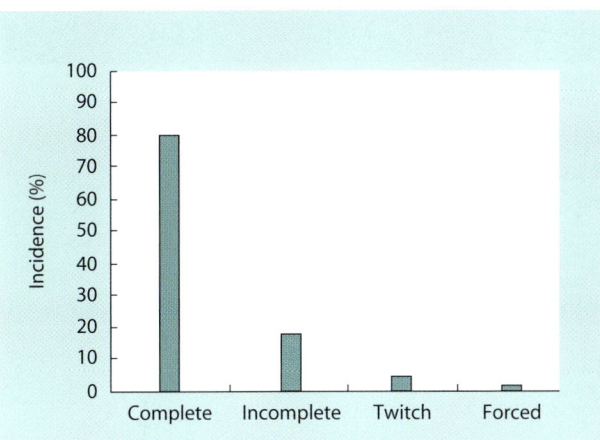

Figure B.8 • Frequency of occurrence of various normal blink types.

Also, as a result of a reflex blink, contact lenses may become mislocated or become dislodged from the eye. Both soft and rigid lens wear causes the spontaneous blink rate to increase. In rigid lens wear this change may be more related to reflex blinking rather than spontaneous blinking; that is, the increased blink rate may be a result of continual irritation caused by the lens edge buffeting against the lid margin. Such alterations to blink rate are not thought to be permanent. Contact lenses can also affect the pattern of blinking. A decrease in the frequency of occurrence of long duration interblink periods occurs in association with rigid lens wear but not with soft lens wear. Neither rigid nor soft lens wear alters the proportion of complete, incomplete, twitch and forced blinks (Figure B.8). Infrequent or incomplete blinking with contact lenses can cause a number of problems, including lens surface drying and deposition, epithelial desiccation, post-lens tear stagnation, hypoxia and hypercapnia, and 3 and 9 o'clock staining. Faults in lens design and fitting can interfere with proper blink-mediated lid-lens interaction.

There are essentially two options when faced with a clinical problem relating to non-pathologic disorders of spontaneous blinking activity associated with contact lens wear, such as incomplete and/or infrequent blinking. These options are to train patients to modify their blinking activity, and/or to alter the lens type or lens fit.

Practitioners should remain alert to the possibility that apparent anomalies in the type or pattern of blinking activity in a contact lens wearer may be attributable to unrelated disease states. Interruptions to the neural input and/or muscular systems of the eyelids can adversely affect normal spontaneous blinking activity. For example, patients with Parkinson's disease exhibit a low blink rate. Increased mechanical resistance to eyelid movement, as in Grave's disease, can also reduce blink frequency. Local pathology of the eyelids, such as ptosis, chalazia and carcinomas, can alter eyelid function and movement, and hence interfere with normal blinking activity. It is therefore essential to rule out the possibility of unrelated pathology before ascribing blinking dysfunction to contact lens wear.

Botulinum toxin

Botulinum toxin is a potent neuro-toxin that selectively binds to cholinergic synapses, blocking the conduction of the nerve impulse. Since its introduction in the 1970's, Botulinum toxin has proved effective in the management of patients with strabismus and other disorders affecting skeletal muscles.

In non-paralytic strabismus, Botulinum toxin is injected into the medial rectus of the squinting eye in esotropia and into the lateral rectus in exotropia. The injected muscle is weakened and lengthened following the injection. In most cases of non-paralytic strabismus, Botulinum toxin is used diagnostically, in the expectation that the strabismus will recur when the effect of the toxin has completely worn off.

Botulinum toxin has been used to treat a variety of disorders. Those of interest in the ophthalmic field include:

- Muscle spasm involving the facial muscles
- Strabismus
- Nystagmus
- Corneal ulceration
- Exposure keratitis.

The main indications for the use of Botulinum toxin in strabismus are listed in Table B.1.

The medial rectus, lateral rectus and inferior rectus muscles are most frequently treated with Botulinum toxin. The overacting inferior oblique muscle can be injected in superior oblique palsy. Treating the superior rectus muscle results in ptosis and is therefore not recommended. The superior oblique muscle is not treated with Botulinum toxin.

Bowman's layer

- See *Anterior limiting lamina of the cornea*.

Boxing system

The eyesize of spectacle frames can be specified using the boxing system. According to this system, a spectacle frame can be enclosed by a theoretical rectangular box, with the horizontal and vertical sides of the box 'touching' the horizontal and vertical aspects of the frame at their widest and tallest dimensions, respectively. The horizontal lens size is equal to the horizontal length of the rectangle. The purpose of this system is to facilitate specification of the dimensions of the eye size of a spectacle frame (or of a lens in a rimless pair of spectacles) which can be of any regular or irregular shape.

BOZD

- See *Back optic zone diameter of a contact lens*.

BOZR

- See *Back optic zone radius of a contact lens*.

Bridge, spectacle frame

This is the part of the spectacle frame that 'bridges' the nose and serves to join the lenses or spectacle frame rims between the two eyes. The spectacle rim and bridge often form a single continuous structural element of the spectacle frame. The bridge rests on the nose via small pads or a continuous 'saddle'. For a given frame design, a number of bridge sizes may be available to accommodate different

Table B.1 • Indications for the use of Botulinum toxin in strabismus.

Diagnostically

- To reduce the angle of strabismus and allow sensory investigation in free space
- In the investigation of patients at risk of post-operative diplopia
- To investigate the presence or absence of fusion before deciding on surgical treatment
- In patients with sixth-nerve palsy who cannot abduct past the midline; improved abduction after injection indicates a partial palsy, failure to improve indicates a complete palsy
- To help predict the effect of surgery on patients with incomitant deviations
- In combination with electro-micrography recording to confirm the presence of neural 'miswiring' in Duane's syndrome
- As a means of further investigation when a slipped or paretic muscle is suspected.

Therapeutically

- To restore fusion, especially in patients with decompensating strabismus and partially recovered sixth-nerve palsy
- In the rehabilitation of patients with cosmetic strabismus
- As an adjunct to strabismus surgery and in the management of acute surgical undercorrections and overcorrections
- In acquired nystagmus to dampen the amplitude of the ocular oscillation and improve visual acuity

facial and nasal dimensions, although additional adjustments may be made by altering the positions of the pads.

British Contact Lens Association (BCLA)

The BCLA's mission is 'to promote excellence in contact lens research, manufacturing and clinical practice'. Membership is drawn from all sectors involved in the field of contact lenses, including optometrists, ophthalmologists, dispensing opticians, and professionals working in the contact lens and contact lens care product industry. The BCLA hosts a major conference and exhibition in May/June each year, runs numerous lectures and courses, and publishes the journal Contact Lens & Anterior Eye. Website: www.bcla.org.uk

British Universities Committee of Contact Lens Educators (BUCCLE)

This is an association of contact lens educators from university-based teaching institutions in the United Kingdom. Its aim is to nurture high standards of contact lens education in British universities. There are two full members from each institution, plus associate members. BUCCLE meets three times each year to discuss and share ideas and developments in UK contact lens education. It is sponsored by the contact lens industry.

BUCCLE

- See *British Universities Committee of Contact Lens Educators*.

Bullous keratopathy

- See *Dystrophies of the corneal epithelium, therapeutic lenses for; Degenerations of the corneal epithelium, therapeutic lenses for*.

Bundling of contact lens systems

- See *Contact lens delivery systems*.

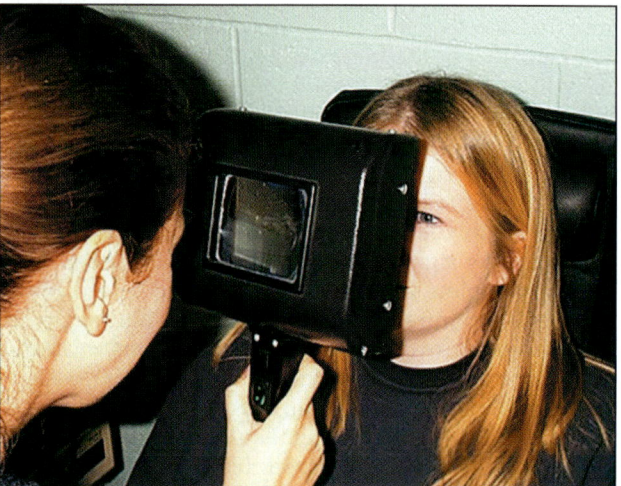

Figure B.9 • Burton lamp.

Burton lamp

A number of manufacturers make a special hand-held magnifying device for contact lens work. This device is usually referred to as a 'Burton lamp' (Figure B.9), after the company that manufactured the original version (Burton Manufacturing Co., USA). The Burton lamp is essentially a large magnifying lens of about +5.00D housed in a broad frame, within which are mounted a combination of 4-W white-light and ultraviolet-light fluorescent tubes, each about 11cm long. The operator can switch between the two light sources for white-light and fluorescein-stain examinations. A key advantage of this instrument is that both eyes of the patient can be viewed simultaneously, which facilitates inter-ocular comparisons in the course of contact lens fitting. The Burton lamp is also useful for conducting an initial screening examination.

BVP

- See *Back vertex power of a contact lens*.

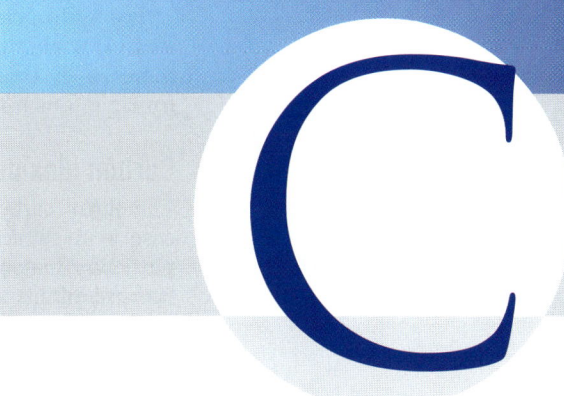

CAB
- See *Cellulose acetate butyrate.*

Calcium deposition on contact lenses
- See *Deposits, lens.*

Canaliculus
- See *Lacrimal drainage system.*

Captive bubble measurement of contact lens surface wettability

This is one of three key techniques for measuring lens surface wettability; the other two are the sessile drop and Wilhelmy plate techniques (Figure C.1). The captive bubble method of measuring surface wettability is often preferred to the sessile drop measurement when assessing contact lenses because the lens does not undergo dehydration during the procedure. When contact lenses are examined the probe liquid is usually water, which has led to the method often being referred to as the 'air-in-water' technique. See *Sessile drop measurement of contact lens surface wettability.*

With the lens immersed in water, a droplet of a second liquid (or air) is introduced at the lower (submerged) sample surface. The contact angle is then measured in the same way as described for the sessile drop technique, i.e. by direct measurement or calculated from the dimensions of the bubble. The contact angle measured is conceptually similar to that obtained when a receding angle is measured with the sessile method.

This method, however, like all methods used for contact angle analysis, is not without its difficulties. If air is introduced, care needs to be taken to avoid bubble distortion. The size of the bubble will also affect the contact angle obtained. Optical effects arising from a multiple layer optical path make it difficult to locate the precise point where the air bubble meets the solid surface. As a result, the exact determination of the tangent to the droplet at its point of contact with the lens is as problematic as for the sessile method, and will inevitably introduce a level of variability into the results.

Manufacturers have been known to quote contact angles using this method, but instead of water they use wetting or soaking solutions. The contact angle produced, however, has no fundamental significance either to surface characterization or to the prediction of eye-lens wettability. Its use in this way serves only to lower the contact angle obtained, presumably for marketing purposes.

Carbon dioxide permeability of contact lenses

This term describes the ease with which carbon dioxide may pass through a particular material under standard conditions. It is thus a property of a

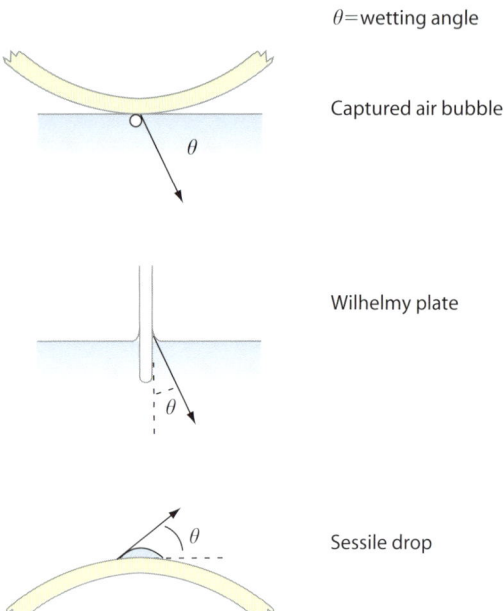

Figure C.1 • Techniques for assessing lens wetting angles.

material, and not of a finished contact lens. Carbon dioxide permeability of a material is a function of the diffusivity (D) and solubility (k) of carbon dioxide in that material, and is represented by the term Dk. Since this term is usually associated with oxygen permeability, $Dk(CO_2)$ is used to denote permeability to carbon dioxide. The diffusivity (D) refers to the speed at which carbon dioxide molecules can pass through the material, and the solubility (k) refers to the number of carbon dioxide molecules that can be absorbed into a given volume of material.

In order to determine the carbon dioxide permeability of a material at a given temperature, it is necessary to measure the rate (volume per unit time) at which carbon dioxide passes through a sample of membrane of given dimensions (area and thickness) for a given gas pressure. The units of Dk take these variables into account, and are quite complex. It is common therefore to quote the value in 'Fatt units' (after Irving Fatt, who pioneered contact lens carbon dioxide permeability measurement) or, more formally, 'Barrer', whereby:

$Dk(CO_2)$ in Barrer (or 'Fatt units')
$= 10^{-11}$ $(cm^2 \cdot mlCO_2)/(s \cdot ml \cdot mmHg)$

The international standard unit for pressure is the pascal (Pa). Because the term mmHg is now becoming obsolete internationally, it is being advocated that the closest accepted metric unit of pressure – 100Pa, or hectopascal (hPa) – should replace the term mmHg. This approach is specified in the international standard ISO 8321-2 (2000). When hPa is used, $Dk(CO_2)$ is quoted as:

$Dk(CO_2) = 10^{-11}$ $(cm^2 \cdot mlCO2)/(s \cdot ml \cdot hPa)$

The difficulty here is that converting from the traditional Barrer or Fatt units to ISO units involves multiplying $Dk(CO_2)$ by the constant 0.75. Thus a lens quoted with a traditional $Dk(CO_2)$ of 40×10^{-11} $(cm^2 \cdot mlCO_2)/$ $(s \cdot ml \cdot mmHg)$, for example, will have a revised ISO $Dk(CO_2)$ of 30×10^{-11} $(cm^2 \cdot mlCO_2)/(s \cdot ml \cdot hPa)$.

For hydrogels, the ratio of $Dk(CO_2):Dk(O_2)$ is 21:1; that is, CO_2 is able to permeate through hydrogels 21 times more easily than O_2. The ratio of $Dk(CO_2):Dk(O_2)$ is 7:1 for rigid lens materials and 8:1 for silicone elastomer.

Carbon dioxide transmissibility of contact lenses

The term 'carbon dioxide transmissibility' describes the ease with which carbon dioxide may pass through a particular material of given thickness. The carbon dioxide transmissibility of a lens is a function of the carbon dioxide permeability (Dk) of the material from which the lens is made, divided by the thickness of the lens (t). Thus, 'carbon dioxide transmissibility' is represented by the term $Dk/t(CO_2)$, and describes the passage of carbon dioxide through a finished contact lens.

The units of $Dk/t(CO_2)$ are as follows:

$Dk/t(CO_2)$ in Barrer/cm = 10^{-9} $(cm \cdot mlCO_2)/(s \cdot ml \cdot mmHg)$

When hPa is used, $Dk/t(CO_2)$ is quoted as:

$Dk/t(CO_2)$ in Barrer/cm = 10^{-9} $(cm \cdot mlCO_2)/(s \cdot hPa)$

To convert from the traditional Barrer or Fatt units to ISO units, Dk/t must be multiplied by the constant 0.75.

Contact lens carbon dioxide transmissibility can be expressed in terms of either central or average transmissibility. The central lens $Dk/t(CO_2)$ is derived by dividing $Dk(CO_2)$ by the centre thickness of the lens. The average lens $Dk/t(CO_2)$ is derived by dividing $Dk(CO_2)$ by the average thickness of the lens over a defined lens radius. The average $Dk/t(CO_2)$ is always less than the central $Dk/t(CO_2)$ for minus powered lenses (which become progressively thicker from the centre to the edge of the lens), and the converse is true for plus powered lenses.

Because the ratio of $Dk(CO_2):Dk(O_2)$ is 21:1 for hydrogels and 7:1 for rigid lenses, the $Dk/t(CO_2)$ of a hydrogel contact lens will be about three times that of a rigid lens of the same $Dk/t(O_2)$ as the hydrogel lens.

Carrier, minus contact lens

- See *High plus power contact lens design*.

Case history

In order to carry out a full eye examination, it is essential to establish exactly why a patient has attended. This will act as a critical initial guide to the set of procedures undertaken in the course of the examination, with a view to meeting the visual requirements of the patient. The necessity to acquire accurate information about both the optical and ocular status of the patient demands that careful, specific questioning precedes the ocular examination. The case history is individual to each patient but should cover the main areas listed below.

- Reason for attendance. It is generally considered that an appreciation of why the patient has attended for an eye examination should be gained from the outset. Whether it is a routine two-yearly recall or to address a specific concern regarding a particular problem, all

Table C.1 • Common presenting symptoms and suggested follow-up questions.	
Headaches	which part of the head both sides or one nature of the pain (sharp, throbbing, dull, cluster and so on) associated nausea and vomiting nature of associated visual disturbance (migraine as opposed to possible ischaemic incident) medication being taken for headache association with any task, visual or possibly other activity
Eye pain	constant or intermittent nature of the pain (severe or otherwise) associated with eye movement onset and duration
Floaters	location in view size moves with the eye solid or web-like associations, such as trauma
Photopsia	one or both eyes persistent or transient associated with onset of floaters onset and duration
Redness	one or both eyes any associations (outdoors, light, season and so on) nature of any discharge
Diplopia	Double as opposed to blurred (many patients may be confused by the difference so the practitioner must be careful to help in the distinction) monocular or binocular vertical or horizontal

Table C.2 • Some useful probing questions.	
History	When was it first noticed, had it before?
Onset	Sudden or gradual?
Timing	Specifically when does it happen?
Causative factors	Does anything start or stop it?
Duration	How long does it last?
Frequency	Constant or intermittent?
Associations	Other symptoms with it?
Change	Getting better or worse?
Other	Does your GP know? Family history?

subsequent questions and actions by the practitioner may follow on from this premise.

- Current ocular and optical status. Details about the patient's current visual status, correction, and symptoms should be established. Closed questions with one specific answer may be appropriate. Furthermore, while the practitioner should be aware of the pitfall of sounding as though they are reading a list of pre-written questions, it is often important to ask questions of a patient to rule out certain possibilities. For example it is common practice to establish that the patient has not experienced photopsia or headache; without asking such questions, it cannot be assumed that such symptoms have not been experienced. Some common presenting symptoms and follow-up questions are shown in Table C.1.
- The general pattern for clinical questioning is one of an initial open question followed by more specific, possibly closed, questions about the presenting symptoms, which is sometimes called a 'funnel approach'. A list of questions of similar form or depth is sometimes called a 'tunnel approach'. The probing types of questions appropriate for most symptoms are summarized in Table C.2.
- Patient ocular history. Details regarding last eye examination (if record cards of this are not available), history of optical correction, injury or trauma, surgery, orthoptic or refractive treatment, or known eye disease or strabismus should be established.
- Family ocular history. Visual problems (e.g. high myopia, amblyopia), squints and eye diseases (particularly glaucoma) in the patient's immediate family need to be ascertained.
- General medical history. This is one particular area where the use of a leading question may confuse the issue. To ask of a patient "Is your health good at the moment?" may elicit a definite "Yes, thank you" from a patient who has just been through a period of poor health which has just recently stabilized. A well-controlled insulin-dependent diabetic may feel in the best of health. More useful approaches might include the following questions: How is your health at the moment? Do you have to visit your doctor for any reason? Are you taking any medication at present (or have been recently)? Are you being treated for diabetes or hypertension? Some indication as to patient compliance, e.g. use of glaucoma drops or control of sugar levels in diabetes, may be obtained through careful questioning. With some conditions, such as hypertension, further questioning may be appropriate to ensure that the patient is being monitored regularly and that they are aware of the importance of adequate control of their condition. With diabetes in particular some more detail may be of direct relevance to the optometrist and may influence the nature of the subsequent correspondence with the general practitioner. Follow-up questions might include: duration of the disease, nature of the disease (Type 1 or 2), nature of the control and whether this has changed, whether it is stable, who monitors the disease and if other eye examinations are included, and when was the last medical check and when will the next check be performed.
- Family medical history. Any family history of hypertension, stroke or diabetes may be of importance, and should be recorded.
- Lifestyle and occupation details. The presenting complaint in many eye examinations may be directly

related to problems such as difficulties in the workplace, driving or carrying out a hobby. Asking about the nature of a patient's work is more useful than just knowing a job title, which may be misleading. Use of a visual display unit may lead onto a whole host of further questions. The need to drive may influence a final consideration of results and there are obvious legal implications here. The practitioner may be able to infer the possible requirement for safety spectacles or advice relating to eye health and safety.

A good concluding question might be "Is there anything else about your eyes or vision which concern you?" or "Is there anything else about your eyes or health that I should know?" This should fill in any missing detail so that the practical examination may begin with a detailed appreciation of the patient's appraisal of their own ocular status and related issues.

Case history for low vision

This has been described as the most important part of a low vision assessment. It is essential to find out exactly what each patient needs and wants, and what they are expecting to be done for them. In addition it is important to assess the patient's adaptation to their visual loss since this will have a major effect on motivation. The clinician must establish a relationship with the patient, and find out about them and their carers. Visual disability is defined by the lifestyle of the patient and the society in which they live, and their families and friends are an integral part of that picture: they can also provide important practical and psychological support. Direct observation of the patient can reveal physical infirmities, such as tremor, or limited movement, which may limit the range of tasks in which the patient is interested, or suggest handling difficulties with some low vision aids. The patient may be seen to be eccentrically viewing (since they do not look directly at the clinician) and can be questioned to find out if they are aware of using this strategy. Their use of tinted lenses, sunglasses, or a hat may also suggest problems with glare.

The clinician should encourage the patient by words or sounds, rather than gestures such as head nodding, which may not be seen. If the conversation includes others in the room, then a touch on the hand or arm of the patient will let them know when a question is addressed to them.

Topics to be discussed should include:
- Duration of condition, and speed of onset.
- Stability of condition, and difference between the eyes. If vision is changing, it may be necessary to change aids frequently.
- Patient's knowledge of condition and prognosis. The better the patient understands the eye condition, the more realistic their expectations will be. It also gives a guide to the capacity of the patient to remember accurately what they are told, which may be relevant for instructions given on the use of magnifiers.
- Ongoing hospital monitoring and/or treatment. If medical assessment of visual impairment has not been carried out, or there has been significant recent deterioration, the patient should be (re)referred.
- Registration status. If not registerable, the patient can be encouraged to self-refer to the local Social Services department for assessment by a rehabilitation officer. See *Registered visual impairment*.
- Education and/or employment, in the past, at present and in the future. This will be a major factor in defining the patient's requirements.
- Present aids and spectacles; their use, and usefulness; any problems experienced with them.
- General health and medication
- Referral route. If referred by another professional (general practitioner or social worker, for example), a report should be sent back to them.
- Current visual status. The questions will obviously be adapted according to circumstances, but need to cover the patient's daily activities, home circumstances and travel abilities. The answers will define what tasks the patient needs or wants to perform, and what the current difficulties are with those tasks.
- Identifying patient requirements and establishing priorities. The patient must be encouraged to identify specific activities which they would like to improve. It is essential to establish whether the activities identified are those for which a low vision aid would be suitable. It may be impossible to help with some requirements, and others may be more appropriately tackled by non-visual means. If it appears that a magnifier would be useful, the assessment can proceed to prescribe this. See *Prescribing magnification*.

Case history for prospective contact lens wearer

A full ocular history, including age of first optical correction and spectacle wearing habits, will help to gauge general suitability in patients who have never previously worn contact lenses ('neophytes'; see Table C.3). For example, a prospective wearer who only wears spectacles intermittently may not be an obvious choice for contact lens wear. However, if that intermittent wear is driven by a dislike for the cosmetic effect of spectacles, then contact lenses become a more obvious choice. Existing use of spectacles for distance and near vision may give some indication of whether the patient will have to adapt to significant changes in accommodation and convergence once contact lens wear is initiated. This may be particularly relevant to early presbyopic myopes who may either take their spectacles off to read or have insufficient reserves of accommodation to cope with the additional accommodative demands in contact lenses compared to spectacles.

Previous ophthalmologic, orthoptic or general practitioner eye treatment will give clues about past ocular status that might influence the clinical decision-making process. General health and use of medication are also significant. A positive family ocular or general health history also gives additional information about future potential risks that may relate to contact lens wear or more general patient management. It may be appropriate to ask whether the patient is a smoker, since this seems to be associated with a higher risk of microbial keratitis.

Table C.3 • Initial history taking for the previous or existing lens wearer and non-lens wearer.

Patient new to contact lenses	Previous or existing contact lens wearer
age at first correction	as new patient plus:
use of spectacles	date of first contact lens correction
full time/part time	type of lens worn
current or present prescription	at initial fitting
ocular history	currently
medical treatment	modality recommended
hospital treatment	daily or overnight wear
orthoptic treatment	replacement frequency recommended
general health history	care system recommended
medication	compliance with recommendations
prescribed or 'over the counter'	average/maximum wearing time
family ocular history	number of nights worn without removal
family general health history	hours of continuous wear at time of visit
smoker – yes/no	primary complaint
allergies	other symptoms/signs
motivation for lens wear	reason for discontinuation of previous care
expectations of lens wear	date of last appointment
occupational/recreational activities	

Questioning about specific allergies will help to guide choice of lens modality, the frequency of replacement and the care system.

Symptoms with the present spectacles will also give information that may in future help to differentiate specific contact lens symptoms from pre-existing problems.

Contact lens-specific questions will include why the patient wants contact lenses, what he or she knows about contact lenses, and what is expected from lens wear. Questions regarding leisure activities and occupation will help to determine the most suitable type of lens, and will also provide an opportunity to offer advice on eye protection if appropriate. With more complex fittings, such as bifocal or toric lenses, it may also help to determine whether an acceptable visual outcome is likely to result from a particular lens type.

This information, when taken in conjunction with observed ocular health, refraction and binocular vision findings obtained during the initial examination, will lead to informed advice being offered to the patient on suitability for lenses generally, and on the most appropriate lens type, wearing modality and care system.

Case history for previous or existing contact lens wearer

When the patient is a previous or existing contact lens wearer, the questioning used for the non-wearer is still appropriate (see *Case history, non-lens wearer*; also Table C.3). However, additional lens-specific information is also required. The type of lens worn, the time since fitting and changes in lens type (e.g. from rigid to soft lenses or from spherical to toric lenses) all start to build a picture of the lens-wearing history. When such changes have been made, it is useful to determine the patient's understanding as to why they were necessary. It is important to determine what modality of wear, frequency of replacement and choice of care system was recommended by the previous practitioner, and whether the patient actually complied with those recommendations.

Average daily wearing time, the number of nights of overnight wear and the number of hours wear at the time of consultation all help to determine the significance of any clinical signs seen during the present and subsequent ocular examination. In particular, it is important to understand the primary complaint of the patient (if any) and any other symptoms that are present at the first consultation. It may also be instructive to inquire as to the reasons why care is no longer being provided by the original practitioner. Knowing the length of time since the last contact lens assessment will help in the judgement of the severity of any ocular changes as well as indicating likely future patient compliance; however, patients are notoriously poor at estimating the time course of previous management.

As with all history taking, it is important to use follow-up questions so as to extract as much information as possible relevant to understanding the patient history and making informed clinical decisions. This is particularly true where there are presenting patient problems, whereby history taking will follow the same pattern as for a general aftercare examination.

Cast moulding of contact lenses

This has become the dominant technology in high volume soft lens manufacture. As with spin casting, a series of highly polished steel tools is used to fabricate polypropylene moulds. The steel master tools are used to make millions of matching male and female moulds, typically in groups of six or eight (Figure C.2).

Cast moulding generally takes place in a continuous, automated production line. Monomer in liquid form is introduced into a concave female mould, which defines the shape of the lens front surface. An ultraviolet-

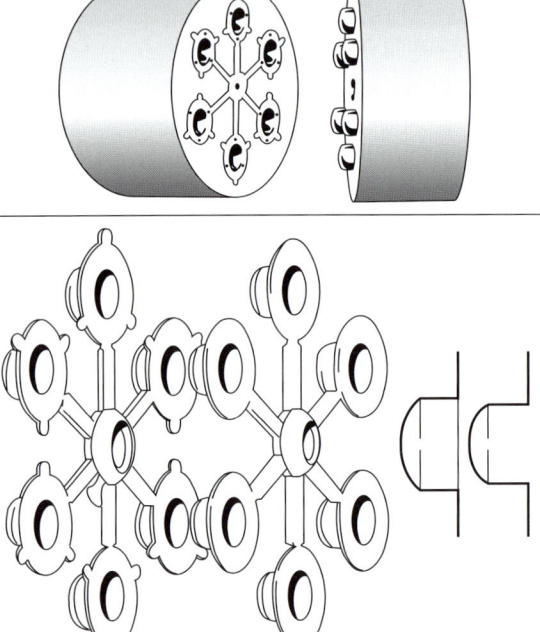

Figure C.2 • Matching male and female steel tools (top) are filled with liquid polypropylene and fitted together. Once the polypropylene has set, the tools are pulled apart to leave a 'flower' of six identical female moulds. An identical procedure (with opposite-shaped tools) is used to make the male moulds. The male and female moulds are filled with the contact lens polymer and brought together (bottom) until polymerization is complete.

transparent male mould is mated to the female mould, and the two are clamped together in a carefully controlled environment. The contact lens edge is formed when the two sides of the mould come together. There is considerable science and art in the control of the polymerization process and the pressure applied to the mould to form the lens. The crucial part is to arrange for the excess polymer (so-called 'flash') to be squeezed out while leaving the edge intact.

Once the polymer is encapsulated in the mould, it is 'cured' – a process in which the assembled moulds are irradiated with ultraviolet light to effect polymerization so as to form the dry contact lens. Most cast moulding processes are designed so that when the dry lens is removed from the mould there is no need to polish the edge. The moulds are disassembled and discarded, and the lens that is released – still in rigid form – is hydrated in saline. Inspection is undertaken either manually or using automated video-based, computer-controlled image analysis. Finally, the lens is packaged and autoclaved.

It should be recognized that the above description is a highly simplified account of a sophisticated engineering process. Various manufacturers have introduced a number of unique variations, such as wet-state polymerization, the employment of re-usable glass moulds, and use of the male half of the mould for final lens packaging. Toric and bifocal lenses can be manufactured using cast moulding technology by engineering the master tools to contain the desired lens forms; these design elements are faithfully transposed to the moulds and then to the final lens.

Cataract

Cataract refers to any opacity within the crystalline lens. Opacities may be acquired or congenital, focal or generalized, large or small, multiple or singular, and may affect any layer of the lens, nucleus or cortex, anterior or posterior. In a mature cataract the whole lens is opaque, whereas a hypermature cataract has a loss of fluid from the lens causing shrinkage with wrinkling of the anterior capsule. Finally, in a Morgagnian cataract the cortex has liquefied and the totally sclerotic nucleus sinks within the capsular bag. Cataract can pose a marked threat to sight if left to develop rather than being operated. It is particularly a problem in developing countries with limited access to surgery.

Senile changes within the lens are the result of accumulation and compaction of lens fibres with age, as well as precipitation of lens proteins, particularly the alpha-crystallins. Solar UV exposure may contribute to senile cataract, particularly posterior subcapsular changes. Nuclear sclerosis occurs with hardening and brunescence of nucleus. Cortical cataract leads to typical white, spoke-like opacities often with associated vacuoles or 'water-clefts'. A posterior subcapsular cataract (PSC) occurs at the posterior capsule as a result of posterior migration of equatorial lens epithelial cells. It has a severe effect on vision. Direct penetrating trauma of the lens usually leads to rapid cortical opacification; rarely this may remain isolated to the area of trauma. Blunt non-penetrating trauma can result in an anterior subcapsular opacity; typically a flower-like appearance. Electrical shock, ionising radiation and microwaves can also lead to cortical and PSC changes. Other causes include nutritional deprivation, toxicity from substances including topical or systemic corticosteroids, inflammatory effects from chronic uncontrolled anterior uveitis or atopic keratoconjunctivitis, and inherited disorders. Congenital cataracts will typically be localized to delineated nuclear layers.

Lenticular opacities lead to a number of symptoms, the most common of which is blurring of vision. Cataract also leads to glare, particularly with cortical cataract and patients may report haloes around headlights especially with night driving. Nuclear sclerotic cataract may lead to a myopic shift and may also alter colour perception as it acts as a yellow filter. The incidence is age-related. By 90 years of age everyone has some lens opacity and in developed countries approximately 25% of 80 year olds have had a cataract extraction.

If the cataract is functionally or clinically significant, in the absence of other pathology or refractive error, then consideration of surgery should be made. One common functional criterion is a deficit of 3 or more lines in visual acuity. The Wilmer Institute Cataract Grading System criteria are a nuclear cataract of grade 2.0 or greater (Figure C.3), cortical cataract affecting more than 4/16ths of the pupillary area, or a posterior subcapsular cataract of more than $1mm^2$. Disproportionate symptoms may also be an indication for surgery in patients with mild cataract. The most common surgical technique for cataract removal is now small incision phacoemulsification and intraocular lens implantation. This technique is performed in day surgery and usually allows a rapid recovery for the patient.

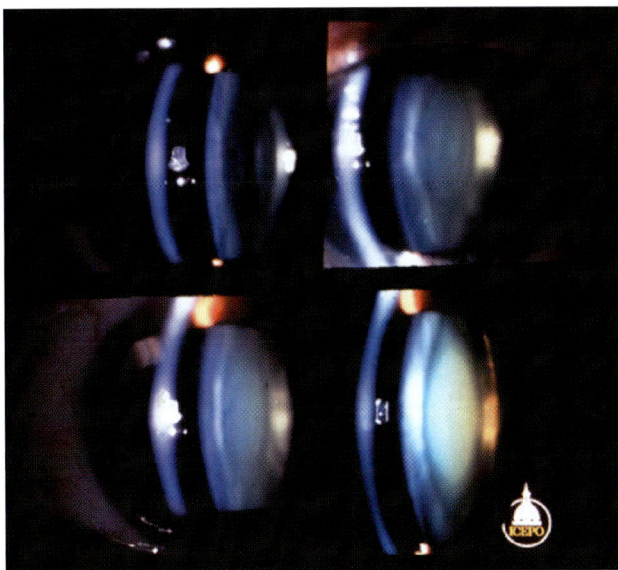

Figure C.3 • Grading of nuclear sclerosis using the Wilmer Institute Cataract Grading System. (Reproduced with permission from H.R. Taylor, S.K. West (1989) The clinical grading of lens opacities. Aust. NZ. J. Ophthalmol. 17: 81–86.

CCLRU grading scales
- See *Grading scales*.

Cellulose acetate butyrate
This was one of the original gas-permeable rigid contact lens materials. Cellulose acetate butyrate (CAB) is a cellulose ester that is less rigid and less brittle (i.e. 'tougher') than polymethyl methacrylate (PMMA). The oxygen permeability of CAB is about 20 times greater than that of PMMA (which is still very low), and is capable of being fabricated by moulding techniques. Because CAB lacks the dimensional stability of other rigid lens materials, it is seldom used for making contact lenses.

CE mark
- See *Antimicrobial efficacy; Medical Devices Directive*.

Centration distance, ophthalmic lenses
The horizontal distance between the centration points of a pair of ophthalmic lenses in a spectacle frame is termed the centration distance. This distance coincides with the interpupillary distance in the absence of prescribed prism.

Centration point, ophthalmic lens
This is the point at which the optical centre of an ophthalmic lens is to be located in front of the pupil of the eye in the absence of prescribed prism.

Centration, soft contact lens
- See *Fitting soft contact lenses*.

Centre thickness of a contact lens
- See *Contact lens thickness*.

Charges, contact lens
- See *Fees and charges, contact lens*.

Chemical bond tinting of contact lenses
In this soft lens tinting process, a strong covalent chemical bond is formed between the dye chromophore and the polymer. The technique involves soaking the lens in a dye solution, in the presence of a catalyst, for a fixed time at a specified temperature. The lens then needs to be put through a series of extraction processes to remove any residual unreacted agents. The result, as with vat dye tinting, is a stable, uniform translucent tint. See *Tinted contact lenses*.

Chemical injuries
Most chemicals harm the eyes by direct contact with the external ocular tissues; these are amongst the most urgent ocular emergencies. Concentrated sulphuric acid from exploding car batteries, household bleaches, detergents, disinfectants, and lime are examples of chemicals that can cause burns to the eyes. In general, chemical eye injuries can be categorized as being caused by acids or alkalis.

The severity of an acidic chemical burn depends on the concentration of the chemical, the duration of the exposure, and the pH of the solution. All solutions are irritating to the eye but are rarely serious if their pH is 2.5 or above. Diluted acids produce redness, oedema, and small conjunctival haemorrhages. However, if the acid is strong, then stromal opacification and corneal vascularization will occur. The tissues may even be charred by concentrated nitric or sulphuric acids and, in the severest cases, complete destruction of the cornea and anterior structures will result. The damage caused by acids depends upon the protein affinity of the acid anion and the concentration of the acid. The acids act by combining chemically with the protein of the more superficial tissues to form an insoluble acid proteinate. This acts as a buffer, which limits the penetration of the acid through the ocular tissues. Acid burns are generally less severe than alkali burns and they tend to improve with treatment and time.

Alkalis penetrate tissues rapidly. They act by combining with the lipoid cells of the membranes and produce total disruption of cells with softening of the tissues. Once the alkali has gained entry to the corneal stroma, it progresses to Descemet's membrane by the cations combining temporarily with the mucoproteins and collagen. The mucoproteins are then denatured rapidly and the released cations attach themselves to even deeper stromal proteins. The initial appearance of the eye after trauma may be deceiving, showing little apparent damage, but it may become worse with time, leaving a totally opaque cornea. The ocular effects of alkalis can be divided into 3 stages:

- Acute stage – ischaemic necrosis of the conjunctiva, loss of the corneal epithelium, oedema, opacification of the subconjunctival tissue and acute iritis.
- Reparation stage – epithelial regeneration, vascularization and the iritis subsides.
- Late complications – symblepharon, dry eye, an opaque vascularized cornea with recurrent ulcerations, uveitis, secondary glaucoma and cataract.

As the hydroxyl ion concentration increases, the severity of the effects increases; a pH above 11 is exceedingly dangerous. However, as alkalis have different fat solubilities, there is variation ability of different alkalis to penetrate the cornea. Ammonium hydroxide has the greatest ability to dissolve fats and it penetrates the cornea rapidly, to produce deep injury. Lime burns are also very serious and commonly occur in the building trades. Calcium oxide is a major ingredient of substances such as cement, lime, mortar, whitewashes, and numerous other compounds used in this industry. When water or tears are added to calcium oxide, heat is created, causing a thermal burn. In addition, calcium hydroxide is produced, which increases the damage to the eye.

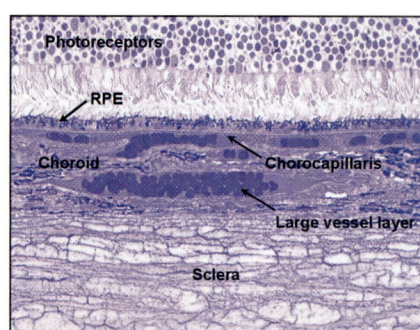

Figure C.4 • Transverse section through the choroid.

Chemical injuries, therapeutic contact lenses for

Much has been written about the use of contact lenses in the management of chemical injuries, especially alkali burns. However, research into the role of the limbal stem cells in the genesis of the corneal epithelium indicates that contact lens coverage of the chronic epithelial defect cannot prevent the colonization of the cornea by conjunctivally-derived epithelial cells. There are, however, some situations in which a contact lens can assist healing, supported by topical medications, although intensive care is required.

Children, contact lenses for

- See *Paediatric contact lenses*; *Paediatric contact lens examination*; *Paediatric contact lens fitting*.

Chlorhexidine-thimerosal-preserved disinfecting solution for contact lenses

Chlorhexidine is probably the most widely used biocide in antiseptics, especially for hand-washing and oral products. Its action has been closely studied, and it is believed that its uptake by both bacteria and yeast is extremely rapid. Chlorhexidine damages cell walls and subsequently attacks the bacterial cytoplasmic or inner membrane, or the yeast plasma membrane.

Thimerosal is considered to be a less effective antimicrobial agent overall, although its action against fungi is better than that of chlorhexidine. Due to this, a combination of chlorhexidine gluconate and thimerosal became common in disinfectants for soft contact lenses. However, owing to the absorption of these agents onto soft lenses, toxic and hypersensitivity reactions were reported when they were used clinically. The build-up of these preservatives, and the subsequent leeching onto the ocular surface over time, had the potential to cause discomfort and discontinuation of lens wear. These products were ultimately superseded by others that offered a similar level of convenience and antimicrobial efficacy, but a lower adverse reaction rate.

Chlorine disinfecting solution for contact lenses

Chlorine-releasing agents have long been established as disinfection systems for swimming pools, baby-feeding equipment and medical instrumentation. In the 1980s, chlorine-releasing systems were developed for the disinfection of soft contact lenses. These were seen as being highly convenient because of their ease of use, portability and low adverse reaction rate. In markets that did not have access to multipurpose solutions when planned replacement lenses were introduced at the end of the 1980s, these systems became very popular.

Two chlorine-releasing systems achieved market success. Alcon introduced the Softab product in the early 1980s. This was a tablet of sodium dichloroisocyanurate, which was dissolved in saline to form three parts per million (ppm) chlorine. Sauflon developed the Aerotab product in the mid-1980s which released 8ppm chlorine. These solutions were effective at killing a range of micro-organisms, including bacteria and fungi; the killing action was thought to be due to the direct effect of the chlorine on some vital constituent of the cell of the micro-organism, such as its protoplasm or enzyme system. However, these products became associated with an increase in contact lens-related microbial keratitis – for example, the 'optimal' use of a chlorine system was associated with an approximately 15-fold increase in the likelihood of Acanthamoeba keratitis compared with hydrogen peroxide or other solutions.

The association of ocular infections with chlorine solutions, despite satisfactory laboratory performance, suggests that there were problems with the efficacy of these systems with normal day-to-day usage. One issue was that the overnight dissipation of chlorine resulted in a loss of disinfecting power, so prolonged storage was not appropriate with these products. There was also evidence that the antimicrobial performance was severely reduced when lenses were soiled. The negative publicity generated by the high incidence of microbial keratitis among users of chlorine disinfection systems, and the widespread availability of multipurpose solutions which were also very easy to use, led to a great reduction in the use of chlorine-releasing systems throughout the 1990s.

Choroid

The choroid is the middle of the three coats of the eye. It is principally a nutritive layer, which serves the outer layers of the retina. It extends from the ora serrata to the margins of the optic nerve head. The choroid consists of four distinct layers (Figure C.4):

- The suprachoroid (lamina suprachoroidea), adjacent to the sclera
- The vessel layer (lamina vasculosa), often composed of an outer layer of large vessels (Haller's layer) and an inner layer of vessels of smaller calibre (Sattler's layer)
- The choriocapillaris (choroidocapillaris)
- Bruch's membrane adjacent to the retina.

The vessels of the choroid are unique in having a single capillary layer of large densely packed, freely anastomosing, fenestrated capillaries disposed on one side of the vascular bed. The organization and distinctive structure of the choriocapillaris ensures maximal metabolite access to the outer retina.

Choroidal vessels are embedded in a loose connective tissue consisting of collagen, a few randomly disposed elastic fibres, numerous fibroblasts and melanocytes. Connective tissue density is greatest in the suprachoroid adjacent to the sclera, where it consists of several layers of flattened fibroblasts and melanocytes. Ciliary nerves and the two long posterior ciliary arteries pass forward within the suprachoroid to the anterior uvea.

Bruch's membrane lies between the choriocapillaris and the pigment epithelium of the retina. It is a double layer consisting of a fenestrated elastic outer lamina and an increased density of collagen fibrils forming an adjacent inner lamina. It is common practice to refer to Bruch's membrane as a five-layered structure by adding an outer collagen layer, and the basement membranes of the choriocapillaris and pigment epithelium. A number of structural and chemical changes occur in the membrane with age, of which debris accumulation (drusen) is the most obvious. It occurs on both sides of the elastic lamina but particularly on the retinal side, and consists of coarse, dense granular and vesicular material. Accumulations develop more rapidly in the sub-macula area and it has been suggested that they may be by-products of retinal pigment epithelial metabolism and/or products of focal degeneration of cells that have failed to disperse.

ChromaGen lenses

ChromaGen lenses are available in the form of tinted soft contact lenses or tinted ophthalmic lenses. The contact lens is prescribed for either one or both eyes, depending on the type and severity of the colour deficiency. A variety of tints are available, and a trial and error method is used to determine the combination that gives the best subjective response in terms of an apparent enhancement of colour vision. Colour deficiency cannot be corrected with filters or by any other means. It is claimed that these lenses can assist people with dyslexia and migraine. Most of these claims have been either challenged or rejected, and a great deal of further research is necessary in order to prove the efficacy of this product. See *X-Chrom lens*.

Chromatopsias

Chromatopsias (coloured vision) are transient phenomenon associated with intracranial pathology in which whole or part of the environment appears suffused with colour (Table C.4). Some patients have described the environment as partially covered in 'snow' or 'gold paint'. Chromatopsia may occur in drug toxicity such as high plasma concentrations of digoxin or chloroquine. Electrical stimulation of the occipital lobe produces transient chromatopsias or the sensation of coloured phosphenes. This condition is associated with intracranial pathology.

Table C.4 • Terms used to describe chromatopsia.

Term	Colour sensation
Cyanopsia	Blue
Chloloropsia	Green
Xanthopsia	Yellow
Erythropsia	Red

Cicatricial conjunctivitis, therapeutic contact lenses for

No type of contact lens can prevent conjunctival shrinkage, but a scleral lens or ring can support the fornices during the healing process following mucous membrane transplantation. More usually, contact lenses are fitted to protect the cornea from the hostile environment created by the disease. See *Eyelid pathology, therapeutic lenses for*.

CIE

- See *Commission Internationale d'Eclairage*.

CIE chromaticity diagram 1931

The CIE established a universal colour measurement and specification system in 1931. Any colour can be specified algebraically and displayed graphically. Specifications are based on the trichromatic colour matching characteristics of a standard observer in a 2° field. However, addition of 3 primary red, green and blue wavelengths, in appropriate amounts, produces white and some colour matches are too desaturated, or mixed with white, to match a given test colour. This leads to negative amounts in some colour matching equations. In order to avoid negative values the CIE adopted a measurement system based on theoretical primaries or tristimulus values, designated X, Y and Z, which produce white when mixed in equal amounts. The relative amounts of each tristimulus value required in any colour match are x, y and z respectively. Since the sum of these quantities is always equal to unity only two quantities, x and y, need be specified and the resulting gamut of colours can be represented in a two dimensional graph, the CIE chromaticity diagram (1931), for each specified luminance level (Figure C.5).

The values of x and y are known as chromaticity coordinates. Wavelengths are positioned on the curved border of the diagram representing the spectral locus. The limits of the visible spectrum are joined by a straight line which locates the fully saturated non-spectral purples. The locus for different colour temperature whites, including standard light sources A, B and C, is positioned in the centre of the diagram. A fundamental property of the chromaticity diagram is that mixtures of two colours always lie on a straight line joining their chromaticity coordinates. Specifications of dominant wavelength, complementary colour and purity (quantity of colour) can be obtained graphically. Equal numerical differences do not represent equal perceptual differences in the 1931 CIE chromaticity diagram. The 1960 CIE UCS diagram has more uniform colour spacing. In this system the tristimulus values are designated U, V and W. The new chromaticity coordinates, u and v, can be calculated from x, and y and vice-versa.

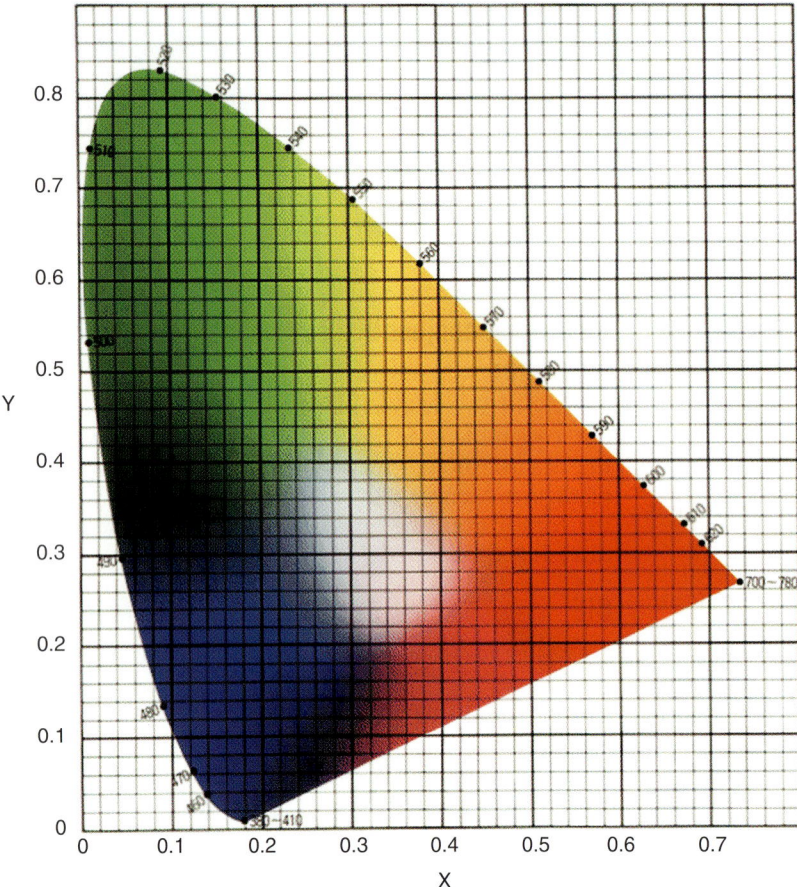

Figure C.5 • CIE Chromaticity Diagram 1931.

Normal hue discrimination ability is determined from psychophysical measurements and displayed in a series of ellipses (MacAdam Ellipses) in the 1931 CIE chromaticity diagram. The unequal dimensions of the ellipses emphasize that colour differences vary within the diagram. Colours with x, y chromaticity co-ordinates within an ellipse cannot be distinguished as long as there is no perceived lightness difference. MacAdam ellipses can therefore be used for colour reproduction and colour manufacturing tolerances. In colour deficiency hue discrimination ellipses are distorted and transformed into enlarged isochromatic (same colour) zones which are characteristic of the type and severity of colour deficiency. Colours which have x, y chromaticity co-ordinates within an isochromatic zone cannot be distinguished by a colour deficient person of that type if there is no perceived luminance contrast.

Knowledge and careful reproduction of isochromatic colours is crucial to the successful design of colour vision tests. Isochromatic lines are drawn through the long axis or mid-point of an isochromatic zone and converge to average co-punctal (convergence) points in each type of congenital dichromacy (Table C.5). The isochromatic line through the x, y chromaticity coordinates of the reference white point bisects the spectrum locus and the purple line. The points of intersection identify 'neutral wavelengths' or colours that appear achromatic (without colour or grey) in that type of colour deficiency. The average neutral wavelengths for protanopes and deuteranopes are 494nm and 499nm respectively. Tritanopic neutral wavelengths are at about 572nm and in the extreme violet part of the spectrum. A range of desaturated neutral colours, with the same dominant wavelength, occur within dichromatic isochromatic zones. These are calculated mean data for dichromats with average macular pigment density. Individual differences in macular pigment alter the co-punctal point and neutral wavelength. The variation is greater for deutans than for protans and tritans. Neutral colours are frequently used in pseudoisochromatic designs intended to classify the type of colour deficiency.

Table C.5 • Dichromatic convergence or co-punctal points in the CIE Chromaticity Diagram 1931.

Type of dichromatism	x	y
Protanopia	0.75	0.25
Deuteranopia	1.40	−0.40
Tritanopia	0.17	0

Cilia
- See *Eyelids*.

Cilliary body

The ciliary body has the common uveal characteristics of rich vascularity and dense pigmentation and it has the distinctive features of a thick smooth muscle (ciliary muscle), responsible for the induction of accommodation, and an extensive surface epithelium generating the circulating aqueous humour. It is continuous posteriorly

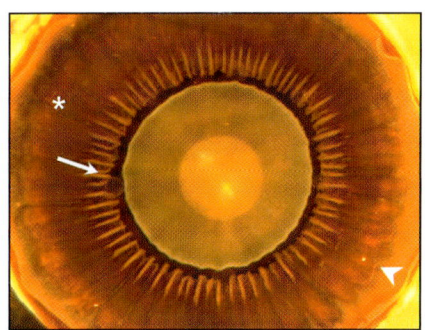

Figure C.6 • Gross view of the inner surface of the ciliary body. Note the radially orientated ciliary processes of the pars plicata (arrow). The pars plana (asterisk) is featureless and uniformly pigmented. The ora serrata (arrow head) marks the posterior aspect of the ciliary body.

with the choroid and retina at the ora serrata and anteriorly with the iris and trabecular meshwork. Externally, it is bound to the sclera and internally it has a free surface, to which the suspensory ligaments of the lens are attached. The ciliary body can be divided into two anatomically distinct regions (Figure C.6):

- Pars plicata: represents the anterior one-third of the ciliary body, and is characterized by 70 to 80 radially oriented ridges, which project into the posterior chamber. These ridges are termed ciliary processes, and represent the primary site of aqueous formation.
- Pars plana: represents the posterior two-thirds of the ciliary body. It is characterized by a smooth and uniformly pigmented surface.

Histologically, the ciliary processes consist of a core of loose connective tissue that contain numerous fenestrated capillaries. The overlying epithelium is a double layer of cuboidal cells. The inner layer, which lies adjacent to the posterior chamber, is non-pigmented and the outer layer is pigmented. The pigmented epithelium (PE) is continuous with the retinal pigment epithelium posteriorly and contains numerous round or elliptical pigment granules (melanosomes). The basal surface of these cells is highly convoluted, to facilitate solute uptake from the stroma. Moreover, numerous gap junctions occur between PE and non-pigmented epithelial cells (NPE) that allow the inter-cellular exchange of ions and metabolites. The NPE, which is the forward continuation of the neuroretina, contains greater numbers of mitochondria and a more pronounced endoplasmic reticulum than the PE. These morphological differences, together with a higher concentration of $Na^+K^+ATPase$, have led to the suggestion that the NPE plays a more important role in aqueous formation. Tight junctions are found between adjacent NPE cells. These junctions are the primary site of the blood–aqueous barrier, and also maintain the transepithelial potential difference across the ciliary epithelium.

Much of the bulk of the ciliary stroma is composed of tightly packed smooth muscle fibres of the ciliary muscle. The muscle forms a complete ring and is approximately wedge-shaped when seen in meridional section, with the sharp end of the wedge pointing backwards. Fibre orientation varies in a manner suggesting the muscle has three parts – meridional (longitudinal), radial (oblique) and circular. The three divisions of the ciliary muscle act together in contraction, and due to its strong attachment to the scleral spur, the muscle is drawn forward and inward towards the anteroposterior axis of the eye, increasing the anterior bulk of the muscle. Meridional fibres appear to be displaced forward towards the spur creating a pull on the retina/choroid. The shortened radial fibres also pull forward towards the spur. Circular fibres are displaced inwards by reducing the diameter of their annulus on contraction, facilitated by the anterior thickening of the other divisions. Consequently, the muscle is sometimes referred to as the 'ciliary sphincter'. In this manner, the muscle parts cooperate in displacing the ciliary body towards the ocular axis, relaxing tension in the suspensory ligaments and permitting the lens to adopt its accommodated form.

City University tests for colour deficiency

There are 3 different editions of the City University tests. The first and second editions have 10 plates. Each plate displays a central hue and 4 peripheral hues derived from the Farnsworth D15 sequence with the addition of grey (Munsell N5). Three of the peripheral hues are typical isochromatic colour confusions, with respect to the central hue, in protan, deutan and tritan deficiency. The fourth hue is an adjacent hue in the D15 sequence. Subjects select the peripheral hue which appears 'most like' the central hue. The second edition differs from the first edition in that 4 of the plates have hues with Munsell value 5 and chroma 2 (as in the Adams desaturated D15 test) and also have smaller subtends. These two editions are both derived from the D15 test but have a different format and visual task. The tests are not designed to identify colour deficiency but are used to grade the severity of colour deficiency when the Ishihara plates are failed. Protan/deutan classification is frequently equivocal because the selected isochromatic hues are very similar. The third edition replaced the second edition in 1998 and contains new untried designs intended for screening (identifying) abnormal colour vision. In these plates the visual task is to select the hue which appears to be different from two other hues. There are only 6 grading plates with the original format and only 4 of these are included in the previous test editions. This test has not been shown to be fit for purpose and is not recommended.

CJD

- See *Trial contact lens set disinfection*.

Cleaning of contact lenses

- See *Surfactant cleaning of contact lenses*.

Clinical records

- See *Record keeping*.

Closed circuit television for low vision

The earliest type of electronic vision enhancement system to be used for low vision was first introduced commercially in the 1970s. A camera is mounted over the material to be viewed, and a magnified image is produced on a monitor display placed above (in-line) or adjacent to the camera (side-by-side). Closed circuit television (CCTV) systems are usually used for near tasks (particularly reading and writing) which may have manual or automatic focussing, with the object positioned directly under the camera, and placed on an X-Y platform to allow control of its movement. Electronic magnification is aberration-free, and the patient can view the screen binocularly from their preferred distance. The user must learn effective 'page-navigation': moving along one line of text, then back to the beginning of the next line, making sure that nothing is missed. This requires at least 15 characters visible on screen simultaneously. If this proves difficult when there is a requirement for high magnification, the patient can be encouraged to use a close viewing distance: this will maximize 'relative distance magnification' whilst using the minimum real image magnification on the screen, and hence optimizing the field-of-view. For example, the same retinal image size will be produced by viewing a screen with 10× magnification at 40cm, as by viewing a screen with 5× magnification from 20cm. In the second case, however, twice as many letters will be visible on screen simultaneously.

Comparison of CCTV to optical magnifier for near vision

Advantages

- Magnification up to > 50×, compared to 20× with optical systems.
- The universal use of zoom lenses permits a rapid change of magnification without altering focus. This allows the use of low magnification for overall assessment of the task before higher magnification is selected for examination of detail.
- The systems all have magnification adjustable over a wide range, so patients can use it for a wide variety of tasks, and can continue to use it if their vision changes.
- Binocular viewing of the screen from a 'normal' working distance is possible, so there are no unusual posture, or extreme convergence, requirements.
- CCTVs can usually be used for longer durations than optical aids of equivalent magnification without fatigue, although the maximal reading speeds obtained may be similar, due to the difficulties of page navigation. However, it is now possible for some CCTVs to scan and capture the full page of text under the camera, and allow the user to choose the way in which it is displayed: in a column just wide enough to fill the screen; in a single continuous horizontal scrolling line; or one word at a time. Each of these is likely to be considerably faster than the traditional manipulation of an X–Y platform.
- The CCTV is psychologically more acceptable than an optical aid, particularly in a school or work environment where VDU terminals are commonplace (and models are available which have a display split between the computer program and the camera image).
- Patients with severe field defects will find it very easy to use eccentric viewing and steady eye strategy.
- The CCTV will be able to provide a higher contrast image than an optical system. This will be particularly beneficial for patients with poor contrast sensitivity for whom the optical aid provides insufficient 'contrast reserve'; see *Reading requirements, low vision*.

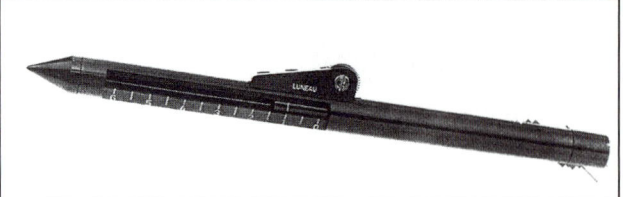

Figure C7 • Cochet–Bonnet aesthesiometer

- Contrast reversal is available (electronic alteration of the polarity of the image on the screen which can be selected with a simple switch) which transforms black-on-white text to a white-on-black screen image. This is particularly useful for patients with media opacities because the average intensity of the image is considerably reduced, and thus light scatter within the eye is decreased, although the majority of CCTV users prefer viewing using contrast reversal mode. See *Contrast enhancement for low vision patients*.
- Some systems with a colour monitor allow a wide choice of background and text colour combinations: there is no rational strategy to the selection of these, but some users claim to find them beneficial.
- Text can be underlined on the screen, and electronic windows can be created to blank out unwanted areas of the image.

Disadvantages

- A patient will require more practice with a CCTV than with optical aids to become proficient in its use.
- In comparison to optical aids, all these systems are bulky, not easily transportable, and obtrusive.
- CCTVs are expensive to buy and require regular maintenance and servicing: in the event of a breakdown, the patient may be unable to continue working.
- The systems are sometimes provided 'off-the-shelf' without a full low-vision assessment. They do need to be prescribed like any other aid to ensure that they are suitable, and to be backed-up by optical aids for the tasks for which the CCTV is unsuitable.
- The depth of field is limited, and scanning across the page of a thick book can cause the image to go out of focus. It is suggested that a glass sheet is placed over the book to produce a flat surface.

See *Magnification for low vision, electronic vision enhancement systems*.

Cochet-Bonnet aesthesiometer

Measurement of corneal sensitivity in the clinical setting has traditionally been achieved by using a Cochet-Bonnet aesthesiometer (Figure C.7). This device can be hand held or mounted on a slit lamp, and uses a single nylon thread to produce various forces by varying its length in 0.5-cm steps (the longer the thread, the lighter the force). The filament is placed lightly onto the cornea by the clinician, using a support that allows manipulation in the x-y-z planes, whilst being viewed through the slit-lamp biomicroscope. The subject reports when the thread can be felt on the ocular surface, and the length of thread at which this occurs is recorded. The corneal touch

Table C.6 • Classification of colour appearance (CIBSE 1994) (courtesy of The Chartered Institution of Building Services Engineers).

Correlated colour temperature	CCT Class	Examples of fluorescent lamps
Less than 3300K	Warm	Colour 93, Warm white
3300–5300K	Intermediate	Polylux, Natural 25
>5300K	Cold	Artificial daylight, Northlight 55

threshold is defined as the length of the nylon filament at which the subject responds to 50% of the number of stimulations. This length is converted into pressure using a calibration curve, and the reciprocal of this value gives the corneal sensitivity. Using this technique it has been demonstrated that corneal sensitivity varies with surface location and is altered by age, iris colour, ambient temperature, time of day, contact lens wear and pregnancy.

A number of factors complicate the use of such a device and can result in variations in the results obtained. These include physical aversion to the approach of the device, problems with mounting the device accurately in the slit lamp, and the impact of ambient humidity on the stiffness of the thread.

Cogan's microcystic dystrophy
- See *Recurrent erosion syndrome, therapeutic lenses for*.

Collagen fibrils
- See *Corneal stroma*.

Collagen lamellae
- See *Corneal stroma*.

College of Optometrists

This is the professional, scientific and examining body for optometrists in the UK. It was formed in 1980 from an amalgamation of the British Optical Association and the Scottish Association of Opticians, and took over the examining role of the Spectacle Makers Company. It is a registered charity incorporated by Royal Charter as a public benefit body.

The stated objects of the College are:
- The improvement and conservation of human vision.
- Advancement for the public benefit of the study of and research into optometry and related subjects and the publication of the results thereof.
- Promotion and improvement for the public benefit of the science and practice of optometry.
- The maintenance for the public benefit of the highest possible standards of professional competence and conduct.

The College publishes a learned Journal 'Ophthalmic and Physiological Optics', a continuing education publication 'Clinical Optometry Update', and a regular newsletter 'In Focus'. The College is administered by an elected council and has approximately 12 500 members.

In support of the College's Code of Ethics, a 'Guidance for Professional Conduct' has been published. The code states: 'An optometrist shall always place the welfare of the patient before all other considerations and shall behave in a proper manner towards professional colleagues and shall not bring them or the profession into disrepute.'

The guidance is divided into sections covering ethics and clinical practice and is a comprehensive coverage of the work of an optometrist. As new techniques develop and clinical and public thinking and expectations change the guidance is updated and revised.

Colour agnosia

Colour agnosia is failure to remember colour names and occurs with other aphasic conditions such as loss of topographical memory, the inability to recognize familiar faces (prosopagnosia), alexia and agraphia. This condition is associated with intracranial pathology.

Colour appearance

The colour appearance of a light source depends on the range of wavelengths emitted. It is generally described as being warm, intermediate, or cold. Cold colours have a blueish tinge, while warm colours are at the red end of the spectrum. Filament lamps have a warm appearance, whilst high pressure mercury lamps have a cool appearance.

The colour appearance of a light source is classified according to the correlated colour temperature (CCT). The colour temperature of a radiator is the absolute temperature (K) of a full radiator (black body), which emits radiation of the same chromaticity as the radiator under consideration. A full radiator is a theoretically perfect absorber of all incident radiation and if it is heated to sufficient temperatures it will emit visible radiation, the wavelength of which depends on the temperature. For filament lamps, the colour temperature approximates to the temperature of the filament itself.

The correlated colour temperature is the term given to the temperature of a full radiator having the chromaticity nearest to that of the light source being considered. For example, the colour of a full radiator at 3500 K is the nearest match to that of a white tubular fluorescent lamp. Each lamp has its own specific CCT but, for practical purposes, these have been divided into three classes, as previously mentioned: warm, intermediate, and cold. It can be seen from Table C.6 that light sources that have a cold appearance have a high CCT and those that have a warm appearance have a low CCT.

The colour appearance of a surface changes when one spectral content of the light source used to illuminate it changes. See *Colour rendering*.

Colour constancy

Colour constancy refers to the ability to ascribe correct colour names to objects in spite of changes in illumination. This is achieved through the combined effect of

Table C.7 • Colour rendering classification (CIBSE 1994) (courtesy of The Chartered Institution of Building Services Engineers).

Colour rendering group	CIE colour rendering index (R_a)	Typical application	Examples of lamps
1 A	$R_a \geq 90$	Accurate colour matching required, e.g. colour printing inspection	Artificial daylight
1 B	$80 \leq R_a < 90$	Accurate colour judgements are necessary or good colour rendering is required for reasons of appearance, e.g. shops	Kolor-Rite 38
2	$60 \leq R_a < 80$	Moderate colour rendering is required	Warm white
3	$40 \leq R_a < 60$	Colour rendering is of little significance, but marked distortion is unacceptable	Colour 35
4	$20 \leq R_a < 40$	Colour rendering of no importance	

adaptation within retinal receptor fields and by neural matrices in areas V1 and V4 of the visual cortex which allow individual colours to be recognized within the context of the surrounding colour.

Colour constancy occurs over a wide range of photopic (daylight) illumination levels for the same light source but is limited for complex scenes composed of small colour differences, such as patterns which resemble paintings by Mondrian, if the spectral content of the light source is changed. In a relatively simple colour pattern an object which looks yellow in white light will look reddish when illuminated by tungsten light but may still be described as yellow because all other objects in the scene have undergone the same transformation. This is known as 'relation colour constancy'.

Colour contrast

Colour appearance is modified by the state of adaptation of the retina. The appearance of a small area of colour is shifted towards the complementary colour of the surround or background colour. For example a yellow object appears 'greenish' when superimposed on a red background and 'reddish' superimposed on a green background due to simultaneous contrast. Simultaneous colour contrast affects the accuracy of some pseudo-isochromatic designs by shifting the desired colours away from the intended isochromatic zone. This is minimized by including a range of lightness differences in the design. Successive contrast changes occur when intense coloured lights or pigments are viewed sequentially. The first colour viewed produces an afterimage, composed of the complementary colour, which is then superimposed on the next colour altering the intended appearance. The accuracy of colour naming in Lantern tests, which display paired colours, is affected by both simultaneous and successive contrast effects.

Colour mixing

Superimposed wavelengths and incandescent light sources are mixed additively because the resulting colour contains all the spectral elements of the components. Pigments are mixed subtractively and the resulting colour is derived from the combined absorption of the components. Red, green and blue are the three (trichromatic) primary colours needed for additive colour mixing. All perceived colours can be obtained by mixing suitable amounts of these three colours. Fundamental colour mixture curves based on precise colour matches can be obtained psychophysically. Magenta, yellow and cyan (blue-green) are the three primaries needed for subtractive colour matching. The appearance of pigment colours depends on the spectral content of the illuminant. For example green and blue appear black when illuminated by red light because the light source only contains long wavelengths which are not reflected by these pigments.

Colour properties of lamps

- See *Colour rendering; Colour appearance*.

Colour rendering

This expression describes the appearance of colours under a given light source compared with their appearance under a reference source. Good colour rendering implies similarity of appearance under an acceptable light source, such as daylight. However, the colour appearance of light from a source is not a guide to its colour properties, as it is possible for the light from two lamps to be apparently identical in appearance but to have different colour rendering properties.

The Commission Internationale d'Eclairage (CIE) has developed a method of indicating the colour rendering properties of a light source. The colour rendering index ranges from 0 to 100, where 100 represents no colour distortion (Table C.7). The Chartered Institute of Building Service Engineers (CIBSE) Code 1994 also provides a classification of colour rendering for light sources. It defines 5 groups ranging from 1A to 4, where 4 represents very poor colour rendering. Accurate colour matching requires good colour rendering. Hence, light sources from Group IA should be used. These have a high CIE general colour rendering index, being greater than or equal to 90.

Colour vision deficiency

Congenital colour deficiency is caused by inherited cone photopigment abnormalities. These arise in several

Table C.8 • Classification and terms used to describe different types of congenital colour deficiency.

Dichromats (2 photopigments types)		Anomalous trichromats (3 photopigment types but one has abnormal spectral sensitivity)	
Protanopia	No long wavelength ("red") sensitive photopigment	Protanomalous trichromatism	A range of abnormal long wavelength ("red") sensitive photopigments
Deuteranopia	No medium wavelength ("green") sensitive photopigment	Deuteranomalous trichromatism	A range of abnormal medium wavelength ("green") sensitive photopigments
Tritanopia	No short wavelength ("blue") sensitive photopigment	Tritanomalous trichromatism	Abnormal partial expression of the short wavelength ("blue") sensitive photopigment gene

different ways. The retina may be lacking functional cone receptors or there may be only one cone photopigment type. These individuals are without hue discrimination ability in photopic viewing and are truly 'colour-blind'. See *Monochromatism*. Normal trichromatic colour vision is derived from three cone photopigment classes and there are 3 types of colour deficiency in which hue discrimination is present but abnormal. There are differences in severity in each of the three types depending on whether a photopigment is absent or has abnormal spectral sensitivity. People with only two photopigment types are described as dichromats and are able to match all spectral hues using 2 colour matching variables. All dichromats have severe colour deficiency and confuse a wide range of colours. Alternatively three photopigment types are present but the spectral sensitivity of one of these differs significantly from that of the normal photopigment. These individuals are described as anomalous trichromats. In this case three colour matching variables are needed to match all the spectral hues but colour matching is abnormal. A range of abnormal photopigments, with different peak wavelength sensitivities, occur in red-green colour deficiency (Table C.8). If an abnormal photopigment is only slightly different from that of the normal the person has slight colour deficiency but if the peak sensitivity is very different the person has severe colour deficiency similar to the corresponding dichromat. Differences in type and severity of colour deficiency lead to different practical difficulties with colour codes at home and in the work place.

Protan, Deutan and Tritan are group terms, derived from Greek words meaning first, second and third, used to include both dichromats and anomalous trichromats derived from absence or abnormality of the same photopigment group.

Protan and deutan defects are described collectively as red-green colour deficiency. Red-green defects share the same X linked mode of inheritance. All colour deficient people see a smaller number of spectral hues than people with normal colour vision. Abnormal colour matching results in colour confusions. Some colours which are distinguished as different by people with normal colour vision look the same to people with colour deficiency and are confused or identified incorrectly if there is no perceived lightness difference (Table C.9). Red-green colour deficiency is characterized by colour

Table C.9 • Colours which look the same and are confused in protan, deutan and tritan colour deficiency if there is no perceived lightness difference.

Colours Confused	Protan	Deutan	Tritan
Red/Orange/Yellow/Green	*	*	
Brown/Green	*	*	
Threshold saturation discrimination: Green/White	*	*	
Threshold saturation discrimination: Red/White	*	*	
Blue-Green/Grey/Red-Purple (*neutral colours*)	*		
Green/Grey/Red-Purple (*neutral colours*)		*	
Red/Black	*		
Green/Black		*	
Violet/Grey/Yellow-Green (*neutral colours*)			*
Red/Red-Purple			*
Dark Blue/Black			*
Yellow/White			*

confusions in the red/orange/yellow/green colour range. Dichromats and severe anomalous trichromats confuse saturated colours whereas anomalous trichromats with slight colour deficiency only confuse dark or pale colours. The relative luminous efficiency of the eye is altered in colour deficiency. Either the wavelength of maximum sensitivity is changed or sensitivity to wavelengths at the limits of the visible spectrum is reduced. The latter leads to differences in relative colour contrast, or lightness, compared with normal values. The largest changes occur in protan colour deficiency. In protans the wavelength of maximum luminous efficiency is at 535nm compared with 555nm in the normal and there is reduced sensitivity at the long wavelength limit of the visible spectrum. Long wavelength red light is not seen. This is known as "shortening of the red end of the spectrum" and is the reason why many occupational colour vision standards specifically exclude protans.

Neutral colours are wavelengths or desaturated pigment colours which appear achromatic and are confused with grey. These colours are frequently used in pseudoisochromatic plates intended to classify the type of congenital colour deficiency.

The retina and visual pathway are not fully developed at birth. Congenital colour deficiency can be identified with electrophysiological tests, such as colour electro-retinogram and visually evoked cortical potentials, when sufficient maturity is achieved at about 3 months of age. Preferential looking, with a pseudoisochromatic 'vanishing' design and a control design, is the principle examination technique for investigating the colour vision of babies and infants. Since colour deficiency is genetically determined both eyes are affected and type and severity remain constant throughout life. Colour vision examination is carried out binocularly.

The term 'Daltonism' is synonymous with colour deficiency and commemorates the 18th century polymath John Dalton who described the characteristics of his own colour deficiency.

Colour vision standards, occupational

Normal colour vision is needed for work involving colour matching, colour reproduction and colour quality assurance in manufacturing industries. As well, employment of colour deficient people is restricted in a number of other occupations. Careers and occupations known to require normal colour vision include:

- Workers in occupations which require accurate colour matching and colour quality assurance
- Commercial airline pilots and air traffic controllers
- Aircraft pilots and engineers in the armed services
- Technical and maintenance ground staff at airports
- Naval officers on surface ships and all submarine personnel
- Masters and watch-keepers on merchant marine vessels
- Customs and excise officers
- Train drivers, railway engineers and track maintenance staff
- Electrical and electronic engineers using complex colour coding without redundancy.

Several occupational colour vision standards are currently under review to ensure that recent equal opportunity of employment legislation is not infringed. The onus is on employers to demonstrate that colour deficient people, or people with certain types of colour vision deficiency, represent a significant safety hazard or are unable to work as effectively as people with normal colour vision. There is an extensive literature on this topic. Psychophysical tests provide objective information about the colour discrimination capabilities of colour deficient people but members of the public are often reluctant to accept that these data are relevant in the workplace and request an 'occupational test'. Unfortunately individually constructed colour matching, naming and sorting tests such as the Holmgren Wool test and informal 'resistor wire tests' are rarely effective even for identifying dichromats. These tests were discarded in the past in favour of reliable clinical colour vision tests, such as the Ishihara plates and the Farnsworth D15 test which are based on isochromatic colour confusions. The preferred approach is for employers to evaluate the importance and characteristics of any colour coding used in the occupation and assess whether swift accurate interpretation is important to maintain efficiency. It may be possible to assist colour deficient users by careful colour selection, segmenting areas of different colour, increasing luminance contrast or adding redundant features. Blue/yellow two-way colour codes can be distinguished by all colour deficient people.

Colour codes convey information connotatively or denotatively. Connotative colour codes provide specific information through colour recognition alone. Connotative colour codes are used for signals in maritime, aviation and railway transport and for electrical and electronics components. The prime example is the three-way signal light code: red for 'stop or danger', orange (amber) for 'caution' and green for 'go or all clear'. Connotative codes are also used in industry to designate the function of pipelines, gas cylinders and chemical containers. Failure to recognize connotative codes correctly and swiftly is a safety hazard. Connotative colour codes are common in the construction, rail and shipping industries which all have a high incidence of accidents involving personal injury.

Denotative colour codes include another means of providing information such as text, shape difference or relative position. In this case colour is said to be used 'redundantly' because information can be retrieved without colour recognition. When considering the effect of redundancy in colour coding it is important to ascertain if redundant features are available in all viewing conditions and all light levels or whether the code becomes connotative in some circumstances. For example, reliance on the relative position of lights in road traffic signal displays may not aid recognition in the dark when only one light is illuminated. The pairing of traffic light signals also varies within the European Community so that anticipation of the next colour may be incorrect. Denotative codes are widespread in business and industry and are an integral feature of geographical maps. Failure to recognize a denotative colour code swiftly may lead to inefficient working practice and may have financial implications.

People with slight colour deficiency may be employed in occupations which do not accept people with severe colour deficiency. Occupations which accept applicants with slight colour deficiency include:

- Fire-fighters (protans excluded)
- Police officers
- Some ranks in the armed services
- Merchant marine engineers and seamen not involved in lookout duties
- Electricians using domestic colour codes or simple industrial colour codes with redundant features.

Table C.10 • CIE Colour vision standards for international transport.

Standard	Colour vision	Test	Association
1	Normal Colour Vision	Ishihara plates	High risk occupations which include the recognition of distant signal colours and other safety critical colour codes
2	Slight colour deficiency but all protans are excluded	Ishihara plates An approved lantern test* A spectral anomaloscope (to exclude protans)	Low risk activities but must be able to recognize signal colours at moderate distance
3	Slight/Moderate colour deficiency	Ishihara plates Farnsworth D15	Low risk activities involving the recognition of pigment colour only

*The Holmes-Wright A lantern in photopic viewing at high brightness, the Beyne lantern and the Spectrolux lantern. The Farnsworth lantern is approved in the USA only.

This policy can be justified because people with slight colour deficiency confuse a smaller range of colours. Use of both the Ishihara plates and the Farnsworth D15 test is usually recommended but a more comprehensive test battery, which includes either a lantern test or the Farnsworth-Munsell 100 hue test, may be specified.

People with protan colour deficiency are excluded from more occupations than deutans because failure to respond to a coded red message due to 'shortening of the red end of the spectrum' may be a safety hazard. This exclusion particularly applies to occupations in transport and is endorsed by the CIE (Table C.10). Since protans may not be clearly identified by the Ishihara classification plates and may pass the D15 test, an additional test such as the Nagel anomaloscope, is needed to obtain this standard. Lantern tests are a traditional means of selecting employees in the armed services (Table C.11) as well as in civilian transport but have a poor reputation for reliability.

Colour vision standards for occupations in the UK armed services are currently under review. The aim is to set uniform standards and examination methods in all the services. This is not straightforward because there is a need to consider career advancement and the requirement for personnel to be multi-skilled in a particular service. Colour deficient people may find that their career progression is limited if a more strict colour vision standard is applied to related work on promotion.

Table C.11 • Colour perception standards in the UK armed services.

Colour perception (CP) classification	Standard
CP1: Superior colour vision	No errors on the Holmes-Wright A lantern at LOW luminance in the dark
CP2: Normal colour vision	Pass Ishihara plates
CP3: Slight colour deficiency	No errors on the Holmes-Wright A lantern at high luminance in the dark
CP4: Moderate colour deficiency	Unable to obtain CP3 Recognition of coloured wires (Royal Navy only)
CP5: Severe colour deficiency	Unable to obtain CP4 (Royal Navy only)

Coloured lenses
- See *ChromaGen lenses; Tinted contact lenses; Tinted ophthalmic lenses; X-Chrom lens.*

Comfort drops for contact lenses
- See *Re-wetting solutions, soft lens; Wetting solutions, rigid lens.*

Comfort, soft contact lens
- See *Fitting soft contact lenses.*

Comitant deviations
A comitant (or concomitant) deviation is one where the eye deviation remains the same in all positions of gaze and/or when it is the same when one or the other eye fixates, although the deviation may vary with the fixation distance.

Comitant strabismus classification is complex and deviations can be categorized in many different ways: primary, secondary to another condition, or consecutive; latent or manifest; constant or intermittent (relates to manifest strabismus only); eye position and direction of eye movement during the cover-uncover and alternate cover test; with respect to fixation distance; effect of accommodation; compensated or decompensated (relates to heterophoria only); and with respect to time (see Figure C.8).

Commission Internationale d'Eclairage (CIE)
The CIE is an international standards organization which has a wide brief in setting colour standards for industry and transport. These include systems for colour measurement, specification of standard light sources and signal lights, and occupational colour vision standards.

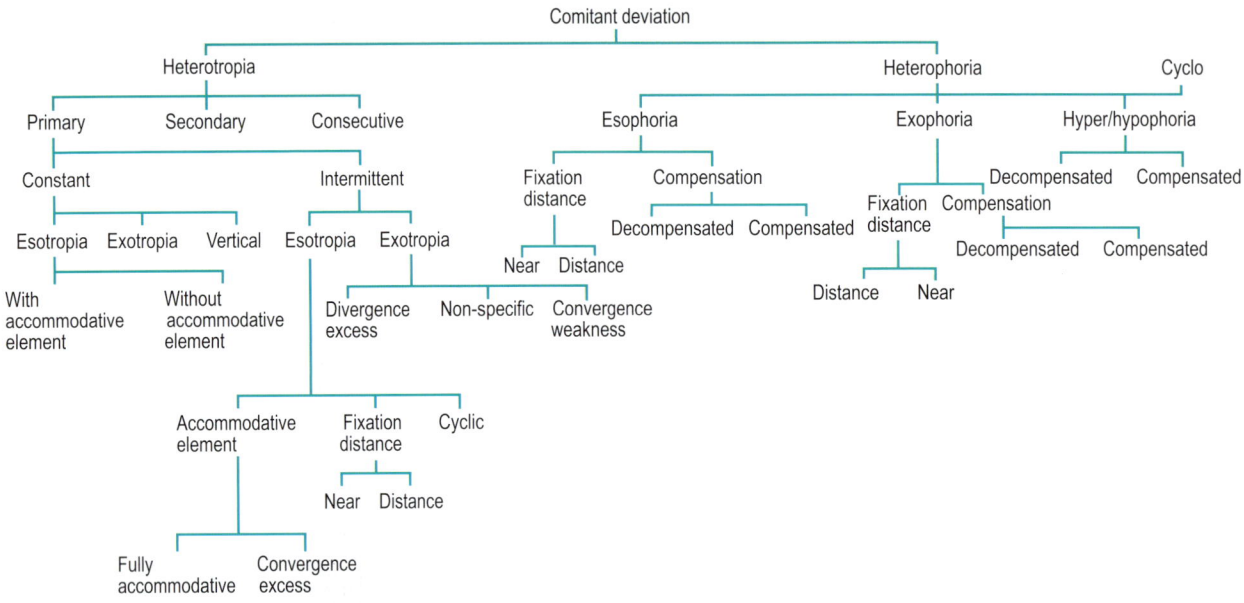

Figure C.8 • Summary of comitant eye deviation classification.

Compensated rigid bitoric contact lens

These are lenses that, like spherical lenses, do not correct for any residual astigmatism. They are bitoric because the front surface contains a cylinder solely for the correction of the induced astigmatism. A compensated bitoric can be thought of as a lens designed to correct all of the refractive cylinder created due to the corneal toricity. If the corneal toricity is equal to the spectacle astigmatism, then the cylinder will be fully corrected when a compensated bitoric lens is worn. A compensated bitoric lens can rotate on the eye without visual disturbance because the effect of the rotation is counteracted by an equal change in the cylinder power of the tear lens. See *Cylindrical power equivalent rigid toric lenses; Induced astigmatism with rigid toric lenses; Residual astigmatism with rigid toric lenses; Stabilization of rigid toric lenses; Toric lens design, rigid; Toric lens, rigid*.

Complementary colours

Complementary colours are colour pairs which, when mixed together in suitable amounts, produce grey or an achromatic sensation. Complementary colour pairs can be demonstrated within the CIE Chromaticity diagram by drawing straight lines across the diagram bisecting the x, y chromaticity coordinates of the reference illuminant. Complementary colours are also seen as after-images following adaptation to intense coloured stimuli. Observation of complementary colours was instrumental in promoting Hering's Colour Opponent theory in the 19th century. This is based on the observation that white is opponent to black, red is opponent (complementary) to green and yellow is opponent (complementary) to blue. See *Simultaneous and successive contrast*.

Compliance with contact lenses

- See *Non-compliance with contact lenses*.

Compliance enhancement with contact lenses

The general principles of enhancing patient compliance with instructions and guidelines issued by an eye care practitioner are encapsulated in the following guidelines:

1. *The clinic*. The clinic must have the following qualities:
- staff should be informed and aware of key issues
- advice given should be consistent over time and between personnel
- appointment times should be individualized (as opposed to 'block booking')
- waiting times should be minimal
- there should be continuity of care wherever possible
- the clinical environment should be warm and friendly.

2. *The practitioner*. Important qualities of the practitioner are to:
- project (rather than internalize) a devotion to eye care
- listen effectively to what the patient has to say
- use minimum jargon
- emphasize key points, especially following delivery of a long and perhaps complex set of instructions
- set specific and realistic goals for patients to aim at
- adopt strategies to motivate patients.

3. *Aftercare*. Strategies for optimizing the effectiveness of the aftercare visit include:
- sending appointment reminders
- advising patients of the importance of regular check-ups
- providing feedback and reward to patients
- repetition of key information
- stimulating the patient's interest in vision
- providing in-practice information via leaflets and posters, videos etc.

4. *The patient*. A valuable approach to learning patient attitudes is to explore the health beliefs using a compliance 'decision tree' (see Figure C.9). The

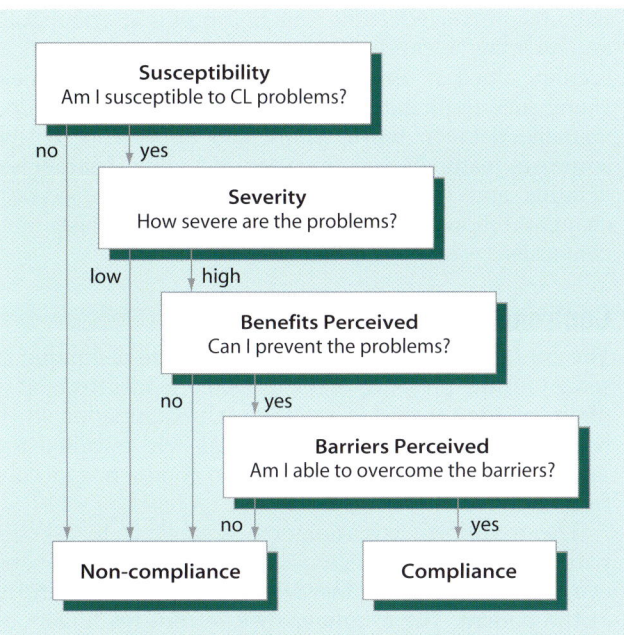

Figure C.9 • 'Decision tree' for exploring patient health beliefs.

answers to the sequence of questions posed in the decision tree will indicate whether or not the patient is likely to be compliant with a contact lens system. If it is determined that the health beliefs of the patient are likely to lead to non-compliance, steps should be taken to modify the erroneous beliefs. This can be achieved via a variety of strategies, such as talking persuasively, supplying pertinent information, or utilizing a health care contract that emphasizes the responsibilities of the patient for achieving safe and comfortable ocular health during lens wear.

5. *The advice.* Care systems should be simple and easy to understand, tailored for the individual, ritualized, and not too expensive. Advice given to patients should be verbal and written. Printed material should be readable and well illustrated. Clearly illustrated sequential steps with minimum wording will aid understanding and interpretation. Written material should also contain warnings; obviously, a balance must be found whereby patients are alerted to possible dangers but are not frightened away from wearing lenses.

6. *The contact lens industry.* An important role is played by the contact lens industry in compliance enhancement, and this role falls into three broad categories:

- pricing policy – it is self-evident that prohibitive pricing will produce a general disincentive to purchase all of the required products and to use them as required, and the contact lens care industry thus has an obligation to contain prices as far as economically possible
- product support – clear and unambiguous packaging and simple instructions are thought to be important contributing factors to compliance enhancement, and such issues are the sole responsibility of the contact lens industry; many companies also provide attractive 'starter packs' which motivate patients
- research and development – contact lens care systems should be designed to be effective, as distinct from the usual practice of designing systems that are merely efficacious. An efficacious system is one that can be demonstrated to work under ideal situations – that is, assuming full patient compliance – whereas an efficient system is one that will work in a 'real world' scenario, allowing for a certain level of inevitable non-compliance. Full compliance does not exist; all patients will be at least partially non-compliant in some aspect of their care regimen. If this argument is accepted, then it behoves the contact lens industry to develop effective contact lens care systems. See *Non-compliance*.

Conditioning solutions for contact lenses
- See *Wetting solutions, rigid contact lens.*

Confirmation set
To facilitate the performing of a subjective refraction – and in particular confirming the end point of refraction – lens pairs of different power can be placed alternately before the eyes of the patient for comparison purposes. This can be achieved using a confirmation set. This consists of two pairs of lenses mounted on either side of a central bar that is continuous with a finger grip. By rolling the finger grip between the thumb and forefinger by 180°, the position of the lenses can be reversed. A confirmation set is usually comprised of two pairs of lenses of the same numeric power but opposite sign e.g. a pair of +0.25D lenses on one side of the central bar and a pair of –0.25D lenses on the other side. A confirmation set configured in this way would therefore allow a change of ±0.50D to be demonstrated to the patient. Confirmation sets are also available with alternating lens powers of 0.50D and 0.75D.

Confocal microscope
The confocal microscope (Figure C.10) is unlike conventional microscopes because defocus causes the image

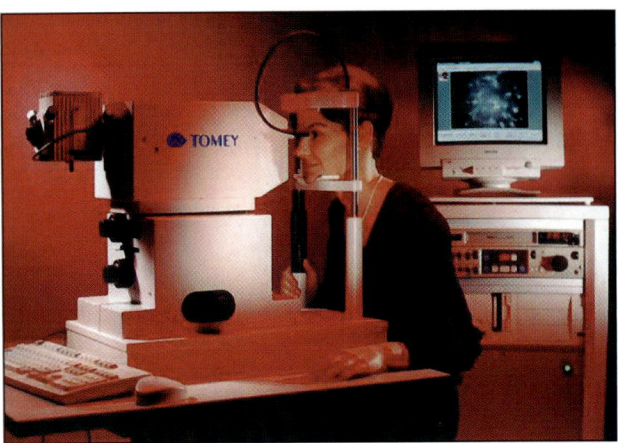

Figure C.10 • Confocal microscope.

to disappear rather than appear as a blurred image. The properties of the confocal microscope stem from its ability to focus the illuminating light and the focal plane of the microscope objective on precisely the same point. In most modern clinical confocal microscopes a point light source is focused onto a small volume within the specimen and a confocal point detector is used to collect the resulting signal. This results in a reduction of the amount of out-of-focus signal from above and below the focal plane, producing a marked increase in both lateral (x, y) and axial (z) resolution. Because only one tiny area of the specimen is observed by each point source, a useful full field of view must be gained by mechanically scanning the area of interest. By varying the plane of focus of both the source and detector within the tissue, the specimen can be optically 'sectioned' non-invasively and detailed information on corneal structure determined.

The microscope objectives most commonly used are non-applanating water immersion objectives that are optically coupled to the cornea using a methyl-cellulose gel. To obtain the maximum axial resolution (and hence optical sectioning), it is necessary to use a microscope objective with a large numerical aperture (which describes the light-gathering ability of the objective). However, there is a compromise in that such devices have a reduced field of view and shorter free working distances, which reduces the distance that the microscope can focus into the specimen from the surface.

The variable-slit, real-time, scanning confocal microscope has two independently adjustable slits that are located in conjugate planes. A rapidly oscillating two-sided mirror is used to scan the image of the slit over the plane of the cornea to produce optical sectioning in real time. This design has the advantages of optimal image contrast, enhanced clarity and decreased scan time, but it is more expensive than Nipkow-based systems, and z-axis quantification is not currently possible.

An adaptation of this technique, known as confocal microscopy through focusing (CMTF), rapidly moves the focal plane of the objective lens through the entire cornea at a speed of approximately 80µm/s while x-y images are acquired at the focal plane. This means that approximately 450 sequential images (which are separated by approximately 1µm) are acquired over the time taken to traverse the cornea (approximately 15s). The cornea is then reconstructed using image-processing techniques and an image is produced that is similar to a histological section, albeit in three-dimensions in a living cornea. Using such techniques confocal microscopy has provided valuable data on the structure and appearance of the cornea in many disease processes, including dystrophies, keratitis and endothelial disease. In addition, corneal changes following refractive surgery, keratoplasty and contact lens wear have been documented.

Confrontation test

The confrontation test is a relatively crude technique to screen for the presence of unsuspected field defects. It is often included as part of a routine eye examination when no formal examination of the visual field is called for. There are 2 different strategies for conducting a confrontation test.

The traditional confrontation strategy is to ask the patient, who has one eye occluded, to fixate either the eye or nose of the examiner who sits opposite within 1m of the patient. The examiner then introduces fingers or hand held targets into the patient's field from the periphery in a plane approximately equidistant from the patient and practitioner. The patient is asked to report when the target can be seen or, in the case where different numbers of fingers are being held up, how many fingers can be seen. The test is a comparison of the visual field of the practitioner with that of the patient, and is intended to establish whether or not there is any significant constrictions or a scotoma. A variant of this technique, kinetic boundary testing, involves moving the stimulus along an arc from behind the patient's head. This variant allows the practitioner to estimate the peripheral limits for the target, which will often extend beyond the reach of the practitioner with the traditional test. A combination of these two tests can be applied when examining a patient.

The suprathreshold comparison strategy involves presenting a suprathreshold target – that is, one that is bright enough to be easily seen – in the 4 different quadrants. The patient asked if it appears brighter or dimmer in any of the quadrants. If a coloured target is used then the patient would be asked if the colour appears different. This strategy is fundamentally different to the traditional strategy in that patients are being asked to compare the appearance of the target as it is transferred from one quadrant to the another rather than simply reporting whether or not it can be seen. A variant of this type of test, the 'red dot test', uses a card with a ring of 8 red dots and a central black fixation point. When held at 30cm, the red dots fall at an eccentricity of 25°. The task of the patient is to look at the fixation point and to count the number of red dots. Missing dots implies the presence of an absolute scotoma. The patient is also asked if any of the dots appear washed out in order to detect relative scotoma.

Confrontation tests have been reported to have sensitivities ranging from 7% for small 'patchy' defect to 100% for altitudinal defects. Their sensitivity to early glaucomatous loss is generally low.

Congenital colour vision deficiency

Red-green colour deficiency (protan and deutan deficiency) is inherited as an x-linked trait. Genes

Table C.12 • Prevalence of red-green colour vision deficiency.		
Type of colour deficiency	Prevalence in men (%)	Prevalence in women (%)
Protanopia	1	0.01
Protanomalous trichromatism	1	0.03
Deuteranopia	1	0.01
Deuteranomalous trichromatism	5	0.35
Total	8	0.40

specifying the long wavelength L ('red') and middle wavelength M ('green') sensitive cone photopigments are located on the X chromosome at Xq 28. Photopigment genes are positioned in a tandem head-to-tail array in sequence from the locus control region at the head of the array. Gene expression is governed by the downstream order. The first gene is usually expressed at the highest level and genes further along the array are expressed in progressively smaller numbers of cones or not expressed at all. In normal colour vision, the L photopigment gene is always first in the array and is therefore expressed at the highest level resulting in a greater number of long wavelength sensitive cones than medium wavelength sensitive cones. An M photopigment gene is normally second in the array followed by more M genes or hybrid genes. There are a number of different genetic mechanisms which result in red-green colour deficiency and it is not always possible to predict the phenotype from the genotype. Dichromatism may arise from a mutation in either the first or second gene in the array which prevents expression. Alternatively one of the genes normally positioned at the head of the array may be lost due to misalignment and unequal crossover at meiosis. Anomalous trichromatism is caused by hybrid genes. The structure of both the L and M photopigment genes consist of chains of 364 amino acids which differ at only 15 sites. Hybrid L/M or M/L genes, which combine regions of the L and M structure, can readily occur at meiosis. These genes code for photopigments which have different peak wavelength sensitivity compared with normal photopigments. However if two hybrid genes, which code for photopigments with the same spectral sensitivity, are present at the head of the array the person will be a dichromat.

Large population studies show that approximately 8% of males and 0.4% of females have red-green colour deficiency. There is no convincing evidence that the prevalence varies in different ethnic groups except in native Australians. The prevalence remains the same in different geographic locations except when the gene pool is limited and frequent intermarriage occurs. The different types of red-green colour deficiency do not have equal prevalence. Deuteranomalous trichromatism has the highest prevalence in both males and females (Table C.12). Some colour deficient females confuse a wide range of colours which suggest that they have combined protan/deutan colour deficiency. This is thought to be due to 'lyonization'. Females inherit duplicate arrays of X chromosome photopigment genes and either maternal or paternal genes may be expressed in different photoreceptors in the cone mosaic. Sufficient abnormal photopigment may be present for some heterozygous females (carriers of colour deficiency) to be identified as minimally colour deficient with psychophysical tests.

Tritan colour deficiency is inherited as an autosomal dominant trait with an equal number of males and females affected. The gene for the short wavelength (blue) sensitive photopigment is on chromosome 7. Expression of the abnormal gene varies and some affected family members are tritanopes and others are tritanomalous trichromats. Hence the term 'incomplete tritanopia' is synonymous with tritanomalous trichromatism. The exact prevalence of tritan colour deficiency is unknown. Tritanopia is estimated to occur in about 1 in 13,000 and tritanomalous trichromatism in about 1 in 500.

Blue cone monochromatism is linked to an abnormality at the locus control region at Xq 28 which prevents expression of all red-green photopigment genes. This type of monochromatism is rare and is inherited as an X linked trait which affects males rather than females. The prevalence is unknown.

In the case of typical (rod) monochromatism, the gene for the rod photopigment (rhodopsin) is located on chromosome 3. Abnormalities of this gene result in retinal dystrophies which primarily involve the rod receptors. Abnormalities of individual genes on chromosomes 2, 8 and 11 have been identified in producing typical (rod) monochromatism in different families. Inheritance is autosomal recessive and consanguinity is a predisposing factor. Prevalence varies worldwide but is estimated to be about 1 in 35 000 in European populations. An equal number of males and females are affected.

Congruity and macular sparing of the visual field

As visual signals pass along the visual pathway from the retina to the cortex, the nerve fibres undergo a considerable amount of sorting and alignment. The nerves that represent corresponding points in the two eyes (points which view the same object) get closer together. Lesions of the visual cortex, therefore, often produce perfectly congruous (identical in both eyes) visual field defects (Figure C.11), while those from the optic tracts often produce incongruous defects (Figure C.12). This characteristic can be valuable in helping to localize the position of a lesion. Congruity only applies to the binocular part of the visual field. Perimetrists must be careful not to label field defects as incongruous simply because they extend into a monocular region of the visual field.

Macular sparing is when the central 5 to 10° of the visual field is unaffected in an otherwise hemianopic

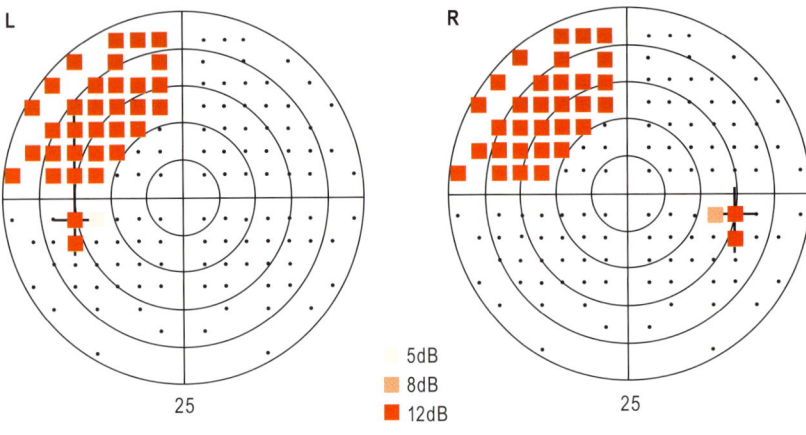

Figure C.11 • Congruous field defect. With the exception of the locations representing the optic disc, in the temporal region of each field chart, the visual field defects are exactly the same in both eyes.

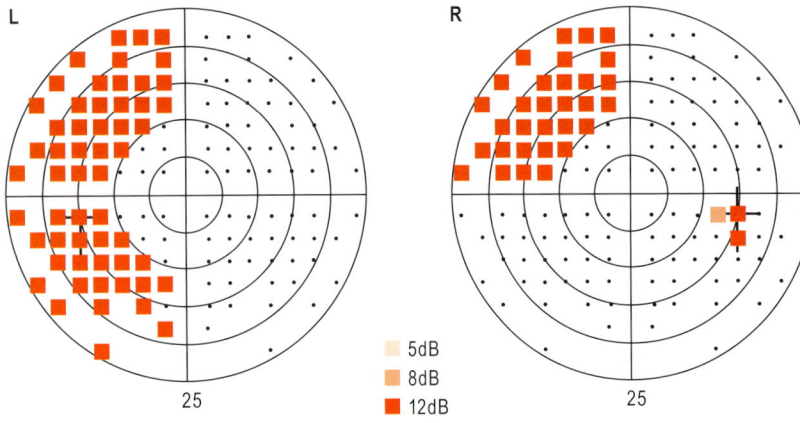

Figure C.12 • Incongruous field defect. The field defect in the right eye is larger, extending to the inferior visual field, than of the left eye.

defect (a defect that affects one half of the field). It is a common characteristic of visual field defects arising from supra-geniculate lesions. Numerous explanations have been put forward to account for macular sparing, many of which have now been refuted as new evidence has come to light. Currently, there are three plausible theories:

1. Shifts in ocular fixation – Patients with hemianopic defects may learn to view objects of interest eccentrically in order to ensure that half of the object is not lost within the field defect. In fact, such techniques are regularly taught to partially sighted patients with macular lesions. The theoretical basis for this approach is that these patients, when asked to look at the fixation target of the perimeter, continue to view slightly to one side, which results in an apparent macular sparing. Some recent work using a fundus perimeter – an instrument that allows the operator to view the fundus during perimetry and to locate the stimuli at a given retinal site – has demonstrated macular sparing in patients who do not show a shift in fixation. This theory cannot, therefore, explain all cases of macular sparing.

2. Separate blood supply – The separate blood supply theory is based upon two observations: a) in some individuals the occipital pole of the visual cortex is supplied by the middle cerebral artery rather than the posterior cerebral artery, and b) in some patients, there is a horizontal border at the macula between the areas supplied by the posterior temporal artery (a branch of the posterior cerebral artery) and the area supplied by the middle cerebral artery. Both these findings could explain macular sparing. If an occlusion occurs in either the posterior cerebral artery in a patient whose macular area is supplied by the middle cerebral artery, or in a branch of the posterior cerebral artery which does not supply the macular area, then some macular sparing would result. The separate blood supply theory must not be confused with an earlier theory based upon the belief that there is a dual blood supply to the visual cortex. There is no anatomic evidence of a dual blood supply to the visual cortex.

3. Extent of macular representation – The final theory to explain macular sparing states that the macular area has such a large cortical representation that in any incomplete lesion there is a high probability that some of the macular fibres will be left intact.

Conjunctiva

The conjunctiva is a thin, transparent mucous membrane that extends from the eyelid margins anteriorly, providing a lining to the inside of the lids before turning sharply upon itself to form the fornices, from where it is reflected onto the globe, covering the sclera up to its junction with the cornea. It thus forms a sac that opens anteriorly through the palpebral fissure. The conjunctiva is conventionally divided into the following regions (Figure C.13):

- marginal
- tarsal
- orbital
- bulbar
- limbal
- fornical.

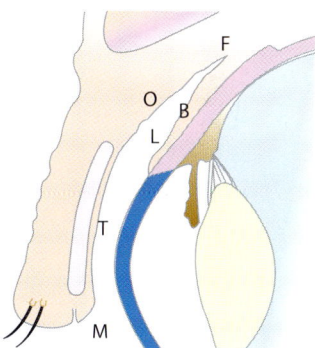

Figure C.13 • Schematic representation of cross-section through the eyelid and conjunctival sac, showing the following regions: M = marginal, T = tarsal, O = orbital, B = bulbar, L = limbal, F = fornical.

Conjunctival blood vessels

The arterial supply of the conjunctiva derives from two sources; palpebral branches of the nasal and lacrimal arteries, and the anterior ciliary arteries. Palpebral vessels serve two vascular arcades within the eyelid. The inferior (marginal) arcade sends branches through the tarsal plate to the eyelid margin and tarsal conjunctiva. The superior (palpebral) arcade supplies the tarsal, orbital, fornical, and bulbar conjunctiva. The limbal zone, in contrast, is served by anterior ciliary arteries. The anterior ciliary arteries travel along the tendons of the rectus muscles and give off branches at the episcleral level prior to dipping down into the sclera to link with the major iridic circle. Episcleral branches pass forward and loop back a few millimetres short of the cornea to become conjunctival vessels. Forward extensions of these vessels form the limbal arcades (limbal loops), which is a complex network of fine capillaries. Conjunctival veins are more numerous than arteries. They can be readily differentiated from arteries due to their larger calibre, darker colour and more tortuous path.

Conjunctival epithelium

The superficial layer of the conjunctiva. In the marginal zone, the conjunctival epithelium is stratified and squamous with few goblet cells. A sub-population of these cells, which lie close to the mucocutaneous junction, may be acting as stem cells for the palpebral conjunctiva. Approaching the tarsus, the epithelium thins to two to three layers of cuboidal cells with scattered goblet cells. The epithelium of the orbital zone is slightly thicker (two to four cells), with more numerous goblet cells. The number of goblet cells declines over the bulbar conjunctiva, and at the limbus the epithelium is again stratified squamous, and goblet cells are absent. The limbus contains a unique array of connective tissue ridges (the palisades of Vogt) that project into the overlying epithelium. The palisades are the repositories of stem cells, and therefore act as the regenerative organ of the corneal epithelium. The conjunctival epithelium additionally contains several non-native cells, including dendritic cells, melanocytes and lymphocytes.

Conjunctival goblet cells

These cells provide the mucus component of the tear film. They arise in the basal cell layers and migrate to the surface, becoming fully differentiated. Mature goblet cells are larger than the surrounding epithelial cells and contain a peripherally placed nucleus. The cytoplasm is packed with membrane-bound secretory granules, which discharge from the apical surface in an apocrine manner. The number of goblet cells shows a marked regional variation in density (Figure C.14), and they are occasionally seen lining intra-epithelial crypts (of Henle).

The apices of many surface epithelial cells of the conjunctiva contain numerous carbohydrate-containing secretory vesicles, which are seen to migrate to the cell surface where they fuse with the plasma membrane. It is likely that this represents a mechanism for recycling the cell-surface glycocalyx rather than a secondary source of secretory mucin.

The marginal, tarsal and orbital conjunctiva collectively form the palpebral conjunctiva. The marginal zone extends from a line immediately posterior to the openings of the tarsal glands and passes around the eyelid margin, from where it continues on the inner surface of the lid as far as the sub-tarsal fold (a shallow groove that marks the marginal edge of the tarsal plate). The tarsal conjunctiva is highly vascular and is firmly attached to the underlying fibrous connective tissue. From the convex border of the tarsal plate, the orbital zone extends as far as the fornices. Over this region the conjunctiva is more loosely attached to underlying tissues, and so readily folds. Elevations of the conjunctival surface in the form of papillae and lymphoid follicles are commonly observed here.

The transparency of the bulbar conjunctiva readily permits the visualization of conjunctival and episcleral blood vessels. Here, the conjunctiva is freely movable due to its loose attachment to Tenon's capsule (the fascial sheath of the globe). As the bulbar conjunctiva approaches the cornea, its surface becomes smoother and its attachment to the sclera increases. The limbal conjunctiva extends approximately 1–1.5mm around the cornea. Its junction with the cornea is ill defined, particularly in the vertical meridian, due to a variable degree of conjunctival/scleral overlap. The limbus has a rich blood supply, and in the majority of individuals a radial array of connective tissue elevations – the palisades of Vogt – can be seen adjacent to the corneal margin. The palisades are most prominent in the vertical meridian, and their visibility is enhanced in pigmented eyes.

The conjunctiva contributes the mucin component of the pre-ocular tear film, and plays an important role in the defence of the ocular surface against microbial infection. Mucins are a family of high molecular weight glycoproteins, which includes membrane-bound and secretory varieties. Conjunctival goblet cells are the primary source of secretory mucin, whilst surface epithelial cells of both the conjunctiva and cornea possess mucin-like molecules within their glycocalyx. The conjunctiva also forms part of a common mucosal defence system, which is an important component of the defence of the human body against micro-organisms. The conjunctiva possesses the immunological capacity for antigen processing, and cell-mediated and humoral immunity. Humoral immunity is provided by specific antibody (particularly IgA) produced by transformed B-cells (plasma cells) in the stroma. T-lymphocytes form the basis of cell-mediated immunity.

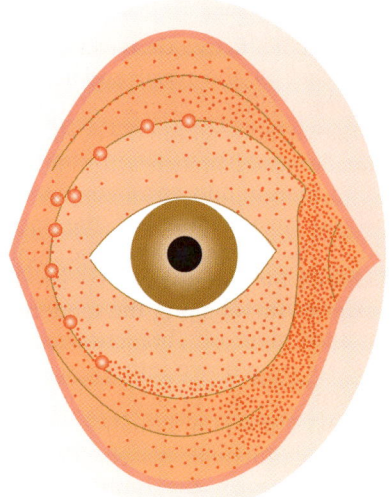

Figure C.14 • Regional variation in goblet cell density in the conjunctiva.

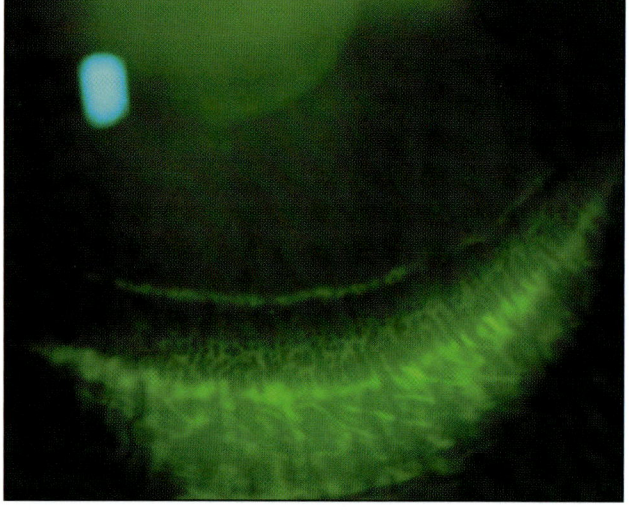

Figure C.15 • Conjunctival and corneal ring staining caused by defects in the edge and periphery of a soft lens.

Conjunctival nerves

The conjunctiva receives nerves from sensory, sympathetic, and parasympathetic sources. Sensory nerves, which are trigeminal in origin, reach the conjunctiva via branches of the ophthalmic nerve. The principal function of these fibres is to equip the conjunctiva with the ability to detect a variety of sensations – for example, touch, pain, warmth and cold. Sensory nerve terminals include both free (unspecialized) nerve endings and the more complex corpuscular endings (classically referred to as Krause end bulbs). Conjunctival blood vessels receive a dual autonomic innervation. Parasympathetic fibres (issuing from the pterygopalatine ganglion) and sympathetic fibres (from the superior cervical ganglion) are responsible for vasodilation and vasoconstriction, respectively.

Conjunctival redness, contact lens induced

The clinical presentation of a 'red eye' can be one of the most difficult cases to solve due to the numerous possible known causes. This problem may be even more complex in a contact lens wearer because of the wide variety of causes of contact lens-related red eye. Conjunctival redness in lens wearers is generally asymptomatic, but patients may complain of itchiness, congestion, non-specific mild irritation, or a warm or cold feeling. The existence of pain usually indicates corneal involvement or other tissue pathology (e.g. uveitis or scleritis).

The conjunctiva contains a rich plexus of arterioles, which comprise of a thick layer of smooth muscle that is richly enervated with sympathetic nerve fibres. The smooth muscle, as well as being under central autonomic control, can be influenced by numerous local changes. Vasodilation refers to enlargement in the circumference of a vessel due to relaxation of its smooth muscle layer, which leads to decreased resistance and increased blood flow through the vessel (active hyperaemia). Since blood vessels can be observed directly through the transparent conjunctiva; this leads to an appearance of increased redness (less white sclera is visible).

A contact lens can have a local mechanical effect on the conjunctiva, resulting in increased redness. A contact lens is a device that a) can interfere with normal metabolic processes of the cornea and conjunctiva, and b) is used in association with various solutions, and can therefore affect the level of conjunctival redness via a local chemical or toxic effect. Local infection and inflammation can cause eye redness. Accordingly, treatment options fall into four broad categories:

1. Alterations to the type, design and modality of lens wear
2. Alterations to care systems
3. Improving ocular hygiene
4. Prescription of pharmaceutical agents.

In general, removal of any noxious stimulus (including a contact lens) will lead to a very rapid recovery of eye redness to normal levels. Recovery from chronic contact lens-induced redness after removal of lenses and cessation of wear takes about 2 days. Syn. conjunctival hyperaemia, conjunctival injection.

Conjunctival staining, contact lens induced

This manifests as areas or spots of increased fluorescence observed following the instillation of fluorescein into the eye and observation using cobalt blue light. About 60% of contact lens wearers exhibit conjunctival staining greater than Grade 1, versus about 10% of non-lens wearers. Small streaks of linear staining parallel to the limbus are a normal finding; this is due to pooling of fluorescein in natural conjunctival folds. The symptom of dryness is associated with increased conjunctival staining.

An imprint can be created on the conjunctiva as a result of chafing or physical compression by the edge of a soft lens. Chafing may be due to a lens edge design that causes the edge to 'dig in' to the conjunctiva. Defects in the lens edge can cause increased conjunctival staining (Figure C.15). Fitting a lens with a different edge design and a 'defect-free' edge will alleviate this problem.

Compression staining will usually be accompanied by a tight fitting and/or a decentred lens, and manifests as a broad ring of heavy conjunctival staining corresponding to the lens edge, which is clearly evident following lens removal. Conjunctival vessels distal to the lens edge may be engorged. The patient is usually asymptomatic. This condition can be solved by refitting the patient with a lens of greater back optic zone radius.

Instillation of fluorescein in a dry-eye patient may reveal the presence of desiccation staining on the conjunctiva, which manifests as a series of diffuse punctate lesions within the interpalpebral zone. The condition will return to normal soon after removing the lens, but long-term resolution may require a combination of treating the underlying cause of the dry eye and refitting the patient with lenses that will facilitate complete conjunctival wetting.

Compromise to the conjunctiva as revealed by fluorescein staining is of concern because of recent demonstrations of morphologic changes to the conjunctival epithelium associated with lens wear. These changes include alterations to conjunctival cell shape, nuclear morphology and chromatin condensation, and are reported to be more prevalent in symptomatic lens wearers. Soft lens wear is also associated with a reduction in goblet cell density; this could lead to a reduction in mucus production, which in turn could explain and perhaps further exacerbate pre-existing symptoms of dryness.

Conjunctival stroma

The conjunctival stroma (substantia propria) lies beneath the conjunctival epithelium, and is variable in thickness. It can be resolved into two distinct layers; a superficial adenoid layer and a deeper fibrous layer. The adenoid layer contains numerous lymphocytes with local accumulations in the form of lymphoid follicles. Follicles represent aggregates of predominantly B-cells, which form part of the so-called 'conjunctiva-associated lymphoid tissue' (CALT). The adenoid layer also contains a large number of mast cells, which play a major role in ocular allergy. The deep fibrous layer is generally thicker than the adenoid layer, and contains the majority of conjunctival blood vessels and nerves.

Conjunctivitis

Conjunctivitis is a non-specific term signifying inflammation of the conjunctiva, with dilation of the conjunctival blood vessels giving the characteristic red eye appearance. There are many different forms of conjunctivitis, the most common being simple bacterial conjunctivitis. One of the main distinguishing features between acute bacterial infections and other causes is its chronicity, because a chronic conjunctivitis (greater than 2 weeks) is uncommon with bacterial and simple viral infections.

Simple bacterial conjunctivitis is a common, usually self-limiting condition, usually occurring in childhood. There is a wide range of causative organisms, both Gram positive and Gram negative. The most common are Staphylococcus aureus, Staph. Epidermidis, Streptococcus pneumoniae, and Hemophilus influenzae.

Conjunctivitis occurs in a number of pathological conditions:

Infective:
- Bacterial: acute, hyperacute and chronic (Figure C.16)
- Viral: including adenovirus, herpes simplex, molluscum

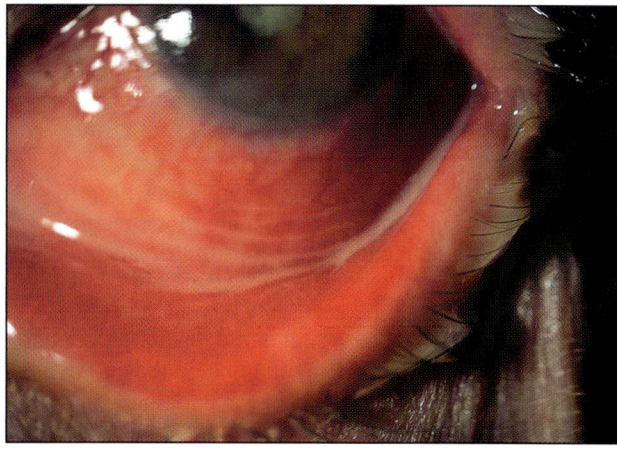

Figure C.16 • Conjunctival injection, papillary conjunctivitis and mucopurulent discharge in bacterial conjunctivitis.

- Chlamydial: ophthalmia neonatorum, trachoma, adult inclusion conjunctivitis
- Lice: phthiriasis palpebrarum.

Allergic:
- Seasonal conjunctivitis, giant papillary, vernal and atopic.

Ocular surface disease:
- Blepharitis
- Keratoconjunctivitis sicca, Sjogren's syndrome, lacrimal and lipid layer anomalies (dry eye).

Immune:
- Ocular cicatricial pemphigoid, Stevens-Johnson syndrome.

Toxic:
- drop sensitivity, chemical injury, photokeratopathy.

Mechanical:
- from eye rubbing, mucous fishing syndrome, artifactual conjunctivitis or contact lens usage.

Nasolacrimal duct obstruction:
- chronic dacryocystitis.

Neoplastic:
- some invasive ocular surface neoplasias such as conjunctival intraepithelial neoplasia can mimic conjunctivitis.

The patient presents with red eyes and may also notice a purulent or watery discharge. A watery discharge is associated with a viral conjunctivitis while a purulent discharge is associated with a bacterial infection. Chlamydial conjunctivitis can have a mixed presentation that may suggest a bacterial or viral aetiology. Both of these conditions tend to be unilateral initially, then bilateral, although herpes simplex disease tends to stay unilateral. A foreign body sensation is common with most causes of conjunctivitis although itch will tend to suggest an allergic aetiology. The discharge in bacterial conjunctivitis increases over 1–2 days and often becomes a significant problem. Patients often report matting of lashes or of their eyes being stuck together on waking.

Conjunctivitis can be associated with numerous signs, such as the following:

- Follicles consist of lymphoid hyperplasia within the palpebral conjunctival stroma, more pronounced inferiorly. Clinically they appear as multiple small 'grains of rice' embedded in the tarsal conjunctiva. There are surrounding accessory blood vessels. Possible causes include viral or chlamydial infections, as well as a hypersensitivity to topical medication.
- Papillae are focal elevations of the conjunctiva, particularly on the superior palpebra and are best highlighted on lid eversion by using fluorescein. Papillae consist of a central blood vessel, with conjunctival epithelial hyperplasia and stromal oedema. There may also be a diffuse white infiltrate of chronic inflammatory cells. Giant papillae are greater than 1mm diameter; conversely normal papillae can occur on the superior edge of the tarsal plate (inferior edge when everted). Papillae can occur in bacterial conjunctivitis, blepharitis, atopic conjunctivitis, giant papillary conjunctivitis and vernal conjunctivitis.
- Membranes/pseudomembranes consist of coagulated exudate firmly or loosely adherent to the conjunctiva. Consider acute bacterial conjunctivitis, including gonococcal, and severe adenoviral conjunctivitis among others.
- Discharge and hyperaemia.
- Chemosis is the term given to sub-conjunctival oedema and is seen especially with acute allergic conjunctivitis.
- Sub-conjunctival haemorrhages. Multiple small haemorrhages can occur in viral and bacterial conjunctivitis.
- Scarring. An uncommon sign in developed countries, and requires differential diagnosis from trachoma, ocular cicatricial pemphigoid and atopy.
- Lymphadenopathy. Enlarged lymph nodes in the pre-auricular and sub-mandibular regions are often seen with viral or chlamydial infections.
- Keratopathy. Associated corneal infiltrates may be seen with some infective forms of conjunctivitis such as chlamydial and adenovirus.

In bacterial conjunctivitis, the conjunctiva shows chemosis, with velvety oedematous papillary changes on the superior and inferior tarsi. The mucopurulent discharge leads to crusting along the lids and matting together of the lashes. The cornea frequently has features of a toxic epitheliopathy with scattered punctate erosions on fluorescein staining.

Conjunctivitis tends be associated with mild to moderate cosmetic concern and discomfort, although some of the less common causes such as ocular cicatricial pemphigoid can be sight threatening. Bacterial conjunctivitis is usually not sight threatening unless complicated with bacterial keratitis or unusually membranous conjunctivitis with symblepharon formation.

Treatment ranges from advice for simple viral conjunctivitis through to biopsy and treatment with systemic immunosuppressive agents for ocular cicatricial pemphigoid. Simple bacterial conjunctivitis is usually a self-limiting disease resolving in 10 to 14 days, but it is usually treated with topical antibiotics to shorten the course of the disease.

Active cleaning of the lids, lashes and eye to remove the discharge is important to decrease symptoms, improve penetration of topical drugs and decrease infectivity. It also helps to protect the ocular surface by removing toxic lytic enzymes present within the discharge. Although not as highly contagious as adenoviral conjunctivitis, care should still be taken not to spread the disease. This usually occurs by direct contact with infected mucous and can be avoided by strict personal hygiene.

Antibiotics with a broad spectrum of activity against known Gram positive and Gram negative pathogens can be used 4 times a day for 1 week. Commonly used antibiotics include chloramphenicol, gentamicin, tobramycin, framycetin and ciprofloxacin.

Constringence

The constringence value (V) is sometimes known as the 'Abbe number' and relates the refractive index of the material in the yellow green region of the visible spectrum to the values at the blue and red ends. An ideal material would have a constant refractive index right across the visible spectrum. Unfortunately, all practical materials have a refractive index which varies with the wavelength.

In BS EN ISO 7944:1998, constringence is determined by measuring the values shown in Table C.13:

The constringence value (V_d) is then defined as:

$$V_d = n_d - 1 / n_f - n_c$$

Table C.13 • Values used to determine constringence.

Source	Line	Symbol	Wavelength (nm)
hydrogen (red)	C	n_C	656.27
helium	d	n_d	587.56
hydrogen (blue)	F	n_F	486.13

In technical optics, it is more common to use the term 'dispersive power', which is the reciprocal of constringence.

The constringence of a material tends to decrease as the refractive index increases. The practical significance of a low constringence is that it indicates a wide range of values for refractive index across the visible spectrum, giving rise to chromatic dispersion in a prism. In a lens, there are two types of recognized chromatic aberration: axial and transverse, depending on whether the incident light is parallel to the optical axis or oblique.

To a first approximation, axial chromatic aberration (ACA) can be expressed (in dioptres) as:

$$ACA = F/V$$

Thus, for a +10.00DS lens with a V of 60, the ACA would 1/6D, and for a V of 30, 1/3D. It might be asked how accurate this approximation is. Consider a lens made of ophthalmic crown glass having a value of n_d as 1.523, and a BVP of +10.00DS as above; an accurate ray trace yields typical values for the blue and red refractive indices of $n_F = 1.5256$ and $n_C = 1.5169$. These values give a lens power of +10.054D for blue light and +9.886D for red, an overall axial chromatic aberration of 0.177D. The approximate formula gives a value of 0.167D.

Axial chromatic aberration does not constitute much of a problem in spectacle lenses because it is generally masked by considerable ACA exhibited by the human eye, which is of the order of 0.75D.

In a similar fashion, transverse chromatic aberration can be calculated from the expression:

$ACA = Fy/V$

where 'y' is the distance from the optical centre in centimetres. The value calculated is in prism dioptres, and the expression is analogous to Prentice's rule for finding the prismatic effect of decentration. Thus in the case of a +5.00DS lens, $V = 60$, at point 20mm from the optical centre (OC), the TCA would be 0.167^Δ, and at 30mm from the optical centre 0.25^Δ. Again, if the value of V was halved to 30, then the resulting TCA would be doubled.

To give an idea of the accuracy of this approximation, an accurate ray trace can be carried out again. CR39 plastics material has a V of 59.3, thus at 20mm from the OC, the TCA for a +5.00DS lens by the expression given above would be 0.167^Δ. Taking a +5.00DS lens of 5.0mm thickness, and rotating an eye 35° at 27mm behind the rear surface, this would give an intersection distance with the front surface of 19.94mm. The difference in deviation for the blue and red indices of 1.5040 and 1.4956 respectively gives a deviation of 0.181^Δ.

Clinically, the effects of TCA are to increase the blurring of images viewed through the periphery of a lens, and in severe cases to cause coloured fringing at high contrast boundaries in the visual field – window frames being a typical example. It is very difficult to predict the subjective acceptability of materials showing high dispersion. Many wearers accept the chromatic effects as a trade off in having a thinner lens in a higher refractive index material. BS 3062:1985 sets tolerances on constringence of ±0.5 for values up to 45, and ±1.0 for values over 45.

Consumer Protection Act 1987 (UK)

The Consumer Protection Act introduced the right to anyone injured by a defective product to sue a supplier without proof of negligence whether or not the product was sold to them. Action may be taken against the manufacturer of the product, the importer into the European union, or in the case of branding, the supplier who puts their name to the product. Wholesalers or retailers are not liable unless they are unable to identify the producer, importer or own brander. It is not possible to exclude liability by means of any contractual arrangement.

A defective product in relation to this Act is defined as a product where the safety is not such as persons generally are entitled to expect. Within this a product will not be considered as defective solely because of its poor quality or because a safer version becomes available. For a case to be proven it must be shown that such a defect in the product was responsible for any damage suffered.

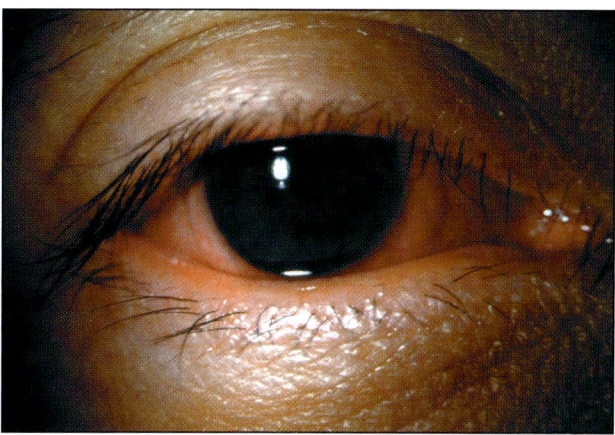

Figure C.17 • Contact lens acute red eye (CLARE) with the causative bound soft lens still in place.

Contact aesthesiometry

- See *Cochet-Bonnet aesthesiometer*.

Contact lens

A transparent optical device with dioptric power that is applied directly to the surface of the eye for the purpose of correcting defects of vision.

Contact lens hygienist

- See *Patient education*.

Contact lens induced acute red eye (CLARE)

Previously referred to as 'acute red eye reaction' and 'tight lens syndrome', CLARE is an acute complication of extended soft lens wear. In its mild form the patient notices problems upon waking naturally; when severe the patient may be awakened by the symptoms, which include ocular pain, tearing and photophobia. The patient then quickly discovers that he or she has a red eye (Figure C.17). Clinical signs include conjunctival and limbal hyperaemia, and small corneal infiltrates near the limbus.

The lens may display little or no movement upon initial examination of a patient suffering from CLARE, and debris can sometimes be seen trapped beneath the lens. Corneal epithelial staining may be detected following lens removal. Other transient clinical signs include anterior chamber flare, endothelial bedewing and guttata, low-grade corneal neovascularization, foci of swollen epithelium, and small non-staining areas on the corneal surface (dry spots). About 10% of cases of CLARE are bilateral, and the mean time to the first occurrence of CLARE after being fitted with extended wear soft lenses is about 10 months.

Contact lens peripheral ulcer (CLPU)

This condition, which is typically seen in soft lens extended-wear patients, is characterized by the presence of one or two small, round, full-thickness epithelial

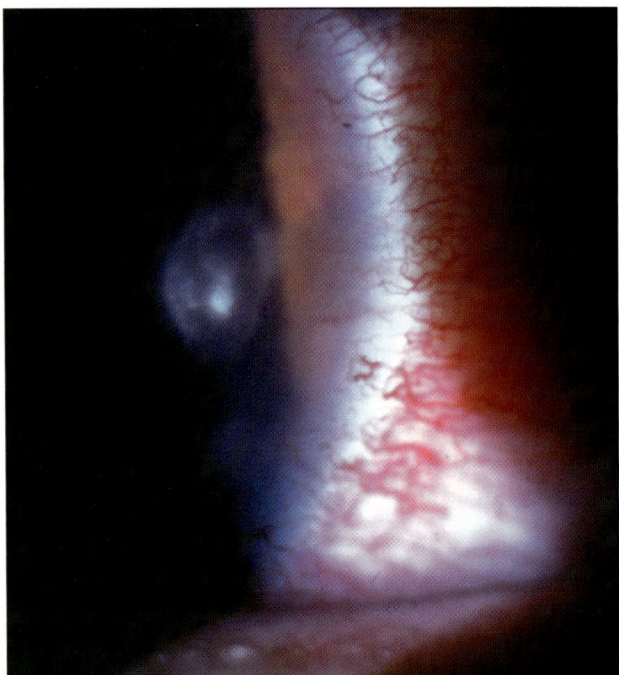

Figure C.18 • Contact lens peripheral ulcer.

lesions (without raised edges) in the peripheral or paracentral cornea (Figure C.18). There is an absence of severe ocular pain, mucopurulent discharge or anterior chamber reaction. However, the patient may experience mild to moderate ocular discomfort or foreign body sensation, mild photophobia and increased tearing. Associated signs may include conjunctival and limbal hyperaemia, and infiltrates beneath or surrounding the epithelial lesion. This condition is typically uniocular, and the mean time to the first occurrence of CLPU after being fitted with extended-wear soft lenses is 26±22 months. If a culture from a scraping of the ulcer fails to reveal the presence of micro-organisms, the condition may be termed a culture-negative peripheral ulcer (CNPU).

The clinical notion that infiltrative events of low clinical severity are more likely to be observed in the corneal periphery has a sound physiological basis. However, anecdotal observations purporting to support this hypothesis have been confounded by the fact that there is much more 'peripheral cornea' than 'central cornea' by way of area. For example, assuming a mean human corneal diameter of 12mm and taking a large zone of 6mm diameter as representing the central region of the cornea, the peripheral corneal represents 75% of the total area of the cornea (treating the cornea as a flat surface viewed from the front). Thus, if infiltrative events were to occur at random locations across the cornea, 75% of such events would be characterized as occurring in the peripheral cornea. It is for reasons such as this that the concept of CLPU is rapidly losing favour in the literature, and being replaced by a model that considers all contact lens associated corneal infiltrative events as being part of a continuum of disease severity.

Contact lens supply routes

The issue of non-optical-practice supply now affects virtually all contact lens types, although disposable lenses are particularly susceptible to third party distribution, given the brand awareness that many of these products have with the public. The critical issue here is that it is in the public interest to have a system of lens supply that guarantees the ongoing preservation of the ocular health of lens wearers. A system that provides no disincentives to patients continuing to purchase lenses for many years without having their eyes examined poses a significant public health risk.

Notwithstanding the role of regulatory authorities in discharging their responsibilities of public health and safety, there are strategies that practitioners can employ to retain control of lens supply and to link this to patient care. Fee splitting – where materials are charged at relatively low mark-ups on cost, and these charges are separated from professional fees – helps demonstrate to patients that most of the cost involved in wearing contact lenses is attributed to the professional time involved. Home delivery plans, perhaps operated on behalf of the practice by a supplier, enable practitioners to match the perceived convenience of mail order and Internet supply companies. Many large practices or group practices are able to come to an arrangement with manufacturers so that lenses and solutions supplied by that manufacturer are 're-branded' prior to delivery. The re-branding (or so-called 'own-labelling' or 'private labelling') facilitates an association of the products with the practice, and thereby serves to enhance patient loyalty. See *Delivery systems, contact lens*.

Contact lens thickness

The thickness of a contact lens can be specified as the thickness at the geometric centre or edge of the lens. The average thickness over a specified diameter (typically that of the central optical zone) can also be specified. Soft lens centre thickness is relevant to ease of lens handling and susceptibility to dehydration. Mid-water lenses (50–59%) are generally manufactured with centre thickness in the range 0.06–0.10mm, while high water content lenses (>60%) generally have centre thickness in the range 0.10–0.18mm. Determination of the average thickness of a soft lens can be useful when considering the physiological impact of a lens on the eye, because the ability of oxygen to permeate through a lens to the eye is inversely related to thickness.

Due to poor measurement repeatability, soft lens peripheral thickness is not the subject of an international standard, and is not always routinely verified during lens manufacture. Nevertheless, variations in peripheral thickness can have a significant effect on lens fit and comfort. Contrary to expectations, lenses with a thicker edge often show a looser fit and are less comfortable than lenses of similar basic design with a thinner lens edge.

If rigid lenses are made too thin not only is there greater risk of breakage but the lenses also tend to flex on astigmatic corneas, leaving residual astigmatism. Flexure is a function of lens thickness and is therefore more problematic with low minus powered lenses. Fluoro-silicone acrylate polymers tend to show more flexure than silicone acrylate materials of similar oxygen permeability (Dk). Also, for a given material type, flexure tends to increase with increasing Dk. It is therefore necessary to increase lens centre thickness with higher Dk materials.

Contact shell

A transparent optical device without dioptric power that is applied directly to the surface of the eye for the purpose of correcting defects of vision by neutralizing an abnormal corneal shape (e.g. as in keratoconus).

Continuous contact lens wear

- See *Extended contact lens wear.*

Contrast enhancement for low vision patients

Many low vision patients have very poor sensitivity to low contrast targets, and object visibility can be improved by increasing the contrast of the object in the environment, and hence of the retinal image. In addition to making an object easier to see, it is often possible to add a tactile back-up to give extra help in recognition – for example, 'Bump-ons' are self-adhesive plastic dots which are clearly visible and easily-felt when used as markers, and there are many other 'home-made' examples.

High illumination is necessary to optimize the available contrast, but care must be taken to avoid glare: for those patients with media opacities, contrast sensitivity is often particularly impaired in the presence of a glare source which leads to scattering of light within the eye and a consequent reduction in retinal image contrast (see *Glare*). The theoretical limit of contrast is 100%, and the highest quality ink print is approximately 90%, with newsprint only reaching 70%. For patients with very poor contrast sensitivity it may be impossible to achieve sufficient contrast reserve (see *Reading requirements, low vision*) unless electronic magnifying systems are used. Contrast approaches 100% and electronically manipulating the text to create white-on-black images reduces the overall luminance of the object and can reduce scattering of light within the eye. See *Typoscope*. Additional electronic edge enhancement of images can also be performed to improve visibility. This appears to be beneficial for tasks such as face recognition, but the results for reading are equivocal.

It is possible to have chromatic contrast within an image in addition to, or instead of, luminance contrast, and this can easily be manipulated electronically using electronic vision enhancement systems. Although some patients express strong subjective preferences, it appears that maximizing luminance contrast as well is the only way to optimize performance.

Optimizing both luminance and colour contrast would appear to offer the best practical approach in the built environment. Consider that in the normal visual system the peak of photopic sensitivity is at 555nm, with less sensitivity to the spectral extremes. Even if there is no specific colour vision defect associated with the visual impairment, one would expect the patient to lose the ability to detect the red and blue wavelengths as sensitivity overall diminished. It is also likely that the ability to discriminate between similar hues of equal luminance will become impaired: patients often report a difficulty in distinguishing between black and blue, or between white and yellow. To maximize luminance contrast needs a bright object and a dark background, or vice versa, and chromatic contrast requires selection of colours widely separated in the spectrum. If choosing a colour from mid-spectrum and one from a spectral extreme, it makes sense to have that from the extreme at low luminance (so if sensitivity is lost it appears even darker), with the brighter one chosen from mid spectrum. Thus, a 'good' combination would be bright yellow and dark blue, but bright red and dark green is a poor choice. Other poor choices would be those hues close together in the spectrum (such as green and turquoise) or pastel shades where hue is indistinct (such as yellow and grey). In these cases, detection would be especially difficult if the two colours were of equal brightness.

Strategies for enhancing contrast in everyday tasks include:

Luminance contrast

- Writing with a fine felt-tip or fibre-tip pen produces higher-contrast letters, which are more visible than those written with a ball-point pen, even though the two are the same size.
- Using lined paper with lines which are thicker and darker than 'normal'. Various writing frames can also be used which provide the patient with a dark elastic marker along which to write, thus keeping the words in straight lines.
- Dark contrasting door knobs will be more easily seen on a light surface, and may stop the patient bumping into the door.
- Vegetables should be peeled or chopped against a light work surface, whereas pastry should be rolled out on a dark board.
- Pale crockery will be seen best against a dark tablecloth or, if using a white tablecloth, crockery with a dark edge band should be used.

Colour contrast

- Food should be arranged on a plate of contrasting colour, such as carrots on a white plate, or fish on a blue plate. Green vegetables placed between fish and mashed potatoes on the plate will aid in the location of each.
- The handles of garden tools could be painted bright yellow to make them easy to locate.
- Coloured electrical sockets and/or plugs can be used. The colour contrast makes each easier to see, and can be used for identification (red for kettle, blue for microwave, for example).
- Toothpaste and shaving cream should be bought in different coloured tubes, and dangerous substances like bleach or white spirit in a distinctively coloured bottle so that these are not mistaken.
- Crockery could be selected from non-matching sets: the shape of cups, milk jugs and sugar bowls is often similar, so choosing such items from crockery sets of different bright colours, preferably with a different shape, will make them easier to see.

Contrast sensitivity testing

The ability to resolve a target varies significantly with the contrast of the target. The visual world a patient inhabits is one of varying target size and contrast and, furthermore, diseases affecting vision may affect the ability to resolve these targets in a selective manner. Therefore, the

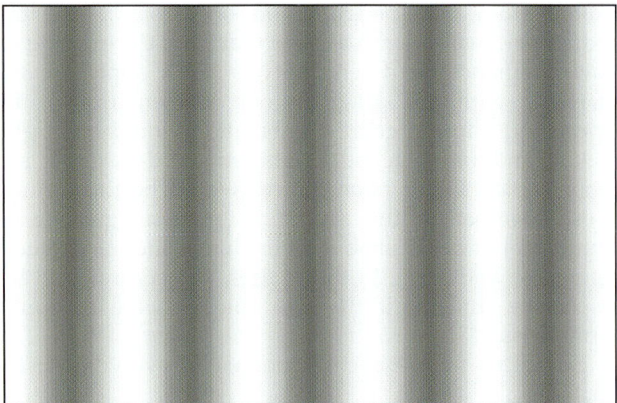

Figure C.19 • A sine-wave grating.

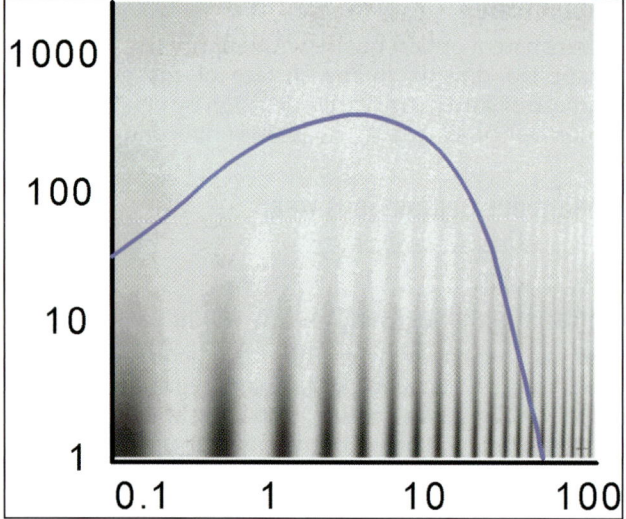

Figure C.20 • Contrast sensitivity function.

use of high contrast targets for acuity testing has been criticized as non-representative of the visual world and less than sensitive at reflecting visual reduction due to disease. If a patient is shown a sine-wave grating of a constant spatial frequency, as shown in Figure C.19, their ability to resolve the grating reduces as the contrast is reduced until a point is reached when it can no longer be resolved. This point, the contrast threshold (the reciprocal of which is called the contrast sensitivity), is different for different spatial frequencies and the plot of the threshold values against spatial frequency is described as the contrast sensitivity function (CSF) as shown in Figure C.20.

Snellen visual acuity relates to the resolution of a high contrast target of maximum spatial frequency and is therefore represented as the cut-off point on the horizontal axis on this curve. This is sensitive to conditions affecting mainly high spatial frequencies, such as refractive error, but less sensitive if lower spatial frequencies are affected, as with cataract, corneal disturbance and contact lens wear.

Increasingly, clinicians are using targets of different contrast to assess the influence upon acuity. LogMAR charts are available in different contrasts, so facilitating the ability of patients to resolve increasing spatial frequencies at a given contrast value. Computerized visual acuity charts, such as the City2000 shown in Figure C.21, allow any contrast value to be preset.

Other charts, such as the Pelli-Robson, incorporate letters of constant size (approximating to one cycle per degree if viewed at 1m) and gradually reducing contrast. In theory, varying the working distance would allow the whole contrast sensitivity function to be assessed with a Pelli-Robson chart, but in practice this is rarely needed as high and low contrast acuity scores combined with contrast sensitivity at 1m with a Pelli-Robson is usually sufficient to suggest any visual compromise. The relationship between the charts and the CSF is shown in Figure C.22.

Contusion injuries

Contusion injuries may result from a variety of causes, including flying blunt objects (for example a squash ball), falling objects, explosions or compressed air accidents, fluid under pressure escaping from burst pipes and water jets from fire hoses, or air bag inflation as a result of a car accident.

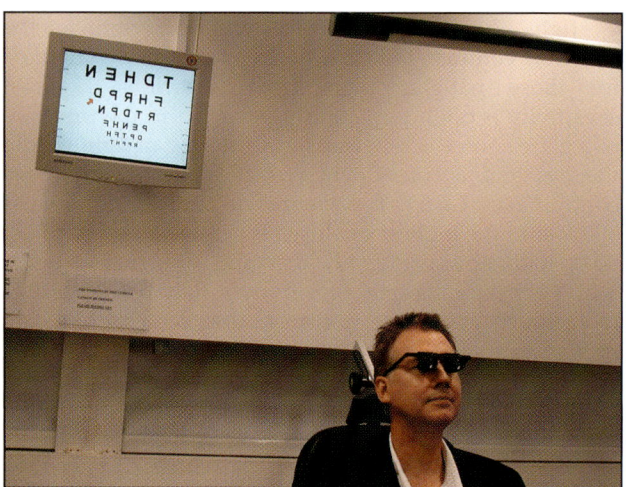

Figure C.21 • The City2000 computerized visual acuity chart.

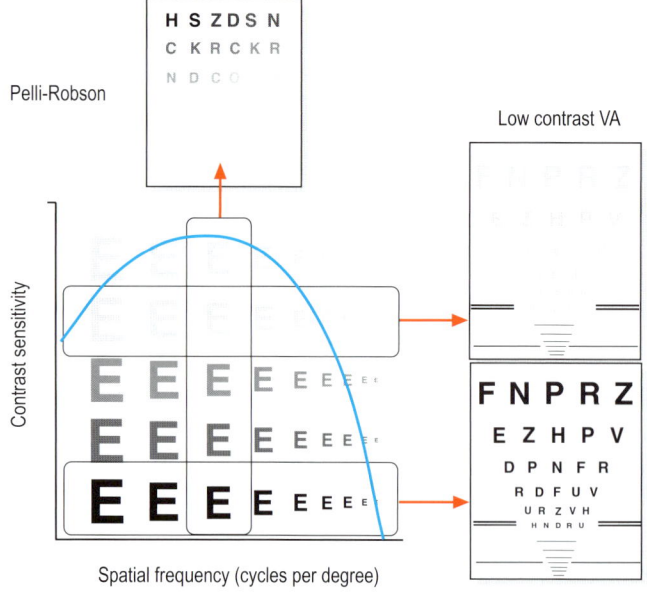

Figure C.22 • Relating high- and low-contrast visual acuity and Peli-Robson contrast sensitivity to the contrast sensitivity function.

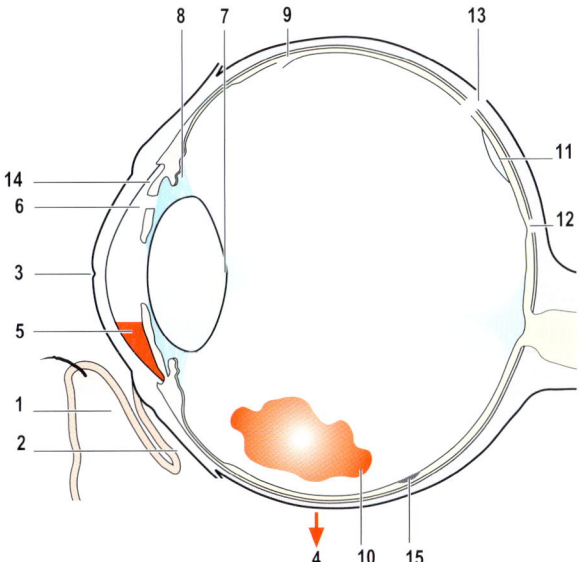

Figure C.23 • Composite diagram of the possible ocular effects of a contusion injury: 1 = black eye; 2 = subconjunctival haemorrhage; 3 = corneal abrasion; 4 = blow-out fracture; 5 = hyphaema; 6 = iridodialysis; 7 = cataract; 8 = lens subluxation due to torn zonules; 9 = retinal tear/detachment; 10 = vitreous haemorrhage; 11 = commotio retinae; 12 = chorodial rupture; 13 = scleral rupture; 14 = angle recession; 15 = retinal haemorrhage (modified from Coakes and Holmes Sellors, 1985, and courtesy of Butterworth-Heinemann, Oxford).

The resultant ocular damage is due to a pressure wave traversing the fluid content of the eye. As the fluid is incompressible the blow will act as an explosive force in all directions from the centre outwards, resulting in the ocular contents being flung against their outer coat. The globe expands around the equator to take up a vertically oval shape. Any part of the eye may be affected as shown in Figure C.23.

Damage to the lids and orbit may result in a black eye, ptosis or an orbital floor fracture. Fractures of the floor of the orbit may occur after a heavy blow and are known as blow-out fractures. The blow increases the intraorbital pressure, which causes the very thin bone of the maxilla to collapse into the maxillary sinus and the orbital contents then prolapse into the antrum. Elevation of the eye will be defective because the tissues surrounding the inferior rectus and inferior oblique muscle become trapped in the fracture. Double vision will also be present in one or more directions of gaze. The herniation of the orbital contents results in a sinking or recession of the eye within the orbit (endophthalmos) with a narrowing of the palpebral fissure. There will also be loss of feeling on the same side of the face due to damage of the infraorbital nerve. Anterior segment damage may result in corneal abrasions, subconjunctival haemorrhages, hyphaema and associated damage to the ciliary body, iris, or lens.

Hyphaema is due to the rupture of a vessel in the iris or ciliary body. The chamber is generally only partially filled and the blood settles inferiorly. It will usually be reabsorbed without any serious consequences. However, in some cases, the anterior chamber may completely fill with blood (total hyphaema). If the blood is not reabsorbed after a few days, its colour changes from red to purple to black. This occurs due to a lack of oxygen from the aqueous and is sometimes referred to as an 'eight ball' hyphaema. This is a serious condition, as the intra-ocular pressure is generally elevated, resulting in secondary glaucoma and possible blood staining of the cornea. Re-bleeding may also occur, resulting in secondary glaucoma, blood staining of the cornea, and permanent loss of vision.

Damage to the iris may result in dilation or constriction of the pupil, this is known as traumatic mydriasis or traumatic miosis, respectively. Depending on the severity of the blow, the paralysis may be temporary, last only a few days, or be permanent. Ruptures may occur to the sphincter pupillae, leaving a permanently irregular, semi-dilated pupil, which will not react to light or accommodation. The iris can be torn from its insertion to the ciliary body; this is known as iridodialysis. It is a permanent condition, usually accompanied by hyphaema, and results in a distortion of the pupil. Both conditions will cause symptoms of glare, especially in the case of iridodialysis where a second pupil has formed that will also result in monocular diplopia.

Traumatic angle recession of the anterior chamber can lead to the development of unilateral glaucoma months or years later. It occurs when the ciliary body has been torn from the sclera. The site of the recession can be predicted from the presence of traumatic mydriasis. The affected area of the pupil is atonic – neither fully dilating nor constricting, and corresponds to the position of the angle recession

The zonular fibres that attach the crystalline lens to the ciliary body can be torn in a contusion injury. As a result, the lens may have become totally dislocated from its attachment, or partially dislocated (subluxated). The dislocated lens may fall either posteriorly into the vitreous, where low grade ophthalmitis may occur, or enter the anterior chamber, causing corneal endothelial damage. There will be a marked hyperopic shift in the refraction and a tremulous iris (iridodonesis) may be seen due to the loss of support by the lens. A subluxated lens produces a prismatic effect upon vision, with the upward displacement of objects. This may cause symptoms such as diplopia, nausea, and vomiting.

Various types of lens changes can be listed as follows:

- a circle of iris pigment, known as the Vossius ring may be seen on the lens after impaction of the iris, usually occurring in the young
- sub-epithelial disseminated opacities; these are small, discrete punctate or flake-like opacities, located beneath the anterior epithelium which may be transient, disappearing within a few days or weeks, or permanent
- traumatic rosette-shaped cataract, occurring anteriorly or posteriorly; the onset may be delayed
- diffuse cataract, which is rare and is usually associated with a tear of the lens capsule
- zonular cataract, which is also rare and consists of a series of concentric, thin sheets of opacities surrounded by clear lens

Damage to the posterior segment may initially be obscured from direct view by a hyphaema. The damage that may occur to the retina includes:

- retinal oedema and atrophy, macular cysts and holes
- retinal haemorrhages
- tears of the choroid and retina
- retinal detachment.

Conventional contact lenses
- See *Non-planned contact lens replacement*.

Convergence

Convergence is mainly a reflex activity but can be initiated voluntarily. Reflex convergence is controlled by the occipital cortex and is considered to have four components:

- Tonic convergence – the convergence brought about by the tonus in the extraocular muscles in an individual who is awake. With age, there is a decrease in tonus and therefore a tendency towards divergence.
- Proximal convergence – the convergence induced by an awareness of the nearness of the object. It is innate and independent of accommodation.
- Accommodative-convergence – the convergence elicited on accommodation. Most convergence is accommodative-convergence and the relationship between the amount of accommodative-convergence produced per dioptre of accommodation is expressed by the AC/A ratio.
- Fusional convergence – the convergence that makes the final adjustment to gain binocular single vision. The stimulus for fusional convergence is disparate retinal images and the response may be positive (convergence) or negative (divergence). Any inelasticity of fusional convergence will give rise to a heterotropia. Fortunately, fusional convergence is the component of convergence that is the easiest to train.

Voluntary convergence is the ability to converge without a near stimulus and is controlled by the frontal oculomotor area of the cortex. Voluntary convergence is always accompanied by pupillary constriction and is probably dependent on accommodation. Reflex convergence and voluntary convergence use a common final pathway resulting in the co-contraction of the medial recti. In the main, reflex convergence is used, but if fusional convergence is reduced for any reason, voluntary convergence can be used to prevent further decompensation.

Optometrists are concerned with the aspects of convergence that are measurable and, preferably, treatable. These are normally the near point of convergence and the amplitude of convergent fusion. The near point of convergence is normally 6 to 8cm; if over 10cm, it is considered to be low, that is, insufficient. A typical method of measurement is:

- Use a RAF rule, ask patient to look at the dot in the middle of the line and advance it until one eye loses fixation – the objective measurement of convergence.
- The subjective measurement of the near point of convergence will be given by one of two responses at the break point:

- The line appears double – the eye that turns out is the non-dominant eye.
- The line is seen to jump towards one side indicating suppression at the break point; the line will appear to jump towards the side of the suppressing eye.

The measurement is normally repeated three times to detect fatigue, which is often indicative of poor convergent fusion.

Fusional convergence is measured in prism dioptres. See *Fusional range/reserves*. This measurement of convergent fusion is also called 'the amplitude of positive fusional reserves'. A typical method of measurement is:

- Use either a prism bar or a rotary prism: ask the patient to look at an accommodative target while increasing prism base-out in front of the eye with the better acuity.

The significant measurements are:

- Blur point. The measurement when accommodation can no longer keep the image clear. The convergent blur-point norm is 17^Δ base out (BO) at near and 9^ΔBO at distance.
- Break point. The measurement when one eye loses fixation. The non-dominant eye will diverge and diplopia will be present if there is no suppression at the break point. The normal convergent fusion range is 30^Δ to 40^ΔBO at near and 14^Δ to 16^ΔBO at distance.
- Recovery point. The measurement when fusion is recovered when the prism base-out is reduced. This measurement should be as least as large as the blur point.

Blur and break points tend to reflect the quantity of fusion, whereas the recovery point indicates the quality of fusion, i.e. the ease of change of fusional demands (the facility), and the ability to maintain fusion (the stamina).

Convergence demand with contact lenses

Contact lenses move with the eyes, and hence convergence demands when viewing near objects are identical to those applying in the uncorrected state. In contrast, myopes with a negative spectacle correction for distance observe near objects through base-in prisms, since they are no longer looking through the optical centres of their lenses. The base-in prismatic effects reduce the convergence requirement, as compared to the naked eye or contact lens situation. Spectacle-corrected hypermetropes, however, experience a base-out effect at near, which increases the convergence demand. Allowing for a typical interpupillary distance of 65mm and the centre of rotation of each eye being about 12mm behind the cornea, application of Prentice's rule shows that, for an object distance of 33cm, the convergence demand for each eye is reduced by about ($0.25\times$ lens power) prism dioptres for a negative spectacle correction and similarly increased for a positive correction. In most cases, then, the change in convergence demand is small as compared with the fusion reserves. Since both accommodation and convergence demands are higher for myopes with contact lenses, and lower for hypermetropes, the accommodation-convergence links are minimally disturbed.

Convergence insufficiency

This is the most common convergence anomaly. Convergence insufficiency is the inability to converge to a normal distance from the nose. Insufficient fusional convergence is an inability to make a convergent movement to attain and to maintain fusion. Therefore convergence insufficiency is almost always accompanied by insufficient fusional convergence. If convergence is treated without attention to fusional convergence, the benefit is likely to be only temporary.

Convergence insufficiency is both treatable and, usually, curable. The patient normally attends with symptoms to discover that the treatment is not the prescription of spectacles (or a change of spectacles), but orthoptic exercises. A course of exercises provides total relief of symptoms, not just for the short-term but probably permanently.

The aetiology of convergence insufficiency may be primary, secondary or consecutive.

Primary – This is not associated with any obvious heterophoria, but often occurs or becomes symptomatic following a change of visual demands at near. It occurs mainly in teenagers or college students or in older people following a change of occupation to one with higher near demands. The symptoms are aggravated by poor health, anxiety or lack of sleep.

Secondary – Convergence insufficiency may be secondary to:

- Intermittent exophoria/tropia of divergence-excess type (divergence greater at distance); true or pseudo
- Exophoria/tropia of convergence weakness type (divergence greater at near) with/without a low AC/A ratio
- Vertical muscle defect
- Disuse of the accommodative-convergence mechanism, for example in:
    i) Uncorrected high myopia
    ii) High hypermetropia
    iii) Newly corrected presbyopia causing a reduced need for accommodative-convergence
    iv) Antimetropia or significant anisometropia
    v) Reduced accommodative facility (i.e. ability to change accommodative demand)
    vi) Accommodative insufficiency
- Poor general health (also associated with loss of accommodation)
- Paresis, such as loss or diminution of contraction of the medial recti through a midbrain lesion
- Drugs/medication – for example, tranquillizers
- Head trauma (particularly whiplash injuries) affecting accommodation and convergent fusion

Consecutive – The post-operative patient may be left with over-liberal recession of one/both medial recti and/or a low AC/A ratio.

In a patient with convergence insufficiency, symptoms normally comprise frontal headaches, blurred near vision, occasional horizontal diplopia at near, aching eyes, and grittiness associated with close work or towards the end of the day. These patients often close one eye while reading.

Reduced convergence and decreased fusional convergence at near may be indicated by the following tests:

Table C.14 • Treatment plan for convergence insufficiency.

1. Correct any refractive error
2. Treat to overcome the suppression
3. Treat to improve the convergence
4. Treat to increase the convergent fusion range at near
5. Teach voluntary convergence to prevent regression

- Cover test – no squint. There may be an exophoria for near with a slow recovery
- Near point of convergence is lower than normal
- Convergent prism fusion range for near is reduced
- Voluntary convergence is absent
- Bar reading is often reduced demonstrating an abnormal (usually a low) AC/A ratio
- Stereoacuity may be reduced.

The prognosis is very good for primary convergence insufficiency. With rare exceptions, convergence insufficiency responds to orthoptic exercises. The prognosis of secondary and consecutive convergence insufficiency depends on cause. In attempting exercises it is important that the patient is told at the outset that there will be homework. The practitioner should give clear (preferably written) instructions, and should also explain that a course of exercises is necessary to prevent future regression, with four to six visits to the practice at two-weekly intervals (weekly if a child). Thereafter, the exercises should be undertaken two or three times a day for three to five minutes. The eyes need to be relaxed after each session by looking in the distance or closing them for a few seconds. A suggested treatment plan is shown in Table C.14.

An ideal outcome of exercises would result in the patient being symptom-free. The patient should have a near prism fusion range of approximately 45^Δ base out to 14^Δ to 16^Δ base in. In addition, the patient should display voluntary convergence, so there should be no risk of regression. It is very rare that primary convergence insufficiency does not respond to exercises, but in cases where exercises are not possible or practicable (e.g. because of age or infirmity), other options include base-in prism or surgery.

Co-polymers, contact lens

- See *Polymers, contact lens*.

Cornea

The cornea is the transparent structure at the front of the eyeball that allows light to enter the eye. It is elliptical when viewed from in front, with its long axis in the horizontal meridian. This asymmetry is produced by a greater degree of overlap of the peripheral cornea by opaque limbal tissue in the vertical meridian. The surface area of the cornea is a $1.1 cm^2$, which represents about 7% of the surface area of the globe. Topographically, the cornea is conventionally divided into four zones; central, paracentral, peripheral and limbal. The central zone, which covers the entrance pupil of the eye, is spherical,

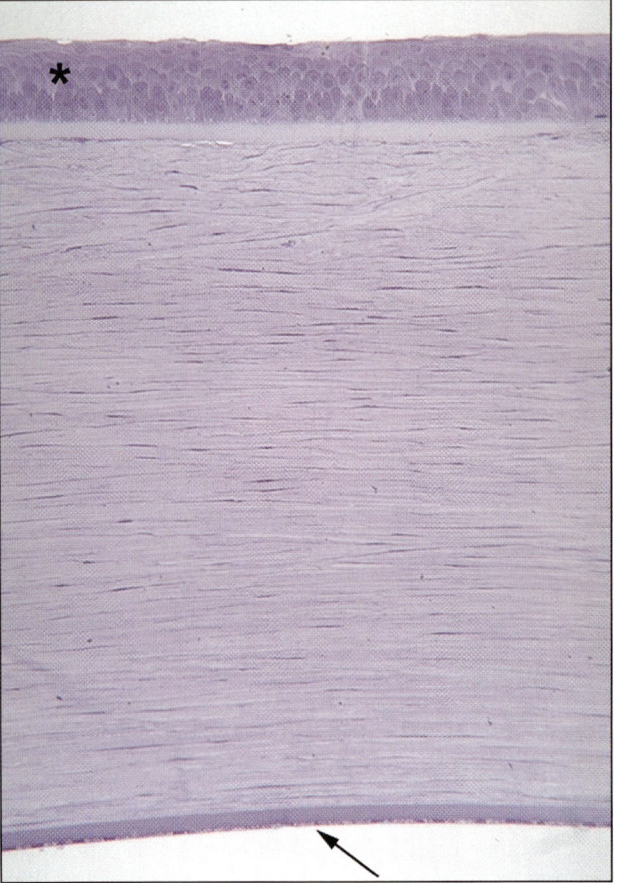

Figure C.24 • Transverse section through the cornea. The stroma, which represents 90% of the thickness of the cornea, is bounded by the epithelium (asterisk) and endothelium (arrow).

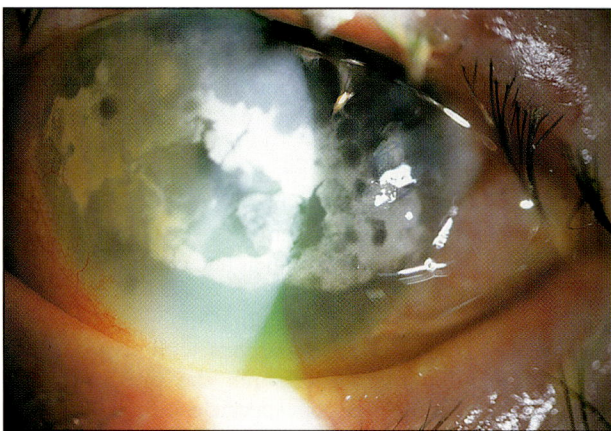

Figure C.25 • Epithelial breakdown in long-term band keratopathy.

approximately 4mm wide, and principally determines high-resolution image formation on the fovea. The paracentral zone, which lies outside the central zone, is flatter and becomes optically important in dim illumination, when the pupil dilates. The peripheral zone is where the cornea is flattest and most aspheric. Owing to differences in curvature between its posterior and anterior surfaces, the cornea shows a regional variation in thickness. Centrally the thickness is approximately 0.52mm, increasing towards the periphery to 0.67mm.

The cornea consists of the following layers (Figure C.24), working from the outermost layer: epithelium, anterior limiting lamina (also referred to as Bowman's membrane), stroma, posterior limiting lamina (also referred to as Descemet's membrane) and endothelium.

Corneal abrasion
- See *Relief of pain, therapeutic lenses for.*

Corneal distortion
- See *Corneal warpage.*

Corneal dystrophies, degenerations and depositions

These are common types of corneal opacifying disorders. Corneal dystrophies are non-inflammatory, progressive, usually bilateral and mostly inherited disorders. They tend to affect the central cornea, be avascular and have an onset early in life. The mode of inheritance is usually autosomal dominant, although inheritance of keratoconus is not so clearly defined.

An anatomical classification of the main dystrophies is as follows:

- Anterior: epithelial basement membrane dystrophy (Cogan's, map-dot fingerprint), Meesmann's epithelial dystrophy, Reis-Buckler's dystrophy
- Stromal: granular stromal dystrophy, lattice stromal dystrophy, macular stromal dystrophy
- Posterior: Fuch's endothelial dystrophy, posterior polymorphous dystrophy, congenital hereditary endothelial dystrophy
- Ectatic: keratoconus and keratoglobus, pellucid marginal degeneration.

Corneal degenerations may be unilateral or bilateral, may be asymmetric, are most often located peripherally and tend to manifest later in life. The degenerations tend to occur in relation to processes such as aging, trauma or disease. Degenerations related to inflammation can be vascularized.

Corneal degenerations can be classified as follows:

- Age related: corneal opacities – peripheral (arcus senilis, Vogt's white limbal girdle), crocodile shagreen and corneal mosaics, Terrien's marginal degeneration
- Inflammation-related: band keratopathy (Figure C.25), Saltzmann nodular degeneration, lipid keratopathy, pseudogerontoxon in vernal disease
- UV radiation and exposure related: climatic droplet keratopathy (spheroidal degeneration), pterygium (although a conjunctival degeneration, it manifests at the corneal periphery).

Depositions in the cornea are usually due to metabolic disturbances or are drug related. Those in the corneal periphery include the Kayser-Fleischer ring, Wilson's disease and copper deposits. Vortex keratopathies can be induced by chloroquine and amiodarone. Fabry disease also results in a vortex keratopathy.

Some of the corneal dystrophies are associated with acute painful episodes due to recurrent erosions. Fuch's dystrophy is associated with glare and blurred vision, particularly on awakening. Some of the corneal degenerations can be associated with significant symptoms in terms of ocular discomfort and effect on vision. The age-related degenerations such as arcus and shagreen tend to be asymptomatic.

The principal sign of a corneal dystrophy or degeneration is the development of an opacity in any layer of the cornea. The opacity is most often white in colour, but may be yellow or other colour. A dystrophy will tend to affect the central cornea and have an earlier onset in life, whereas degeneration more frequently affects the peripheral cornea and onset is in middle age or later. Despite the possible appearance of an opacity that may resemble corneal infiltration, there is an absence of associated signs of infection including conjunctival hyperaemia, anterior chamber reaction, and discharge. The epithelial surface is usually intact with no fluorescein staining.

Dystrophies are uncommon to rare (approximately 1/1,000 to 1/10,000) across all age groups. Degenerations are very common (greater than 1/10) in the older age groups. Most of these conditions are chronic and progressive. Whilst to do nothing and review is an option, management or treatment at some point in time is likely to be required, sooner for some conditions than others. For the conditions related to UV, general advice about the use of sunglasses is helpful. Topical lubrication can be helpful for ocular surface irritation. Either incisional or laser surgery may be indicated for some conditions, and some of the more significant dystrophies may require corneal grafting. See *Recurrent erosion syndrome, therapeutic lenses for*.

Corneal endothelium

The endothelium is a monolayer of squamous cells that lines the posterior surface of the cornea (Figure C.26). As it has a limited capacity for mitosis to replace damaged or effete cells, there is a progressive reduction in the number of endothelial cells with age. At birth the cornea contains a total of approximately 500 000 cells, which represents a mean density of 4500 cells/mm^2. During infancy cell loss is particularly marked, and a 26% reduction occurs in the first year. Thereafter the rate of loss progressively declines into old age. Since grafted corneas appear to maintain transparency and functional normality with an endothelial cell density of less than 1000 cells/mm^2, it would seem that the normal cell density represents a considerable 'physiological reserve'. The endothelium appears as a mosaic of polygonal (typically hexagonal) cells. In response to ocular and systemic pathology, trauma, age and prolonged contact lens wear, the endothelial mosaic becomes less regular, and shows a greater variation in cell size (polymegethism) and shape (pleomorphism), as cells spread to fill gaps caused by cell loss. The lateral borders of the cells are markedly convoluted, and adjacent cells are linked by tight junctions (with less frequent gap junctions). The complement of organelles seen in endothelial cells reflects their high metabolic activity, with numerous mitochondria and a prominent rough endoplasmic reticulum.

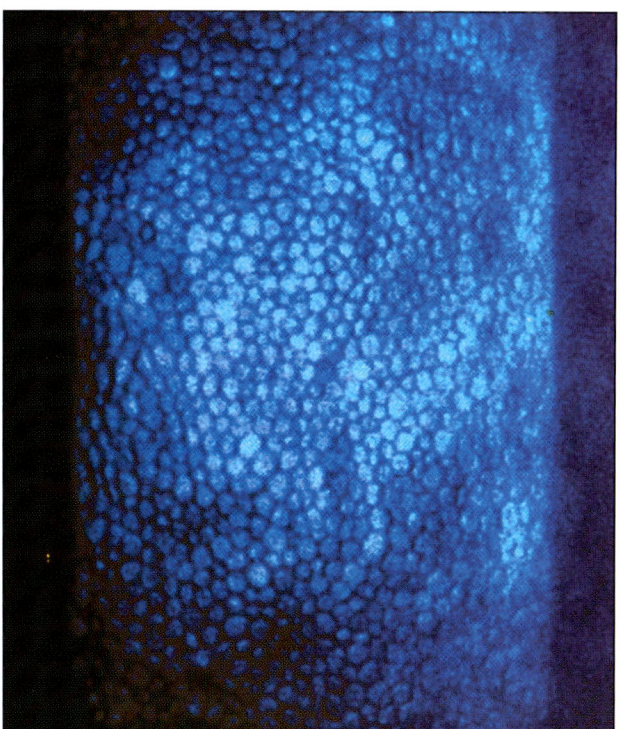

Figure C.26 • Normal human corneal endothelium.

Corneal epithelial wound healing

A smooth and intact corneal epithelium is necessary in order for the cornea to maintain clear vision. However, due to its exposed position the cornea is potentially vulnerable to a variety of external insults, including contact lens wear. The cornea possesses several protective mechanisms to avoid injury, but should tissue damage occur it is capable of an effective wound healing response. Corneal epithelial repair is a complex process involving an orchestrated interaction between cells and extracellular matrix, which is co-ordinated by a variety of growth factors. The process can be divided into three phases:

1. Initial covering of the denuded area by cell migration
2. Cell proliferation to replace lost cells
3. Epithelial differentiation to reform the normal stratified epithelial architecture.

Following a full-thickness epithelial defect, fibronectin, an adhesive glycoprotein, is synthesized and covers the surface of the bared stroma, where it serves as a temporary matrix for cell migration. The adhesion between fibronectin and the epithelium is mediated by integrin-matrix interactions (integrins are a family of cell surface receptors which bind to certain extracellular matrix proteins). Several growth factors have been implicated in the control of the wound healing response, including epidermal growth factor (EGF), transforming growth factor beta (TGFb), platelet-derived growth factor (PDGF) and fibroblast growth factor (FGF). Growth factors, which are produced by a variety of sources (e.g. ocular surface epithelia and the lacrimal gland), are able to regulate the process of epithelial migration, proliferation

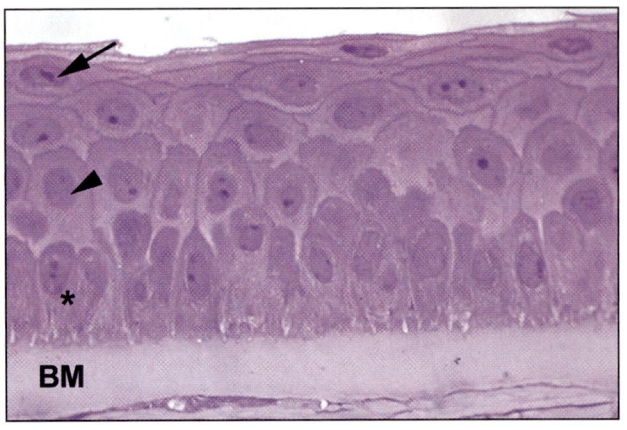

Figure C.27 • Corneal epithelium in cross-section. Three cell types can be distinguished: basal cells (asterisk), wing cells (arrowhead) and squamous cells (arrow). BM= Bowman's membrane.

and differentiation. Epithelial-stromal interactions play an important role in corneal wound healing. Epithelial injury triggers keratocyte apoptosis (programmed cell death) in the anterior stroma via the release of apoptosis-inducing cytokines from epithelial cells. Keratocyte apoptosis subsequently triggers a wound healing cascade, which influences epithelial repair.

Regeneration of the corneal epithelium is highly dependent on the integrity of the limbus. A proportion of limbal basal epithelial cells possess the properties of stem cells, which are ultimately responsible for corneal epithelial replacement. Stem cells have several unique characteristics – they are poorly differentiated, long-lived, and have a high capacity for self-renewal. When these cells divide, one of the daughter cells replenishes the stem cell pool whilst the other is destined to undergo further cell divisions before differentiating. Such a cell is referred to as a 'transient amplifying' (TA) cell. Transient amplifying cells undergo several rounds of cell division before fully differentiating. These cells play an important role in epithelial wound healing, where their proliferative capacity is increased by shortening cycle times and increasing the number of times that the TA cells can divide before maturation.

Corneal epithelium

The epithelium is the outermost layer of the cornea, and represents approximately 10% of the thickness of the cornea (50μm). It is a stratified squamous non-keratinized epithelium, consisting of five to six layers of cells. Three distinct epithelial cell types are recognized (Figure C.27); a single row of basal cells, two to three rows of wing cells and two to three layers of superficial (squamous) cells. In addition, several non-epithelial cells are present (e.g. lymphocytes, macrophages and Langerhans cells). The epithelium forms a permeability barrier to small molecules, water and ions, as well as forming an effective barrier to the entry of pathogens. Further epithelial specialization enhances adhesion between cells, to withstand shearing and abrasive forces.

Superficial cells are structurally modified for their barrier function and interaction with the tear film. Scanning electron microscopy of surface cells shows extensive finger-like and ridge-like projections (microvilli and microplicae). Light, medium and dark cells can be distinguished, depending on the number and pattern of surface projections. It has been suggested that dark cells, which are relatively free of these surface features, are close to being desquamated into the tear film. By contrast, the newly arrived light cells possess a more extensive array of surface projections. In high power transmission electron micrographs, microvilli and microplicae show an extensive filamentous covering known as the glycocalyx. The glycocalyx is formed from membrane-bound glycoconjugates, and is important for the spreading and attachment of the pre-corneal tear film. In accordance with their barrier function, a complex network of tight junctions links superficial cells.

Wing cells are so named because of their characteristic shape, with lateral extensions and a concave inferior surface to accommodate the apices of the basal cells. Their nuclei tend to be spherical or elongated in the plane of the cornea. The cell borders of the polygonal wing cells show prominent infoldings, which interdigitate with adjacent cells, and numerous desmosomes. This arrangement results in a strong intercellular adhesion. The cytoplasm contains prominent cytoskeletal elements (predominantly actin and cytokeratin intermediate filaments), and although the usual complement of organelles is present, they are few in number.

Basal cells consist of single layer columnar cells with a vertically orientated oval nucleus. Ultrastructurally, they are similar in appearance to wing cells. The plasma membrane similarly shows pronounced infolding, and the cytoplasm contains prominent intermediate filaments. A variety of cell junctions are present, including: desmosomes, which mediate adhesion between cells; hemidesmosomes, which are involved in the attachment of basal cells to the underlying stroma; and gap junctions, which allow for intercellular metabolic coupling. Basal cells form the germative layer of the cornea, and mitotic cells are often seen at this level.

Corneal erosion
- See *Recurrent erosion syndrome, therapeutic contact lenses for.*

Corneal exhaustion syndrome, contact lens-associated

This is a condition in which patients who have worn contact lenses for many years suddenly develop a severe intolerance to lens wear, and is characterized by:
- ocular discomfort
- reduced vision
- photophobia
- excessive oedema
- distorted endothelial mosaic
- moderate to severe polymegethism.

The suggested aetiology of this condition is that the corneal endothelium has become 'exhausted'; that is, it has suffered a reduced capacity to keep excess fluid from entering the corneal stroma. The evidence to support this concept is that patients with corneal exhaustion syndrome display marked endothelial polymegethism, which is in turn associated with an impaired capacity of the cornea to recover from excess stromal oedema (the endothelium being responsible for corneal hydration control).

Corneal graft, contact lens fitting following
- See *Post-keratoplasty, contact lens fitting.*

Corneal hydration control

The state of corneal hydration is an important determinant of corneal transparency. The hydrophilic properties of the stroma are to a large part determined by proteoglycans, which contribute to the fixed negative charge of the stroma and produce a passive gel swelling pressure through electrostatic repulsion. Physiologically, corneal hydration is maintained at approximately 78%. If the cornea is allowed to swell by ±5% of this value, it begins to scatter significant quantities of light.

Mechanisms for the maintenance of physiological corneal hydration are located in the corneal endothelium; these mechanisms comprise a barrier function and a metabolically driven pump. The endothelial barrier to the free passage of molecules from the aqueous is formed principally by focal tight junctions between adjacent endothelial cells. However, in contrast to other barrier epithelia, these junctions are of low electrical resistance and allow the passage of ions and small molecules. This 'leak' is offset by the metabolically-driven pumping of ions out of the stroma by the endothelium, which maintains a transcellular potential difference (aqueous side negative) to balance stromal swelling pressure. Disruption of this osmotic gradient will result in stromal fluid imbibition.

A flux of bicarbonate ions is the predominant component of the endothelial ion transport system. The bicarbonate is generated either by a Na^+/HCO_3^- co-transporter located on the basolateral plasma membrane, or via the intercellular conversion of carbon dioxide by the enzyme carbonic anhydrase. Bicarbonate leaves the cell via an apical bicarbonate ion channel. The driving force for the bicarbonate flux is generated by a sodium-potassium ATPase, which resides on the basolateral endothelial membrane. The energy associated with subsequent sodium re-entry (via Na^+/H^+ and Na^+/HCO_3^- transporters) is coupled to active HCO_3^- flux.

The epithelium also contributes to corneal hydration control. The tight junctions between superficial epithelial cells form an effective permeability barrier to ions and polar solutes. For example, the anionic molecule sodium fluorescein does not penetrate an intact epithelium. Damage to the superficial epithelial cells allows fluorescein to enter the epithelium, with resulting corneal staining. In addition to its barrier properties, the epithelium also possesses active ion transport systems for Na^+ and Cl^-. Since these pumps contribute to the tonicity of the tear film, it is likely that they are involved in the maintenance of stromal hydration.

Corneal infiltrates

Corneal infiltrates are focal accumulations of inflammatory white blood cells (leukocytes), debris such as proteins, cells and oedema (Figure C.28). They represent localized areas of inflammation within the cornea that if persistent can lead to loss of corneal tissue (keratolysis). The major concern with an infiltrate is whether it is infectious; however, they can also be caused by non-infectious processes.

Microbial keratitis describes the situation in which bacteria, viruses, fungi or protozoa have infected the cornea, leading to an inflammatory reaction characterized by corneal infiltrates, usually with an overlying epithelial defect. The inflammation often extends to the anterior chamber, causing cells in the aqueous (flare), focal keratic precipitates on the posterior corneal surface around the site of keratitis, and in severe cases, hypopyon and posterior synechia.

A focal sterile inflammatory reaction can occur in response to either microbial or non-microbial antigens. They are usually less dense and smaller than infiltrates from infectious causes, and the overlying epithelium may be intact. Infiltrates can be associated with soft contact lens wear, especially with poor lens care or extended wear. People with posterior blepharitis can also develop corneal infiltrates adjacent to the lid margin. These are referred to as a marginal keratitis.

When corneal infiltrates are associated with significant corneal inflammation, the eye becomes red and sore, photophobic, and often the vision is blurred. There is also increased lacrimation. A discrete opacity is seen usually within the anterior corneal stroma. The centre of the infiltrate is often densely opaque and white to grey in colour. Surrounding this central dense area there is often a halo of less intense stromal infiltration, such that individual inflammatory cells can be seen on slit-lamp examination. There is usually also some degree of limbal or conjunctival hyperaemia. The lesion should be assessed for the presence of an associated epithelial defect.

Infectious and sterile infiltrates may be able to be differentiated by their location and size, as well as the presence of associated signs. The PEDAL mnemonic can be helpful in distinguishing the two conditions – an infected ulcer is more likely to be associated with any of the following: pain, epithelial defect, discharge, anterior chamber reaction and a more central location. In general, corneal infiltrates are uncommon, however they are more common in at-risk groups such as contact lens wearers and people with rosacea-associated blepharitis.

If there is doubt about the diagnosis, then the infiltrate should be treated as a microbial keratitis. Microbiological investigation and treatment with the appropriate antimicrobial agents is indicated if the condition is thought to be infectious e.g. bacterial, herpetic. These require urgent treatment.

If the corneal infiltrate is non-infectious, the following management strategies may be adopted:

- Application of a mild topical steroid will usually lead to rapid resolution of the lesion. This is often covered with a broad spectrum topical antibiotic.
- If contact lens associated then withdrawal of contact lens use and increased lens hygiene are indicated. Changing to daily disposable soft contact lenses may be indicated if the condition is thought to be related to hygiene and/or problems with lens care.

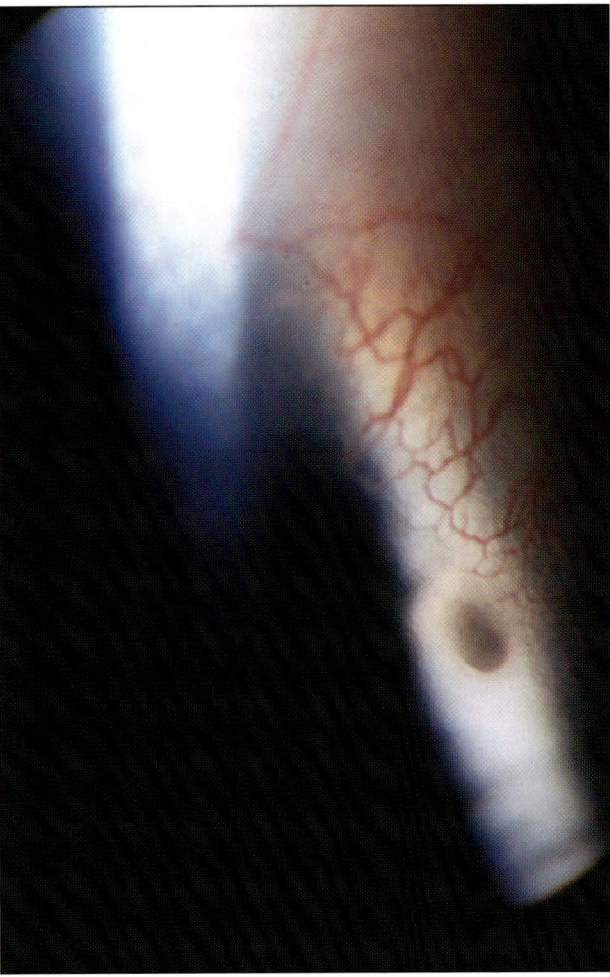 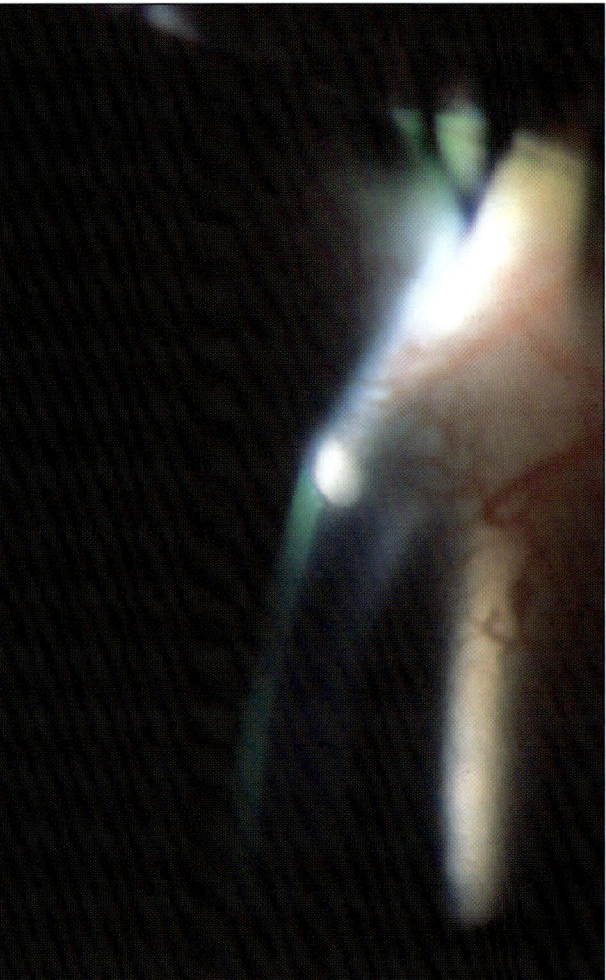

Figure C.28 • Two views of a focal sterile corneal infiltrate in a marginal keratitis. Left: infiltrate observed in retroillumination. Right: negative sodium fluorescein staining where the epithelium is raised and not ulcerated.

- If associated with blepharitis then treatment of the lid disease with lid hygiene and oral tetracyclines may be indicated.

Review is indicated usually within 1 to 2 days to ensure resolution and lack of progression that may indicate an infection.

Corneal metabolism

In order to perform its vital functions, the cornea requires a constant supply of oxygen and other essential metabolites (e.g. glucose, vitamins and amino acids). However, its avascularity dictates that alternative routes must exist for the provision of its metabolic needs. There are three possibilities:

1. Perilimbal vasculature
2. Tear film
3. Aqueous humour.

In open-eye conditions, the bulk of the oxygen required for the cornea is obtained from the atmosphere via diffusion across the pre-corneal tear film. Under steady state conditions it can be assumed that the tears are saturated with oxygen, and are therefore at an oxygen tension corresponding to the atmosphere (155mmHg at sea level). The oxygen tension of the aqueous lies between 30 and 40mmHg. The cornea depends on tear-side oxygen to avoid oedema and maintain normal function. During eye closure the oxygen level in the tears is in equilibrium with the palpebral vasculature (55mmHg).

Significantly, corneal thickness increases by approximately 2–4% during sleep, and returns to baseline levels within 1 hour of eye opening. This is due primarily to reduced oxygen availability, but is also related to changes in tear film tonicity, temperature, humidity and pH. The oxygen flux into the cornea as a whole is in the region of $6\mu l/cm^2$ per hour, although the consumption rate for its composite layers is not equal. Consumption rates have been estimated as 40:39:21 for the epithelium, stroma and endothelium respectively.

The aqueous is the primary source of glucose and essential amino acids for the cornea. The glucose concentration of the tears is low compared to that of the aqueous, and the insertion of nutrient impermeable implants into the stroma results in degeneration of the tissue lying anterior to the implant. Although exogenous glucose is primarily utilized, glycogen stores are present in all corneal cells to provide glucose in conditions of metabolic stress. The role of the perilimbal vasculature in

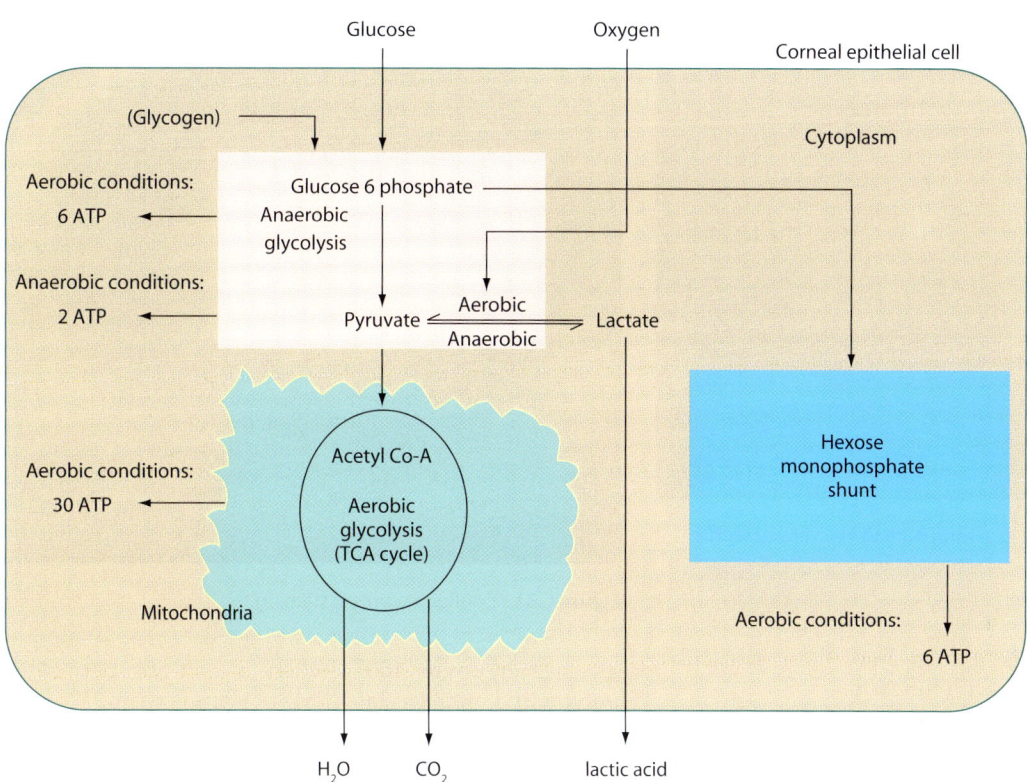

Figure C.29 • Metabolic processes in a corneal epithelial cell.

the provision of oxygen and nutrients is limited, and is only significant for the corneal periphery.

The cornea derives its energy principally from the oxidative breakdown of carbohydrates (Figure C.29). Glucose, which is the primary substrate for the generation of adenosine triphosphate (ATP), is catabolised by three metabolic pathways:

1. Glycolysis
2. Tricarboxylic acid TCA (Krebs) cycle
3. Hexose monophosphate shunt.

Anaerobic glycolysis accounts for the majority of glucose metabolism. In this pathway, glucose is first oxidized to pyruvate and then subsequently reduced to lactate, with a net yield of two molecules of ATP. The TCA cycle results in a greater energy yield (36 ATP). This pathway is most active in the corneal endothelium, which has the greatest energy requirement.

Metabolic waste products can be potentially damaging if allowed to accumulate. Although carbon dioxide can readily diffuse out of the cornea across its limiting layers, lactate is less easily eliminated. Under normoxic conditions, lactate is able to slowly diffuse across the endothelium into the anterior chamber. However, during periods of hypoxia the proportion of glucose that is metabolized anaerobically increases. The resulting accumulation of lactate causes stromal oedema via an increased osmotic load and localized tissue acidosis.

The hexose monophosphate shunt (also known as the pentose phosphate shunt) plays a significant role in the epithelium and endothelium, where it accounts for 35–65% of glucose utilization. It fulfils several important functions, including the generation of intermediates for biosynthetic reactions and the prevention of oxidative damage by free radicals.

Corneal moulding, contact lens induced

- See *Corneal warpage, contact lens induced*.

Corneal nerves

The cornea is the most richly innervated surface tissue in the body, and it receives its predominantly sensory nerve supply from the nasociliary branch of the trigeminal nerve. There is also evidence for the existence of a modest sympathetic innervation from the superior cervical ganglion. Branches from the nasociliary nerve either pass directly to the eye as long ciliary nerves, or traverse the ciliary ganglion, leaving as short ciliary nerves that enter the eye close to the optic nerve. Nerves destined for the cornea travel initially in the suprachoroidal space, before crossing the sclera to advance radially towards the cornea.

Most of the 50–80 precorneal nerve trunks, which contain a mixture of myelinated and unmyelinated fibre bundles, enter the cornea at mid-stromal level. Myelin is soon lost, and the unmyelinated nerve fibre bundles divide repeatedly and move anteriorly to form a rich plexiform network in the anterior one-third of the stroma (Figure C.30). Axons are particularly dense immediately beneath the anterior limiting lamina (Bowman's layer). From this sub-epithelial plexus, axons pass vertically through the anterior limiting lamina, losing their Schwann cell sheath in the process. Upon entering the epithelium, axons turn through 90° and divide into a series of fine branches that course between the basal cells. Some branches pass into the more superficial layers before terminating. Corneal nerves display a complex neurochemistry. A variety of neurotransmitters and neuromodulators have been identified, including acetyl choline, substance P, and calcitonin gene-related peptide

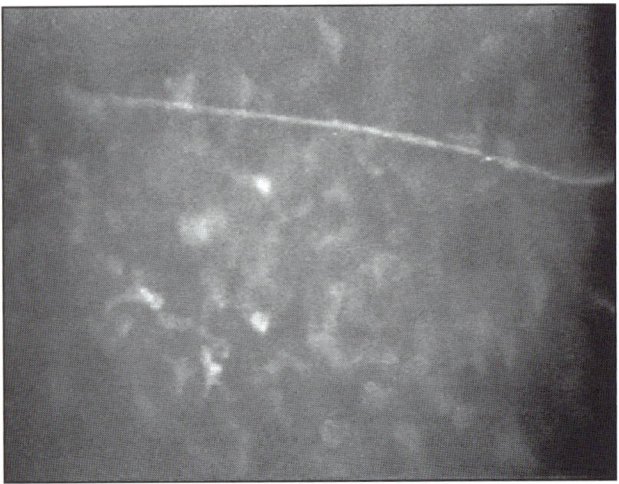

Figure C.30 • Corneal nerve in a living human eye viewed with a confocal microscope.

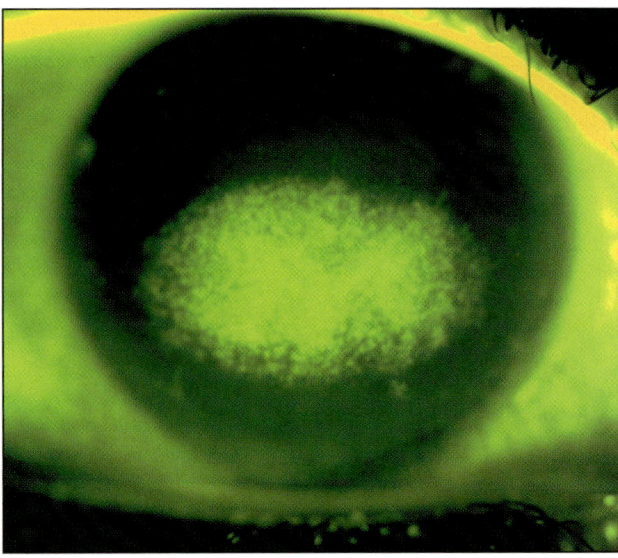

Figure C.31 • Confluent corneal staining.

(CGRP). However, it is unclear how these particular neurochemicals correlate with function.

Corneal nerves serve important sensory, reflex and trophic functions. Damage to corneal sensory nerves by surgery, trauma or infection produces neuroparalytic keratitis – a condition that is characterized by progressive epithelial cell loss and oedema. The mechanism of this trophic role is not fully understood, although the release of neuropeptides (e.g. substance P and CGRP) may be a factor. Sympathetic nerves also play a role in epithelial maintenance by regulating ion transport processes, and cell proliferation and migration during wound healing.

Corneal sensitivity

Carefully controlled corneal stimulation with a variety of mechanical, chemical and thermal stimuli evokes only sensations of irritation or pain. By contrast, electrophysiological studies of corneal afferent neurones have identified neurones that respond to mechanical, chemical and thermal stimulation. However, since the conscious perception of these sensations has not been demonstrated, it is likely that such specificity of modality is lost during central nervous system processing. Electrophysiological recording also allows for the mapping of receptive fields. These are often large and overlapping, which explains the inability of the cornea to localize a stimulus accurately. The sensitivity of the cornea to mechanical stimulation is particularly acute, and acts as a trigger for the protective blink and lacrimal reflexes. Cold receptors may be important in signalling evaporative cooling, which is a major determinant of spontaneous eye blink frequency.

Corneal sensitivity is measured as its touch threshold, and the classic technique for determining corneal touch threshold is with the Cochet-Bonnet aesthesiometer. Corneal sensitivity varies according to corneal location, with the central cornea being the most sensitive. The corneal touch threshold has proven to be a very sensitive measure of corneal health, with the cornea being perhaps the most sensitive organ (to touch) in the body. This has been shown to be a particularly useful measurement in contact lens wear, where the touch threshold may increase by over 100% when a non-gas permeable polymethyl methacrylate (PMMA) lens is worn.

Corneal staining, contact lens-associated

Strictly speaking, 'corneal staining' is not a condition in itself; rather, it is a general term that refers to the appearance of tissue disruption and other pathophysiological changes in the anterior eye as revealed with the aid of one or more of a number of dyes, such as fluorescein, rose bengal, lissamine green, fluorexon or alcian blue. Fluorescein has by far the greatest utility in contact lens practice, so the term 'corneal staining' is generally taken to mean staining with fluorescein unless stated otherwise.

Corneal staining following instillation of fluorescein is observed under cobalt blue light as a bright green fluorescence, which can be described as 'punctate' (spot-like), 'diffuse' (spots merging together) and 'coalescent' (large regions of confluence) (Figure C.31). The staining pattern may be described according to the following groups of type descriptors:

- arcuate, linear or dimpled
- superior, inferior, temporal, nasal or central
- deep or superficial.

Staining 'syndromes' include:

- inferior epithelial arcuate lesion (smile stain)
- superior epithelial arcuate lesion (SEAL; otherwise known as epithelial splitting)
- exposure keratitis
- epithelial plug – a large, coalescent field of full-thickness epithelial loss
- superficial punctate keratitis (SPK).

Observed areas of fluorescence indicates one of three phenomena:

1. Fluorescein entering damaged cells
2. Fluorescein entering intercellular spaces
3. Fluorescein filling the gaps in the epithelial surface that are created when epithelial cells are displaced.

Depending on the cause of the problem, severe staining (Grades 3 and 4) may be accompanied by:
- bulbar conjunctival redness and chemosis
- limbal redness
- excessive lacrimation
- stromal infiltrates.

Visual acuity is generally unaffected by corneal staining, although a slight loss might be expected in extreme cases (Grade 4). There is no clear relationship between the severity of staining and the degree of ocular discomfort.

There are numerous contact lens-related causes of corneal staining, which can be broadly classified into six aetiological categories:

1. Mechanical
2. Exposure
3. Metabolic
4. Toxic
5. Allergic
6. Infectious.

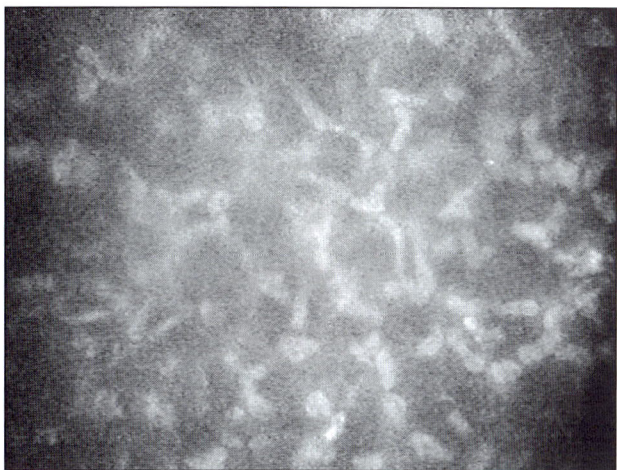

Figure C.32 • Stromal keratocytes appear as irregular white spicular shapes when viewed with a confocal microscope (only the cell nuclei are visible).

In many cases the pattern of staining, and whether the condition presents in one or both eyes, can provide a clue to the cause. Low level staining (less than Grade 2) does not necessarily require action to be taken. Such staining is commonly observed in contact lens wearers; it is typically transient, and in a daily lens wearer will have disappeared by the following morning. However, persistent minor staining forming a characteristic or repeatable pattern, as well as staining greater than Grade 2, may require intervention.

Management strategies are generally self-evident if the cause can be discerned. For example, mechanical trauma due to a foreign body trapped beneath a rigid lens can be resolved by removing and rinsing the lens and rinsing the eye; exposure keratitis causing 3 and 9 o'clock staining in a rigid lens wearer can be resolved by fitting soft lenses; epitheliopathy due to metabolic disturbance can be solved by fitting a lens of higher oxygen transmissibility; staining due to toxicity or allergy can be resolved by eliminating the toxic or allergic agent; and staining associated with an infection is treated by applying the appropriate antimicrobial therapy. Recovery from corneal staining generally occurs within hours or days of removal of the offending source, but will be more prolonged if lenses are worn during the recovery period.

Corneal stroma

This structure is approximately 500μm thick, and accounts for 90% of the thickness of the cornea. It is composed predominantly of collagen fibrils (68% dry weight) embedded in a highly hydrated matrix of proteoglycans. A variety of different collagen types have been identified. Type I is the major stromal collagen, and there are lesser amounts of types III, V and VI. Collagen fibrils are arranged in 200–250 layers (lamellae) running parallel to the surface. Lamellae are approximately 2μm thick and 9–260μm wide, and extend from limbus to limbus. Fibrils of adjacent lamellae make large angles with each other. In the superficial stroma angles are less than 90°, but they become orthogonal in the deeper stroma. This particular arrangement of collagen imparts a high tensile strength for corneal protection, which is important given its exposed position. Within lamellae, all collagen fibrils are parallel, with uniform size and separation. The mean fibril diameter in the human cornea is 31nm, with an interfibrillar spacing of 55.3nm. This narrow fibril diameter and constant separation, which is a characteristic of corneal collagen, is a necessary prerequisite for transparency.

The interfibrillar space contains a matrix of proteoglycans (approximately 10% of dry weight). Keratan sulphate and dermatan sulphate are the major corneal proteoglycans. These molecules are highly sulphated and, along with bound chloride ions, create a polyanionic stromal interfibrillar matrix, which induces osmotic swelling. As well as playing a major role in the maintenance of fixed levels of corneal hydration, collagen-proteoglycan interactions are important in determining the spatial arrangement of collagen fibrils.

Collagen and proteoglycans are maintained by keratocytes (Figure C.32). These cells occupy 3–5% of stromal volume and lie between collagen lamellae, flattened in the plane of the cornea. Keratocyte density is non-uniform; density decreases from superficial to deep stroma and increases from the centre to the periphery. Keratocytes display a large central nucleus, and long slender processes extend from the cell body. Processes from adjacent cells sometimes make tight junctions with each other. Cell organelles are not numerous but comprise the usual complement of organelles, including, endoplasmic reticulum, Golgi apparatus and mitochondria.

Corneal topographic analysis

The aim of corneal topography (also termed 'keratoscopy' or 'videokeratography') is to accurately describe the shape of the corneal surface in all meridians. In most cases the technique uses a similar principle to keratometry, in that it determines the size of the image of a target reflected in the corneal surface, the primary difference relating to the fact that for keratoscopy a series of circular concentric targets are used (a Placido-disc image; see Figure D.13). This arrangement allows both central and peripheral

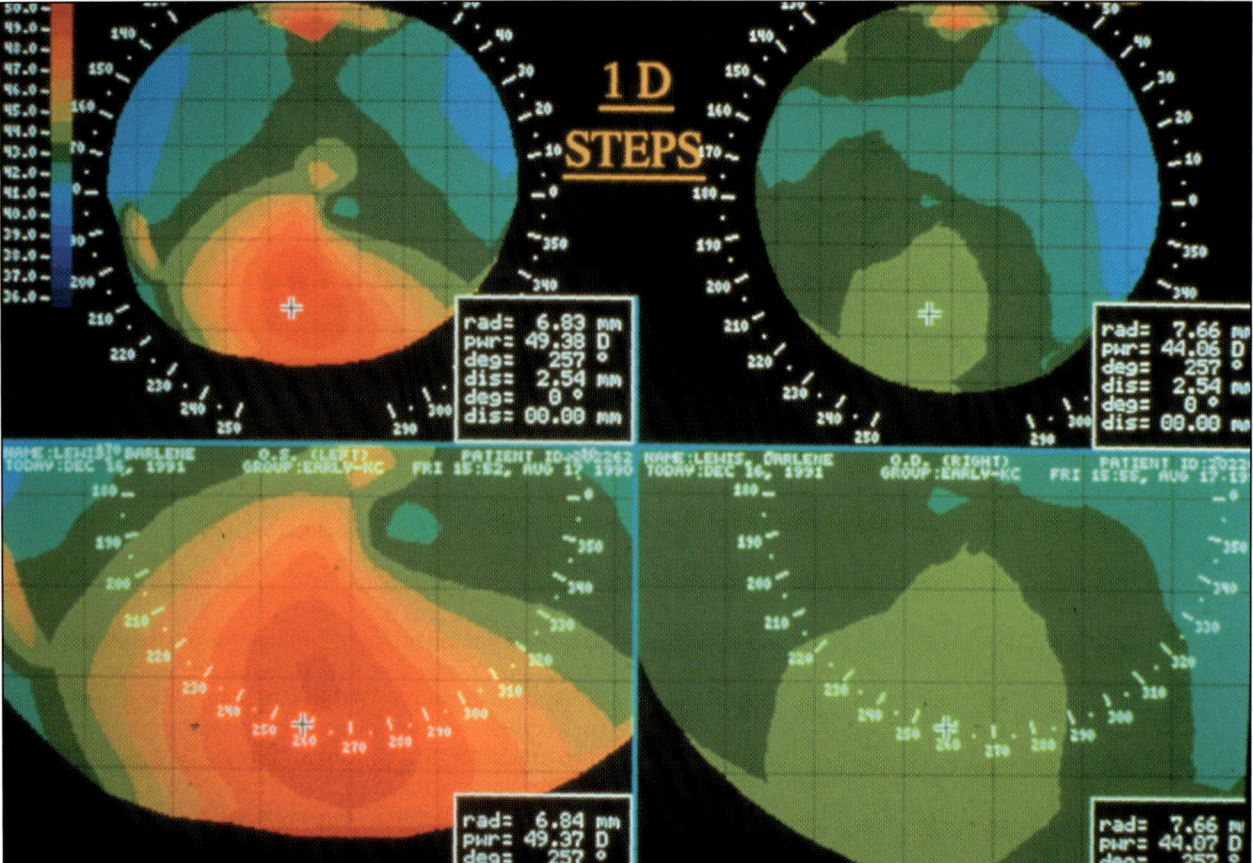

Figure C.33 • Topography maps of a patient with advanced keratoconus in one eye (left images) and possible early keratoconus in the other eye (right images).

curvature to be determined. The topographer captures the image electronically on a computer, and uses sophisticated image-processing software to provide immediate analysis of the reflected image (video-keratoscopy). Using this technique it has been clearly demonstrated that the cornea is aspheric, and can best be described as a flattening ellipse whose rate of flattening is asymmetrical about its centre.

Modern topographers can be categorized into two distinct forms; reflective devices and slit-scanning devices. Reflective devices measure topography based on the reflection of mires from the anterior surface tear film, which is essentially identical in shape to the corneal surface. The images are captured with a video camera, and a computational approach is adopted to analyze the data and derive a description for the corneal shape. The choice of computational method is important, as this will largely dictate the accuracy and validity of the keratoscope. The most frequently utilized computational method is the 'slope of surface' method. Basically, devices that use this technology measure slope directly as a function of distance from a central reference axis, and derive curvature from these results. It is important to note that these distance-based instruments are only estimating the average shape of the cornea, since the algorithms are based on a radially symmetric surface, which does not accurately describe the cornea. These axial or sagittal measurements result in an underestimation of the radius of curvature in areas that may be steeper than the central cornea, and an overestimation in areas that are flatter. More recently the algorithms have been modified, and are now generally based on the radius of curvature in an attempt to provide a better estimate of the local shape of the cornea.

The images (or 'maps') produced by reflective or placido-based keratoscopes display the power distribution of the corneal surface using colour-coded displays, in which greens and yellows represent powers characteristic of those found in normal corneas, blues or cooler colours represent flatter areas (low powers), and reds or hotter colours represent steep areas (high powers; Figure C.33). These maps permit recognition of corneal shape through pattern recognition, and swiftly reveal the presence of abnormal powers. All devices display simulated keratometry (SimK) values, which are analogous to standard keratometry values, and simultaneously display the power and axis of the flattest meridian. A number of manufacturers now produce hand-held topographers. These portable devices can prove very useful for examining children, the elderly and the infirm, and for 'off-site' consultations.

The Orbscan II™ device uses a slit scanning method to obtain topographic measurements of both anterior and posterior corneal surfaces, in addition to the anterior lens and iris. The instrument scans across the anterior corneal surface, obtaining 40 sequential slit images, whilst simultaneously recording eye movements and reflection data from a placido-disc device. The data are then reassembled into a three-dimensional reconstruction of the anterior and posterior corneal surfaces. The advantage of this system is that it allows for the measurement of multiple ocular surfaces. The instrument differs from traditional keratoscopes in that it uses a combination of slit scan triangulation and surface reflection to determine corneal shape. Specifically, this instrument unifies triangulated and reflective data to obtain accurate measurements of corneal elevation, slope, curvature and thickness. In addition to conventional axial and tangential maps, shape data can be displayed as an elevation map in which the relative height of the cornea is compared to a spherical reference surface. Elevations above the reference sphere are coloured red, and depressions below the reference sphere are coloured blue.

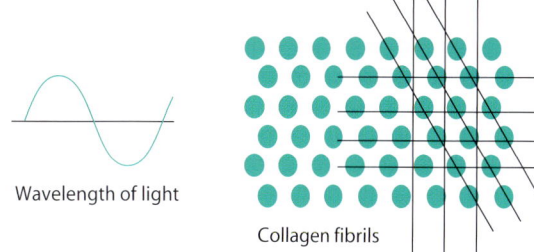

Figure C.34 • Collagen fibrils have an orderly structure and a spacing that is less than the wavelength of light.

Corneal topography

The topography of the anterior cornea is of particular interest since, as the dominant refractive surface, its form has a major influence on overall refractive error and ocular aberration. In contact lens work, it is of enormous importance to the fitting geometry.

The radius of curvature over the central region, as measured by conventional keratometers, shows considerable individual variation, and it has been recognized for more than a century that many corneas display marked astigmatism. Corneal astigmatism is not necessarily equal to the total ocular astigmatism, since additional astigmatism (residual astigmatism) may be contributed by the crystalline lens.

Earlier work on corneal topography using modifications of traditional keratometers concentrated on approximating the form of the corneal surface by a conicoid, in which each meridian is a conic section. In this approach the anterior corneal surface can be described by the equation:

$$x^2 + y^2 + pz^2 = 2r_0 z$$

where the coordinate system has its origin at the corneal apex, z is the axial coordinate, r_0 is the radius of curvature at the cornea apex, and the shape factor p is a constant parameter characterizing the form of the conic section for the individual eye. Values of p<0 represent hyperboloids; p=0, paraboloids; 0<p<1, flattening (prolate) ellipsoids; p=1, spheres; and p>1, steepening (oblate) ellipsoids. The same equation is sometimes written in terms of the Q-factor or the eccentricity e of the conic section, where:

$$p = 1 + Q = 1 - e^2$$

Mean human r_0 and p values are 7.72±0.27mm and 0.74±0.18 respectively. Thus the typical general form of the cornea is that of a flattening ellipsoid, with the curvature reducing in the periphery; however, not all corneas will have this form.

In recent years, corneal topographic analysis has been facilitated by the development of a range of instruments that marry optical with electronic and computer technology. These instruments show that the conicoidal model is only a first approximation to corneal shape, and that individual eyes show a wide range of individual asymmetries. In particular, the rate of corneal flattening is often different in different meridians, while the corneal cap of steepest curvature may be displaced with respect to the visual axis, on average lying about 0.8mm below. Currently the most popular form of output for the topographic data is the colour-coded map of the cornea, showing regions of different power. This may be a little misleading, since each local area of the cornea is toroidal rather than spherical.

Corneal transparency

Under normal conditions the cornea is highly transparent, transmitting more than 90% of incident light. Structurally the cornea is a typical connective tissue, consisting principally of a matrix of collagen and proteoglycans. Under normal circumstances such an arrangement would favour light scatter, with consequent loss of transparency. However, corneal transparency can be explained on the basis of the small diameter and regular separation of the stromal collagen – the collagen fibrils of the stroma are disposed in a regular crystalline lattice, and light scattered by the fibrils is eliminated by destructive interference in all directions other than the forward direction. This situation holds as long as the axes of the collagen fibrils are arranged in a regular lattice with a separation less than the wavelength of light (Figure C.34).

The factors involved in the maintenance of collagen fibril size and spatial order are not fully understood. It has been proposed that collagen fibril diameters may be controlled by the incorporation of minor collagens (e.g. type V) into the predominantly type I fibrils, and that their spatial separation is a function of proteoglycan-collagen interactions. Proteoglycans are a family of glycoproteins that consist of a protein core to which are attached sugar chains of repeating disaccharide units termed glycosaminoglycans (GAG). In the corneal stroma two major proteoglycans have been identified; keratan sulphate and dermatan sulphate. Several keratan sulphate isoforms have been described in the cornea of different species. In the human cornea an isoform predominates that has been termed lumican. There appears to be a link between the keratan sulphate content of the cornea and transparency; transgenic mice that lack the gene for lumican fail to develop a clear cornea.

Corneal transplantation, contact lens fitting following

- See *Post-keratoplasty, contact lens fitting for.*

Corneal warpage associated with contact lens wear

Videokeratographic corneal mapping techniques reveal that all forms of contact lens wear are capable of inducing small changes in corneal topography. These shape changes, which are generally referred to as 'warpage', are primarily mediated by the stroma, which is the main structural entity of the cornea (the epithelium and endothelium offering little mechanical resistance to deforming forces).

The degree of irregularity of corneal surface shape can be expressed by various mathematical indices. For example, the surface asymmetry index (SAI) provides a quantitative measure of the radial symmetry of the four central videokeratoscope mires surrounding the vertex of the cornea. The higher the degree of central corneal symmetry, the lower the SAI. Mean SAI values (± standard error of mean) associated with various forms of lens wear are as follows: non-lens wear, 0.35±0.03; PMMA, 0.86±0.22; daily wear rigid, 0.48±0.09; daily wear soft, 0.48±0.11; extended wear soft, 0.46±0.08.

The surface regularity index (SRI) is a measure of central and paracentral corneal irregularity derived from the summation of fluctuations in corneal power that occur along semi-meridians of the 10 central photokeratoscope mires. The more regular the anterior surface of the central cornea, the lower the SRI. The SRI is highly correlated with best spectacle-corrected visual acuity. Mean SRI values (± standard error of mean) associated with various forms of lens wear are as follows: non-lens wear, 0.41±0.04; PMMA, 1.17±0.34; daily wear rigid, 0.93±0.18; daily wear soft, 0.52±0.08; extended wear soft, 0.51±0.06.

All known forms of contact lens-induced warpage can be explained in terms of three underlying pathological mechanisms that primarily act on the stroma. These mechanisms are:

1. Physical pressure on the cornea exerted either by the lens and/or eyelids
2. Contact lens-induced stromal oedema
3. Mucus binding beneath rigid lenses.

The relative contributions of these factors will govern the type and extent of topographical alteration.

Rigid lenses can induce clinically significant warpage, which may be especially evident in patients with higher prescriptions requiring thicker lenses or unusual lens designs. Such lenses will impart greater physical and hypoxic stress on the cornea compared with thinner lenses made of the same material. Altering the parameters of a rigid lens can reduce the physical impact of the lens on the cornea and thus minimize corneal shape changes. Of course in any case of rigid contact lens-induced warpage refitting into soft lenses will usually provide a cure, because soft lenses are known to have little or no effect on corneal topography.

The prognosis for recovery of normal corneal topography is highly variable and is dependent upon the cause, magnitude and duration of the lens-induced deformation. The time course of recovery from physical forces on the cornea is difficult to predict. Recovery from chronic lens-induced oedema is known to occur within 7 days of cessation of lens wear, and thus recovery from oedema-mediated warpage would be expected to follow a similar time course.

Corneal wrinkling associated with contact lens wear

- See *Wrinkling, contact lens induced.*

Cornea plana

- See *Distorted corneal shape, therapeutic lenses for.*

Corticosteroids

When stimulated by the adrenocorticotropic hormone, the cortex of the adrenal gland synthesises three types of steroids:

- Mineralocorticoids – mainly aldosterone and desoxycorticosterone, which maintain the electrolyte balance of the body
- Androgenic (sex) steroids – androgens and oestrogens, which are important in the development of secondary sex characteristics
- Glucocorticosteroids – cortisol and corticosterone, which promote the conversion of fats and proteins to glucose, play an important part in the homeostasis of glucose metabolism, and fulfill a minor role in the control of the excretion of salt and water. The glucocorticosteroids are strongly anti-inflammatory, inhibit the manifestation of cell-mediated immunity and stabilize lysosomal enzymes.

Cortisone and hydrocortisone (cortisol), which are naturally occurring glucocorticoids, depress the production of antibodies and reduce the inflammatory response of tissues without affecting its cause. Synthetic analogues of cortisone and hydrocortisone have been developed in order to exploit and enhance their anti-inflammatory property. Cortisone is rapidly absorbed after oral administration and converts to hydrocortisone. Since cortisone is inactive until it is metabolized, it is of no value for topical application but was utilized in the treatment of conditions such as Addison's disease. Hydrocortisone is similarly employed as replacement therapy in adrenocortical insufficiency. In contrast to cortisone, hydrocortisone is active topically and is used not only to suppress ocular inflammation, but also in the treatment of mild inflammatory skin disorders (e.g. eczema).

The anti-inflammatory and immunosuppressant actions of corticosteroids include:

- Decreasing the numbers of leukocytes
- Inhibition of leukocytic functions
- Alteration of vascular functions (i.e. permeability and constriction)
- Reduction of the effects of complement, cytokines, etc.

Betamethasone is a synthetic corticosteroid with high glucocorticoid activity and insignificant mineralocorticoid activity. It has increased anti-inflammatory action that allows its use at a relatively low dose with reduced side

Table C.15 • Topical corticosteroids: preserved multidose preparations.

Non-proprietary name	Proprietary name	Formulation	Preservatives
Betamethasone sodium phosphate	Betnesol® Vista-Methasone®	Drops 0.1% Drops 0.1%	Benzalkonium chloride 0.02%* Benzalkonium chloride 0.01%*
Dexamethasone	Maxidex® Maxitrol® Sofradex® Tobradex®	Drops 0.1% with hypromellose 0.5% Drops 0.1% with hypromellose 0.5%, neomycin sulphate 0.35% & polymyxin B sulphate Drops 0.05%, with framycetin sulphate 0.5% and gramicidin 0.005% Drops 0.1% with tobramycin 0.3%	Benzalkonium chloride 0.01%* Benzalkonium chloride 0.04% Phenylethyl alcohol 0.6% Benzalkonium chloride 0.01%*
Fluoromethalone with polyvinyl alcohol	FML®	Drops 0.1% with polyvinyl alcohol 1.4%	Benzalkonium chloride 0.0046%*
Prednisolone acetate	Pred Forte®	Drops 0.1%	Benzalkonium chloride 0.006%*
Prednisolone sodium phosphate	Predsol® Predsol-N®	Drops 0.5% Drops 0.5% with neomycin sulphate 0.5%	Benzalkonium chloride 0.04%* Benzalkonium chloride 0.01%*
Rimexolone	Vexol®	Drops 1%	Benzalkonium chloride 0.01%*

* with disodium edetate

Table C.16 • Topical corticosteroids: unpreserved single dose preparations.

Non-proprietary name	Proprietary name	Formulation
Dexamethasone sodium phosphate	Minims® Dexamethasone sodium phosphate	Drops 0.1%*
Prednisolone sodium phosphate	Minims® Prednisolone sodium phosphate	Drops 0.5%*

* with disodium edetate

Table C.17 • Topical corticosteroid: ointments.

Non-proprietary name	Proprietary name	Formulation
Betamethasone sodium phosphate	Betnesol®	Ointment 0.1%
Dexamethasone	Sofradex®	Ointment 0.05% with framycetin sulphate 0.5% & gramicidin 0.005%

effects. With the exception of Addison's disease, it can be used in all inflammatory allergic and other conditions in which corticosteroid therapy is indicated.

Dexamethasone has similar characteristics and uses to betamethasone and has the greatest propensity of all steroids to raise intraocular pressure.

Prednisolone is a glucocorticosteroid, and although its actions and uses are similar to those of hydrocortisone, it is effective at much lower doses. It is regarded as the preferred corticosteroid for oral administration.

Both rimexolone and fluoromethalone have a surface-limited action due to poor solubility in the cornea or to metabolic breakdown within it with the consequence that they are associated with a reduced risk of inducing an increase in intraocular pressure or other side effects.

Loteprednol etabonate is described as a 'site-specific' agent that has a minimal effect on intraocular pressure. It is available in the USA and other countries but not currently in the UK.

Topical corticosteroids in multidose, single dose and ointment forms are listed in Tables C.15–17, respectively.

Inflammation of the anterior segment, together with that caused by surgery, can be treated with topical corticosteroids administered as drops, ointment or by sub-conjunctival injection, or they may be administered orally. Although the topical instillation of corticosteroids impairs wound healing by diminishing fibroplastic and keratocytic activity, they can be used following ophthalmic surgery (e.g. cataract extraction). In penetrating keratoplasty, steroids both suppress inflammation and help to prevent graft rejection. Topical steroids are effective in the treatment of anterior uveitis and for many years prednisolone was regarded as the 'gold standard' for this purpose. Severe, refractory cases of allergic ocular disease such as vernal or atopic keratoconjunctivitis that have failed to respond to less toxic anti-inflammatory agents such as antihistamines can also be treated with steroids. Combinations of steroids with antibiotics are available and considered by some to be appropriate for the treatment of the immune-type marginal corneal ulceration caused by staphylococci.

Both topical and systemic treatment of ocular conditions with corticosteroids is associated with the risk of inducing 'steroid cataract' which first affects the posterior subcapsular region and later the anterior subcapsular region. While the risk is very low in patients receiving less than the equivalent of 10mg of systemically administered prednisolone per day and in those treated for less than four years, it increases with higher doses or a longer duration of treatment. Unfortunately, asthmatics and patients with chronic obstructive pulmonary disease may require long-term treatment with steroids which, even if administered by inhalation, are associated with an increased risk of the development of cataract.

Other adverse side effects from long-term use of corticosteroids are corneal thinning, known as 'corneal melt', or perforation. A small proportion of the population, about 1 per cent, is susceptible to raised intraocular pressure following long-term topical or systemic treatment with steroids. If the raised pressure is unrecognized, these 'steroid responders' will develop open angle 'steroid glaucoma' and in some cases this condition proves to be intractable despite the discontinuation of steroid therapy. Since topical corticosteroids reduce local tissue immunity, they are capable of aggravating an eye infection particularly if it was viral or fungal in origin. They may also facilitate opportunistic infection especially by bacteria. If a steroid were used to treat the inflammation accompanying a *Herpes simplex* ulcer, viral replication would be encouraged leading to a much larger area of ulceration. Accordingly, steroids should *not* be used in the treatment of a 'red eye' if the exact aetiology has not been established.

Patients taking oral steroids equivalent to 5mg prednisolone or more daily for longer than three months are at risk of developing osteoporosis. Accordingly, all patients commencing oral steroids should receive advice regarding this potential problem together with a calcium supplement in their diet. Hormone replacement therapy should be considered in the case of post-menopausal women. Patients' general medical practitioners should be suitably informed and, if the course or treatment is likely to be prolonged, bone densitometry should be undertaken.

Cosmetic tinted contact lenses

A cosmetic tinted lens can be defined as a lens that is designed to beautify an otherwise normal appearance. This can amount to enhancing eye colour with translucent tints, modifying eye colour with a combination of translucent and opaque tints, or completely changing eye colour with opaque tints. Cosmetic tinted lenses are considered to be a fashion accessory, and as such they are often worn by emmetropes. Indeed, most tinted lenses are produced for their cosmetic effect. The most frequently used tints are aquamarine, blue, green and amber. As is the case with handling tints, cosmetic tints do not appreciably affect vision or colour perception, although patients may report an initial transient effect. The light transmission through cosmetic tinted lenses is usually in the range of 75–85%.

Figure C.35 • Four basic combinations of cosmetic tint.

Selective distribution of a tint across the surface of lenses designed for cosmetic use allows four basic combinations (Figure C.35). The variables are whether or not to leave a 1.5-mm band clear of tint around the lens edge, and whether or not to have a clear pupil. A full tint covering the pupil appears more natural; however, this creates a small but constant tinting effect on vision. A clear pupil eliminates the visual effect but introduces problems of obtaining good alignment and size-matching between the clear pupillary zone of the lens and the natural pupil of the eye, which of course will vary with ambient lighting . Tints that extend to the edge of the lens are cosmetically unsatisfactory because they are visible against the white sclera at the limbus. See *Tinted contact lenses*.

'Cost per wear' (CPW) model for contact lenses
- See *Pricing of contact lenses*.

Cost to patient, contact lens
- See *Pricing of contact lenses*.

Costume contact lenses
- See *Theatric tinted contact lenses*.

Cover test
The cover test (or cover-uncover test) is an objective dissociation test to determine the presence of a

heterophoria or heterotropia. The practitioner makes a judgement on the behaviour of the eyes whilst the patient fixates a target at a predetermined distance and each eye is covered and uncovered in turn. Practitioners typically estimate the magnitude of any movement with a cover test, and hence the amount of heterophoria present. Checking the approximate amount of movement is easy. At 6m the 6/12 Snellen line is approximately 12cm long. Looking from one end to the other will give the approximate movement of 2^Δ. While estimations are useful, practitioners should beware since it has been shown that cover tests give under-estimations of results, especially at near, by as much as 11^Δ of exophoria and 13^Δ of esophoria. Ten useful tips on the cover–uncover test are:

- Ensure the patient looks at a letter size slightly larger than the letter representing the threshold acuity to ensure that fixation is easily maintained.
- Distance testing is recommended at 6m but if intermittent divergent strabismus for distance is suspected, it is better to test at 20m. Near testing is performed at either 30cm or 40cm. Ideally, the test should be conducted at the habitual near working distance of the patient.
- Make sure the illumination level in the room is high and that the patient's face is well lit (but not so bright as to cause glare or discomfort).
- Remove the cover vertically.
- Hold the cover in place long enough to get a good result. Some authorities suggest one second, some two seconds. Recent research suggests that four to five seconds may be required for optimum performance of the test. It has been suggested that the speed of recovery movements are good predictors of symptoms but that the number of movements are not.
- If amblyopia is suspected, take a little longer before removing the cover, as the amblyopic eye takes longer to take up fixation.
- Do not assume there is no strabismus if you see no movement. There could be a microtropia with abnormal retinal correspondence so consider a 4^Δ suppression test and the Bagolini lens test.
- Use the alternating cover test if you are unsure of the direction of movement and to see how easily the binocularity breaks down. There should be no difference in the amplitude of the heterophorias in each eye for normal subjects.
- When the patient will not pay attention, consider using multiple targets a few centimetres apart and watch for a versional movement to re-fixate.
- Do not use additive prisms with their bases in the same direction to measure the heterophoria or strabismus angle. They do not add arithmetically; for example, adding a 40^Δ and 5^Δ prism gives 58^Δ.

Repeating a cover test will inevitably interfere with fusion and increase the risk of binocular breakdown. This will exaggerate the amplitude of heterophoria or heterotropia measured. The least number of attempts at measuring will yield the most accurate results. A useful tool for assessing what goes on under the cover is an opaque occluder. It allows the observer to see the eye

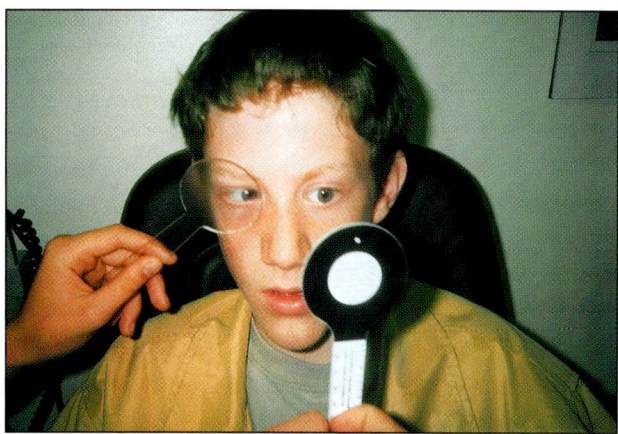

Figure C.36 • Semi-opaque occluder.

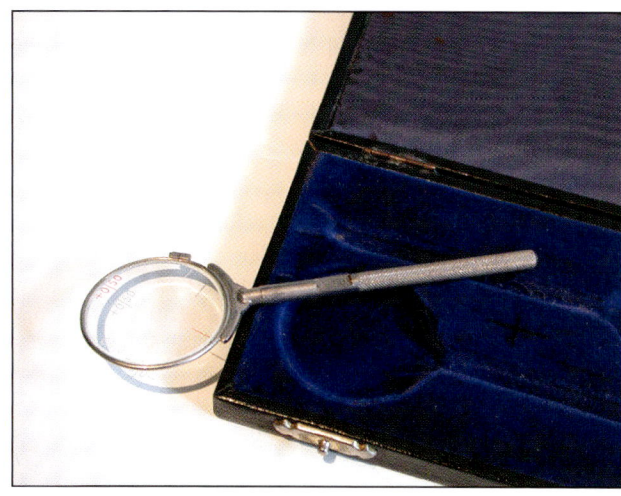

Figure C.37 • Jackson cross cylinder.

being occluded but prevents the patient from seeing more than 6/60 equivalent and thus suspending normal binocular vision almost as if the occluder was opaque (Figure C.36).

Crazing, contact lens

- See *Surface damage, contact lens*.

Cross-cylinder technique

The Jackson cross-cylinder (JCC) technique is the most common method of determining the astigmatic component of a refractive error. The cross-cylinder lens has a positive cylinder worked onto one surface with an equal power negative cylinder on the opposite side at ninety degrees to the first. The axes are marked (usually with a red dash for the negative axis, black for the positive) and the lens is held in a housing with a handle orientated along a line at 45 degrees to the two perpendicular axes (Figure C.37).

The lens most commonly used is a ±0.25D lens (which is the equivalent therefore of a +0.25D sphere with a –0.50D cylinder); this lens generally allows the patient to notice appreciable differences in target quality when held in different positions before an eye with reasonable acuity (6/12 or better). For reduced levels of acuity, however, ±0.50D and ±1.00D lenses are available.

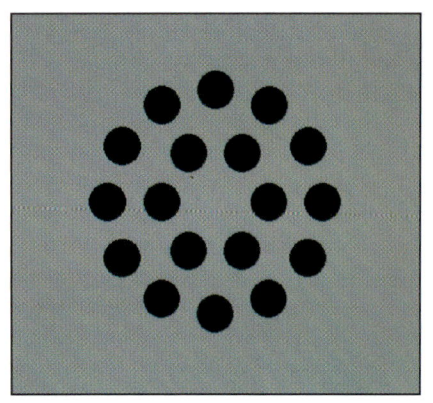

Figure C.38 • Suitable visual target of dots for performing the cross-cylinder technique.

Having established the best sphere, the patient should be directed to look at a target, preferably circular or an array of dots (Figure C.38), which should be large enough to be seen by the patient.

The first step is to establish or confirm the axis of the cylinder in the patient's refractive error. Where no cylinder has yet been established, the JCC should be held before the best sphere with the axes at 90 degrees and 180 degrees; the handle of the cross cylinder is then rolled between the thumb and forefinger so that the cross cylinder lens rotates, effectively transposing the positions of the cylinder axes. The patient is asked in which position ("one or two") the target appears clearer. This is then repeated with the axes at 45 and 135 degrees. If there is no difference in the target quality between these four presentations, it may be assumed that there is no cylinder present.

A negative cylinder should then be introduced with its axis between the two negative JCC axis positions where the clearer target was seen. For example, if the target is clearest when the negative JCC axis is at 90 and 135 degrees, the lens introduced should have its axis somewhere between these two values. The axis may then be modified by lining the handle of the JCC with the axis of the trial cylinder lens such that the positive and negative JCC axes are 45 degrees either side of it. The JCC is then flipped and the trial lens axis rotated in the direction of the negative JCC axis where the better image was found. The amount of rotation is dependent upon the degree of difference in image quality between the two positions. If, for example, the image is much clearer in the first presentation to when the JCC is flipped over, then the trial cylinder should be rotated by 10 or 15 degrees towards the position of the JCC negative axis in the first presentation, but rotated less for more ambiguous responses. This is repeated until there is no reported difference between the images for the two presentations. The axis may be checked by repeating the exercise after deliberately rotating the trial lens axis away from the value established to hopefully arrive at the same result. In cases of patient uncertainty with a range of trial lens orientations eliciting no clear response from the patient, then exaggerated movement away from the objective refraction result should be introduced to 'force' a response; the final selected axis will be halfway between the two extreme points (a technique described as 'bracketing').

Having established the axis, the cylinder power is found by aligning the positive then negative JCC axes over that of the trial lens and finding which offers the clearer image. The trial lens should then be adjusted to reflect the better image position (e.g. increasing by +0.25D if the image was better when the positive JCC axis was over the trial lens axis) until a point is reached when neither the plus nor minus JCC axis results in a preference. If the trial cylinder is changed by 0.75D or more, then the sphere needs to be adjusted by half this amount but in the opposite sign in order to maintain the circle of least confusion upon (or just behind) the retina. Large cylinder changes should also always be followed by a second check of the best vision sphere.

Culture-negative peripheral ulcer (CNPU)
- See *Contact lens peripheral ulcer.*

Cycloplegics

A cycloplegic is a drug that is used to paralyze the ciliary muscle which results in a loss of accommodation and its action is accompanied by mydriasis. Cycloplegics are most commonly used as an aid in refraction to disclose latent hyperopia and their use is mandatory at the first examination of a child presenting with concomitant esotropia in order to establish to what extent it is accommodative in origin.

Cycloplegics are also used as adjunctive therapy in the treatment of anterior uveitis or bacterial keratitis. By relaxing the ciliary body and immobilizing the iris, cycloplegics alleviate the patient's discomfort and also help to prevent posterior synechiae.

Cycloplegia results in the blocking of muscarinic receptors that are normally stimulated by the release of acetylcholine from the nerve endings of the parasympathetic system. Drugs having this mode of action are known as antimuscarinics, anticholinergics, cholinergic antagonists, muscarinic antagonists, parasympathetic antagonists or parasympatholytics. Since the pupil sphincter muscle is also innervated by the parasympathetic system, mydriasis invariably occurs with cycloplegia.

Indications for cycloplegic refraction include the following:

- Children with constant or intermittent esotropia on their initial presentation and sometimes subsequently
- Children and young adults with asthenopia and esophoria, especially when a latent refractive error is suspected
- When retinoscopy suggests that accommodation is fluctuating significantly
- When retinoscopy findings differ significantly from the results of subjective refraction
- In cases of anomalies of accommodation such as accommodative insufficiency, accommodative fatigue, accommodative inertia and spasm of accommodation
- In cases where retinoscopy along the visual axis is difficult due to lack of patient co-operation or intellectual handicap
- Candidates for refractive surgery.

Since it is most unlikely that cycloplegia will be necessary in presbyopic adults, the usual contraindications in respect of the concomitant mydriasis are unlikely to apply, with the principal exception of an abnormally shallow

Table C.18 • Comparative performance of cycloplegics commonly used in refraction.

Cycloplegic	Time to maximum cycloplegia after instillation of drops	Duration of cycloplegia	Residual amplitude of accommodation (D.)
Atropine 1%	36 h	Up to 7 days	Nil
Cyclopentolate 0.5%	60 min	24 h	1.00
Tropicamide 1%	30 min	6 h	2.00

anterior chamber. Cycloplegia is contraindicated where there is dislocation or subluxation of the crystalline lens.

Preservative-free single dose drops are the most convenient and appropriate presentation for use in optometric practice and the drugs available in this form are:

- Cyclopentolate hydrochloride – this is an anticholinergic and is the drug of first choice for the cycloplegic examination of children. Up to the age of 12 years, one drop of the 1% solution is sufficient but if the amplitude of accommodation has not reduced adequately after 15 minutes, a further drop can be instilled. The 0.5% concentration may be sufficient for children with very light iris pigmentation. Above the age of 12 years, one drop of the 0.5% solution is used and repeated after 15 to 20 minutes if there has been no significant reduction in the amplitude of accommodation. Dark iris pigmentation necessitates the use of the 1% solution. With either concentration, retinoscopy is performed when the cylcoplegia is maximal, which is usually 40 to 60 minutes after instillation of the drops. Due to individual variation in the time required to achieve maximum cycloplegia, the amplitude of accommodation should be monitored at intervals or dynamic retinoscopy used to establish the accommodative state. Residual accommodation with cyclopentolate is about one dioptre.
- Tropicamide (bistropamide) – this is used at 0.5% as a mydriatic and at 1% as a cycloplegic. For the latter purpose, two drops are instilled with a five-minute interval between each one. In general, tropicamide is unsatisfactory for use with children and its relatively short duration of action makes it more convenient for young adults.
- Atropine 1% – although this can provide the most effective cycloplegia with no residual amplitude of accommodation, it is rarely used in optometric practice due to (a) the length of time required to achieve its maximal effect, (b) the long duration of cycloplegia, and (c) the greater risk of ocular and systemic adverse reactions.

The comparative performance of cycloplegics commonly used in refraction is shown in Table C.18.

The following precautions should be observed when using cycloplegics during refraction:

- Explain to the patient or parent the reason for undertaking a cycloplegic examination.
- Patients or parents should be forewarned that photophobia is likely and that it can be alleviated by wearing sunglasses and/or a broad-brimmed hat. They

Table C.19 • Cycloplegics: unpreserved single dose preparations.

Non-proprietary name	Proprietary name	Formulation
Atropine sulphate	Minims® Atropine Sulphate	Drops 1%
Cyclopentolate hydrochloride	Minims® Cyclopentolate Hydrochloride	Drops 0.5% or 1%
Tropicamide	Minims® Tropicamide	Drops 1%

should also be warned that near vision, and possibly distance vision, will be blurred. Adults should also be told that riding a motorcycle or driving a car should be avoided.

- Anterior chamber depth should be evaluated and cycloplegia avoided, or undertaken with extreme care, in patients with narrow angles.
- Ask whether the patient has previously undergone cycloplegia and whether there was any adverse reaction to the drug used.
- Issue a note which identifies the cycloplegic used and provides advice on what action the patient should take in the event of an adverse reaction.

Other cycloplegics that are not used in optometric practice include homatropine, lachesine and hyoscine.

A method of amblyopia treatment known as pharmacological penalization employs atropine cycloplegia of the fixing eye of strabismic infants and children in order to promote the use of the amblyopic eye in near vision. Loss of visual acuity in the good eye has been reported because of non-compliance with this treatment regime.

Examples of cycloplegics are shown in Table C.19.

Cycloplegic refraction

Refraction, both objective and subjective, may be carried out after the suspension of accommodation with a cycloplegic drug, such as cyclopentolate, atropine or tropicamide. Some suggest that a cycloplegic examination should be carried out on all new child patients. However, it is possible to highlight certain groups of children on whom a cycloplegic refraction is essential: those in whom a satisfactory standard of acuity or stereopsis is not demonstrated; those who present with a manifest squint, particularly an esotropia or where an esophoria appears significant or unstable; those with a family history of squint, amblyopia or high hypermetropia; those in whom pseudomyopia is suspected; those who have anisometropia of greater than 1D; and those in whom poor accommodation is found. A cycloplegic agent also may be used as an aid to refraction for a patient who shows poor co-operation during a standard routine refraction.

Cycloplegic refraction reveals latent hypermetropia, aids fundus examination and makes accurate fixation for static retinoscopy is less crucial. Disadvantages of using a cycloplegic drug include photophobia due to dilated pupils, decreased ability in close work tasks after the examination due to paralysis of accommodation, distress to the patient on instillation of drops, and a risk of adverse and allergic reactions (particularly with atropine). The dilation also introduces increased spherical aberration so it should be remembered that often the best acuity achieved during a cycloplegic refraction will not be as good as during the non-cycloplegic state.

Following a refraction with atropine, the final correction may need to be adjusted to take into account the natural tonus of the ciliary muscle. When cyclopentolate has been used, the full correction found under cycloplegia should be prescribed where there is an esophoric state or where adaptation to the full plus correction is not an important consideration.

Cylindrical ophthalmic lens

The simplest astigmatic lens form is the 'cylindrical' lens. Note that the spherical radius of curvature of the lens is the same for all sections perpendicular to the axis of symmetry, and that along the axis of symmetry the thickness is constant (Figure C.39). Cylindrical lenses can also be produced in negative form (Figure C.40).

A cylindrical lens will produce a line image from a point object, the line being parallel to the axis of symmetry. Object and image positions can be found by using the same equations as for spherical surfaces and lenses. Although plane cylindrical lenses as described can be used in spectacles, it is more common to use a cylindrical surface in combination with a spherical surface, in order to provide a sphero-cylindrical lens. A lens with purely cylindrical power would be described as, for example, –6.00DC (Dioptres Cylindrical) in order to differentiate from the spherical case which would be described as –6.00DS (Dioptres Spherical).

Because cylindrical surfaces are not rotationally symmetrical about the mid-point, a notation is required for their positioning in front of the eye. This is achieved by specifying the angle between the axis of symmetry of the cylinder (which is always simply referred to as the 'axis') and the horizontal. The universally used 'standard' axis notation uses a protractor that reads anti-clockwise when looking at the face of a lens wearer (Figure C.41). Angles up to 180° are used for the axes of cylinders, the full 360° protractor only being required for the base direction of prisms. When describing a horizontal cylinder axis, it is conventional to use the angle 180, rather than zero. Note that degree signs are not used when writing the specification of cylinder axes.

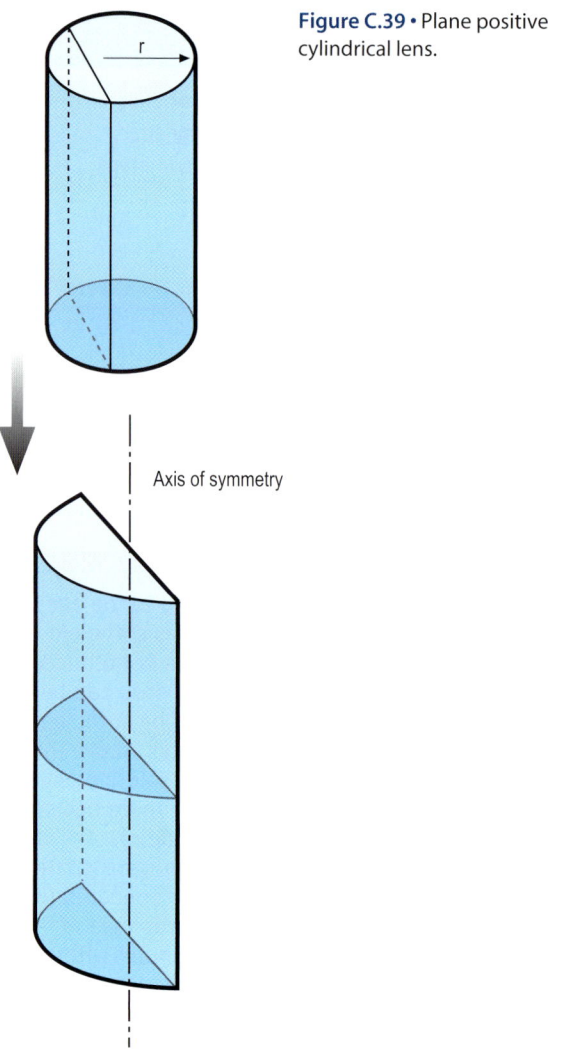

Figure C.39 • Plane positive cylindrical lens.

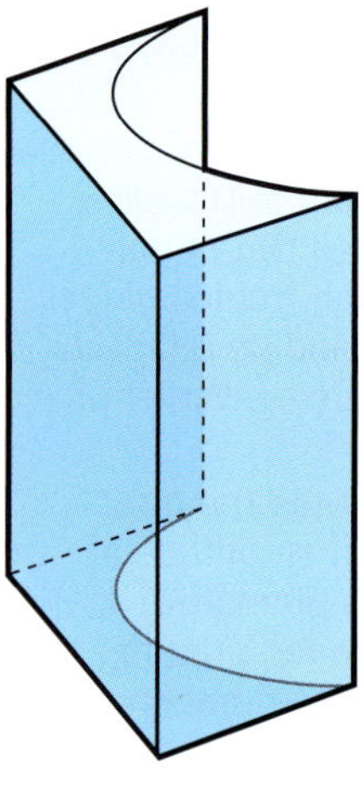

Figure C.40 • Plane negative cylindrical lens.

From Figure C.39 it should be apparent that the curvature of a cylindrical surface of radius r is at a maximum perpendicular to the axis of symmetry, and a minimum (with infinite radius) parallel to the axis. Thus if a surface of radius +100mm is worked on material of refractive index 1.5, then the surface power will vary from zero along the axis, to a maximum of:

$$F = 1000(n-1)/r = 500/100 = +5.00D$$

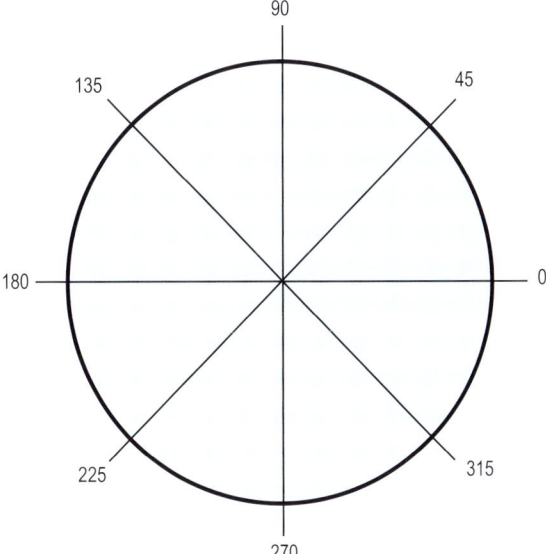

Figure C.41 • Standard axis notation.

Indeed the maxima and the minima will be the only two powers that can be optically resolved.

Cylindrical power equivalent rigid toric contact lenses

All types of rigid toric lenses (apart from compensated rigid bitoric lenses) come under this classification, and the unifying feature that these lenses have in common is that they incorporate a correction for residual astigmatism. This type of lens can be further categorized as follows:

- Alignment bitoric lenses (also known as parallel bitoric lenses). Both the front and back surfaces are toroidal. The front surface incorporates correction for residual astigmatism as well as for the induced astigmatism. In addition, the axes of the spectacle refraction over the lens correspond with the principal meridians of corneal curvature, so the correction for the residual astigmatism will be along one of the principal meridians of the lens (hence the name 'alignment bitoric'). As such, the use of the term 'alignment bitoric' here should not be confused with alignment in regard to lens fitting.
- Back surface toric lenses. These lenses have a toroidal back surface but a spherical front surface. The design principle is similar to that for alignment bitoric lenses. As with alignment bitoric lenses, the front surface incorporates correction for residual astigmatism as well as for the induced astigmatism, and the axes of the spectacle refraction over the lens correspond with the principal meridians of corneal curvature, so the correction for the residual astigmatism is along one of the principal meridians of the lens. In the case of a back surface toric lens, however, the correction for the residual astigmatism is equal and opposite to the correction for the induced astigmatism. Hence, the two required cylindrical corrections cancel each other out, meaning that the front surface can be left spherical. Very occasionally, a case of induced and residual astigmatism cancelling out one another is encountered in practice. A back surface toric design is only possible if the correction for the residual astigmatism is equal and opposite to the correction for the induced astigmatism. A back surface toric design is therefore only worth considering if the ocular astigmatism of the patient is greater than the corneal astigmatism. The residual astigmatism must also be of a magnitude such that it will be neutralized by the resultant induced astigmatism. The likelihood of both of these requirements being met is low, so only in a small percentage of cases will a back surface toric design be appropriate. Indeed, in most cases the induced astigmatism usually exaggerates the effect of the residual astigmatism.
- Front surface toric lenses. Residual astigmatism frequently needs to be corrected in cases where the patient is fitted well, physically, with a lens utilizing a spherical back optic zone. Such a lens therefore requires a toroidal front surface, but lens rotation must be avoided, otherwise visual disturbance will result. When the corneal astigmatism is less than 2.00D a toric back surface will not generally prevent lens rotation, and so other forms of lens stabilization, such as prism ballast or truncation, are required.
- Oblique bitoric lenses. As with alignment bitoric lenses, oblique bitoric lenses have toroidal front and back surfaces. With oblique bitoric lenses, however, the principal meridians of the toroidal back and front surfaces are not parallel, due to a difference between the axes of the spectacle refraction and the principal meridians of corneal curvature. The specification and manufacture of these types of lenses is very difficult. One solution is to use a fitting set of lenses, all of which have a toroidal back optic zone and a spherical front surface. A refraction is performed over the appropriate trial lens and then the oblique cylinder obtained from this refraction is incorporated onto the front surface of the lens. These lenses are rarely prescribed. See *Compensated rigid bitoric lenses; Induced astigmatism with rigid toric lenses; Residual astigmatism with rigid toric lenses; Stabilization of rigid toric lenses; Toric lens design, rigid; Toric lens, rigid*.

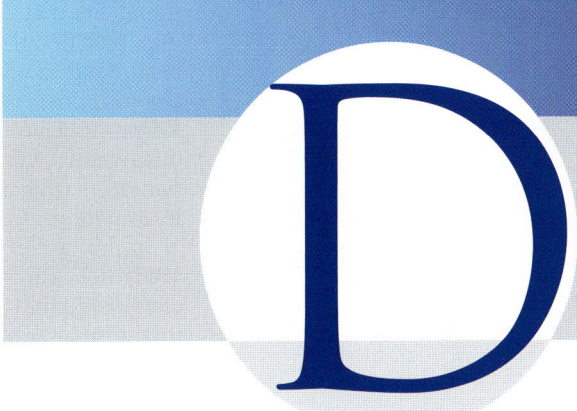

Daily disposable contact lenses

Daily disposable lenses are one of the two versions of true, single-use only, disposable lenses, the other being disposable extended wear lenses. Three brands of daily disposable lenses were launched into major contact lens markets from the mid-1990s. These three brands are known today as Soflens 1 day (Bausch & Lomb), Focus Dailies (CIBA Vision) and 1 Day Acuvue (Johnson and Johnson). Unlike monthly replacement lenses, which tend to be worn on most days, daily disposable lenses tend to be worn on a part-time basis (Figure D.1).

The clinical benefits of daily disposable lenses include fewer symptoms, fewer deposits, better vision, better comfort, fewer tarsal abnormalities, fewer ocular complications, and better overall satisfaction compared with conventional lenses. The obvious advantage offered by daily lens disposal is a fresh, sterile pair of lenses for wear each day. If cost and parameter availability were not limiting factors, then it could be argued that all daily-wear soft lens patients should be using this modality. The expansion of available parameters and lens types continues as signalled by the launch of daily disposable lenses for astigmatism and daily disposable multifocal lenses for presbyopic patients.

Specific advantages of daily disposable lenses from the standpoint of the practitioner include the following:

- less patient education time is required; virtually no advice needs to be given about lens care
- the absence of a lens storage case from the regime is beneficial, given the role that a lens case can play in the development of ocular infection
- less professional 'chair time' is required because there are no problems relating to lens care solutions (e.g. toxicity or sensitivity reactions) or to patient non-compliance with use of solutions
- less ancillary staff time is required because there is no need for discussions and sales relating to lens care products
- there are no disputes concerning wearing frequency (e.g. some patients might argue that a lens designed for monthly replacement, but only worn once a week, can last for 3 months)
- daily disposability is more hygienic for intermittent wearers, as long-term storage problems are eliminated (making daily disposability the replacement modality of choice for such patients).

Advantages of daily disposable lenses from the perspective of the patient include:

- there is no need to be concerned with lens care systems (although it is desirable for daily disposable lens wearers to have a supply of sterile saline

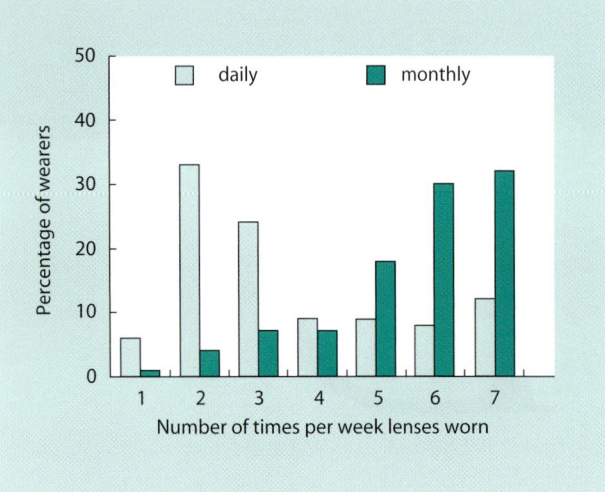

Figure D.1 • Number of times per week patients wear monthly- versus daily-replacement lenses.

or multipurpose solution for lens rinsing if there is discomfort during, or soon after, lens insertion)
- there are no anxieties about lost or damaged lenses
- daily disposable lenses are convenient and compact for travel; there is no need to carry bulky lens care solutions
- daily disposable lenses are highly cost effective in that lens wear is directly linked to lens cost (unlike, say, a monthly disposable lens that may, for example, only be worn five times during the month)
- daily disposable lenses are excellent for monovision correction of presbyopia, as it is easy to alternate between various lens combinations (e.g. two distance lenses versus monovision, depending on the need)
- daily disposable lenses are easy to discard ('any time, any place, without a case')
- compliance is easier because there are fewer instructions to remember.

Daltonism
- See *Colour vision deficiency*.

Data Protection Acts 1984 and 1998 (UK)

The increasing use of computers to hold personal data led to the introduction of the Data Protection Act in 1984. The Act gave new rights to people to enable them to view information about themselves, challenge it if appropriate, and in certain circumstances, claim compensation. The order was enacted for health records SI 1987/1093 Data Protection (Subject Access Modification) (Health) Order in November 1987. Subsequently these rights were extended to hard copy records by the 1998 Act.

The following are allowed access to personal data held on computer:
- The person directly involved (data subject).
- A person authorized by the data subject.
- A person authorized to act on behalf of the data subject.
- A person having a power of attorney.

On making a written request and payment of a fee, any of the above may be supplied with a copy of any personal data held about a data subject. Any such request must be responded to within 40 days and failure to do so entitles the applicant to complain to the Data Protection Registrar. The information may be supplied as a print-out, written text or typed and should have any accompanying explanations that are required to understand the information.

In the case of health care records held on computer SI 1987/1093 allows for modified access to data where it is considered that disclosure is likely to cause serious harm to the physical or mental health of the data subject or another person or where disclosure of data could lead to identification of another individual other than a health professional involved in the health of the patient.

A register of data users complying with this Act (and it is a criminal offence not to be registered unless you are in one of the exemption groups) is held by the Data Protection Registrar's Office. The entry in the Registrar contains the data user's name and address together with:
- Description of the personal details which the data user holds.
- Outline of the purposes for which the data are to be used.
- Data sources.
- To whom the data may be disclosed.
- Any overseas countries or territories to which the data user may wish to transfer the data.

The Registrar can refuse registration should the information given prove inadequate but once registered the data user commits a criminal offence if they knowingly:
- Hold personal data not described in the Register entry.
- Hold or use personal data for purposes other than described in the Register entry.
- Obtain personal data or information to be placed in personal data from a source not described in the Register entry.
- Disclose personal data to a person not described in the Register entry unless covered by a non-disclosure exemption.
- Transfer personal data to an overseas country or territory not described in the Register entry.

Any optometrist keeping patient records or other personal details on computer is likely to require registration with the Data Protection Registrar.

Daylight factor

The extent to which daylight is available at a point inside a room is normally expressed as the 'daylight factor'. This is the illuminance received at a point on a plane in an interior expressed as a percentage of the illuminance outdoors:

$$\text{Daylight factor} = \frac{\text{daylight illuminance at point within room} \times 100\%}{\text{Simultaneous illuminance on a horizontal plane outside from an unobstructed sky}}$$

Table D.1 • Symptoms of decompensated heterophoria.
1. Blurred vision
2. Double vision
3. Distorted vision
4. Difficulty with stereopsis
5. Monocular comfort
6. Difficulty changing focus
7. Headache
8. Sore, tired, aching eyes
9. General irritation

When the average daylight factor is 5% or more, the interior will appear to be well lit, and it should be sufficient for most of the day. If the average daylight factor is between 2 and 5%, then it may be worthwhile to consider using artificial light in addition to the available daylight. When the daylight factor falls below the expected value, supplementary lighting can be used. For values of less than 2%, the interior will be poorly lit and artificial light sources will be required nearly all the time.

Decompensation

Heterophoria can be classified according to whether it is compensated or not. Decompensation occurs when the vergence eye movement system fails to adequately overcome a heterophoria. In practical terms, most clinicians seem to use the term *decompensated* when they consider that the heterophoria requires treatment.

Decompensated heterophoria is sometimes defined as a symptomatic heterophoria. Yet there are rare occasions when a heterophoria might require treatment even if it is not producing symptoms. For example, foveal suppression may exist as a sensory adaptation to heterophoria. In young patients, this, or an enlargement of Panum's fusional areas, might represent an intermediate stage in the development of strabismus (microtropia) and hence treatment may be appropriate, even in the absence of symptoms. Typical symptoms of decompensated heterophoria are listed in Table D.1.

An alternative definition of decompensated heterophoria is a heterophoria that produces clinical signs during a particular clinical test. An obvious problem with this interpretation of the term is that the meaning will be completely dependent on the test and on the precise test conditions.

Decongestants, ocular

Ocular decongestants are essentially weak concentrations of sympathomimetic or α-adrenergic agonists that can be used on an occasional basis for the temporary relief of acute conjunctival hyperaemia caused by minor irritation. A number of these products are available over-the-counter so that cosmetic improvement can be obtained by self-treatment following exposure to an environment that was either polluted by dust, fumes, etc. or simply irritating (e.g. exposure to wind while cycling or swimming pool). Excessive use of a decongestant over a long period can diminish its vasoconstrictive effect resulting in a reactive or rebound hyperaemia.

When examining a patient, it is essential that any self-prescribed use of a decongestant be elicited in the case history so that an appropriate allowance can be made when examining the eyes. It is also necessary to establish what problems prompted the use of these eye drops. Notwithstanding their minimal mydriatic effect, decongestants are considered to be contraindicated in patients with narrow angle glaucoma.

A decongestant should not be used to treat contact lens complications such as the conjunctival hyperaemia in the horizontal meridian that accompanies '3 and 9 o'clock' staining in wearers of rigid contact lenses. Since almost all formulations of decongestants are preserved with benzalkonium chloride, hydrogel contact lenses should not be inserted until at least 15 minutes after instillation of the drops. Historically, adrenaline tartrate or hydochloride 0.1% was instilled in order to constrict conjunctival vessels prior to taking an eye impression in the fitting of moulded scleral contact lenses. This practice, which was of doubtful benefit, is no longer considered to be necessary and more stable drugs have superseded adrenaline.

The principal decongestants are:

- Phenylephrine hydrochloride 0.12% combined with hypromellose 0.5% – this is available as multidose drops that are preserved with benzethonium chloride for use as an ocular lubricant. See *Artificial tears*. Slight mydriasis may occur in patients with light coloured irides.
- Naphazoline, as the nitrate or hydrochloride, about 0.01 % (sometimes combined with the astringent, witch hazel 12.5%) – this formulation constitutes the basis of some over-the-counter products. These do not cause any mydriasis.
- Xylometazoline combined with antazoline sulphate 0.5% – this is available as drops that are preserved with benzalkonium chloride and intended for use in allergic conjunctivitis. See *Anti-histamine drugs*. This product can be obtained from a pharmacy as an over-the-counter preparation. Xylometazoline causes very little mydriasis.

Deep stromal opacities, contact lens associated

Apparently benign, deep stromal opacities (DSOs) are occasionally seen in the corneas of contact lens wearers. The opacities have been variously described as being white, grey, brown, blue and cyan in colour, and cloudy, scar-like, lattice-like and stellate in form. They are sometimes associated with folds and striae in Descemet's layer, and with deep stromal neovascularization. It is possible to distinguish DSOs from infiltrates (which typically reside in the anterior half of the stroma) because DSOs are invariably located deep in the stroma (Figure D.2). However, DSOs can take on a similar appearance to certain forms of posterior stromal dystrophy, and some of the reported cases of DSOs may have been confused with dystrophies. The aetiology of this condition is unknown but probably varied.

Defects, contact lens

- See *Quality, soft contact lens*.

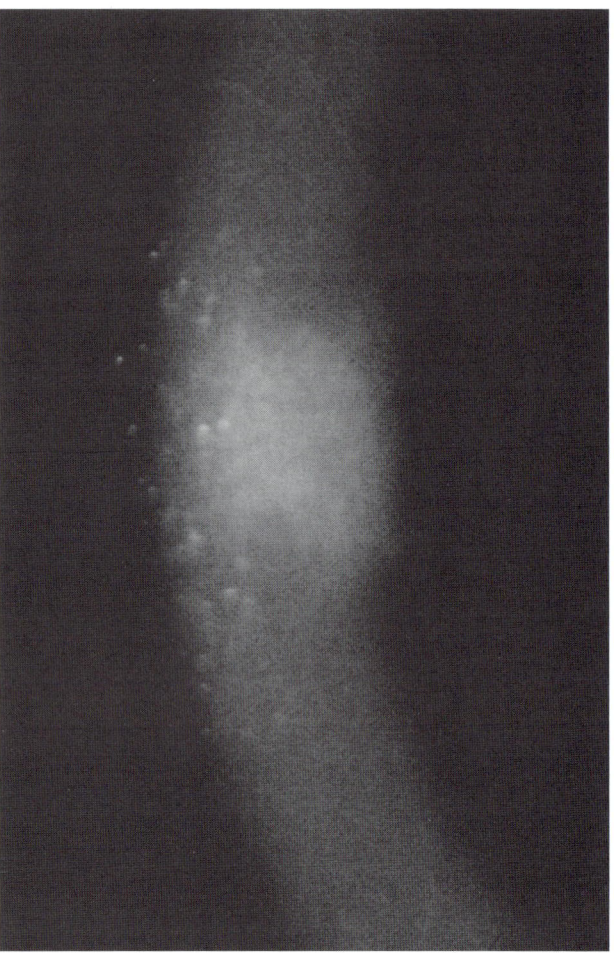

Figure D.2 • Deep stromal opacities.

Degenerations of the corneal epithelium, therapeutic contact lenses for

Conditions such as Salzmann's nodular degeneration, rosacea keratopathy and atopic keratoconjunctivitis (with or without ectasia) can sometimes be so uncomfortable that a therapeutic contact lens is indicated. Such a lens will probably also have visual improvement potential. Concurrent conjunctival disease and tear abnormality may well benefit from the use of a scleral lens. Corneal trauma or surgery that has depleted endothelial functional reserves can lead to epithelial bullous keratopathy, the discomfort of which is often amenable to management with hydrogel lenses. In many cases, a corneal transplant will subsequently provide a cure.

Delivery systems, contact lens

Two main methods for managing the implementation of planned lens replacement systems have evolved; manufacturer-driven and practice-driven systems.

Manufacturer-driven systems are common in the UK. The names of new patients are registered with the manufacturer by the practice, along with relevant prescription details. Depending on the lens type, there may also be an option to select a frequency of lens delivery to the practice; for example, monthly replacement lenses may be supplied to the practice in 3- or 6-month quantities. Once the patient is registered, fresh supplies of lenses will be automatically dispatched to the practice until the manufacturer is advised otherwise by the practice.

Manufacturers have, in some cases, branded their systems to promote the service provided. The main benefit to practices is reduced administration. Simple computer programs run the systems, and the arrival of a new supply of lenses for a given patient acts as a trigger for the practice to recall that particular lens wearer.

In the UK, such systems complement the method by which many patients pay for frequent replacement lenses – namely, monthly direct payment from the bank account of the patient to that of the practice. In this way, both payment and regular lens supply is automated, and compliance with the designated replacement schedule is encouraged.

Some manufacturers have expanded their service to include direct delivery of lenses and possibly lens care products (so-called 'bundling') to the home address of the patient. The increased convenience afforded by this approach is promoted as a means of retaining the custom of the patient for replacement lenses, given the growth of non-practice sources of supply such as direct mail and the Internet.

If a manufacturer-driven system is not employed, an in-house practice-driven system is required to ensure the timely purchase of replacement lenses and recall of patients. With larger patient bases the amount of stock involved can soon become quite large, and adequate storage space is often an issue. On the other hand, bulk purchasing may allow practices to secure preferential terms from suppliers. A practice operating its own system is also in complete control of the process and less vulnerable to any manufacturer supply problems. See *Lens supply routes*.

Denatured protein on contact lenses
- See *Deposits, contact lens*.

Densitometry, contact lens
- See *Specific gravity, rigid contact lens*.

Density, contact lens
- See *Specific gravity, contact lens*.

Deposits, contact lens

The extent of general lens deposition increases over time. Numerous factors, many of which are interactive, are involved in the formation of deposits on the front or back surface of contact lenses. These factors include:

- lens wear modality (daily or continuous wear)
- bulk chemical composition of the lens
- lens water content
- physico-chemical nature of the lens surface (such as ionicity)
- chemical composition of lens maintenance solutions
- adequacy of lens maintenance procedures (a measure of patient compliance)
- hand contamination
- proximity to environmental pollutants
- intrinsic properties of the tears of the patient.

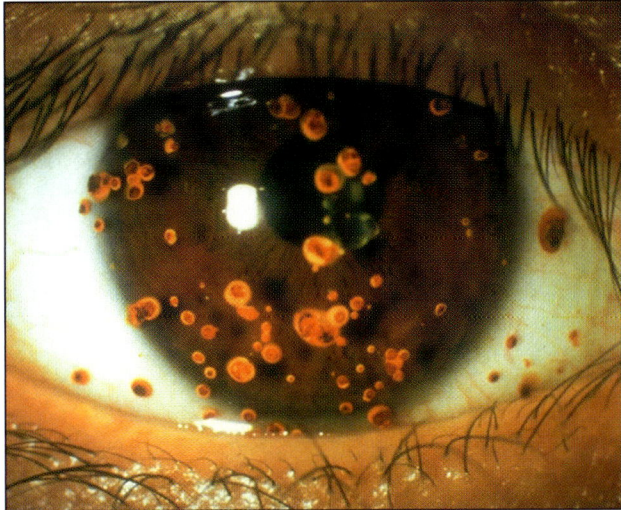

Figure D.3 • Iron deposits on a soft lens worn on a non-replacement basis.

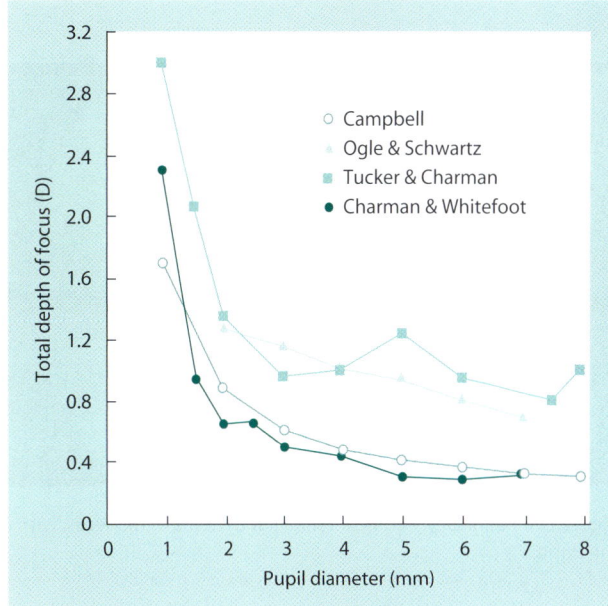

Figure D.4 • Examples of experimental measurements of photopic, total monocular depth-of-focus as a function of pupil diameter.

The most common tear-derived components of lens deposits are proteins, which cannot be detected under normal clinical viewing conditions. A heavy deposition of protein can manifest as a general lens haze on the surface of both soft and rigid lenses, and extensive lipid formation can appear as a clear smear or smudge on the lens surface.

Visible soft lens deposits generally take months or years to form, and are thus only encountered in patients wearing lenses on a non-planned replacement basis. The most common form of visible deposition derived from the tear film is known as 'jelly bumps' or 'mulberry deposits', which consist of various layered combinations of mucus, lipid, protein and, sometimes, calcium. Barnacle-like calcium carbonate deposits, which are also derived from the tear film, can project anteriorly and be a source of discomfort. Iron deposits, which are derived from exogenous sources, appear as small red-orange spots or rings, and form when iron particles become embedded in the lens and oxidize to form ferrous salts (Figure D.3). These deposits were often seen in patients who did not replace lenses regularly and who frequently commuted on trains or trams, as there is a high probability of fine iron particles (which are thrown into the air as the vehicle moves along the steel tracks) coming to rest on the lens surface. Deposits such as those described above are rarely seen on rigid lenses because of the inability of contaminants to become embedded in the lens surface.

It is clear that proteins and lipids from the tears can deposit on soft lenses, and to a lesser extent on rigid lenses, within minutes of insertion; however, such deposits are thought to be innocuous over periods of less than 1 month. Lipid is easily removed with surfactant cleaning. A small amount of protein deposition may be beneficial to the eye, as long as it does not become denatured, because the protein forms a natural biocompatible lens coating. Although these rapidly forming deposits can not be seen and do not generally compromise vision or comfort, they can reduce lens surface wettability.

Long-term protein deposition can be problematic because in time it can become denatured and thus no longer be 'recognized' by the eye, leading to an adverse immunological reaction. Lens surface protein can also absorb (and concentrate) preservatives and other active ingredients in contact lens care solutions, which may be released back into the eye in noxious concentrations, leading to toxic reactions. The physical presence of excess deposits can also cause direct mechanical insult to the anterior eye.

Soft lenses can also become discoloured over time. The cause may be intrinsic or extrinsic. High levels of melanin can lead to a brown discoloration; nicotine can become absorbed into the lenses of patients who smoke or spend time in a smoky environment, leading to an orange-brown discoloration; and exposure to mercury can lead to a black/grey discoloration. Extreme lens discoloration can be cosmetically unsightly to an onlooker.

Depth-of-focus

If the retinal image is gradually defocused, its quality will deteriorate due to defocus blur. Nevertheless, there is a finite range of focus over which this blur causes no appreciable deterioration in visual performance; this range is referred to as the 'depth-of-focus'. The precise value of the total depth-of-focus depends on how it is assessed (Figure D.4). For typical photopic pupil diameters of about 4mm, visual performance will remain relatively unaffected provided that the spherical error of focus does not exceed about ±0.25D.

Descemet's membrane
- See *Posterior limiting lamina of the cornea*.

Design, contact lens practice
- See *Layout, contact lens practice*.

Desmosomes
- See *Corneal epithelium*.

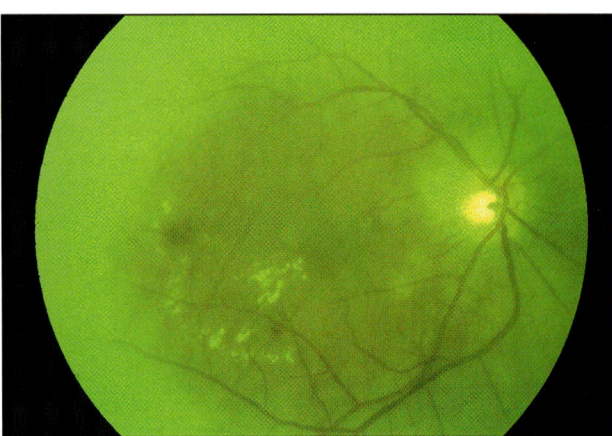 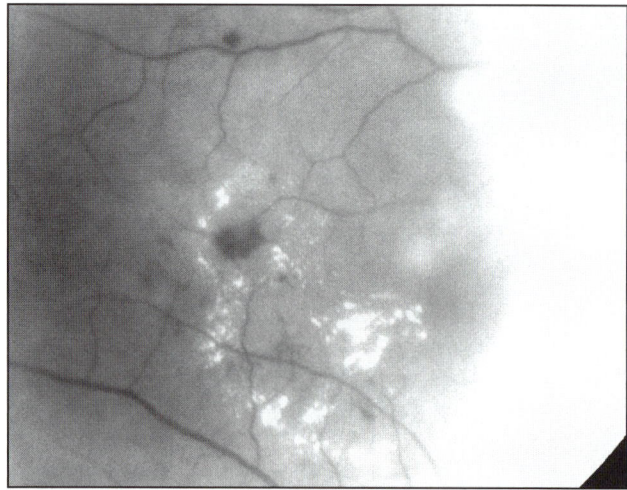

Figure D.5 • Clinically significant macular oedema in diabetes, with red-free view on left and magnified monochrome high contrast view on the right.

Diabetes, contact lenses for

Given the alterations to the anterior segment that accompany diabetes, an important issue to be addressed is whether or not cosmetic contact lenses should be prescribed for diabetic patients. Daily-wear soft contact lenses can be a viable mode of vision correction for patients with diabetes. Practitioners should not expect to see adverse clinical signs in diabetic contact lens wearers that are any different from those seen in non-diabetic lens wearers. If adverse signs are detected in a diabetic lens wearer, they should not be attributed solely to the fact the patient has diabetes. However, the predisposition of the diabetic patient to corneal infection should always be borne in mind.

'Hand grooming' is especially important for the diabetic patient. Roughening of the fingertips caused by home blood–glucose monitoring could lead to damage to the lens surface during cleaning, and patients should therefore be reminded to inspect contact lenses for damage prior to lens insertion. Fingernails should be kept short and smooth to reduce the risk of corneal erosion.

Diabetic retinopathy

Diabetic retinopathy is a microvascular complication of the group of chronic systemic diseases known as diabetes. The elevated blood glucose (hyperglycaemia) adversely affects the wall of the retinal capillaries, leading to increased capillary permeability (leakage), breakdown in the blood–retinal barrier and eventual closure of the retinal or choroidal capillaries. Chronic capillary dysfunction and dropout leads to retinal tissue hypoxia and abnormal new vessels, termed proliferative retinopathy.

Diabetes is commonly classified according to an aetiology, as follows:

- Type 1 or insulin-dependent diabetes mellitus (IDDM) is due to insulin deficiency.
- Type 2 or non-insulin-dependent diabetes mellitus (NIDDM) is due to insulin resistance. These patients may still require insulin treatment, if diet and other medical treatments fail.

There are generally no symptoms in the milder stages of retinopathy. Fluctuations in blood sugar may be associated with transitory increases in myopia and blurring of distance vision due to crystalline lens changes. Blurring of vision may occur in macular oedema (Figure D.5), and significant visual loss or blindness may occur in proliferative retinopathy if untreated.

Pupillary mydriasis and stereoscopic fundus examination are essential for examination. The International Clinical Classification of Diabetic Retinopathy is as follows:

1. No Diabetic Retinopathy: No microaneurysms, haemorrhages, or exudates evident.

2. Non-Proliferative Diabetic Retinopathy (NPDR), also known as 'background retinopathy':

- Minimal NPDR – only microaneurysms are present. These are focal dilations in the retinal capillary wall and appear in the fundus as red dots approximately 100 microns in diameter.
- Mild NPDR – microaneurysms are present as well as occasional 'dot and blot' haemorrhages, or exudates away from the macula.
- Moderate NPDR – microaneurysms are present with some 'dot and blot' haemorrhages or exudates, but no macular oedema. Vision is normal. Occasional signs of retinal hypoxia are present, such as venous beading (VB), cotton wool patches (CWP), and intra-retinal microvascular anomalies (IRMA), but these signs are less severe than in severe NPDR.
- Severe NPDR – extensive microaneurysms, haemorrhages, exudates and vessel changes are evident in all four quadrants; or significant hypoxic signs with VB in at least two quadrants; or IRMA in at least one quadrant (the 4:2:1 rule). Macular oedema and vision loss is likely.

3. Proliferative Diabetic Retinopathy (PDR): Evidenced by any definite neovascularization or vitreous/preretinal haemorrhage. Neovascularization may be either New Vessels on the Disc (NVD) or New Vessels Elsewhere (NVE) in the fundus, iris or anterior chamber. There are usually other fundus changes as in severe non-proliferative retinopathy. In addition, there may be pre-retinal or vitreous haemorrhages and fibrinous strands in the vitreous. Vision is usually affected. If scar tissue

develops due to the neovascularization, it can cause retinal detachment.

4. Macular oedema: Defined as retinal thickening or exudates within two disc diameters of the centre of the macula, arising due to leakage from local capillaries. It is termed Clinically Significant Macular Edema (CSME) if affecting the retina within 0.5 disc diameters or 500 microns of the centre of the macula. Vision may be normal or affected.

Diabetic retinopathy is present in 29% of people with diabetes, and threatens vision in 10%. It is a potentially blinding condition if untreated. Any signs of diabetic retinopathy should be recorded as carefully as possible. In addition, a report should be written to the patient's general medical practitioner and endocrinologist.

Fluorescein angiography can be used diagnostically for demonstrating areas of retinal ischemia or neovascularization. Scanning laser ophthalmoscope testing can allow macular oedema to be quantified. If there is no retinopathy, or minimal non-proliferative retinopathy, then the mainstays of management are regular review and correspondence with the patient's primary care physician. In these circumstances, the review interval may be one or two years. Mild retinopathy may be reviewed with a 6 to 12 month interval, moderate retinopathy every 3 to 6 months and severe retinopathy at least every 3 months.

If macular oedema is present or there is a risk of development, the patient may be asked to report any vision change immediately and be provided with an Amsler grid for home monitoring. If vision becomes reduced, it is important to check the refraction in order to maximize vision. In some instances low vision aids may be required. Tight blood glucose control is effective in minimizing diabetic retinopathy. The patient should be encouraged in this regard, including a healthy diet, reduction in obesity, no smoking, medical therapy and adequate physical exercise.

Prompt laser treatment is indicated for PDR and CSME, and should also be considered for severe NPDR (pre-proliferative). Pan-retinal laser photocoagulation of PDR greatly reduces the risk of severe visual loss. This procedure typically involves the creation of 1200 burns of 500 micron diameter scattered across all quadrants of the peripheral retina, outside the temporal vascular arcades. Focal or grid laser of CSME also reduces the risk of visual loss. This procedure involves the creation of mild laser burns of 100–200 micron diameter on focal areas of macular oedema or in a grid pattern across diffusely thickened areas but remaining at least 500 microns from the macula. Surgical removal of the vitreous (vitrectomy) may benefit patients with severe persistent vitreous haemorrhage or tractional retinal detachment.

Diffuse wide-beam illumination, slit-lamp technique of

A ground-glass filter is placed in the focused light beam of the slit lamp. This will defocus and diffuse the light to give a broad, even illumination over the entire field of view and is generally used to provide low magnification views of the opaque tissues of the anterior segment, including the bulbar conjunctiva, sclera, iris, eyelid margins and the tarsal conjunctiva of the everted lids (Figure D.6).

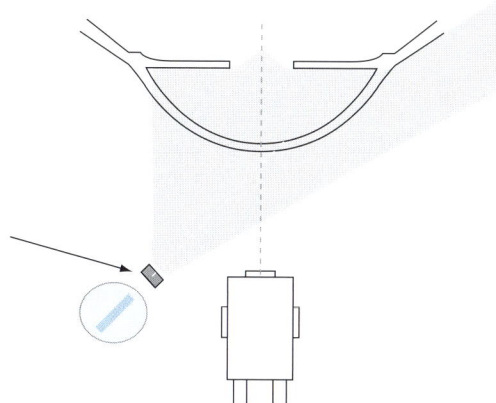

Figure D.6 • Diffuse wide-beam illumination. (Adapted from L.W. Jones, D.A. Jones (2001) Slit lamp biomicroscopy. In: N. Efron (ed.) The Cornea: its Examination in Contact Lens Practice, pp.1–49, Butterworth-Heinemann, Oxford.)

Dimensional stability, rigid contact lens

The ability of a rigid lens to maintain its shape in the presence of deforming forces is referred to as dimensional stability. The problems associated with the use of increasing quantities of siloxymethacrylates to achieve high oxygen permeabilities in rigid lens materials are twofold. First, incompatibility, phase separation and deterioration in mechanical properties – particularly dimensional stability – limit the proportion of such monomers that can be incorporated. Secondly, their use requires the incorporation of hydrophilic monomers containing hydroxyl, carboxyl, amide or lactam groups to improve wettability, and these monomers tend to reduce oxygen permeability and produce low levels of water uptake, which in turn reduces dimensional stability.

In general, rigid lenses of higher oxygen permeabilities tend to suffer from mechanical instability. This manifests clinically as lens flexure (temporary bending) or warpage (permanent bending) whereby, for example, the lens tends to conform to the topography of a toric cornea. Such problems can be overcome by increasing the lens thickness and/or using a material of lower oxygen permeability, but these changes could have an adverse effect on ocular health by restricting corneal oxygenation.

The extent to which a strip of material will either extend or shorten when a force is applied to the material can be predicted from Young's modulus. This is a universally accepted method for quantifying the 'stiffness' of lens materials; a higher Young's modulus indicates a 'stiffer' or less flexible material.

Dimensional stability, soft contact lens

- See *Swell factor, soft lens*.

Diplopia

Diplopia occurs when a patient sees two images of one object. Figure D.7 represents a case of an adult with recent onset left esotropia. The patient is viewing an isolated letter 'A', with no other objects present in the field of view. The letter is imaged on the right fovea (f) but, because the left eye is convergent, it is imaged on a region of the left retina (a), which is not the fovea. The object is imaged on non-

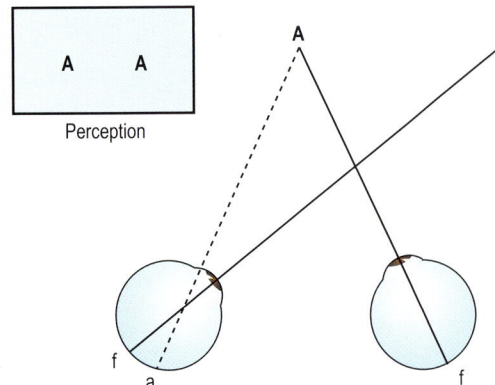

Figure D.7 • Diplopia in left convergent strabismus. From B. Evans, S. Doshi (2001) Binocular Vision and Orthoptics. Butterworth-Heinemann-Optician, Oxford.

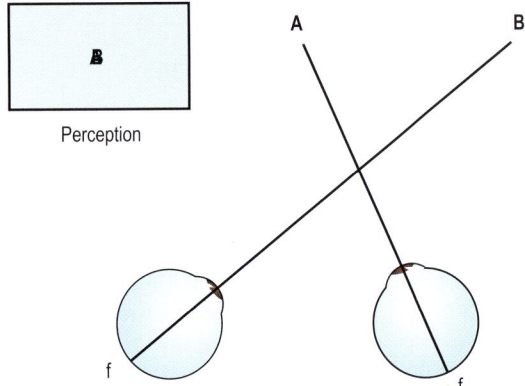

Figure D.8 • Illustration of confusion in left convergent strabismus.

corresponding retinal points. Therefore, it is perceived in two different visual directions, causing diplopia.

Everyday visual scenes are usually much more complicated than that illustrated in Figure D.7. Figure D.8 illustrates the situation, for the same patient, when there are two isolated objects in the visual field. The letter A is imaged on the fovea of the right eye and the letter B is imaged on the fovea of the left eye. If the case is a recent onset strabismus in an adult patient, then the patient is likely to have normal retinal correspondence. This means that both foveae share the same visual direction, so the patient will see the two letters as being superimposed. The visual perception is described as 'confusion'. The diplopia illustrated in Figure D.7 would also be present in the situation illustrated in Figure D.8, so confusion is likely to be accompanied by diplopia. In the unlikely situation in Figure D.7, where there is only one object visible in the field of view, then diplopia alone will occur. But in normal everyday scenes, both diplopia and confusion co-exist. Depending on the magnitude of the separation of the images, diplopia may be more troublesome than confusion.

Patients use the phrase 'double vision' rather more loosely than eyecare professionals. Many different conditions can lead to reports of this symptom and the practitioner needs to follow a logical deductive approach to investigate the cause of diplopia. In particular, a shadowed image is often seen in uncorrected refractive errors (especially astigmatism) and described as 'double vision'.

The investigation of diplopia is a straightforward deductive process, as summarized in Figure D.9. Covering one eye will determine whether the diplopia is monocular or binocular. Monocular diplopia can be due to refractive errors, cataracts, corneal disease, or occasionally retinal disease. Sensory causes of monocular diplopia and polyopia (more than two images) include brain trauma, cerebrovascular accidents, and migraine.

When diplopia is binocular, then orthoptic tests should be used to detect the presence of strabismus, in all positions of gaze. The direction of the diplopia (horizontal, vertical, oblique, torsional) should be determined by questioning the patient. Some authorities argue that torsional diplopia (from cyclotropia) never occurs in isolation but always accompanies vertical or oblique diplopia. By introducing a red filter in front of one eye, or by covering an eye, the practitioner can determine whether any horizontal diplopia is crossed (heteronymous, suggesting an exotropia) or uncrossed (homonymous, suggesting an esotropia). If diplopia occurs after surgery, it should be determined whether it is in accordance with the postoperative deviation or 'paradoxical' (crossed with esotropia and uncrossed with exotropia), in which case there is a persistence of the preoperative sensory adaptation.

Monocular diplopia (seeing two images with one eye) or binocular triplopia (seeing three images with both eyes) can occur through a similar mechanism to paradoxical diplopia because of a persistence of the sensory state preceding a surgical intervention. The strabismic eye sees two images of a fixation point, as a result of competition between the innate normal retinal correspondence and long-standing anomalous retinal correspondence that existed before surgery. During binocular viewing, the normal retinal correspondence in the dominant eye can cause triplopia.

Most cases of strabismus do not have diplopia but have developed binocular sensory adaptations. These adaptations are either harmonious anomalous retinal correspondence (HARC) or suppression. Intractable diplopia suggests that either the patient was unable to develop sensory adaptations (e.g. because they were too old when the strabismus occurred) or that there has been a change in their sensory or motor status.

Rarely, binocular diplopia can result from a change in fixation preference when a previously dominant eye becomes the more myopic, causing a change in ocular dominance. Such cases are resolved by correction of the myopia. A particularly troublesome form of binocular sensory diplopia occurs in non-strabismic patients who have developed a macula or retinal lesion causing metamorphopsia. Bifoveal fusion may be impossible, yet peripheral fusion is likely to be normal.

It is possible that sensory diplopia might also occur as one of the anomalous visual effects accompanying migraine or epilepsy. One theory is that these anomalous visual effects result from hyperexcitability of the visual cortex. Covering one eye halves the sensory input to the visual cortex and thus reduces the probability of such anomalous visual effects. Sensory diplopia from this source could conceivably present as binocular diplopia, which resolves on covering one eye, even though the patient does not have a strabismus.

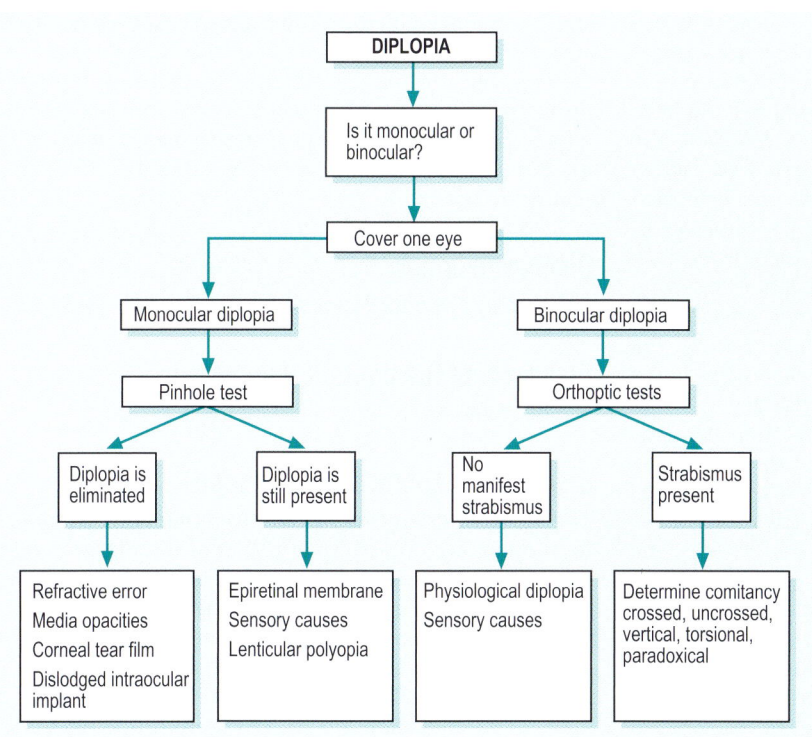

Figure D.9 • Algorithm for investigating diplopia (after von Noorden, 1996).

Direct delivery of contact lenses
- See *Delivery systems, contact lenses*.

Direct focal illumination, slit-lamp technique of
This describes any illumination technique where the slit beam and viewing system are focused coincidentally. The illumination beam is turned up as brightly as possible (ensuring that the patient remains comfortable) and placed at a separation of 40–60° on the side of the microscope corresponding to the same side of the cornea to be viewed. The beam is swept smoothly over the ocular surface and the illumination system moved across to the opposite side as the beam crosses the mid-point of the cornea. Typically a beam width of 2–3mm is chosen initially, and this may be reduced so as to bring more contrast (due to less light scatter) to an area of interest. While scanning the external ocular surface a low-to-medium magnification is initially chosen, and the magnification is increased if any area of interest needs to be examined more closely.

Directorate of Optometric Continuing Education and Training (UK)
The Directorate of Optometric Continuing Education and Training (DOCET) is a committee established at the request of the Department of Health to ensure that funds made available by the Department are used towards meeting the continuing education and training (CET) needs of optometrists. DOCET's aim is to improve the eye health and eye care of the population through CET for optometrists.

DOCET links with the College of Optometrists, which is responsible for the financial budget and training provision policy. DOCET itself has representatives from the various professional bodies, the UK regions and Department of Health, and takes overall responsibility for the programme.

Disability Discrimination Act 1995 (UK)
This Act covers a number of areas including:
- Employment
- Access to goods, facilities and services
- Buying or renting land or property.

Section 21 of this Act is the most relevant to optometrists in practice and lays down requirements to make goods, facilities and services more accessible to disabled people. The intention is to ensure that no person with a disability is discriminated against because of the disability. The regulations require service providers to:
- adopt policies, procedure and practices that make it possible for people with disability to use a service and to overcome physical barriers by providing a service by a reasonable alternative method
- to ensure that there are no physical barriers to prevent a person with disability from accessing services
- to ensure that there are no physical features that make it unreasonable, difficult or impossible for people with disability to use a service.

Disability glare, tests for
When suffering from disability glare, the patient reports that in the presence of high ambient illumination, or a discrete bright source within the visual field, the target appears washed out or faded: the measured acuity for high-contrast letters may remain relatively unchanged, whilst a low-contrast target may disappear completely. In attempting to quantify this phenomenon, no standardized method of measurement has been generally agreed, but the subject is usually required to perform a visual task in

the presence of one or more glare sources. Some tests use controlled (single or multiple) small, bright glare sources at a fixed location relative to the test task, while others use a more extensive glare source surrounding the task. It appears that the former focal sources resemble the conditions of 'night-time' glare experienced when driving towards car headlights, whereas the extended source is more like the high ambient illumination of bright sunny 'day-time', and the luminance of the task itself can be adjusted to simulate these situations even more realistically. Although these different stimuli may help illustrate to patients the practical relevance of the test, there is no evidence to suggest that each would give significantly different results for an individual.

There is reported to be a higher correlation between the measurements of disability glare and everyday functional limitations (e.g. difficulty in night driving), than between 'standard' visual acuity tests and those same disabilities. In driving, detecting pedestrians, the edge of the roadway, or reading signs against a bright sky, sun, or headlights is likely to be difficult if ability to see in the presence of glare is impaired, and it has been suggested that disability glare testing should form a part of the capability assessment of older drivers who may well have minimal lens opacities.

Some of the available tests use a single visual test: e.g. the Miller-Nadler test uses a back-projector to present Landolt rings of variable contrast against a bright background; the Berkeley Glare Test uses low-contrast acuity charts surrounded by a large, bright background; the Vistech MCT 8000 (Vistech Consultants, Dayton, OH, USA) uses sine-wave gratings to measure contrast sensitivity in the presence of either a central or peripheral glare source.

Other tests allow the clinician to choose the specific test task (e.g. high- or low-contrast visual acuity chart, contrast sensitivity). This applies to the OPTEC 3500 Vision Tester (Stereo Optical Co., Chicago, IL, USA) where the central visual target is surrounded by a ring of 10 point sources of variable intensity. The CSV-1000 HGT Halogen Glare Test (Vector Vision, Arcanum, OH, USA) uses a pair of bright lights either side of a test chart to simulate oncoming halogen car headlights as seen at night from 150 feet. Perhaps the most popular device is the MARCO BAT Brightness Acuity Test (Marco Ophthalmic, Jacksonville, FL, USA) which consists of a 60mm hemisphere held up to the eye of the patient with a 12mm aperture through which the visual target can be viewed. The reflective white interior surface of the hemisphere is illuminated by an integral light source which can be adjusted to one of three levels (low = indoor to high = overhead sunlight): normally-sighted individuals should show only minimal decrease in the performance of any visual test at even the highest glare level.

The research team at the Netherlands Ophthalmic Research Institute has adopted a rather different approach in trying to actually measure the amount of light which is scattered within the eye. An annulus (or ring) of flickering light is the glare source, and a small spot inside the annulus is the target. If there is no scatter of light in the eye, the luminance of the target spot remains the same, whether the glare source is on or not. In the presence of scatter, however, the intensity of the target spot increases when the glare source flickers on, so it also appears to flicker. By making the target flicker in counterphase to the glare source (decreasing the target luminance when the glare source comes on), the point at which the target appears to stop flickering occurs when the luminance change is exactly equal to the intra-ocular scatter. See *Glare*.

Discharge lamps
- See *Gas discharge lamps*.

Discharging the contact lens patient
- See *Patient discharge, contact lenses*.

Discomfort, contact lens induced

The most common patient symptom that will be reported to a contact lens practitioner is that of discomfort, and in particular 'dryness'. Reconciliation of patient symptoms with clinical signs is a constant challenge to all health care practitioners. There is always the potential to devote undue attention to a complaint that bears little significance to the wellbeing of the patient, or conversely to give token consideration to a symptom arising from a potentially serious condition. Furthermore, there are many signs that the clinician detects that will also have a major influence upon patient management, but for which the patient shows no or minimal symptoms. Conditions that may be asymptomatic, such as corneal neovascularization, microcystic oedema and endothelial polymegethism, are important pathophysiologic signs that require some form of management. However, the most rewarding management plans, from the perspective of the patient, are those that alleviate discomfort.

During adaptation to contact lens wear, soft lenses offer a greater level of comfort than rigid lenses. Both soft and rigid lenses are very comfortable once the patient has become adapted to lens wear, but nonetheless occasions will arise when lenses become less comfortable. The neural mechanisms by which the conjunctiva and cornea produce ocular sensibilities during contact lens wear have yet to be elucidated. Certainly, these mechanisms are somewhat imprecise. For example, ocular sensibilities are often poorly differentiated, such that the description and localization of an abnormal event in the eye by a patient is often inaccurate. It is therefore not surprising that patient reports of ocular sensations can be confusing to the practitioner. In the absence of major anomalies of the lens or eye, the comfort of the lens appears to depend upon the interaction between the lid and the lens.

The exact nature of the stimulus that gives rise to the sensation of dryness is also unclear, and the reasons for the high frequency of this symptom in contact lens wearers are a matter for speculation, given that it is the least frequently reported symptom of non-lens wearers. Since there are no specific 'dryness receptors' in human tissue, the ocular sensation of dryness must be a response to specific coding of afferent neural inputs. One may hypothesize that dryness results from an interference with tear physiology and structure by the contact lens, the particular mechanism being an increased tear evaporation and faster break-up of the tear film. The sensation may

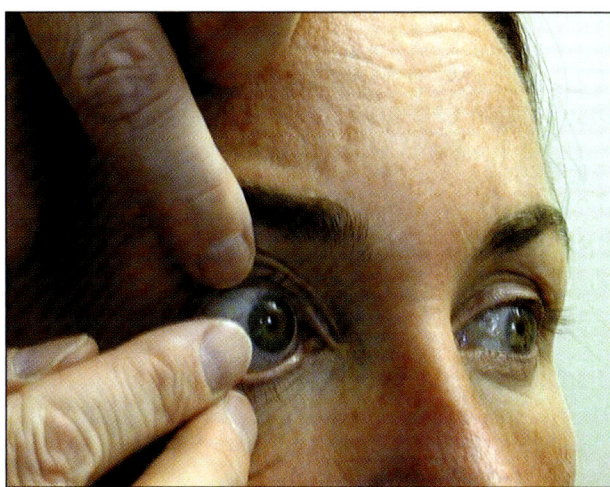

Figure D.10 • Displacing a soft lens to dislodge a foreign body.

also arise from the neural misinterpretation of stimuli seemingly unrelated to dryness, such as direct mechanical interaction of the lens with the ocular tissues, lens dehydration, or vasodilation and the subsequent rise in local temperature. See *Discomfort following lens insertion; Discomfort, investigation of*.

Discomfort following contact lens insertion

Soft lenses can attract debris during lens preparation prior to insertion, and wearers can experience some mild irritation. Patients should be advised that sliding the lens temporally onto the sclera can relieve this, and they can be taught the following procedure. For the right eye, the patient looks directly into the mirror and turns the head to the right whilst maintaining a straight-ahead gaze. This helps to expose a large area of temporal conjunctiva onto which the lens can be displaced. Using the right hand, the patient displaces the inferior lid slightly with the middle finger and uses the forefinger to slide the lens completely off the cornea onto the temporal conjunctiva. The patient will usually experience instant relief from any previous foreign body sensation. At this point, the patient blinks three to five times, which washes tears over the cornea, thereby displacing any unwanted debris. The lens can be manually repositioned onto the cornea, or alternatively the patient can look temporally and execute a couple of blinks, which will achieve the same result. If a foreign body sensation persists after this technique has been tried, the lens should be removed, rinsed and inspected for any signs of damage; the lens can then be reinserted if all looks well, or replaced if it is damaged. If foreign body-type discomfort is experienced on insertion of a rigid lens, the lens should be removed, rinsed and reinserted. The above procedures can also be undertaken by a practitioner if the patient experiences discomfort following lens insertion during a fitting/evaluation examination (Figure D.10). See *Discomfort, contact lens induced; Discomfort, investigation of*.

Discomfort, investigation of contact lens

Patients can employ one or more of a myriad of descriptions to describe symptoms of discomfort during contact lens wear. Terms that may be used include:

- scratchy
- uncomfortable
- cold
- watery
- hurting
- tired
- gritty
- painful
- hot
- dry
- sore
- burning
- itchy
- aching
- irritated
- stinging

A systematic approach can be applied to quantify the level of subjective discomfort experienced during lens wear. Specifically, the severity of discomfort can be described in three ways, known as:

1. Nominal – purely descriptive terms are used, such as mild or severe.
2. Ordinal – the level of severity is ranked on a scale of discrete steps, e.g. grades 0, 1, 2, 3 or 4. Descriptors may be employed for the extreme grades as a guide, e.g. grade 0 means 'no sensation' and grade 4 means 'extreme pain'.
3. Analogue – the level of comfort is indicated on a continuous scale. A popular technique employed in contact lens research is the 'vertical analogue scale'.

The following strategies can be used to determine whether the discomfort is eye- or lens-related:

- always be on the lookout for concurrent ocular pathology that may be unrelated to lens wear (e.g. glaucoma)
- consider the laterality of the discomfort – for example, discomfort due to a toxic reaction to a contact lens solution would be expected to be bilateral, whereas discomfort due to a damaged contact lens would be expected to be unilateral
- remove the lenses – persistent discomfort following lens removal suggests an ocular problem that may or may not have been caused by the lens; relief of discomfort following lens removal suggests a lens problem
- swap the lenses between the eyes – an ocular problem is indicated if unilateral discomfort remains in the same eye after the lenses have been swapped; a lens-related problem is indicated if unilateral discomfort transfers to the other eye after the lenses have been swapped
- prescribe ocular lubricants – relief after an ocular lubricant has been instilled into the sore eye suggests a mechanical or abrasive source of the discomfort.

There are many possible causes of lens-related discomfort. These causes, and strategies for alleviating the problem, include:

- poor fitting lens – change to a better fitting lens; specifically, a lens of larger diameter and/or steeper base curve may move less and therefore be more comfortable
- physical defects in the lens – replace the lens and/or change to a non-defective product
- particulate matter partially embedded in the lens – replace the lens

- foreign bodies beneath the lens – rinse the lens
- higher water content lenses are generally thicker and initially less comfortable than thinner lenses – use thinner lenses
- a toric soft lens might be slightly less comfortable than its spherical equivalent because of thick stabilization zones – employ a toric design with a thinner profile
- dehydration of hyper-thin (<0.04mm) soft lenses can lead to epithelial drying and discomfort – re-fit the patient with standard thickness lenses (>0.07mm)
- older lenses tend to feel more dry – replace lenses more frequently
- lenses with surface deposits can be uncomfortable – replace lenses more frequently.

If a patient complains of lens discomfort but there is no apparent cause after having carefully examined the lens and eye, the lens should be thoroughly cleaned with a surfactant cleaner, rinsed in saline and reinserted into the eye. If the discomfort persists, the lens may contain a sub-clinical defect, or it may have a microscopic foreign body imbedded in the back surface. In either case, the lens should be replaced.

Various forms of contact lens-related ocular pathology can cause discomfort, and it should be noted that the apparent severity of the tissue pathology does not necessarily correlate with the degree of discomfort suffered by the patient. Such conditions include:

- corneal epithelial microcysts – may cause slight discomfort
- corneal stromal oedema – moderate oedema (<5% swelling) can cause mild discomfort; severe oedema (>20% swelling) can be very painful, although the pain may be attributed to associated pathology such as an anterior uveal reaction; oedema associated with the corneal exhaustion syndrome may be very uncomfortable
- acute red eye – occurs in extended wear patients and can be very painful; lens removal often gives immediate relief
- superior limbic keratoconjunctivitis – causes increased lens awareness and itching; symptoms are alleviated by ceasing lens wear
- infectious keratitis – can be extremely painful, especially Acanthamoeba keratitis, even leading to patients becoming suicidal
- tear film dysfunction – discomfort is due to lens surface drying; ocular lubricants can provide short-term relief.

Ocular discomfort during contact lens wear may be due to the use of associated lens care products. Specifically, the discomfort may be related to:

- solution pH
- solution tonicity
- solution toxicity
- solution allergy
- lens denaturation due to heat disinfection (rarely used today)
- residual un-neutralized hydrogen peroxide
- hydrogen peroxide burn.

See *Discomfort, contact lens induced; Discomfort following lens insertion*.

Disinfection of contact lenses

- See *Antimicrobial efficacy; Trial contact lens set disinfection*.

Dispensing visit, contact lens

- See *Patient education, contact lens; Patient discharge, contact lenses*.

Display screen equipment regulations

The European Community issued Directive 90/270/EEC "Council Directive on the Minimum Safety and Health Requirements for Work with Display Screen Equipment." Article 2 in Section 1 provides definitions for the three main terms used:

- Display screen equipment – an alphanumeric or graphic display screen, regardless of the display process employed.
- Workstation – an assembly comprising display screen equipment, which may be provided with a keyboard or input device and/or software determining the operator/machine interface, optional accessories, peripherals including the diskette drive, telephone, modem, printer, document holder, work chair and work desk or work surface and the immediate work environment.
- Worker – any worker as defined in Article 3(a) of Directive 89/391/EEC who habitually uses display screen equipment as a significant part of his normal work.

Section II deals with the employer's obligations and is subdivided into Articles 3 to 9 of which Article 9 relates directly to eyes and eyesight. In essence Articles 3 to 8 require an employer to perform an analysis of workstations to evaluate any risk to workers, in particular as regards eyesight, physical problems and problems of mental stress and take appropriate steps to remedy any risks that may be revealed.

Article 9 relates directly to the protection of workers' eyes and eyesight

- Workers shall be entitled to an appropriate eye and eyesight test carried out by a person with the necessary capabilities (a) before commencing display screen work, (b) at regular intervals thereafter, and (c) if they experience visual difficulties which may be due to display screen work.
- Workers shall be entitled to an ophthalmological examination if the results of the test referred to in paragraph 1 show that this is necessary.
- If the results of the test referred to in paragraph 1 or if the examination referred to in paragraph 2 show that it is necessary and if formal corrective appliances cannot be used, workers must be provided with special corrective appliances appropriate for the work concerned.
- Measures taken pursuant to this Article may in no circumstances involve workers in additional financial cost.

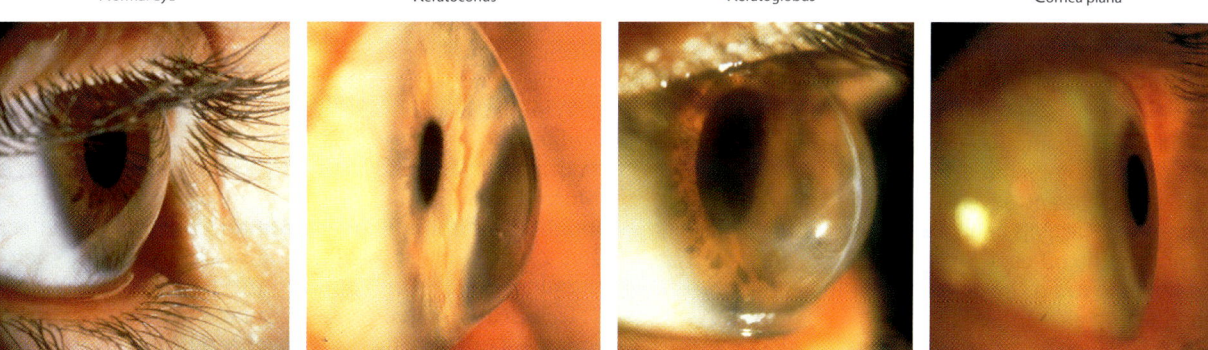

Figure D.11 • Congenital abnormalities of corneal shape.

- Protection of workers' eyes and eyesight may be provided as part of a national health system.

Disposable contact lenses
- See *Planned soft contact lens replacement*.

Distorted corneal shape, therapeutic contact lenses for
Congenital abnormalities of corneal topography, such as keratoconus, keratoglobus and cornea plana (Figure D.11), typically result in vision loss that can only be corrected with rigid forms of contact lenses – usually scleral lenses. Keratoconus occurs in 5.5 out of 10000 in the population, while keratoglobus and cornea plana are extremely rare. Patients suffering from these conditions are usually highly motivated to wear scleral lenses. See *Keratoconus, contact lens correction of*.

Dk, contact lens
- See *Carbon dioxide permeability of contact lenses; Oxygen permeability of contact lenses*.

Dk/t, contact lens
- See *Carbon dioxide transmissibility of contact lenses; Oxygen transmissibility of contact lenses*.

Dot matrix print tinting of contact lenses
This technique of making a coloured contact lens involves applying a matrix pattern of small opaque dots to the front surface of the lens (Figure D.12). The dots are created by bonding an opaquing agent (such as titanium dioxide) and a colouring agent (which may be a pigment or dye) to the lens surface. A binding polymer such as di-isocyanate is used to form a strong chemical bond between the opaque tinted agent and the lens surface. The final cosmetic effect will be a combination of dot matrix pattern and reflections from the natural iris between the opaque matrix dots. See *Tinted lenses*.

Double vision
- See *Diplopia*.

Drainage angle of the eye
- See *Anterior angle of the eye*.

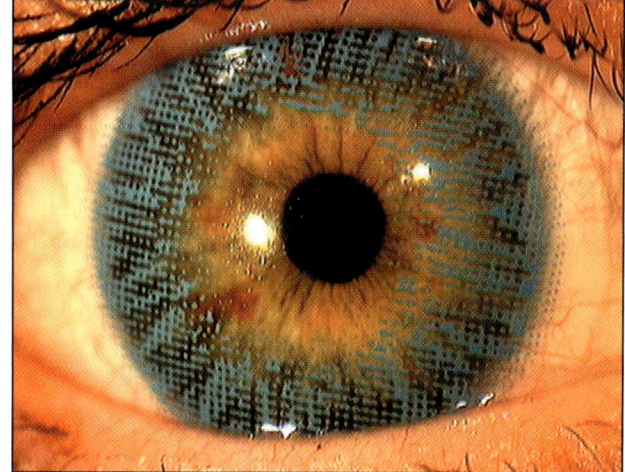

Figure D.12 • Lens with a matrix of opaque blue dots.

Drug delivery, contact lenses for
Hydrogel lenses steeped in pilocarpine solutions (e.g. 4%, unpreserved) are sometimes used in the management of acute closed angle glaucoma. This technique has also been used in the delivery of antibiotics, antiviral agents, epidermal growth factor and fibronectin.

Drugs in optometric practice, safeguards for the use of
The precautions that should be observed in relation to any drugs used or supplied by an optometrist include the following:
- Drugs kept at the practice should be stored securely (e.g. inaccessible to children)
- Follow the manufacturer's recommendations regarding optimal conditions of storage, especially temperature
- Consider the possible interaction of an ophthalmic drug to be used with *any* other medications taken by the patient
- Explain to the patient the reasons for using a drug
- Before using the drug, review the patient's record and confirm that there has been *no* previous adverse reaction to its use both by questioning the patient and by reference to the case record
- Prior to the administration of any drug, inspect the container to confirm that it is actually the one

required, the correct concentration, and it is within the expiry date
- As drops are instilled, the practitioner or patient, as appropriate, should apply a finger firmly over the medial canthal area for about one minute in order to occlude the canaliculi. This procedure reduces the absorption of drops through the nasopharyngeal mucosa so that any adverse systemic effect is minimized. Nasolacrimal obstruction has been shown to improve the efficacy of *some* topically applied drugs and helps to avoid the possibility of the patient experiencing an unpleasant taste
- Write on the patient's record full details of any drug used, supplied or recommended. In the case of eye drops, record the number of drops instilled into each eye
- Ensure that the patient knows what action to take in the event of an adverse response to the drug.

Drugs, ocular side effects of

Prior to receiving a licence to allow drugs to be widely prescribed, they have to be submitted to rigorous clinical trials to demonstrate their therapeutic efficacy and safety. Notwithstanding rigorous regulatory processes, from time to time drugs become available which are subsequently found to have serious systemic or ocular side effects. The most notorious example of the former is thalidomide, which was introduced in the late 1950's as a sleeping pill and as a treatment for morning sickness in pregnancy. A few years later, it was realized that this drug was responsible for foetal malformation of limbs and other defects of the eye, ear, heart, genitals, kidneys, digestive tract and nervous system. Despite these devastating effects, thalidomide remains in use in some countries for the treatment of leprosy and acquired immune deficiency syndrome (AIDS).

Practolol is an example of a drug that was withdrawn from general use as a beta-adrenergic antagonist for the treatment of cardiac arrhythmias after it was recognized in the early 1970's that in some patients it caused an oculomucocutaneous syndrome, which involved the eyes, skin and mucous membranes. Affected individuals complained of ocular irritation and the presence of tenacious, stringy mucous in their eyes; some suffered severe visual loss as a consequence of corneal damage.

Although it has long been acknowledged that long-term administration of high doses of chorloquine can cause keratopathy and maculopathy, this drug continues to be used as an antimalarial agent and in the treatment of rheumatoid arthritis, and systemic and discoid lupus erythematosus. Hydroxychloroquine is regarded as safer than chloroquine in relation to ocular side effects. The advice of the College of Ophthalmologists is that prior to treatment with either of these drugs, patients should be asked whether they have any visual impairment that is uncorrected by spectacles. If impairment or ocular disease is present, the patient should be assessed by an optometrist and any abnormality referred to an ophthalmogist. Near visual acuity is recorded at that stage. Throughout treatment, the College of Ophthalmologists advises annual measurement of near visual acuity together with questioning about any visual symptoms.

Aspirin is the most commonly used drug in the UK. When used in high doses, it can give rise to ocular side effects that include anterior chamber and sub-conjunctival haemorrhages.

While it is likely that a patient experiencing severe ocular side effects of any drug will contact a general medical practitioner, if the only symptom is one such as 'blurred vision', the advice of an optometrist may be sought. Importantly, asymptomatic ocular side effects may only be discovered as the result of an optometric examination.

It is clearly essential in the routine eye examination to enquire about both the state of general health and whether *any* form of medication is taken. The appropriate questions should be phrased in an open form to encourage disclosure of information about prescribed medication, products purchased over-the-counter, including herbal medicines, and any nutritional supplements. Since oral contraceptives may not be regarded by patients as drugs or medicines, it may be necessary to ask specifically about their use in view of the fact that their reported complications include corneal steepening, optic neuritis and occlusion of the central retinal vein or artery. It is important to identify the names of drugs and to know their dosage together with the current duration of treatment.

The association between dose and the occurrence of ocular side effects can be demonstrated with reference to sildenafil citrate, a medication used for male erectile dysfunction, which is universally recognized by its proprietary name, Viagra. The ocular side effects associated with this drug are mydriasis, conjunctival hyperaemia, dryness, ocular pain, blurred vision and a temporary bluish discoloration of vision, and these occur in:

- About 3% cent taking 25 to 50mg (the recommended daily dose is 50mg)
- About 11% taking 100mg (the maximum recommended daily dose)
- About 50% cent taking 200mg
- Nearly all taking 600 to 800mg.

It is impossible for optometrists to be familiar with all the possible ocular effects of the numerous medications that are responsible for them. Since some of the adverse reactions are rare or only occur with unusually high drugs doses, it is necessary to have access to appropriate reference sources in either printed or electronic form (i.e. CD-ROM or Internet). A representative range of ocular side effects of systemic medications is presented in Appendix A.

In addition to their effects on the eye, drugs can create other difficulties of concern to the optometrist. Discolouration of hydrogel contact lenses has been reported in patients using eye drops containing adrenaline or phenylephrine. Systemic medications such as rifampicin, nitrofurantoin, tetracycline and thioridazine have caused orange/pink/red, brown and yellow-brown, and grey-brown discoloration, respectively. The current popularity of daily or monthly disposable lenses should avoid this problem.

It should be borne in mind that agents other than prescribed medication can also produce undesirable ocular effects. For example, excessive intake of vitamin D can result in the deposition of calcium within the cornea and, more seriously, an excess of vitamin A can cause pseudotumour cerebri in which intracranial pressure is raised resulting in papilloedema.

Examples of ocular side effects induced by herbal medicines include mydriasis due to valerian and 5-hydroxy tryptophan, and conjunctivitis associated with propolis and psyllium.

Alcohol and nicotine in tobacco can be considered under this heading and the consequences of their excessive consumption are very well known. The effects of alcohol include blurred vision, mydriasis, conjunctival hyperaemia and diplopia. Smoking appears to be a risk factor in cataract, macular degeneration and contact lens associated keratitis. In alcohol-tobacco amblyopia, reduced vision is accompanied by a visual field defect and impaired colour vision. In some cases there is permanent visual loss due to optic atrophy.

While patients may not admit to the illegal use of drugs, their use may sometimes be suspected. Amphetamines can produce dilation of the pupil and reduced accommodation. Cocaine users may suffer inadvertent trauma of the partly anaesthetized corneal surface resulting in ulceration. Marijuana can lead to conjunctival hyperaemia, mydriasis and visual hallucinations.

Dry eye associated with contact lens wear

Of all the symptoms experienced by contact lens wearers, that of 'dryness' is reported most frequently. A major difficulty in assessing the symptom of 'dryness' is that there may be many stimuli that elicit this sensation; that is, it cannot be assumed that the cause of a patient's symptom of 'dryness' is necessarily due to an absence of moisture in the eye. Because there are no specific 'dryness receptors' in human tissue, ocular dryness must be a response to specific coding of afferent neural inputs. Aside from an actual dry eye, reports of 'dryness' may arise from the neural misinterpretation of stimuli that are unrelated to dry eye, such as vasodilation induced by mechanical irritation of ocular tissues by deposits on the lens surface. Thus, the condition of 'dry eye' may be related to a broad spectrum of tear film abnormalities in addition to a reduced tear volume.

A prudent initial approach in dealing with a tentative diagnosis of contact lens-induced dry eye is to apply a comprehensive dry eye questionnaire that attempts to identify the following:

- other systemic correlates of dryness, such as dryness of other mucous membranes of the body (e.g. mouth, vagina)
- the use of medications
- the effect of different challenging environments
- the times when dryness is noted.

Such questionnaires can help identify a true dry eye situation in prospective or current contact lens wearers, and thus form a clinical rationale for more detailed assessment.

The most fundamental test that a clinician can apply when investigating contact lens related dry eye is to observe the tear film using the slit-lamp biomicroscope. The overall integrity of the tears during lens wear can be assessed by observing the general flow of tears over the lens surface following a blink, as indicated by the movement of tear debris. A 'sluggish' movement may indicate an aqueous-deficient, mucus-rich and/or lipid-rich tear film, and the amount of debris provides an indication of the level of contamination of the tears (for example, from over-use of cosmetics). This can result in increased deposit formation, intermittent blurred vision and symptoms of dryness. Incomplete blinking in soft lens wearers can lead to lens dehydration and consequent epithelial staining of the inferior cornea, corresponding to the position of the palpebral aperture.

The volume of tears in prospective and current contact lens wearers can be assessed by observing the height of the lower lacrimal tear prism. Measurements of tear meniscus radius of curvature and height correlate well with results of the cotton thread test, non-invasive tear break-up time (NITBUT) and ocular surface staining scores, demonstrating the value of such an assessment in diagnosing contact lens associated dry eye. A wide-field, cold cathode light source, which is available as a hand-held instrument known as a tearscope, can be used to assess tear quality during lens wear.

Most of the strategies that are applied to alleviating signs and symptoms of dry eye of the non-lens wearing eye can also be applied to the eye during contact lens wear. The following types of lenses are most suitable for patients experiencing dry eye problems:

- soft lenses, for full corneal coverage (although some patients report relief from dry eye symptoms after changing from a soft lens to a rigid lens)
- high water content lenses, to maximize the volume of water in front of the lens
- lenses that display minimal in-eye dehydration, to prevent ocular surface desiccation
- lenses that are replaced frequently, for optimal, deposit-free surface characteristics.

Numerous other strategies have been advocated for alleviating contact lens related dry eye, including:

- avoidance of preservatives in care solutions
- avoidance of solutions altogether via the use of daily disposable lenses
- use of re-wetting drops
- periodic lens rehydration
- use of nutritional supplements
- control of evaporation
- prevention of excess tear drainage (with punctal plugs)
- use of tear stimulants
- reduction of wearing time, and ceasing lens wear.

Dry eye questionnaire

Perhaps the most widely noted symptom of contact lens wearers is a sensation of dryness. Contact lenses will disrupt the normal tear film, and it is important to pay particular attention to both the quantity and the quality of the tears before offering advice on suitability for contact lens wear. A dry eye questionnaire can be used to identify patients who have a tendency to ocular sicca and those who might develop symptoms associated with provocative factors such as contact lens wear.

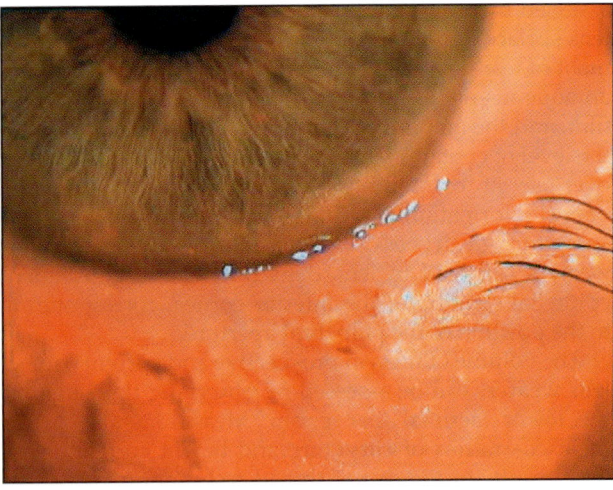 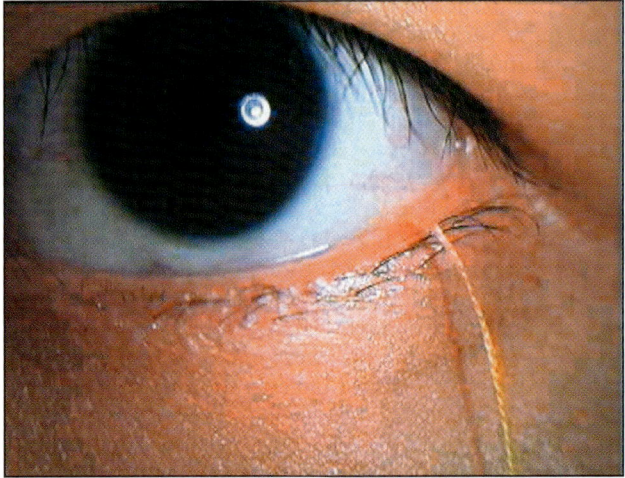

Figure D.13 • Tests for an aqueous deficiency dry eye. Left: scanty tear film meniscus. Right: phenol red cotton thread.

Dry eye syndromes

The cornea and conjunctiva are unique in the body in that they are an exposed mucous membrane requiring constant wetting to maintain their health, and in the case of the cornea, its clarity. Ocular surface wetting is achieved by the action of the tear film, eyelids, lacrimal glands and ocular surface.

The tears consist of an aqueous component from the lacrimal and accessory lacrimal glands and lipid from the meibomian glands. A layer of mucin produced by both the conjunctival goblet cells and the corneal epithelium facilitates wetting of the ocular surface. A deficiency in any one of these components can result in tear film instability and lead to drying of the ocular surface; this is referred to as dry eye.

Dry eye syndromes can be classified as follows:

- Aqueous deficiency: a dry eye resulting from a decrease in the aqueous component of the tear film is referred to as keratoconjunctivitis sicca (KCS). A minor degree of aqueous tear film deficiency is common, especially in post-menopausal women.
- Lipid anomaly: chronic blepharitis with an alteration in the lipid component of the tear film may lead to a dry eye through instability of the tear film.
- Mucous deficiency: this is a rare cause of dry eye and usually leads to particularly severe disease. It results from goblet cell destruction secondary to such causes of conjunctival scarring as chemical burns, vitamin A deficiency and ocular cicatricial pemphigoid.
- Dysfunction of tear film distribution: ocular surface dryness can result from dysfunction of the normal wetting action of the eyelids as occurs with a decreased blink rate (with Alzheimer's disease), lagophthalmos and malposition of the lids. It may also occur with ocular surface irregularities.
- Allergy: The presence of inflammatory cells or other inflammatory components in the tear film as occurs in allergic eye disease also causes instability of the tears. Chronic irritation from other forms of dry eye can also cause ocular surface inflammation, thereby exacerbating the underlying condition.

Symptoms and signs of dry eye may be grouped into seven categories (the seven Ss):

- Symptoms: assessed by asking patients how their eyes feel; patients may report symptoms such as dryness, burning, sandy or foreign body sensation, with varying frequency and severity.
- Stability of the tear film: assessed using fluorescein tear break up time (TBUT) and non-invasive break-up time. A TBUT less than 5 to 10 sec is considered abnormal.
- Surface integrity: assessed using fluorescein staining, rose bengal staining and impression cytology.
- Secretion or quantity: assessed using the Schirmer or cotton thread tests.
- Slit lamp biomicroscopy: assessed by observing tear meniscus height, tear film debris and reflected interferometric patterns in the lipid layer (Figure D.13).
- Surfacing by the eyelids: assessed by observing blink rate and completeness, and surface irregularities.
- Solute levels: assessed by measuring tear osmolality, observing tear ferning patterns, and assaying tear lactoferrin.

Signs common to the various forms of dry eye are (a) fluorescein and rose bengal staining of the inferior interpalpebral corneal and conjunctival epithelium with associated sparse tear film, and (b) rapid break-up of the tear film.

Any underlying cause such as blepharitis or eyelid disturbance should be treated. In addition, the following alternative management strategies should be considered:

- Advice: avoidance of drying situations such as being in hot or cold winds, near dehumidifying air-conditioners or radiant heaters. Protective glasses may be useful in such situations.
- Tear Supplements: tear supplements (also termed lubricants) are available in multi-use bottles for occasional use, ointment form for overnight use, and in unpreserved unit-dose form if required more than several times a day.
- Therapeutics: in any allergic or severe forms of dry eye a mild anti-inflammatory agent may be used.

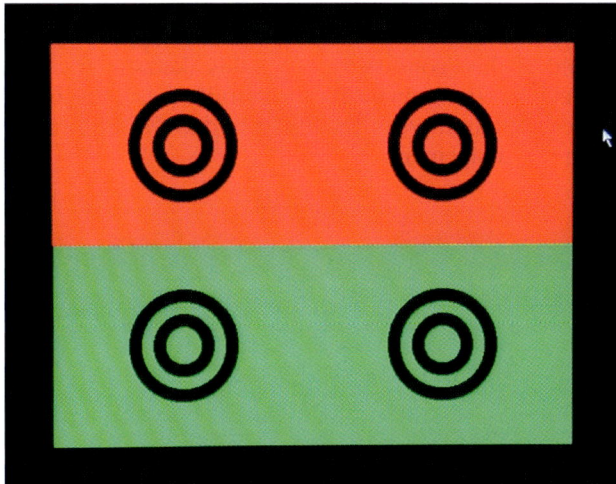

Figure D.14 • Duochrome test.

- Office procedures: maximizing both normal tears and lubricant effect by occluding the puncta, may be appropriate for an aqueous tear deficiency.
- Tarsorrhaphy: reduction of the ocular surface area with a lateral tarsorrhaphy is reserved for severe sight-threatening cases of dry eye that are refractory to more conservative treatments.

Drysdale method of contact lens surface curvature measurement
- See *Radiuscope*.

Duochrome test
The duochrome (or bichromatic) test is a display comprising a red filter above a green filter, each having two sets of ring targets upon them (Figure D.14). The test is usually performed at 6 metres; near versions of the duochrome test are also available.

The duochrome test is used to check for small uncorrected spherical error, particularly as part of the best sphere check or final sphere check during subjective refraction. The test exploits the axial chromatic aberration in the eye. Assuming a best focus in the yellow region of the spectrum (570nm), the red filter (620nm) will focus behind the retina by an equivalent of 0.24D and the green (535nm) in front of the retina by 0.20D. An uncorrected myope (or someone over-minussed) should therefore see the targets on the red background more clearly, and a hypermetrope (or someone over-plussed) those against the green. An end point such as the choice of best sphere is reached when the patient has no preference between the clarity of the ring targets on either colour background.

The ease of use of the duochrome test needs to be tempered by considering the several sources of error using the test. First, many patients express a subjective preference for one colour (commonly stating red to be a "stronger" colour) irrespective of focus. Second, the 0.50D difference between the two foci means that for larger errors (greater than 1.00D or vision worse than 6/9) it is unreliable. Patients over 55 years, particularly with small pupils, have reduced dioptric difference between the foci. Also, yellowing of the crystalline lens with age causes a red shift leading to over-minussing. The test is generally considered to be useful for checking purposes when refracting younger patients – especially verifying refractive status during contact lens wear – rather than a self-contained test for determining a refractive prescription.

Duty of care and negligence
The law of tort covers many areas but the most common to impact on practice is that of negligence. While many people will have their own concept of negligence in law it has been clearly defined as: 'A breach by the defendant of a legal duty of care which is owed to the plaintiff among others and breach of which causes damage to the plaintiff.' At face value this definition seems clear enough and indeed to succeed in an action for negligence the plaintiff is required only to prove the following three conditions:

- A duty of care is owed personally by the defendant to the plaintiff
- The duty of care has been broken
- Harm has been suffered as a result of the breach of duty.

As always with the law, however, it is not quite so easy to prove the conditions. To prove a duty of care is owed it is necessary to show that a defendant could reasonably have been expected to have seen that a person such as the plaintiff might have been affected by his act or failure to act.

D-value
- See *Antimicrobial efficacy of contact lenses*.

Dye dispersion tinting of contact lenses
This technique is used primarily to create a translucent tint in rigid lenses. A dye or pigment is mixed into the polymer matrix by adding the dye to the monomer mixture prior to polymerization, or by adding the dye to the polymer and then mixing to disperse the colour. This results in an evenly distributed, stable dye. The disadvantages of this process are that it is not possible to vary the distribution of tint across the lens (e.g. to create a clear pupil), and that the density of tint is proportional to lens thickness. This process is unsuitable for soft lenses because the dye, which is non-water-soluble, can leach out from the polymer during hydration. See *Tinted lenses*.

Dynamic stabilization
- See *Stabilization of soft toric lenses*.

Dystonia
- See *Filamentary keratitis, therapeutic contact lenses for*.

Dystrophies of the corneal epithelium, therapeutic contact lenses for
Epithelial basement membrane dystrophy is by far the most common epithelial dystrophy, but other dystrophies

that can involve the corneal epithelium are also often the cause of pain that can be relieved with soft lenses. They include Reis-Bückler's dystrophy, Meesmann's dystrophy, lattice dystrophy, and Fuchs's dystrophy, in which the failing corneal endothelium cannot prevent stromal oedema and bullous keratopathy in the epithelium.

Thygeson's superficial punctate keratopathy is not considered to be a dystrophy, but it is appropriate to consider this condition here; this keratopathy can sometimes be managed successfully with hydrogel lenses, although weak topical steroid is the more usual form of management.

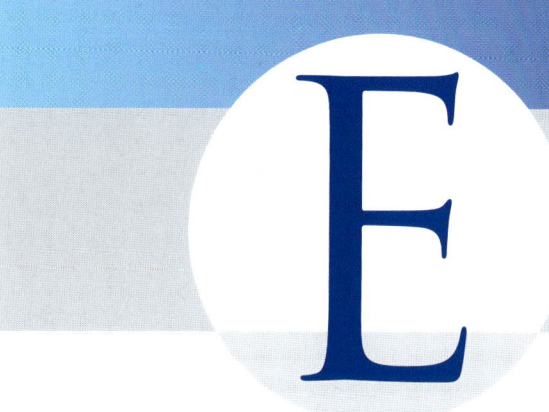

Eccentric fixation

Eccentric fixation is a monocular sensory adaptation and exists when a non-foveal point is used for fixation in an amblyopic eye. As retinal sensitivity is reduced parafoveally, there is always reduced acuity in an eye which fixates eccentrically. With the inclusion of graticules in ophthalmoscopes it has become apparent that eccentric fixation is not a rare but common feature of amblyopia. The angular subtense of the graticule can be found either by direct measurement of its projection on to a screen or by estimation compared to the size of the optic disc.

Strabismus is known to influence eccentric fixation as follows:

- Eccentric fixation is more common in strabismic rather than ansiometropic amblyopia.
- The eccentrically fixating point is usually on the side of the fovea to be expected on the basis of the squint, i.e. nasal eccentric fixation in esotropia, and not randomly anywhere around Worth's annulus of best vision.
- Reduction in the angle of squint by surgery sometimes reduces the angle of eccentric fixation.
- In cases where inappropriate occlusion has resulted in amblyopia in the good eye, this occlusion amblyopia sometimes itself has eccentric fixation.

These observations suggest that the position of the eye in the orbit during the habitual strabismic state has some influence on the position the eye takes up when required to fixate monocularly. The clinical significance of eccentric fixation is not clear. Long-standing, deep amblyopia with steady eccentric fixation several degrees from the fovea has a bad prognosis. But the general uncertainties of the success rate in amblyopia therapy make it difficult to argue that the presence or absence of a small angle of eccentric fixation should have a decisive influence on management strategy or the prognosis.

Eccentric viewing and steady eye strategy

The patient who has a central scotoma will need to use eccentric viewing (EV) and deliberately fixate to the side of the object of interest so that it is not obscured. An area of retina other than the fovea will then be used for fixation – the preferred retinal location (PRL). See *Preferred retinal focus*. Some patients have discovered this strategy for themselves, but others are not aware of their scotoma, or do not appreciate why their vision 'comes and goes,' and they need to be taught EV. Even those patients who use EV successfully when looking at static targets, have often not learnt to apply this to a dynamic task (such as reading) without guidance. Reading involves maintaining fixation on a word for a period, before making an accurate saccade to the next word. If this same sequence of saccades and fixations is to be achieved using EV throughout, it means that the PRL must have effectively replaced the fovea as the 'centre' of oculomotor control, and the saccades are placing the retinal image precisely and consistently on the PRL instead of the fovea. In these cases, the PRL is so well established that the patients actually believe that they are looking straight at the target, but this stage only appears to be reached in a minority of patients. It appears that when patients look at the first word on a line of text they are viewing eccentrically and can resolve the small print, but as they saccade on to the next word they return to central fixation, since it appears that the fovea remains the reference point for their oculomotor system. Their view of the word that they are trying to read is thus obscured by the scotoma and they cannot resolve it. So whilst reading usually involves holding the text still and moving the eyes along the lines when reading, patients with a central scotoma read best by moving the text from right to left whilst being instructed to hold their eyes still and simultaneously adopting EV. Thus, the patients fixate the first letter on the line of print, and are instructed to obtain the clearest possible view of it. This should mean that they are using EV to image the letter on the PRL. As they keep the eye still and move the print, this 'Steady Eye Strategy' (SES) allows each succeeding letter to be imaged in turn on the PRL and for the words to be read accurately, letter by letter.

As patients become more proficient at adopting these strategies, the speed of reading increases, and they are encouraged to appreciate when the end of a word is reached, and to identify what that word is. They must be discouraged from guessing words before the final letter is reached, because this does not speed up their reading. Even if they guess forthcoming letters correctly, these must still be imaged on the PRL and visualized: there is no mechanism in SES for skipping a letter that does not need to be seen. This feature means that extremely high speeds are impossible, but when the technique is mastered, it can support a reading speed which is fast enough for leisure reading (≈160 words per minute) (see *Reading requirements, low vision*) and allows a reasonable duration of reading without undue fatigue.

This new method of reading (EV and SES) is novel to all patients, and unlike their habitual reading. It requires patients to practice for a few minutes each day at home to improve their technique and speed, returning to the clinic every 1–2 weeks to check on progress and to move on to more difficult tasks. The average patient might require 3 to 5 sessions to achieve reading of newsprint. EV training can undoubtedly be very successful in many cases, although it is not universally accepted, and some patients will never master it. It is time-consuming and inconvenient for the patient, who also has to have a clear understanding of the technique, and be prepared to follow the instructions. Advocates of EV would argue that it is a necessary part of dealing with patients with a central scotoma, since such patients cannot be effectively helped by simply using magnification (since a plateau of acuity is reached which cannot be improved no matter what level of magnification is used). SES can be a valuable technique for any low vision reader with a limited field of clear vision: this includes those who are using a high-powered optical magnifier which has a field of view of only a few letters, and those with hemianopia or tunnel vision.

See *Low vision training*.

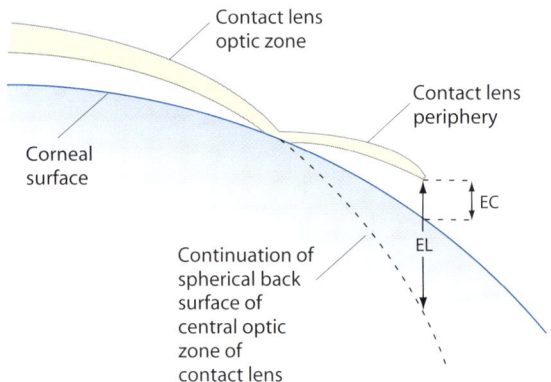

Figure E.1 • Axial edge lift (EL) and edge clearance (EC).

ECDP
- See *Equivalent carbon dioxide pressure beneath contact lenses*.

Edema
- See *Oedema*.

Edge clearance of contact lenses
Without a peripheral gap between the edge of a rigid lens and the cornea, known as 'edge clearance', mechanical pressure from the lens edge leads to superficial corneal damage (Figure E.1). Edge clearance is also important for tear exchange and to enable lens removal using the lids. The edge clearance can be specified axially (as shown in Figure E.1) or radially. A minimum axial edge clearance of 60–80μm when the lens is centred is considered to be the optimal value. Edge lift is measured with respect to the continuation of the spherical lens back curve.

Edge defects
- See *Quality, soft contact lens*.

Edge fluting
- See *Fluting of contact lenses*.

Edge form of contact lenses
The shape of the lens edge is one of the most important factors in minimizing any discomfort. Poor edge rounding in particular can result in greater edge awareness by the upper eyelid. Good rounding of the front surface edge is more important than rounding of the posterior edge. This suggests that the interaction of the edge of the lens with the eyelid is more important in relation to comfort than the interaction with the cornea. Figure E.2 shows examples of edge shapes.

Edge lift of contact lenses
Certain lens fitting philosophies are based on the concept of edge lift. Figure E.3 summarizes the various parameters used to describe edge lift. Edge lift is the distance between a point on the edge of the lens back surface and the circular continuation of the back optic zone. This can be

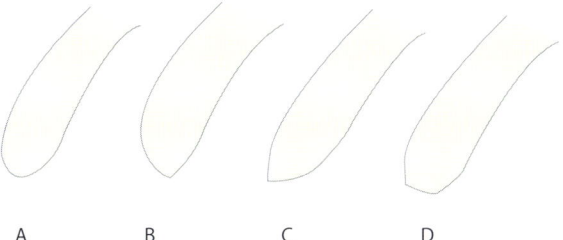

Figure E.2 • Various edge forms on rigid lenses. (A) Well rounded edge. (B) Sharp posterior edge. (C) Sharp anterior edge. (D) Flat edge.

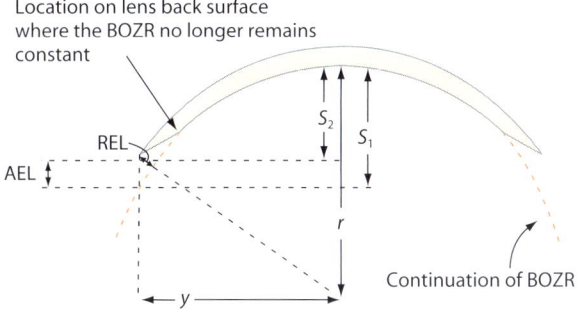

(y = half overall diameter of lens)

Figure E.3 • The form of the edge of a rigid lens can be defined in terms of either axial edge lift (AEL) or radial edge lift (REL).

measured axially or radially. Unlike edge clearance, edge lift is not referenced to the corneal surface.

With reference to Figure E.3, the edge lift can be calculated from the basic geometry of the lens surface as follows:

$$REL = \sqrt{[(r - s_2)^2 + y^2]} - r$$
$$AEL = (s_1 - s_2), \text{ where } s_1 = r - \sqrt{(r^2 - y^2)}$$

where REL is radial edge lift and AEL is axial edge lift. Measuring the overall sag of a finished lens, namely s_2, allows both the axial and radial edge lift to be derived. However, the error in both derivations is dependent upon errors in r and y. The likely magnitude of the final error can be estimated using partial differential equations for the two expressions. For example, consider a lens of BOZR 7.7mm and TD 10mm. If the respective errors in r, y and s_1 were ±0.015mm, ±0.1mm and ±0.01mm, then it can be shown that the errors in REL and AEL would be ±0.053mm and ±0.071mm. These figures represent the precision in the determination of REL and AEL.

Alternatively, for AEL, the sag of a monocurve lens of identical BOZR and TD could be used to directly measure s_1 in an attempt to improve precision. The lens may be placed on a glass plate, and by using a travelling microscope s_2 could be measured. The exact shape and dimensions of the lens edge profile will affect the estimation of edge lift.

Edge shape
- See *Edge form of contact lenses*.

Edge thickness of a contact lens
- See *Contact lens thickness*.

Edging, ophthalmic lens
Ophthalmic lenses are generally supplied in a large circular form. The edge of the lens must then be ground into the shape of the spectacle frame. This process is commonly referred to as 'edging', and is performed by a machine incorporating a grinding wheel and a system for tracing the correct lens shape, known as an 'edger'. The process also involves creating a bevel on the edge of the lens to enable it to be retained by the inner groove of the spectacle frame. A smooth contoured edge is imarted for lenses designed to be used in rimless spectacles.

Education of patients
- See *Patient education with contact lenses*.

EFCLIN
- See *European Federation of the Contact Lens Industry*.

Effectivity
The role of the distance correction is to produce an intermediate image at the far point of the particular eye. Due to the non-zero vertex distance of any spectacle correction, this far point will lie at slightly different distances from the two types of correcting lens. Thus the spectacle and contact lens powers required to correct a particular eye will differ.

From Figure E.4A it can be seen that, using a reduced eye model, if the vertex distance is a (taken as positive) and the ocular refraction is K, giving a far point distance from the cornea k=1/K, the second focal point of the correcting lens lies at a distance a+k. Thus the power, F_c, of the correcting lens is:

$$F_c = 1/(a + k) = 1/(a + 1/K) = K/(1 + aK)$$

For a contact lens, a will be zero so that the required value of F_c equals the ocular refraction in this simple model. This does not apply with a spectacle lens. The result is that a hypermetrope will require a higher-powered contact lens than spectacle lens, the reverse occurring for a myope. The difference between the required powers of correction only becomes significant (i.e. greater than 0.25D) when the magnitude of the ocular refraction exceeds about ±4.00D (Figure E.4B). Appendix B provides a table for vertex distance correction.

Efron grading scales for contact lens complications
- See *Grading scales*.

Eikonometer
The degree of aniseikonia (spectacle-induced binocular spatial distortion) perceived by a patient can be measured using an instrument known as an eikonometer. The direct comparison (or standard) eikonometer involves placing polarized filters before each eye of the patient and asking

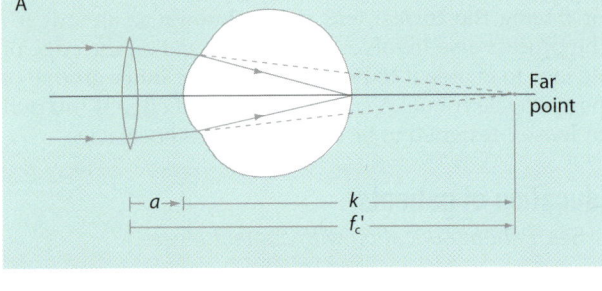
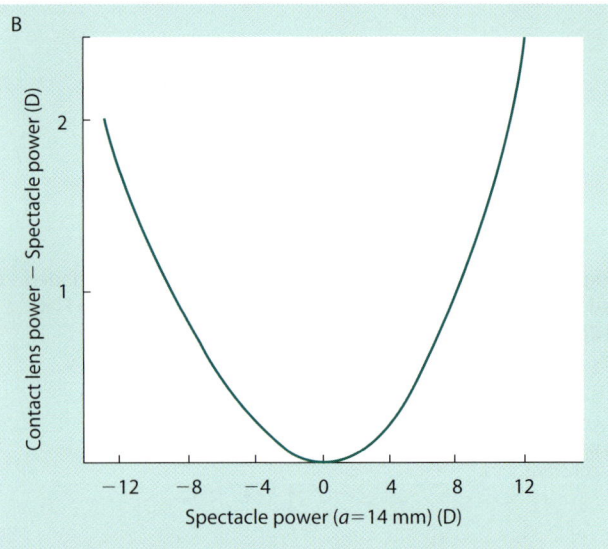

Figure E.4 • (A) Geometry relating the far point of an ametropic eye and the correcting lens. (B) Difference between the required powers of a contact lens and spectacle corrections, as a function of the spectacle correction, assuming that the vertex distance of the spectacle lens is 14mm.

the patient to report where the arrows (seen by one eye) are pointing with respect to a numbered target. Alignment of the arrows and target is achieved by altering an adjustable magnifying device before one eye, which gives a measure of the degree of aniseikonia. A space eikonometer operates by having the patient look at a large three-dimensional field (such as the inside of a large room). The space will appear distorted if the patient is suffering from aniseikonia. Special lenses are introduced in front of the eye until the distortion disappears, thus providing a measure of the degree of aniseikonia.

Aniseikonia is often noticed when a patient is dispensed with a new spectacles prescription, especially when there has been a change in cylindrical axis or power. Since spectacle lens wearers invariable readily adapt to aniseikonia, eikonometers are seldom used in routine clinical practice.

Electrical contact thickness gauge, soft contact lens

Electronic contact systems relying on the electrical conductivity of soft lenses can be used to measure the thickness of soft lenses. The lens is centred on a support dome that has an electrical contact in its surface. Another contact is gradually lowered onto the lens, and its position relative to the first contact is monitored using a vernier scale. On contact with the lens, a flow of electrical current is detected and the vernier scale is read.

Electrolytes in tears

- See *Tear electrolytes*.

Electromechanical thickness gauge, soft contact lens

An electromechanical thickness gauge is operated by lowering a lightweight probe until it touches the surface

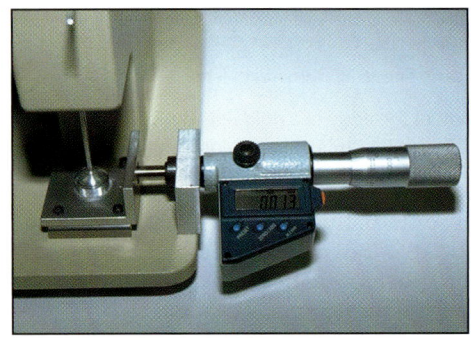

Figure E.5 • Electromechanical thickness gauge modified for measuring central and peripheral lens thickness.

of a soft lens sitting on a support dome (Figure E.5). The force of contact of the probe is extremely low (around 0.015N). Using this technique, thickness can be measured to a resolution of 0.01mm. The device still tends to compress the lens, thus the result is typically a few microns lower than the true thickness.

Electronic vision enhancement systems

Electronic Vision Enhancement Systems (EVES) produce an electronically magnified image of an object such that it can be more easily seen by a visually impaired user. The EVES consists of a camera and a display, plus a power supply (which may be mains or battery depending on the portability requirements of the system). Currently, there are many different configurations of the camera which can be hand-held, stand-mounted, head-mounted, or in the form of a 'mouse' on rollers. Equally varied are the display options, including large table-top monitors, small portable screens, or displays mounted in front of the eyes on a spectacle. Typical examples of such systems are the closed circuit television, the head-mounted video display and the television reader. An EVES uses real-image magnification: that is, there is a direct increase in the linear size of a feature as measured on the display screen, compared to that of the original object, and very high magnification (at least for near) is possible. See *Magnification for low vision*.

Emmetropia

Light from a distant object is perfectly focused on the retina when accommodation is relaxed, resulting in clear distance vision – that is, the absence of a refractive defect of the eye. Antonym: ametropia.

Endothelial bedewing, contact lens associated

Contact lens associated endothelial bedewing (CLEB) is characterized by the appearance of small particles in or on the endothelium in the region of the inferior central cornea, immediately below the lower pupil margin. The area of bedewing can vary in shape. For example, CLEB may appear as an oval cluster of particles or a less discrete dispersed formation. The condition is usually bilateral. The cells invariably display 'reversed illumination' (see *Microcysts* for an explanation of this phenomenon), suggesting that bedewing represents inflammatory cells rather than intracellular endothelial oedema (which would display unreversed illumination). When viewed in direct illumination, CLEB can appear as fine white precipitates or as an orange/brown dusting of cells. The colour of the particles can give a clue regarding the length of time they have been present; newly deposited cells are often whitish in colour, but these become pigmented over time. The cells can become engulfed within the endothelium over time.

The following signs may co-exist with CLEB:

- conjunctival injection
- epithelial erosion
- epithelial oedema
- reduced corneal transparency.

The main associated feature of endothelial bedewing is either total or partial intolerance to lens wear. Some patients may present after having recently abandoned lens wear. Patients may also complain of 'fogging' of vision or of stinging.

On the assumption that CLEB represents a mild inflammatory uveal response, the origin of the inflammatory cells is likely to be the iris and/or ciliary body. During inflammation, vascular permeability is increased and inflammatory cells leave vessels in the iris and ciliary body and float around in the aqueous until they come to rest on the endothelial surface. The reason for the deposition on the inferior cornea relates to the characteristic pattern of aqueous current flow. One would therefore expect occasionally to observe mild aqueous flare in patients with CLEB, but this does not appear to have been reported. This mild inflammatory status probably causes lens intolerance.

Patient management is guided by symptomatology rather than clinical signs. Wearing time should be reduced to a level that represents the balance between the needs of the patient to wear lenses for a desired length of time each day versus the level of discomfort that can be tolerated. The presence of inflammatory cells on the endothelial surface should be viewed with great caution by clinicians, because the condition may not necessarily be related to lens wear. Certainly, all forms of

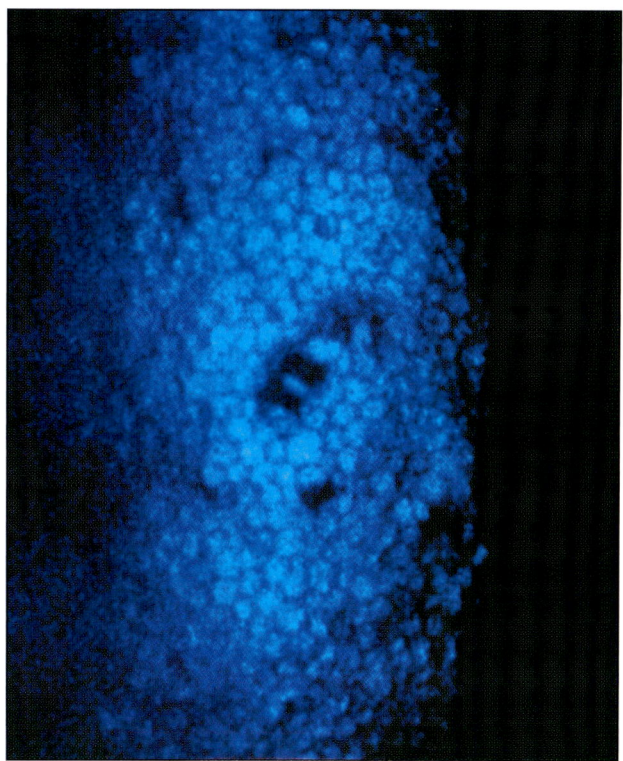

Figure E.6 • Endothelial blebs.

uveitis should be considered and tests should be conducted to exclude such possibilities. In all cases of CLEB intraocular pressures should be measured, because some inflammatory cells may have migrated into the anterior angle, creating a blockage of aqueous outflow. Gonioscopy is also indicated, especially if intraocular pressure is elevated.

The pattern of recovery from CLEB is variable. In some cases bedewing will completely disappear within 4 months, and in other cases it may change little over a much longer time period. Lens intolerance may persist for many months in some patients, even after the bedewing has disappeared.

Endothelial blebs, contact lens associated

The endothelial mosaic undergoes a dramatic alteration in appearance in all lens wearers within minutes of inserting a contact lens. These changes can only just be resolved when observed under the highest magnification possible (×40) using the slit-lamp biomicroscope. When viewed at much greater magnification (×200), a number of black, non-reflecting areas can be seen in the endothelial mosaic corresponding to the position of individual cells or groups of cells. These are called blebs (Figure E.6). There is also an apparent increase in the separation between cells. There is a large variation in the intensity of the response between patients.

Blebs can be seen within 10 minutes of lens insertion. The number of blebs peaks in 20–30 minutes (Grade 3), then decreases to a lower level after about 45–60 minutes. A low-level bleb response (Grade 1) can be observed throughout the remainder of the wearing period. Hydrogel lenses cause a greater bleb response than rigid lenses, and hydrogel lenses of greater average thickness also induce a greater response than thinner lenses.

The appearance of blebs can be explained as follows. When the endothelium is viewed using specular reflection, light rays reflect from the tissue plane corresponding to the interface between the posterior surface of the endothelium and the aqueous humor. This interface acts as the reflective surface because it represents a significant change in tissue refractive index. The light rays that are reflected from this interface give rise to an observed image of an essentially flat (or slightly undulating) and featureless endothelial cell mosaic. Light rays that strike 'blebbed' endothelial cells will be deflected away from the observation path, leaving a corresponding area of darkness. Thus an endothelial bleb is simply an individual endothelial cell (or group of adjacent cells) that has become swollen and bulged in the direction of the aqueous humour, giving rise to the compelling optical illusion that the cell (or cells) has disappeared.

Endothelial blebs are caused by a local acidic pH change at the endothelium. Two separate factors induce an acidic shift in the cornea during contact lens wear:

1. An increase in carbonic acid due to retardation of carbon dioxide efflux (hypercapnia) by a contact lens
2. Increased levels of lactic acid as a result of lens-induced oxygen deprivation (hypoxia) and the consequent increase in anaerobic metabolism of epithelial tissue.

All cells in the human body function optimally when surrounded by extracellular fluid that is maintained within an acceptable range of pH, temperature, tonicity, ion balance etc. The carbonic acid and lactic acid alter the physiological status of the environment surrounding the endothelial cells by shifting the pH in the acidic direction. This induces changes in membrane permeability and/or membrane pump activity, resulting in a net movement of water into certain endothelial cells when the threshold for a change in membrane permeability is exceeded for those cells. The resultant cellular oedema in such cells is observed as 'blebbing'.

Despite their stunning clinical appearance, blebs are asymptomatic and are thought to be of little clinical significance. After removal of a contact lens, blebs disappear within minutes.

Endothelial microscope
- See *Specular microscope*.

Endothelial polymegethism, contact lens associated

The human corneal endothelium is a single cell layer that appears as an ordered mosaic of primarily hexagonal-shaped cells. A significant variation in apparent size of cells is referred to as endothelial polymegethism (Figure E.7). ('Polymegethism' is derived from the Greek words megethos, meaning size, and poly, meaning many.) The extent of polymegethism increases throughout life, and consequently the degree of lens-induced polymegethism should be taken to mean the degree of change in excess of that expected for a given age.

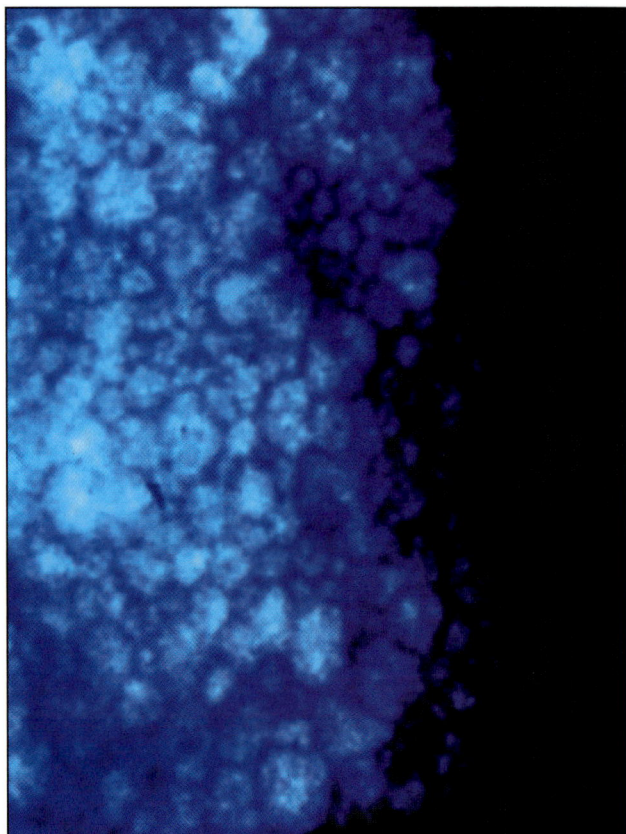

Figure E.7 • Endothelial polymegethism.

It is difficult to assess the integrity of the endothelium using a slit-lamp biomicroscope, because individual endothelial cells are just beyond the limit of resolution. Thus, a normal endothelial mosaic can only be seen as a speckled or textured field. Endothelial polymegethism of a severity greater than Grade 2 can sometimes be detected because some of the larger cells can be seen. Inspection of the endothelium is best undertaken by imaging the cornea through the eyepiece of a slit-lamp biomicroscope, or using instruments designed specifically for high magnification imaging, such as the specular microscope or confocal microscope.

An anecdotal association exists between endothelial polymegethism and a condition termed 'corneal exhaustion syndrome'. This may be related to the link between endothelial polymegethism and impairment of corneal hydration control, whereby recovery from oedema is significantly slower in the corneas of contact lens wearers (who have high levels of polymegethism) compared with corneas of non-lens wearers (who have lower levels of polymegethism).

It is likely that the aetiology of endothelial polymegethism – contact lens induced endothelial acidosis – is precisely the same as the aetiology of endothelial blebs, where the former represents a chronic response and the latter represents an acute response to the same stimuli. Endothelial acidosis may induce changes in membrane permeability and/or membrane pump activity, resulting in water movement that acts to elongate endothelial cell walls. A reconfiguration of cell shape then occurs in order to preserve cell volume, resulting in the appearance of polymegethism at the apical surface of the endothelium.

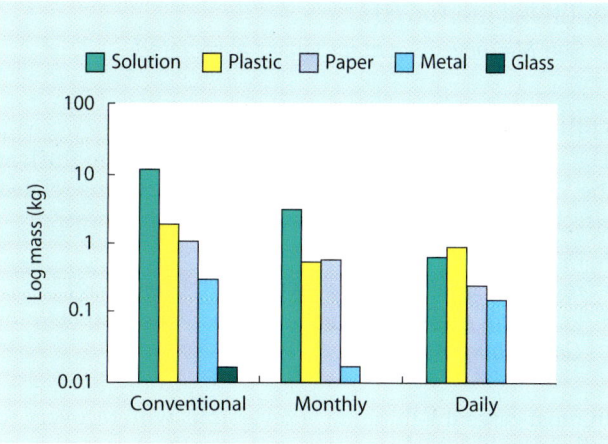

Figure E.8 • Mass of various material components of daily, monthly and 'conventional' (non-replacement) systems used by a single patient over a 12-month period.

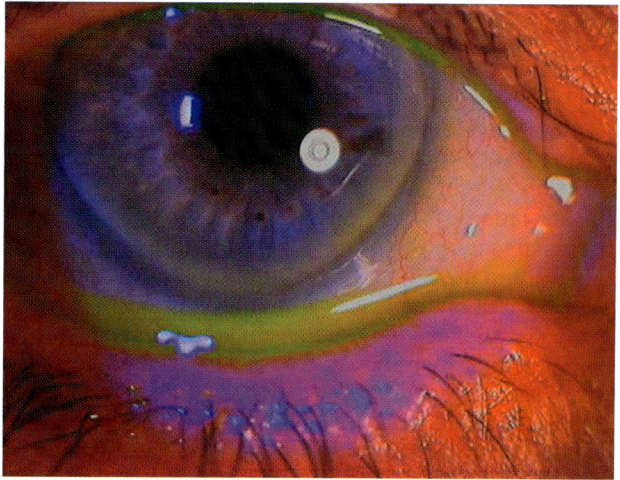

Figure E.9 • Increased marginal tear film stained with fluorescein.

Lenses of lower oxygen performance induce higher levels of polymegethism. From a clinical perspective, it is essential to take note of the presence of significant endothelial polymegethism and to take action to minimize the metabolic stress to the cornea known to be associated with this change. Strategies for alleviating contact lens induced hypoxia and hypercapnia include the following:
- fitting lenses of higher oxygen transmissibility
- sleeping in extended-wear lenses less frequently
- changing from extended lens wear to daily lens wear
- reducing lens wearing time
- fitting rigid lenses with more movement and edge lift (to enhance oxygen-enriching tear exchange).

The prognosis for recovery from endothelial polymegethism is poor. Recovery from polymegethism is likely to take many years, if it occurs at all.

Endothelium
- See *Corneal endothelium*.

Enhancement of compliance
- See *Compliance enhancement with contact lenses*.

Entropion
- See *Eyelid pathology, therapeutic contact lenses for*.

Environmental impact of contact lenses

Concerns have been expressed regarding the possible environmental impact of disposable contact lenses. Specifically, consideration needs to be given to the amount of waste glass, plastic, metal and paper involved in the consumer use of various modalities of contact lenses (solutions can be ignored because they have a negligible environmental impact). Non-planned lens replacement has the highest environmental impact and monthly lens replacement the lowest environmental impact, with daily disposability falling between the two (Figure E.8). It is certain that the overall level of wastage incurred in contact lens manufacture is more significant than that incurred by consumers. From a wider perspective, the environmental impact of wastage in the use of contact lenses and care systems by consumers pales into insignificance when considered against major sources of world environmental pollution (e.g. road construction, general domestic wastage, deforestation etc.).

Enzyme cleaning systems
- See *Protein removal systems for contact lenses*.

EOP
- See *Equivalent oxygen pressure beneath contact lenses*.

Epiphora

Epiphora refers to overflow of tears. They usually run down the cheek from the medial canthus; however, especially in the elderly with lateral canthal tendon laxity, the tears may overflow from the lateral canthus.

Epiphora results from:
- Increased lacrimation: a marked increase in tear secretion occurs with reflex tearing (Figure E.9). This is triggered by emotional or environmental factors or ocular irritation, including underlying dry eye (paradoxical tearing).
- Decreased outflow: physical or functional obstruction of the lacrimal outflow system can occur anywhere from the punctum, through the canaliculi, common canaliculus, lacrimal sac, nasolacrimal duct to the outlet of the nasolacrimal duct in the inferior nasal meatus on the lateral wall of the nose. The most common site of physical obstruction is at the punctum (punctal stenosis), the lacrimal sac and the nasolacrimal duct. In infants failure of the lower end of the nasolacrimal duct to canalise is the most frequent cause of epiphora. This can rarely lead to a congenital dacryocele, a cystic dilation of the lacrimal sac.
- Lacrimal pump failure: the lids normally act to pump the tears medially across the eye towards the puncta and along the canaliculi into the lacrimal sac. Failure of this mechanism as with medial ectropion and facial nerve paralysis can also lead to epiphora.

Patients suffering from epiphora usually complain of a watery eye, slight ocular discomfort and frequent blurring of vision due to an excess tear film. The frequency and extent of epiphora should be determined. Epiphora made worse by cold winds is usually due to anatomical or functional obstruction, whereas epiphora that is worse in hot, dry conditions or after prolonged concentration is often due to dry eye. An increase in the marginal tear strip is observed on slit-lamp examination; this is more obvious with the application of fluorescein. Skin excoriation may occur from the overflow of tears. In general, epiphora is usually only a cause of ocular irritation and frustration at the need to constantly dry the eye. It can however become a more significant problem if skin excoriation or dacryocystitis occurs.

If obstruction of the lacrimal drainage system is suspected the following tests may be useful in defining the cause.

- Dilation and irrigation (syringing): after instillation of a drop of local anaesthetic the punctum is dilated with a punctal dilator and a lacrimal cannula inserted. Sterile saline or water is then injected. If the canaliculus is blocked fluid will reflux through the same punctum. Blockage to the common canaliculus or more distal structures will lead to efflux of fluid through the other punctum. If the drainage system is patent fluid will pass through to the back of the throat.
- Jones dye test: this is a test for functional blockage. Fluorescein is instilled into the tear film. After 5 minutes an anaesthetic soaked cotton bud is placed under the inferior turbinate. If fluorescein is collected the drainage system is functionally patent.
- Dacryocystogram: radio-opaque dye is directly injected into the canaliculi and X-rays are taken immediately and five minutes post injection. This reveals any physical obstruction to the passage of dye.
- Lacrimal scintillogram: a radionuclide (usually technetium-99) is instilled into the tear film and its passage through the lacrimal drainage system is followed radiologically. This provides a more physiologic test of drainage function and can reveal a functional blockage.

Any cause of increased tear production such as ocular surface inflammation or dry eye should be treated. Surgical intervention with either a dacryocystorhinostomy to establish a fistula from the lacrimal sac to the nasopharynx for nasolacrimal duct obstruction, probing for congenital nasolacrimal duct obstruction, or Jones' tube for a blockage to the canaliculi may be indicated. Failure of lid function from an ectropion may need to be surgically repaired.

Epithelial degeneration
- See *Degenerations of the corneal epithelium, therapeutic contact lenses for.*

Epithelial dystrophies
- See *Dystrophies of the corneal epithelium, therapeutic contact lenses for.*

Epithelial microcysts
- See *Microcysts, contact lenses associated.*

Epithelial thinning, contact lens induced
The corneal epithelium is normally about 50 μm thick at the corneal centre. The following contact lens-related effects can cause a reduction in epithelial thickness:
- rigid contact lens wear
- reverse geometry lenses used for orthokeratology
- long-term extended hydrogel contact lens wear (see *Gothenburg Study*).

In most cases the thinning is reversible, with recovery to full epithelial thickness within 1 month of cessation of lens wear.

Epithelial vacuoles
- See *Vacuoles, contact lens-associated.*

Epithelial wrinkling
- See *Wrinkling, contact lens induced.*

Epithelium
- See *Corneal epithelium.*

Equivalent carbon dioxide percentage
- See *Equivalent carbon dioxide pressure beneath contact lenses.*

Equivalent carbon dioxide pressure beneath contact lenses
This represents the partial pressure of atmospheric carbon dioxide (CO_2) at the cornea-contact lens interface beneath a contact lens. Equivalent carbon dioxide pressure (ECDP) values are derived from in vivo human experiments, whereby the efflux of CO_2 from the cornea after application of a contact lens is compared to that following corneal exposure to various environments of known CO_2 content for about 5 minutes (Figure E.10). Efflux of CO_2 is measured by pressing a CO_2 electrode against the cornea and monitoring the build-up of CO_2 in the electrode. A higher rate of build-up of CO_2 indicates higher pre-exposure levels of CO_2.

The pressure of CO_2 in the atmosphere is 0.3mmHg. Because the partial pressure of carbon dioxide in the aqueous is about 40mmHg, and because CO_2 can diffuse rapidly through the cornea, the partial pressure of CO_2 at the corneal surface will never exceed 40mmHg. Thus the ECDP scale effectively ranges from 0–40mmHg. If it is stated that the ECDP beneath a lens is 25mmHgCO_2, it is inferred that the cornea has responded as if it was in a gaseous environment containing 25mmHgCO_2.

Equivalent oxygen percentage
- See *Equivalent oxygen pressure beneath contact lenses.*

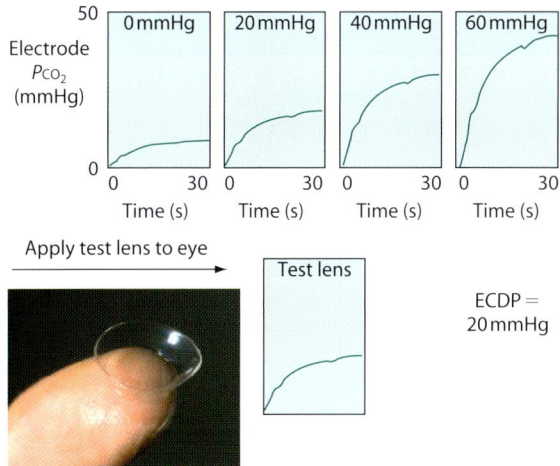

Figure E.10 • Equivalent carbon dioxide pressure technique. The rate of corneal carbon dioxide efflux following lens wear is matched to that following exposure to known carbon dioxide environments.

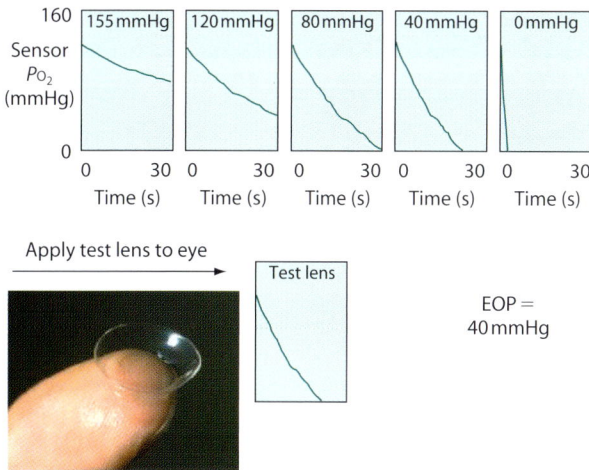

Figure E.11 • Equivalent oxygen pressure technique. The rate of corneal oxygen uptake following lens wear is matched to that following exposure to known oxygen environments.

Equivalent oxygen pressure beneath contact lenses

This represents the partial pressure of atmospheric oxygen at the cornea–contact lens interface beneath a contact lens. Equivalent oxygen pressure (EOP) values are derived from in vivo human or rabbit experiments, whereby the corneal respiratory response ('hunger' for oxygen) after application of a contact lens is compared to that following corneal exposure to various gaseous oxygen environments of known oxygen content. Hunger for oxygen is taken to be the rate at which oxygen is consumed by the cornea from the oxygen-enriched Teflon™ membrane of a polarographic oxygen sensor when the sensor is pressed against the cornea immediately following exposure of the cornea to either a contact lens or a gaseous environment for about 5 minutes (Figure E.11). A higher rate of consumption indicates pre-exposure to a more hypoxic environment.

Under conditions of standard temperature and pressure at sea level, the partial pressure of oxygen in the atmosphere is 159mmHg (or 155mmHg allowing for water vapour pressure); this represents the theoretical maximum oxygen partial pressure at the cornea–contact lens interface beneath a contact lens. If it is stated that the EOP beneath a lens is 30mmHg, it is inferred that the cornea has responded as if it was in a gaseous environment containing 30mmHg O_2.

Whereas the percentage of oxygen (20.9%) remains constant under any conditions and at any altitude within the earth's atmosphere, the oxygen partial pressure falls at increasing altitudes. Some prefer to think in terms of 'equivalent oxygen percentage' rather than 'equivalent oxygen pressure' (the acronym 'EOP' of course remains the same). Thus the EOP scale ranges from 0–155mmHg or from 0–20.9% when thinking in terms of oxygen pressure or oxygen percentage, respectively. Under conditions of standard temperature and pressure at sea level, these two scales are interchangeable; to convert mmHg to %O_2, multiply by 0.1348.

Erosion

- See *Recurrent erosion syndrome*, *therapeutic contact lenses for*.

Esophoria

Esophoria occurs where both visual axes are directed towards the fixation point but deviate on dissociation. On cover testing the eye under the cover moves in. Outwards recovery movements take place when the cover is removed. Eso-deviations can be classified according to whether the size of the deviation varies with fixation distance:

- Convergence excess esophoria – the deviation is greater at near than distance
- Divergence weakness esophoria – the deviation is greater at distance than near
- Non-specific (basic) esophoria – the deviation remains the same at distance and near.

Esophorias may occur as a result of anatomical irregularities such as: enophthalmos, narrow interpupillary distances, and extraocular muscle anomalies. Refractive causes include hypermetropia and anisometropia. A high AC/A ratio and weak divergent fusional reserves can also result in esophoric deviations.

Esotropia

Esotropia occurs when one eye deviates inwards and so its visual axis is not directed to the fixation point. An esotropia may or may not have an accommodative element. The various types of esotropia are discussed below.

Constant esotropia with an accommodative element. This deviation is present under all conditions and increases when accommodation is exerted (Table E.1). Onset is usually between 3 to 4 years of age and is associated with hypermetropia, astigmatism and anisometropia.

A fully accommodative strabismus results from uncorrected hypermetropia and the patient is orthotropic when wearing the full refractive correction (Figure E.12). A partially accommodative strabismus is present without spectacles and is reduced, but not eliminated, by the wearing of a hypermetropic prescription. Constant deviations are normally unilateral and result in the typical secondary defects associated with such a condition; e.g.,

Type of accommodative esotropia	Distance	Near	Treatment
Fully accommodative	Esotropia	Esotropia	Optical
Convergent excess (high AC/A ratio)	Orthophoria	Esotropia	Optical, miotics, surgery
Accommodative plus high AC/A ratio	Esotropia	Esotropia	Optical, surgery
Partially accommodative	Esotropia	Esotropia	Accommodative treatment, surgery

Table E.1 • Types of accommodative esotropias.

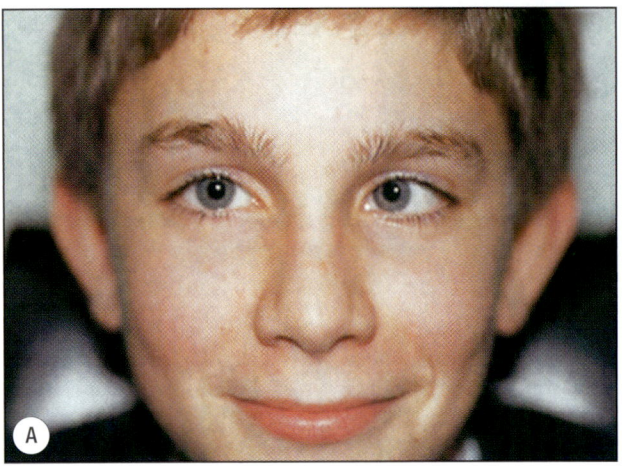
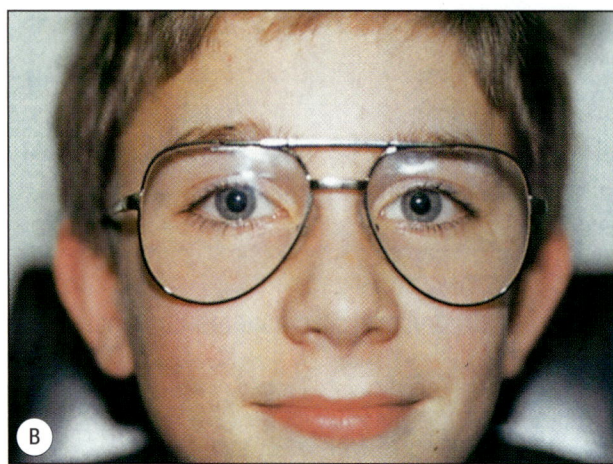

Figure E.12 • (A) Fully accommodative left convergent strabismus that is (B) fully corrected by the hypermetropic correction.

amblyopia and abnormal retinal correspondence. Management involves correction of the refractive error and treatment of amblyopia; surgery may be required for a cosmetic or functional result in cases that are not fully accommodative. Some cases can be straightened at near with bifocals.

Constant esotropia without an accommodative element. A form of non-accommodative comitant esotropia is 'infantile esotropia syndrome', which presents in the first six months of life (Figure E.13). Although it may be associated with hypermetropia, refractive correction rarely reduces the size of the deviation which is usually large, present under all conditions, stable in size and with a limited potential for single binocular vision.

It may be unilateral or alternating; if alternating the deviation will not result in amblyopia. It can be associated with dissociated vertical deviation, oblique muscle dysfunction and latent nystagmus. The aetiology remains controversial and it may be that different mechanisms acting early in life lead to the same endpoint. Management involves correction of any refractive error, treatment of amblyopia and possibly surgery for a cosmetic or functional result.

Intermittent esotropia with an accommodative element. Intermittent convergent deviations often have an accommodative element. The deviation is present only under certain conditions and is therefore unlikely to cause amblyopia. It usually occurs between the age of two and five years and is associated with a moderate degree of hypermetropia and a normal AC/A ratio. The convergent deviation is affected by the state of accommodation and this is the primary factor in the aetiology of the strabismus. Two-thirds of cases of comitant convergent strabismus have an accommodative element, and the angle of deviation will be reduced by a refractive correction for hyperopia (a full correction in some cases, and partial in others).

For intermittent fully accommodative esotropia, binocular single vision is present for all distances when the hypermetropia is corrected. Without refractive correction the patient is usually orthotropic for distance and markedly esotropic for near. When fully corrected, the patient is usually orthotropic at distance and either esophoric or orthophoric for near. Full cycloplegic refractive correction is important even at the risk of reducing the distance visual acuity slightly, to prevent the occurrence of a partially accommodative esotropia and associated amblyopia. Orthoptic exercises can be used with older children to control the manifest deviation.

Intermittent convergence excess esotropia. In this condition the eyes are straight for distant fixation but there is an intermittent near esotropia. There may be some control when fixing on a near non-accommodative target such as a light. An esophoria may be present for distance fixation. Onset is usually between two and five years of age and is more noticeable when the patient is looking at close objects. This condition is often associated with hypermetropia but sometimes occurs with myopia and always with an AC/A ratio of greater than 5:1. Children with this condition can often be managed well with bifocals at least until they reach an age when they can undergo exercises. Often, the strength of the near addition can be gradually reduced with time until the patient is comfortably straight at distance and near with single vision spectacles. Treatment may also involve orthoptic eye exercises and surgery.

Intermittent near esotropia without an accommodative element. Binocular single vision is present for distance

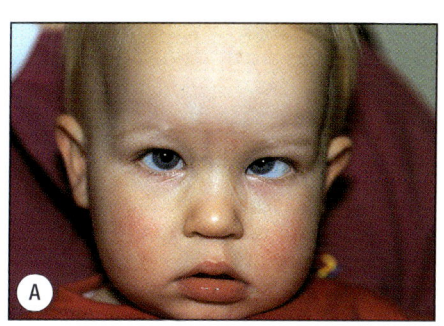 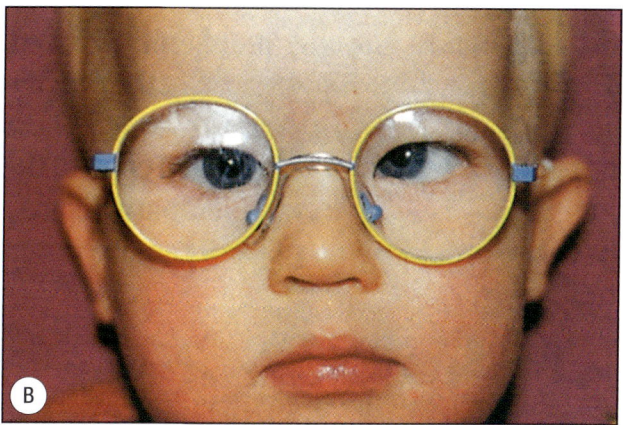

Figure E.13 • (A) A non-accommodative left convergent strabismus that is (B) not corrected by spectacles.

fixation and intermittent esotropia for near fixation, even when any extra accommodative effort due to uncorrected hypermetropia is relieved. Multifocal spectacles are inappropriate as there is no accommodative element. Any refractive error should be corrected and amblyopia treated; surgery is usually indicated. Orthoptic exercises can be difficult in these patients.

Intermittent distance esotropia. These cases exhibit an esotropia on distance fixation and heterophoria on near fixation. Amblyopia, if present, should be treated and prisms can be used if the angle at distance is 10° or less; surgery may be necessary.

Intermittent cyclic esotropia. This deviation relates to time, the anomaly occurring at regular intervals with the most common pattern being an alternate day deviation. It is usually late onset, from four to five years of age. Occasionally, after six months, the alternate day pattern may alter and the deviation becomes constant. On the strabismic day a marked deviation for near and distance fixation is present; on the straight day an esophoria may be present for near and distance fixation. Surgery is usually indicated especially if the deviation becomes constant.

Intermittent non-specific esotropia. This is an intermittent esotropia not conforming to any pattern; the deviation is intermittently manifest at any fixation distance and there is no significant change in the angle of deviation for near or distance fixation or with accommodation exerted. Any refractive error should be corrected and amblyopia treated; surgery may be considered. By definition an intermittent strabismus is not constantly undermining binocular function and therefore immediate treatment may not be necessary; if periodic observation reveals that the deviation is becoming manifest more frequently, treatment becomes urgent.

Nystagmus blocking esotropia. This is another type of early esotropia. It occurs in young children with nystagmus of early onset, typically prior to the age of six months; an esotropia often develops as the patient learns to adduct the fixing eye in an attempt to control the nystagmus. It eventually leads to a large constant unilateral esotropia with an abnormal head posture to maintain the position of the adducted eye. Non-accommodative esotropia is usually treated with surgery, although full refractive correction and treatment of any associated amblyopia is advisable.

Esotropia associated with myopia. When uncorrected some adults with high myopia may demonstrate an esotropia. The mechanism is uncertain but normal retinal correspondence is demonstrated when the deviation is corrected. Visual acuity might be reduced due to degenerative myopic fundus changes. Management involves constant wear of a full myopic correction.

Ethnic variations in ocular dimensions

Ethnic variations in ocular topography may be of relevance to contact lens fitting. In the UK-resident Chinese population, corneas have been noted to be steeper and smaller and to show less corneal flattening than Caucasian eyes. This suggests a requirement for smaller rigid lenses showing less peripheral flattening for such patients. The eyes of American Japanese people show, on average, a smaller HVID but no difference in corneal curvature. It is likely that environmental factors such as nutrition, as well as cultural differences, influence corneal topography and probably account for the mean flattening that has been observed in corneal curvature noted in the Japanese population over a 20-year period. Oriental eyes tend to show a narrower palpebral aperture – on average, about 1.0mm smaller than in Caucasian eyes. Corneas in Afro-Caribbean populations tend to be larger and flatter than corneas of Chinese or Japanese populations.

European Federation of the Contact Lens Industry (EFCLIN)

An organization for European contact lens manufacturers and wholesalers, EFCLIN offers a platform for exchange of information on technical and marketing subjects.

Eversion

- See *Eyelid eversion*.

Exophoria

Exophoria occurs where both visual axes are directed towards the fixation point but deviate on dissociation. On cover testing the eye under the cover moves out. Inward recovery movements take place when the cover is removed. Exo-deviations can be classified according to their change with fixation as follows:

Convergence weakness exophoria – the deviation is greater at near than distance. This is *not* synonymous with convergence insufficiency. The latter is characterized by an unusually remote near point of convergence, and is often but not always associated with an exophoria that is greater at near than distance. Convergence weakness exophoria is often used to describe a decompensated exophoia at near, and the near point of convergence may be within normal range.

Divergence excess exophoria – the deviation is greater at distance than near.

Non-specific (basic) exophoria – the deviation is the same at distance and near.

Exophoria may occur as a result of structural anomalies such as exophthalmos, wide interpupillary distance and extraocular muscle anomalies. Refractive causes include myopia, presbyopia and anisometropia. Weak convergent fusional reserves and age may result in an exophoria.

Exotropia

A patient with exotropia has one eye deviating outwards and so its visual axis is not directed to the fixation point. Like any other tropia it can be classified as: primary, secondary or consecutive; intermittent or constant; occurring at distance or near; true or simulated. The following discussion will relate to primary anomalies only.

Constant exotropia. A divergent deviation constitutes the initial defect that is constantly present under all conditions. Anatomical causes include wide interpupillary distance, exophthalmos, orbital asymmetry, muscle anomalies and craniofacial anomalies. It may be hereditary, and can be associated with myopia. It often commences as an intermittent deviation, which then becomes constant with time. The deviation may increase in size when the patient is in bright sunlight and presentation is with a history of closing one eye and photophobia. If the deviation is alternating visual acuity can be equal. Refractive error should be corrected and amblyopia treated. Surgery is an option but there is a risk of post-operative intractable diplopia and use of Botulinum toxin may be an alternative.

Intermittent exotropia. The eyes may be diverged at times but aligned at others. Intermittent exotropia is often related to fixation distance but there may be no accommodative element. There are three types:

- *Near-fixation type (insufficient convergence).* An exotropia is present on near fixation with binocular single vision on distance fixation, although there may be an exophoria in the distance. Onset is usually late and may be associated with myopia or presbyopia. It is very common among young people with decompensating exophoria who present with diplopia and asthenopic symptoms. Investigation will reveal a remote near point of convergence, a manifest deviation at near, and binocular single vision at distance. Management includes correction of refractive error, orthoptic exercises, base-in prisms and very rarely surgery.
- *Distance-fixation type (excessive divergence).* Associated with high AC/A ratio and anatomical abnormalities, this is a condition in which the patient maintains binocular single vision at near (there may be an exophoria) and has an exotropia at distance. The distance exotropia characteristically increases with greater viewing distances, so it may be useful to test the patient when looking at an object out of a window (greater than 6m). The angle of deviation for near fixation may increase on prolonged disruption of fusion or elimination of accommodation. Patients who demonstrate an increase in angle for near fixation on occlusion or with plus lenses are described as 'simulated distance types'. These are characterized by an increase in angle of greater than 10^Δ for near fixation with +3.00D lenses. The deviation may appear controlled initially for distance but decompensates quickly on dissociation. Onset is usually within the first year of life but small-angle deviations may not be present until later because of the intermittent nature of the deviation. Parents often notice the condition when the child is not concentrating or is fatigued. The patient is usually asymptomatic but may be aware of the divergence from the 'feel of the eye' or notice an increase in the visual field. Like the near-fixation type, the deviation is often larger in conditions of bright sunlight, and photophobia is common. Visual acuity is usually equal while good binocular visual acuity indicates good control of the deviation. Management is by full correction of any myopic refractive error, under-correction of any hyperopia, orthoptic exercises for small deviations (<15^Δ), negative over-correction when the AC/A ratio is high, base-in prisms, tinted lenses when light constitutes a dissociative factor and possibly surgery.
- *Non-specific type.* This is characterized by a manifest divergent strabismus that occurs at any distance and at any time. The size of the deviation does not change with fixation distance and causes can be any of those described for the near and distance types as well as poor fusional ability. Surgery is often the only management option.

Extended contact lens wear

This refers to a contact lens that is worn during the day followed by at least one sleep cycle (overnight) without removal. From a cosmetic standpoint, extended wear offers convenience to patients because there is no need for routine lens cleaning and disinfection. Extended-wear lenses also have important therapeutic applications as bandage lenses for use following ocular surgery and in the treatment of a wide variety of ocular pathology.

During the early development of soft lenses it was suggested that it might be possible to wear contact lenses continuously for many weeks, months or even years without removal; however, it soon became clear that such a practice was not clinically viable.

Various combinations of lens removal and lens replacement have been advocated over the years, and this has been driven to some extent by directions from the USA Food and Drug Administration (FDA). In 1981, the FDA gave approval for certain lenses to be worn continuously for 30 days and nights, after which the lenses had to be removed and cleaned, left out overnight, and reinserted the next day for another 30 day/night cycles, and so on. This recommendation was later revised to 7 day/night cycles in view of the growing body of evidence at the time that the risk of microbial keratitis increased significantly the longer lenses were worn

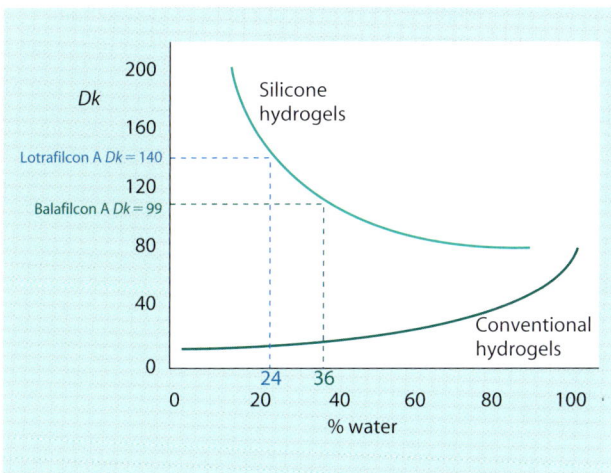

Figure E.14 • Relationship between water content and oxygen permeability (Dk) for conventional hydrogel and silicone hydrogel materials.

without removal. With the introduction of disposable lenses in the late 1980s, lens removal was linked to lens replacement. The Acuvue™ disposable soft lens was designed as a lens that could be worn for 7 day/night cycles and discarded thereafter. Silicone hydrogel lenses have both USA and European regulatory approval to be worn for up to 30 day/night cycles. At the present time, 'extended wear' is taken to mean a 7 day/night cycle of lens wear, and 'continuous wear' is taken to mean a 30 day/night cycle of lens wear.

A primary concern in prescribing lenses for extended wear is that the lenses must provide sufficient oxygen to avoid excess corneal oedema. The Holden-Mertz criterion for the critical lens oxygen transmissibility (Dk/t) to meet this 'no oedema' criterion is 87Barrer/cm. The maximum achievable Dk/t for hydrogel lenses is about 35Barrer/cm. It is therefore not possible for hydrogel lenses to meet this criterion; nevertheless, certain patients appear to have higher thresholds for developing excess oedema and are capable of wearing hydrogel lenses successfully overnight. 'Stress testing' has been advocated as a means of assessing suitability for sleeping in lenses; this involves measuring the oedema response to a standard 'test lens' worn for a specified period with the eyes closed. Such tests have yet to be fully validated.

Silicone hydrogel lenses have oxygen transmissibilities in excess of 100Barrer/cm (Figure E.14); these lenses therefore satisfy the Holden-Mertz criterion and can be advocated for continuous/extended wear. The incidence of severe microbial keratitis with these lenses is 5× less than with conventional hydrogel lenses. Non-sight threatening conditions such as sterile keratitis (which manifests in many forms), superior epithelial arcuate lesions and papillary conjunctivitis appear to be occurring at a similar rate in silicone hydrogel and conventional hydrogel lens wearers.

External hordeolum

This condition presents as a discrete, tender swelling of the anterior lid margin; specifically, it is an inflammation of the tissue lining the eyelash follicle and/or an associated gland of Zeis or Moll. Contact lenses may add to the discomfort of an external hordeolum due to various mechanical pressures exerted by the lens, and patients may prefer to cease lens wear during the acute phase of the condition. *Syn.* Stye.

Extraocular muscles

The six extraocular (extrinsic) muscles of the eye are composed of skeletal (striated) muscle fibres and are so-called to distinguish them from the intrinsic (smooth, unstriated) muscles within the eye. They attach to the bone of the orbit and insert into the sclera of the eye, which they rotate. A seventh striated muscle, the levator palpebrae superioris, also attaches to the orbital wall and inserts into the upper eyelid, which it raises. The six oculorotatory muscles may be grouped into antagonistic pairs imposing opposite rotation on the eye namely, the medial and lateral rectus, inferior and superior rectus, and inferior and superior oblique muscles. Five of the six extraocular muscles and the levator palpebrae superioris have short tendonous origins in a common fibrous ring, the annulus of Zinn. The origin of the sixth, the inferior oblique muscle, is located anteriorly, close to the orbital margin. The oval-shaped annulus lies at the apex of the orbit where it encircles the optic canal.

The rectus muscles have a roughly similar length of approximately 40mm (36 to 43mm) and tendon lengths at insertion vary more than twofold (3.6 to 8.4mm). Muscles lie close to the orbital wall, bowed outwards slightly when relaxed and form an incomplete muscle cone with the apex at the annulus and the base at the globe. The medial orbital wall is in the sagittal plane and the lateral orbital wall is at 45° to it; the lateral rectus therefore has a slightly longer course from origin to insertion than the medial rectus, a greater length in apposition to the globe and a tendon more than twice the length. As the muscle cone diameter increases anteriorly, the approximately strap-like rectus muscles thicken and widen to a maximum of 8 to 11mm at their middle thirds. Their tendons insert in the anterior half of the globe 3 to 8mm from the limbus.

The superior oblique muscle has a narrow 2.5mm wide origin becoming thicker and widening to a maximum of about 5mm. It advances to the trochlea, a U-shaped ring of hyaline cartilage located in the frontal bone at the upper medial angle of the orbit close to the margin. Anteriorly, the muscle thins becoming cylindrical and tendonous, reducing to about 1.5mm in diameter before entering the trochlea. Passing through the trochlea, the tendon is reflected making an angle of approximately 54° with its initial path, thins and widens and passes across the upper surface of the globe beneath the superior rectus muscle and attaches obliquely to the upper lateral posterior quadrant of the sclera. Its length to the trochlea is 32mm, and the distance from trochlea to insertion is 20mm (Figure E.15).

The inferior oblique arises as a short rounded tendon, 1 to 2mm in length, in a shallow depression in the floor of the orbit medially in the same vertical plane as the trochlea. The muscle passes posterolaterally and slightly upwards at an angle of 51° to the sagittal plane, or 75° to the axis of the orbit. Its width quickly increases and

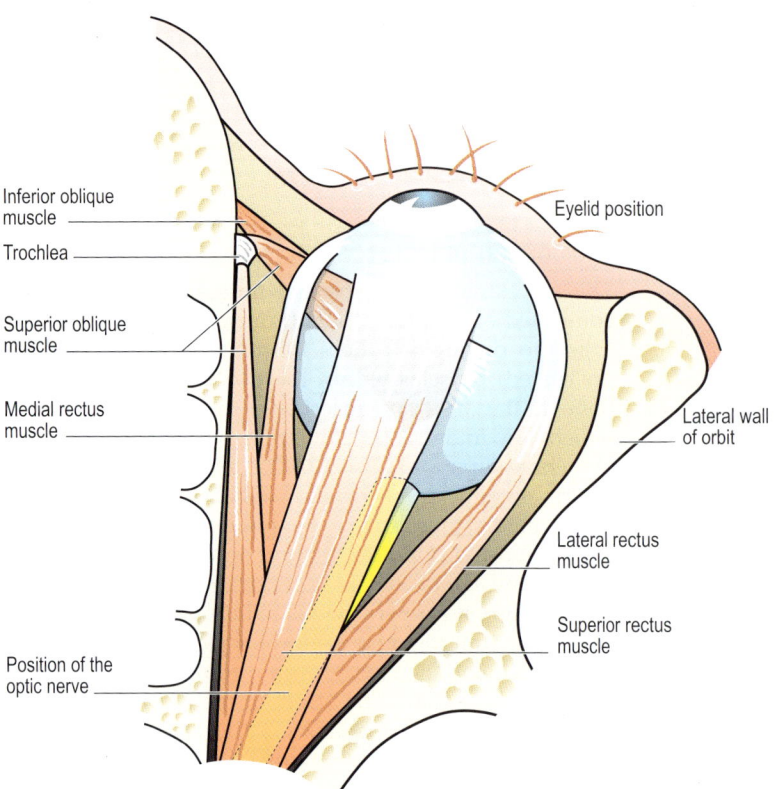

Figure E.15 • Extraocular muscles viewed from above. All but the inferior oblique have their origins in the common annulus of Zinn.

becomes a flat band passing beneath the inferior rectus muscle then curving upwards obliquely in close apposition to the sclera, inserting into the inferior lateral quadrant of the globe posteriorly with a barely discernible tendon 10mm in width. It averages about 36mm in length.

The levator palpebrae superioris arises from the annulus of Zinn above the medial border of the superior rectus, widens slightly at first but then more expansively to completely cover the superior rectus and enter the upper eyelid as a thin aponeurotic band. The transition from muscle to tendon also marks a change in direction from horizontal to almost vertical. It becomes fan-shaped and extends the full width of the eyelid adjacent to the anterior aspect of the tarsal plate to which it has fibrous attachments at intervals along its full length and others penetrate the orbicularis muscle possibly to the skin. At its medial and lateral extremes the aponeurosis has attachments to the orbital margin at the medial and lateral midpoints. A division of the oculomotor branch serving the superior rectus enters the belly of the levator. The transverse ligament of Whitnall is commonly regarded as a check ligament for the muscle.

Eye

The eye (Figure E.16) is a sensory organ of the body responsible for capturing images of the external world and converting these images into neural signals which can be interpreted by the brain. In essence, the eye is an opaque, spherical, fluid-filled sac approximately 24mm in diameter containing a transparent open window at the front (the cornea). Light passes through (and is refracted by) the cornea and into the aqueous humour in the anterior chamber; it then passes through a small round aperture (the pupil of the iris) and is further refracted by the crystalline lens. Light then continues through the clear vitreous humour and hits the retina. The light energy is absorbed by rods and cones in the retina, converted to neural impulses, and transmitted via nerve fibres, via the optic nerve at the back of the eye, to the back of the brain (the visual cortex) where the visual world is perceived. Six extraocular muscles coordinate the movements of the eyes.

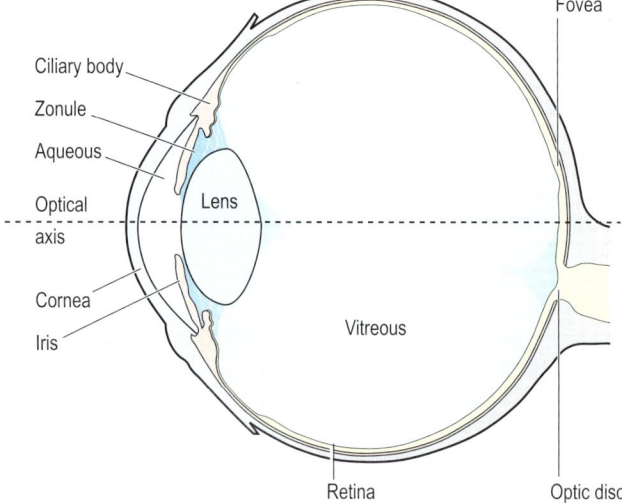

Figure E.16 • Schematic horizontal section of the human eye.

Eye dominance

- See *Ocular dominance*.

Eye protection programme

Eye safety in an industrial environment can be facilitated by implementing an eye protection programme. The main aim of such a programme is to identify potential ocular hazards and then to eliminate or control them. It should include:

- plant environment survey
- vision screening
- implementation of the programme
- maintenance of the programme.

Potential hazards in an industrial plant should be assessed by conducting a plant environment survey. For example, there may be acids, flying particles from a lathe, or radiation from welding, against which the eyes need to be protected. Once the hazard has been identified, a method of eliminating or controlling it must be devised. Hazards may be eliminated at their source by modifying the design of the machinery or equipment, and the layout of the work place. The wearing of eye protectors should always be considered as the last option. Accident records may also be analyzed to determine where and how ocular injuries have occurred in the past.

There is little doubt that poor lighting can be a contributory factor in some accidents. Lighting conditions should be assessed for the various tasks to check that they are appropriate for the job to be performed efficiently. Sites of emergency first aid equipment should be noted and the need for any additional equipment and their placement should also be assessed. For example, where chemicals are being used, a water fountain or shower unit should be installed to provide rapid dilution of any chemicals accidentally splashed on an employee.

About one-third of employees have vision below the standard required for their occupation. Obviously, an employee whose vision is below standard is more likely to be injured and may unintentionally injure colleagues. Vision screening can be carried out and those employees who fail can be referred to a qualified person for a full examination.

Depending on the findings of the plant survey, the following actions may be necessary:

- Elimination or control of ocular hazards.
- Provision of eye protectors. These must be personally issued to make sure that they fit correctly and are of the correct type for the task involved.
- Areas where ocular hazards exist, and where eye protection must be worn, should be marked clearly. Provisions must be made for eye protectors to be readily available for visitors to the hazardous areas.
- First aid facilities. These should be set up so that immediate medical attention can be provided. All employees should be made aware of the first aid centres, and they should be clearly signposted.
- Lens cleaning stations should be made available. These should contain cleaning solutions, anti-fog solutions, and clean cloths with which to wipe the eye protectors.
- A safety committee should be formed, which includes employee representatives.
- Employees should be educated about the hazards involved in their jobs and the need for eye protection.

The maintenance of the eye protection programme is essential for continued safety and cost-effectiveness. It may involve:

- Assessing new manufacturing processes and their potential hazards.
- Continuing education and training for the employees.
- Maintenance of lens cleaning and first aid facilities.
- Vision screening, which should be carried out at regular intervals to maintain the necessary standard of vision.
- Maintaining an active safety committee so that the employees can suggest methods of improving the safety of their environment.
- Maintenance of stocks of replacement eye protectors. Employees should be informed as to the location of these supplies, which should be readily available. Any adjustments to the fitting of the eye protectors should be carried out by trained personnel to provide maximum comfort and protection.
- Recognition of employee achievements regarding their efforts to maintain and create a safer environment.

Eye protectors

Protection against ocular hazards may be provided by:

- spectacles with or without side shields
- goggles – cup and box type
- face shields
- helmets.

The various standards for eye protection include:

- BS EN 165 Personal eye protection – vocabulary
- BS EN 166 Personal eye protection – specifications
- BS EN 167 Personal eye protection – optical test methods
- BS EN 168 Personal eye protection – non-optical test methods
- BS EN 169 Personal eye protection – filters for welding and similar operations
- BS EN 170 Personal eye protection – ultra-violet filters
- BS EN 171 Personal eye protection – infra-red filters
- BS EN 172 Personal eye protection – sun glare filters
- BS EN 175 Personal eye protection – equipment for eye and face protection during welding and allied processes
- BS EN 207 Personal eye protection – filters and eye protectors against laser radiation
- BS EN 379 Personal eye protection – welding filters with switchable luminous transmittance and with dual luminous transmittance.

As far as the majority of optometrists are concerned, the standard that is the most important is BS EN 166. The form of eye protector and the protection that they provide and their markings are summarized in Table E.2.

The test procedures for the level of impact resistance are summarized in Table E.3.

The filter markings are shown in Table E.4. The first number marked on the oculars (before the manufacturers mark) indicates the type of filter that is present.

Table E.2 • Types of eye-protectors and their markings according to BS EN 166.

	BS EN 166		Type of eye-protector		
	Housing	Oculars	Spectacles	Goggles	Face shields
Optical class	–	1	Yes	Yes	Yes
	–	2	Yes	Yes	Yes
	–	3	Yes	Yes	
Mechanical strength					
Increased robustness	–	S	Yes	Yes	Yes
Low energy impact	–F	F	Yes	Yes	Yes
Medium energy impact	–B	B		Yes	Yes
High energy impact	–A	A			Yes
Field of use					
Liquid droplets/splashes	3	–		Yes	Yes
Large dust particles	4	–		Yes	
Gas, fine dust particles	5	–		Yes	
Short circuit electric arc	8	–			Yes
Molten metals/hot solids	9	9		Yes	Yes
Resistance to fogging	–	N	Yes	Yes	Yes
Resistance to surface damage	–	K	Yes	Yes	Yes

Table E.3 • BS EN 166 – grades of impact resistance.

Symbol	Level of impact resistance*		Types of eye-protector
–F	Low energy	45m/s	All types
–B	Medium energy	120m/s	Goggles and face shields
–A	High energy	190m/s	Face shields

*The eye protector must withstand the impact of a 6-mm diameter steel ball of mass 0.86g.

Table E.4 • BS EN166 – code numbers for filters.

Filter code number	Filter property
(no code number)	Welding filters
2	UV filters where colour recognition may be affected
3	UV filters with good colour recognition
4	IR filter
5	Sunglare filter without IR specification
6	Sunglare filter with IR specification

Eyelashes

- See *Eyelids*.

Eyelid eversion

It is often necessary to turn the upper eyelid 'inside out' in order to observe the structures of the tarsal plate on the underside of the eyelid. This procedure is referred to as 'lid eversion'. The procedure is performed as follows. The head of the patient must be secured, either in the chin and brow rest of a slit lamp biomicroscope, or with the head resting on a headrest in an ophthalmic chair. With the patient's head in an upright position, the patient is instructed to direct his/her gaze downwards. A cotton applicator (or any other thin rod-like implement) is placed against the upper canthal fold and the eyelashes are grabbed and lifted up so that the upper lid folds back over the cotton applicator. (In many patients with loose eyelids, a cotton applicator is not required). The lashes and upper lid border can then be held against the brow with the thumb while the tarsal plate is inspected. This technique is used routinely in contact lens practice to check for contact lens induced papillary conjunctivitis or to search for a 'lost contact lens'. Lid eversion is also used to search for foreign bodies when a patient complains 'there is something in my eye'. The foreign body may be a tiny speck of dust or dirt, a small insect or a dislodged eyelash. Patients often report that the discomfort has been relieved following lid eversion even if no foreign body was detected, because the act of everting the eyelid often serves to dislodge a foreign body. A double eyelid eversion can be performed under local anaesthetic to inspect the superior conjunctival fornix.

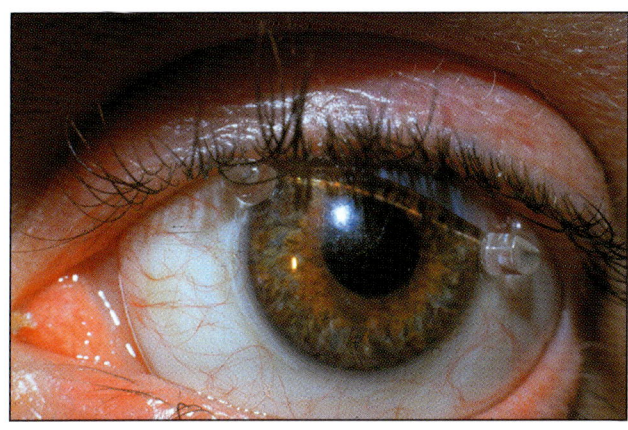

Figure E.17 • Lid support lugs built into a scleral lens to act as a ptosis crutch.

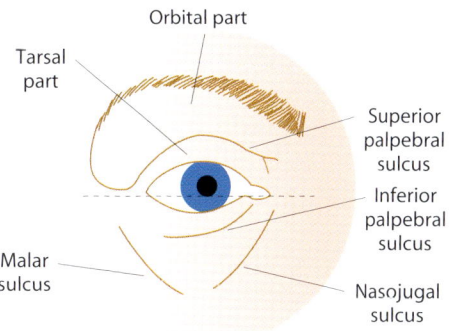

Figure E.18 • Surface anatomy of the eyelids.

Eyelid pathology, therapeutic contact lenses for

If the lids are deficient (for example, congenitally or following trauma or surgery), or immobile (for example, following seventh (facial) nerve disease), part or all of the anterior globe may be exposed and dry. The corneal epithelium will be eroded and undergo dysplasia, and blood vessels will invade the previously clear stroma, unless protection can be given. Possibilities include a temporary or permanent tarsorrhaphy, temporary paralysis of the levator palpebrae superioris muscle using botulinum toxin, and the use of therapeutic contact lenses.

The lids themselves may consititute the challenge. They may be inturned (entropion) so that the lashes touch and traumatize the globe (trichiasis), or the tarsal conjunctiva – especially the area adjacent to the lid margin – may be keratinized. Both situations are found in chronic cicatrizing disease, such as Stevens–Johnson syndrome and cicatricial pemphigoid, and following chemical injury. Keratinization without entropion is a feature of atopic keratoconjunctivitis. Most soft lenses will not survive in this type of environment, rapidly becoming decentred and often falling out of the eye. There is a place for rigid lenses here, but the first choice will often be a scleral lens.

Ptosis results in an unsightly cosmetic appearance and can deprive the eye of vision if severe. A scleral lens with a ptosis crutch is one possible solution (Figure E.17).

When the cornea is insensitive – such as following surgery for acoustic neuroma, in herpes zoster ophthalmicus, and in trigeminal neuralgia – great care must be taken when fitting contact lenses. The danger is that the insensitivity of the eye will result in a situation where the patient is not alerted to otherwise painful complications such as epithelial detachment and infection. Patients with acute corneal problems due to neuroparalytic keratitis are usually best managed with lid taping, tarsorrhaphy or botulinum toxin induced ptosis.

Eyelids

The eyelids are two mobile folds of skin that perform several important functions: they act as occluders, which shield the eyes from excessive light, and through their reflex closure afford protection against injury. The lids also form a pre-corneal tear film of uniform thickness during the upturn phase of each blink. The action of blinking is important for tear drainage.

The eyelids are joined at their extremities, termed the canthi, and when the eye is open an elliptical space, the palpebral fissure, is formed between the lid margins. The position of various folds, or sulci, indicate to the clinician the integrity or otherwise of the anatomical configuration of the eyelids (Figure E.18). In the adult, the length of the fissure is approximately 30–31mm, with a vertical height of 10–11mm. In the primary position, the upper lid, which is the larger and more mobile of the two, typically covers approximately the upper third of the cornea, whilst the lower lid is level with the inferior corneal limbus. The eyelid margins are about 2mm thick from front to back. The posterior quarter consists of conjunctival mucosa, and the anterior three-quarters is skin. The junction between the two is referred to as the mucocutaneous junction. Two or three rows of eyelashes (cilia) arise from the anterior border of the lid margins. These are longer and more numerous in the upper lid. The lashes receive a rich sensory nerve supply, and their sensitivity provides an effective alerting mechanism.

The meibomian (tarsal) gland orifices emerge just anterior to the mucocutaneous junction. About 30–40 glands open onto the upper margin, and slightly fewer (20–40) onto the lower. On eversion of the lids the yellowish meibomian acini are visible as yellow clusters through the tarsal conjunctiva. At the medial angle, the eyelid margins enclose a triangular space, the lacus lacrimalis, which contains the plica semilunaris and the caruncle. Lacrimal papillae are small elevations, located 5–6mm from the medial canthal angle, which have a small aperture (punctum) that forms the opening to the lacrimal drainage system.

Movements of the eyelids occur through the co-ordinated action of several muscles – the levator palpebrae superioris, tarsal muscles, the orbicularis oculi, and the frontalis muscle. The elevation of the upper lid and the control of its vertical position are mediated principally by the levator. In vertical gaze, lid position and eye movements are closely linked. During elevation, the state of contraction of the levator is varied to maximize visibility. In extreme upgaze, lid retraction is augmented by the action of the frontalis, which elevates the eyebrows. In downgaze, co-ordinated lid movements similarly occur through levator relaxation. In periodic and reflex blinks the levator is spontaneously inhibited prior to orbicularis contraction in lid closure. Similarly, in lid opening the orbicularis relaxes, followed by contraction of the levator. Spontaneous eye blink activity is influenced by both central and peripheral factors.

Compared to the upper lid, the lower lid is relatively immobile and has no counterpart to the levator palpebrae superioris. The depression of the lower lid that occurs in downgaze is due to the attachment of the sheaths of the inferior oblique and inferior rectus muscles to the tarsal plate via a fibrous extension.

Eye size

- See *Apparent eye size*.

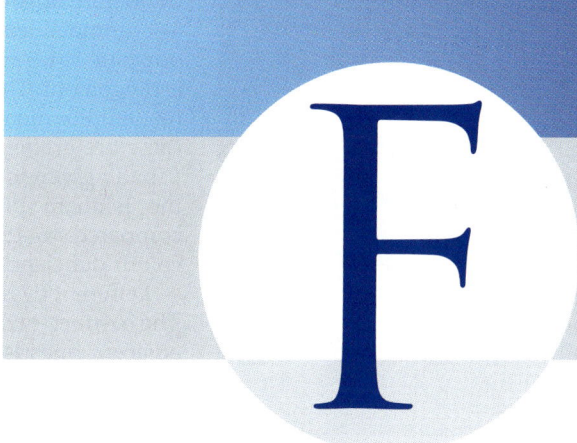

Fan and block technique

Though considered to be less accurate for small cylinders, the fan and block technique is a useful alternative to cross-cylinder for determining the astigmatic component of a refraction, particularly when a patient fails to respond well to or understand the latter. The target consists of a fan of radial lines of typically ten degrees separation spread around a central target with two blocks of straight lines orientated at ninety degrees to each other. The blocks have an arrow head above them and may be rotated so that the arrow head may point at any of the radiating lines in the fan (Figure F.1).

Having established the best vision sphere, an extra +0.50D is added (i.e. the patient is slightly 'fogged') so that one or more of the lines in the fan appears sharper. If this is not the case, further plus power may be added. If no lines become clear it may be that there is no cylinder. If they do, then the arrow is rotated to point to the central clear line such that the block of lines parallel to the clear fan line becomes clear. If the block is not quite clear, further plus power may be added until it actually starts to blur. At this point, a negative cylinder may be introduced with its axis orientated as indicated by the scale next to the clear fan line. The power of the trial lens is then increased until the clarity of the perpendicular block matches that of the first block. If equality is never exactly reached, then the lowest cylinder power at which equality is almost found should be chosen. At this point the fogging sphere should be reduced until best acuity is reached.

Farnsworth colour vision tests

Two hue discrimination tests for use in vocational guidance, the Farnsworth-Munsell 100 hue test (F-M 100 hue test) and the Farnsworth D15 test (D15 test), were introduced by Dean Farnsworth in the 1940's. These tests are not intended, nor designed, for colour vision screening but aim to identify people who make significant colour confusions likely to lead to practical difficulties in occupations which make frequent use of connotative colour codes. Protans are likely to achieve better results on these tests than deutans because differences in colour contrast, due to changes in relative luminous efficiency, lead to perceived lightness differences. Both tests consist of matte Munsell hue samples placed in small caps which subtend approximately 1.5° at a test distance of 50 cm. The x, y chromaticity co-ordinates of all the hue samples used are available from published spectrophotometric data and can be located in the CIE chromaticity diagrams. The person being examined is required to place the caps in what appears to be a natural hue sequence either between two reference hues or beginning from a single reference hue.

Farnsworth tests are frequently used to examine people with acquired colour deficiency because typical isochromatic colour confusions are not included in the test design. Although typical results may be obtained in significant congenital colour deficiency, non-specific hue discrimination

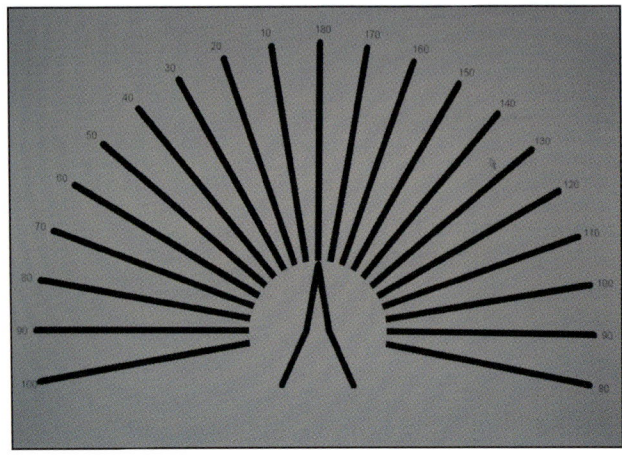

Figure F.1 • Fan target.

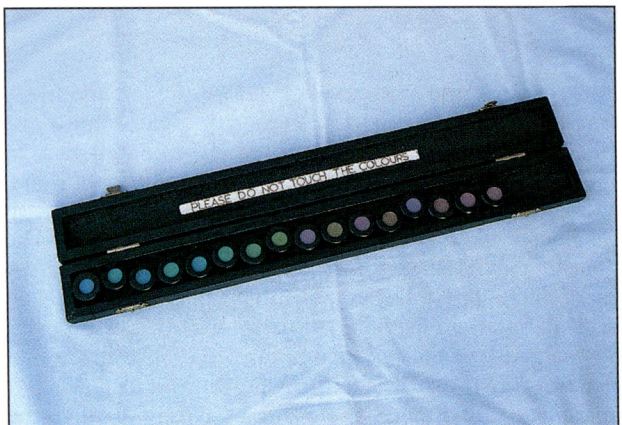

Figure F.2 • The Farnsworth D15 test.

losses can be demonstrated and changes with time monitored. Several other tests have been developed consisting of different hues and/or differences in Munsell value and chroma. See *Lanthony tests*. These tests have different levels of difficulty and different pass/fail levels. However, hue discrimination tests, even composed of desaturated hues, are not reliable for colour vision screening.

Farnsworth D15 test

The Farnsworth (standard) D15 test was developed from a prototype dichotomous test consisting of 20 hues (Figure F.2). The D15 test was originally intended to select people for work in electrical and electronic engineering. There are 16 Munsell hues, selected from an almost complete hue circle, with value 5 and chroma 4. The first or pilot cap is used for reference and the remaining 15 moveable caps must be arranged in sequence. The results are displayed graphically. Isochromatic colour confusions are demonstrated when colours from the opposite sides of the hue circle are placed together in the person's arrangement. The test aims to divide, or dichotomise, people into 2 groups. The first group consists of people with normal colour vision and slight colour deficiency who arrange the hues correctly and pass the test. The second group consists of people with significant (moderate or severe) colour deficiency who demonstrate isochromatic confusion errors by placing hues from opposite sides of the hue circle next to each other in the arrangement. The latter were considered to be unsuitable for employment in the electrical industry. The test therefore grades the severity of colour deficiency and is usually given to people who fail a screening test such as the Ishihara plates. About 5% of men make errors compared to the known prevalence of 8% red-green colour deficiency.

Different pass/fail criteria are applied for the D15 test. The correct arrangement or a single transposition of adjacent hues is considered as a pass. The isochromatic colour difference steps are unequal across the hue circle hence some examiners allow a 'pass' if there are only two isochromatic errors across the hue circle in positions where colour differences are small (Table F.1). This is equivalent to passing people with moderate colour deficiency. When isochromatic errors are made, identification of protan, deutan and tritan defects are achieved by considering typical (isochromatic) arrangement patterns. Protans tend to make fewer errors than deutans because perceived lightness differences may be utilized to obtain more correct placements. Vector analysis and error scores based on the sum of the colour differences between all the adjacent hues in the arrangement have been proposed but these procedures are difficult to equate with the appearance of the results diagram. Error scores are less for tritans than for protans and deutans because a smaller number of isochromatic confusions are available. A version of the D15 test with larger size caps is available for examining acquired colour deficiency in patients with reduced visual acuity.

A number of variants of the Farnsworth D15 test have been devised. The Adams desaturated D15 test has the same hues as the Farnsworth D15 test but with Munsell value 5 and chroma 2. Desaturating the hues reduces the colour difference step between adjacent hues and between isochromatic hues on opposite sides of the hue circle. More colour deficient people make errors with this test. However, desaturating the samples produces a small hue shift and typical isochromatic confusions, demonstrated with the Farnsworth D15 test, are not reproduced exactly with the Adams desaturated D15 test. The Farnsworth D15 and Adams desaturated D15 tests may be used together to obtain more detailed grading of the severity of colour deficiency. The Lanthony D15 test is usually described as 'the desaturated D15' and has the same hues as the Farnsworth D15 test but with Munsell value 8 and chroma 2. People with normal colour vision are likely to make errors. See *Lanthony tests*.

The H16 test does not have the same Munsell hues as the Farnsworth D15 test. The selected hues have value 5 and chroma of 6 or 8. Errors are made by people with severe red-green colour deficiency. The H16 test was intended to fail protanopes and deuteranopes only but some severe anomalous trichromats also fail. The hue circle is incomplete and there is no capacity for identifying tritans.

Farnsworth F2 pseudoisochromatic plate

The Farnsworth F2 pseudoisochromatic plate (F2 plate) is intended to identify tritanopes. Fortuitously the plate

Table F.1 • Combining tests for identifying and grading the severity of red-green colour deficiency.

Screening Test	Grading Tests			
Ishihara plates	Farnsworth D15 test	City University test (2nd edition)	Severity of red-green colour deficiency	AO HRR plates
Fail	Pass	Pass	Slight	Pass, minimal or slight +
Fail	2 Isochromatic errors or incomplete error pattern	4 errors or less*	Moderate	–
Fail	Fail with complete isochromatic error pattern	5 errors or more*	Severe	Moderate or severe +

* Effective for deutans but not protans. + according to the test manual

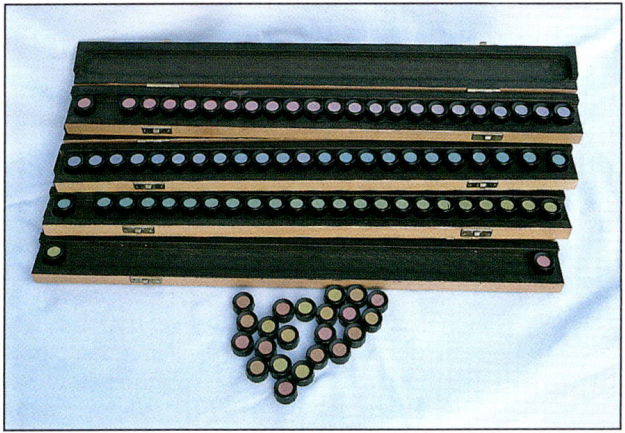

Figure F.3 • The Farnsworth-Munsell 100 hue test.

also has some capability for identifying congenital red-green colour deficiency.

Farnsworth-Munsell 100 hue test

The Farnsworth-Munsell 100 hue test (F-M 100 hue test) consists of 85 numbered colour caps, selected from a complete Munsell hue circle (Figure F.3). These are divided between 4 boxes. The colours in each box must be arranged in sequence between two reference caps, one of these is the first colour in the following box and the other is the last colour of the preceding box. Isochromatic colour confusions cannot be demonstrated because colours from opposite sides of the hue circle are not available at the same time. Test results are scored and the results displayed graphically. Hue discrimination ability is estimated from the total error score and the type of colour deficiency is determined by visual inspection of the results diagram. In congenital colour deficiency characteristic F-M 100 hue plots show concentrations of errors in two well-defined positions which are nearly opposite in the polar diagram representing the circle of hues. These positions occur where isochromatic zones are tangential to the hue circle and groups of adjacent hues are within the isochromatic zone. The combined effect is of an 'axis of confusion' centred around particular hue caps (Table F.2).

The axis is more prominent in severe colour deficiency but dichromats and severe anomalous trichromats cannot be distinguished. Protan and deutan error clusters tend to overlap and classification of the type of colour deficiency may be unclear. Therefore protan/deutan classification is best obtained from pseudoisochromatic designs based on neutral colours. Monopolar distributions of errors also occur. Poor overall hue discrimination is shown by random errors without an axis of confusion. Several computational methods have been proposed to maximize extraction of information from F-M100 hue plots. These methods frequently disregard the clinical nature of the test and the instability of test/retest scores, and assume that typical error clusters are exactly opposite in the results diagram. Proposed scoring techniques include the square root of the error score, Fourier analysis and vector

Table F.2 • Position of centre caps defining the axis of confusion on the F-M 100 hue test for congenital dichromats.

Type of dichromatism	Mean positions of the centre cap defining the axis of confusion	Range of mean values
Protanopia	17	15–26
	64	58–68
Deuteranopia	15	12–17
	58	53–60
Tritanopia	5	4–6
	45.5	45–46

analysis. These methods are rarely helpful. In acquired colour deficiency the total error score may be very large. In this case averaging techniques, which eliminate poor overall hue discrimination, may be useful in determining whether an underlying axis of confusion is present.

Changes in the total error score with time must be considered with caution because facility with the test can be obtained with experience. Total error scores increase slightly with age, especially after about 55 years, because more errors are made in the blue-green segment of the hue circle due to increased ocular lens density. Personal motivation, the encouragement of the examiner and careful review of the initial arrangement all play a part in achieving a low error score. Therefore 'age norms' which suggest the maximum normal score in different age groups, have to be accepted with caution. However, optimum performance occurs at about 20 years of age and the test is not recommended for children under about 10 years of age.

The F-M 100 hue test may be used to select people with normal colour vision for work as colour matchers, or in colour quality control, as well as people with slight colour deficiencies for other occupations. An acceptable error score is specified by the employer. Low error scores demonstrate that the person is motivated to apply effort to the task of arranging the colours correctly. See *Occupational colour vision standards*. The F-M 100 hue has replaced previous scored occupational tests designed to demonstrate colour aptitude or hue memory.

The 28 hue and 40 hue tests consist of approximately every third or every second hue from the F-M 100 hue sequence respectively. The hues are all displayed at the same time and both isochromatic colour confusions and poor hue discrimination, within an isochromatic zone, can be demonstrated. There is a single reference cap. Colour deficient people often find these tests difficult to complete because there are a number of possible alternative arrangements and it is frequently impossible to complete a hue circle beginning and ending with the reference cap. Desaturated 28 and 40 hue tests have also been constructed to examine acquired colour deficiency. The results are displayed graphically.

FDA
- See *Food and Drug Administration*.

FDA soft lens classification
- See *Water content*, *hydrogel*.

Federation of Ophthalmic and Dispensing Opticians (UK)

The Federation of Ophthalmic and Dispensing Opticians (FODO) is an organization that represents the business interests of registered opticians and its membership ranges from the large national corporate bodies to individual dispensing and optometry businesses. FODOs stated objectives are to consider optical employment and business issues with particular reference to:
- Education and manpower
- The regulatory and legislative framework in the UK and Europe

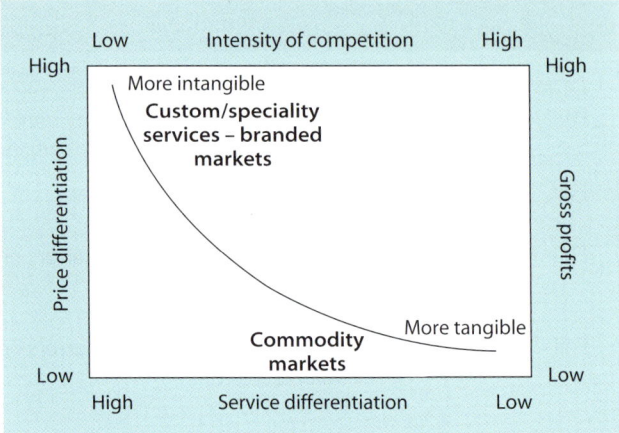

Figure F.4 • The speciality-commodity continuum.

- The National Health Service
- The consumer interest

The organization aims to ensure that the views of its members are taken into account by policy makers, government and the regulatory bodies. FODO is administered by an elected Council.

Fees and charges, contact lens

The very personal and individual nature of both services and products involved in optometry means that 'mass production' approaches cannot be applied without risking negative effects to the practice. When making pricing decisions, three elements normally need to be taken into account: the practice cost base, the patients and customers to the practice, and the competition. The fees and charges of the practice will generally be a compromise between what the business needs to cover costs, what the patients and customers expect to pay for the services and the products, and what the competition charges. Pricing issues are further confounded by the fact that not every practice owner will seek to maximize profits, and nor is detailed information about costs, competition and the potential patient/customer easily available to the practice.

The concept of the speciality-commodity continuum applies to both contact lens products and services. At one extreme is the service product, consisting of a speciality service and highly differentiated from the rest of the competition, whilst at the other extreme is a commodity. Figure F.4 illustrates this speciality-commodity continuum as a conceptual map, describing some of the characteristics of the competition, gross profits, price differentiation and image differentiation associated with the two extremes. Eye care practices would be best served by ensuring that contact lens products and services do not slide to the extreme commodity end. It is worth noting the features of a commodity, which include self-determination of need, self-management of use, being non-invasive with little (perceived) potential for harm, being non-regulated, and price determined by market forces.

Developing a fees and charges schedule is never an easy task. Once one subscribes to the need to move away from the commodity end of the market (where competition relies primarily on purchase decisions based only on price) to the speciality end, then the need for a professional model for fees and charges becomes paramount. One way to do this is to establish the expenses overhead per hour for the practice (chair time). Knowing the actual chair time required for differing types of contact lens services (e.g. spherical rigid lenses, soft lenses, daily/monthly disposable soft lenses, toric and bifocal lenses etc.), allowing for potential unscheduled visits, adding the contact lens material and care system costs (duly marked up at, say, 20–35%), and any other handling charges, this figure can then be used to calculate the fees and charges for any service-product provided by the practice. With the advent of mail-order contact lenses, Internet trading and an increasing trend for contact lenses to be considered as a commodity, it is important to adopt a transparent fees and charges schedule that is competitive on a like-for-like basis without eroding the professional fees dimension.

Fenestrated lenses for optic measurement (FLOMs)
- See *Fitting scleral contact lenses*.

Fenestration of contact lenses
A hole in a lens that has one or more of the following effects:
- facilitating tear exchange beneath the lens
- enhancing corneal oxygenation (alleviating hypoxia)
- alleviating the build-up of carbon dioxide (hypercapnia) beneath the lens
- modifying the extent of positive and negative force (suction pressure) beneath the lens
- allowing air bubbles to form beneath scleral lenses, which aid 'settling back'.

Fenestrations are usually only employed in scleral lens fitting and orthokeratology. See *Fitting scleral lenses*.

Field expanders
Field expanders (also known as reverse telescopes) may be suggested to a patient who has an extreme peripheral field constriction, such that the remaining visual field is approximately 10 to 20° or less ("tunnel vision"). If the field has been lost gradually, the patient may have adapted to it, and be able to function remarkably well by using good scanning eye movements (an organized sequence of small horizontal and vertical saccades) to systematically search the environment: in this way, their dynamic field may be much greater than the static field measured by conventional perimetry.

To assist such a patient it is necessary to minify the retinal image in order to present more information within the limited remaining visual field. As the image size is decreased, however, there is a loss of resolution proportional to the increase in field. The poor acuity means that such systems can rarely be used in spectacle-mounted form. It is more likely to be used as a hand-held system for intermittent spotting: the patient can gain a better appreciation of objects and their relative spatial localization on the threshold of an indoor or outdoor space, or search for mislaid items in the home or work environment. Such systems are in fact 'reversed' Galilean telescopes, consisting of a negative objective and positive eyepiece to create magnification <1.0. See *Telescopes, distance*. A door peep-hole viewer, available from a hardware store, is an inexpensive version of such a device, and can give a monocular field of 90° to 140° (and magnification typically from 0.5 to 0.1). A hand-held minus lens positioned at about 20 to 30cm from the eye allows viewing of an expanded field with a diminished image. Such a device is in fact also a 'reverse' Galilean telescope, with the hand-held minus lens being the objective, and the user's accommodative power providing the positive eyepiece component. The higher the power of the minus lens, and the closer it is held to the eye, then the more accommodation is required. Typically, however, the accommodative demand is modest, and the presbyope may be able to tilt his/her head to view through their multifocal segment. Lens powers up to –50.00D have been suggested which may require the use of Fresnel lenses to give a lightweight, large diameter (approximately 50mm), inexpensive lens: lower powers may be supplied as uncut blanks. A hole can be drilled through the lens near the edge and a cord passed through, so that the lens can be conveniently carried around the neck for intermittent use. Even with intelligent, motivated patients who can develop good handling skills, field expanders can probably only be used for a few specific tasks.

Field of fixation
With a spectacle lens, a prismatic effect associated with the lens periphery results when the eye is rotated to view objects away from the axis of the correction; a larger eye movement, in comparison with the uncorrected eye, is required with a negative spectacle lens and a smaller one with a positive correction. These fixation effects are absent with contact lens corrections, since the lenses follow the movements of the eyes from fixation to fixation.

Field of view
With a spectacle lens a prismatic effect associated with the lens periphery results when the eye is stationary, whereby an annular zone of the visual field is invisible (a ring scotoma) with a positive correction and an annular zone of the visual field is seen diplopically with a negative correction (Figure F.5). The periphery of the field of view may be slightly affected if the lens or its optical zone is small. In the case of rigid lenses, flare or glare may occur due to discontinuities at the edge of the lens or optic zone affecting ray pencils from the periphery of the field.

Field of view, plus lens magnifiers
The field of view (FOV) of a magnifying lens is defined as the angle subtended by the lens periphery at the image of the entrance pupil of the eye. In practice it is more useful to know the linear size of the FOV, since this can be more easily related to the task (e.g. the width of a column of newsprint). If the object is placed at the focal point of the magnifying lens, then

$y = D/aF_M$

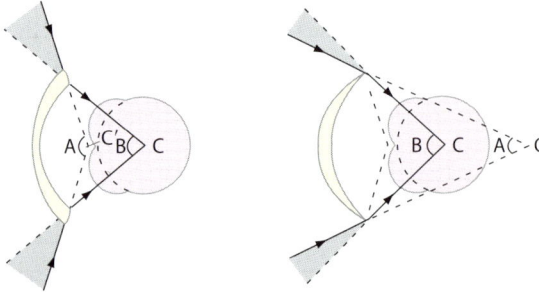

Figure F.5 • Fields of view as seen through spectacle lens corrections. The centre of rotation of the eye is at C, and its image is seen through the spectacle lens at C1. B is the apparent macular field of view and A the actual field.

where y is the linear FOV, D is magnifier diameter, F_M is the equivalent power of the magnifier, and a is the distance of the magnifier from the entrance pupil. For the purpose of clinical comparison, this formula is often approximated to

$$y = D/dF_M$$

where d is the distance of the magnifier from the cornea.

These formulae can be applied to spectacle, hand-held or stand-mounted plus-lens magnifiers, consisting of one or more lenses.

The limited FOV is a very frequent complaint of magnifier users, who remark that only a few letters are visible at a time, and that excessive movement of the magnifier is needed to read a whole line of text. Consideration of the formula shows that opportunities to increase this are limited. Thus the FOV which the patient obtains with a magnifier depends on:

- The lens diameter. This is the parameter which the patient feels should be changed. It must be explained that there are practical limitations of weight, manufacturing capability and peripheral aberrations which limit lens diameter. Low-powered hand magnifiers are often available in a smaller diameter spherical form and a larger diameter (and more expensive) aspheric form, where optimum lens form has allowed the increased diameter whilst maintaining image quality across the enlarged FOV.
- The power of the lens. As lens power increases, FOV decreases, in addition to the secondary effect that more powerful lenses are usually smaller in size. This is one of the reasons for the practice in low-vision work of giving the minimum magnification which allows the patient to perform the task. See Reading requirements, low vision.
- The magnifier-to-eye distance. Halving this, for example, will double the field-of-view, and there is obviously a dramatic increase in the field-of-view when the magnifier is spectacle-mounted. This parameter is the most powerful influence on the area which can be viewed through the lens, and its effect should be demonstrated to the patient, who should be encouraged to hold the magnifier as close to the eye as the task allows. Changes in the magnifier-to-eye distance do not alter the magnification if the object is at the focal point of the magnifier. See Plus lens magnifiers.

Filamentary keratitis, therapeutic contact lenses for

A 'wet' form of filamentary keratitis sometimes occurs without tear volume deficiency in herpes simplex keratitis, recurrent erosion, dystonia, and Theodore's superior limbic keratoconjunctivitis. This condition often responds well to the use of hydrogel lenses. The more usual 'dry' form of filamentary keratopathy occurs in tear deficiency, although contact lenses have little part to play in the management of this form of the disease. Scleral lenses have been used successfully in 'dry' filamentary keratitis.

Filtration angle of the eye
- See Anterior angle of the eye.

Financial considerations
- See Indications and contraindications for contact lens wear.

Financial management in optometry practice

Income to an optometry practice will arise from patients, customers and third party payments (national and private health insurance, driving licence authorities, employers etc.). It is therefore important that records are kept of every transaction and that there is no hindrance to receiving these payments by any method (e.g. cash, credit cards, cheques, direct debit, standing order, electronic transfer of funds etc.). Of these methods, the use of direct debits in pre-paid subscription schemes has proved to be a particularly useful option. Similarly, the practice will need to pay its vendors (e.g. laboratories, prescription houses, various forms of sales tax, telephone, printing and stationery etc.) and its staff.

The provision of optometry services is indeed a provision of professional time. The supply of products is secondary to this, and it is appropriate to adopt an accounting method that mirrors this approach.

Computers are now used almost universally in general practice management, and in particular in the management of practice finances. Many 'off-the-shelf' software options are available and adaptable, whilst others dedicated to optometric practice management and incorporating the special needs for contact lens practice are also available. See Fees and charges, contact lens.

Fitting philosophy, contact lens

This term is generally applied to rigid lens fitting, and refers to any specified approach to achieving a satisfactory lens fit. The fitting philosophy applies primarily to the lens design, but also to desirable aspects of the lens fit, including lens positioning and movement, and appearance of the fluorescein pattern. The concept of 'fitting philosophy' was prominent in the days of exclusively scleral and rigid lens fitting (prior to the introduction of soft lenses), and perhaps related more to the 'art' rather than the 'science' of lens fitting; as such, the term 'fitting philosophy' is seldom used today.

Fitting rigid contact lenses

The conventional method of fitting rigid lenses is by use of trial lenses, although there are two other options: empirical fitting and videokeratoscopic fitting.

Some rigid lens fitting is still undertaken using trial (or 'diagnostic') lens fitting sets in a range of back optic zone radius (BOZR) and total diameter (TD). A set of lenses in a given trial fitting set usually follows a single design concept – for instance, constant edge clearance.

Lenses in a 'standard' trial fitting set are usually available in a single diameter and back vertex power (BVP), with a range of BOZRs in 0.1-mm steps; however, it is preferable to use fitting sets that have lenses available in two diameters (e.g. 9.2 and 9.8mm). Examples of additional useful fitting sets include:

- plus power, e.g. +3.00D, smaller diameter
- high minus power, e.g. –8.00D, larger diameter
- small diameter for interpalpebral fitting, e.g. 8.6mm
- keratoconus, diameter varying with BOZR.

The procedure for selecting an initial fitting of spherical lenses using a trial fitting set is as follows:

1. Select a lens diameter based on corneal diameter, palpebral aperture and lid configuration.
2. Select the BOZR based on the flattest keratometer ('K') reading, adjusting the BOZR to be flatter or steeper than K depending on BOZD. Since relatively steep fitting lenses are easier to visualize with fluorescein, err on the steep side.
3. If more than one power is available, select a lens power closest to the refraction of the patient.

A high degree of success can be achieved by empirical fitting, i.e. ordering initial lenses based on keratometry and refraction. Most contact lens laboratories will supply lenses on a 'per case' basis – that is, a fixed cost for an unlimited number of lens exchanges for a given 'case' (patient) until a final satisfactory fit is obtained. This is an attractive option, especially in some countries, because of concerns about cross-infection. Notwithstanding such concerns, there are occasions when most practitioners would wish to use this method – for example, when wishing to fit a design not covered by an available fitting set, or when an initial trial fitting is inconvenient for the patient.

The procedure for empirical fitting of spherical lenses is as follows:

1. Select a lens diameter based on corneal diameter, palpebral aperture and lid configuration.
2. Select the BOZR based on the flattest K reading, adjusting the BOZR to be flatter or steeper than K depending on BOZD. Flatter radii tend to be used with larger BOZD and vice versa.
3. If the lens is an average diameter, select the BVP based on the sphere power from the refraction (minus cylinder form) corrected for vertex distance. With an average diameter lens no adjustment is necessary; however, an adjustment is necessary if the BOZR is steeper or flatter than K.
4. Order the lens and use this effectively as a trial fitting lens, being prepared to modify or exchange the lens prior to dispensing.

Most videokeratoscopy (VK) instruments incorporate rigid lens fitting software. This enables the practitioners to model different rigid lens designs on an accurate representation of the cornea of the patient. The fitting success rates are relatively low when relying solely on the default settings of the manufacturer of the VK instrument being used, but can be relatively high when a practitioner uses the software to select an appropriate lens.

The main advantages of VK contour maps in rigid lens fitting is that they:

- indicate whether the corneal apex is decentred
- show atypical corneal shapes, e.g. extremes of corneal asphericity
- allow the practitioner to monitor changes in corneal shape
- allow virtual trial fitting of rigid lenses.

The obvious limitation of VK contour maps in trial lens fitting is that they fail to take into account the influence of the lids.

The adequacy of a rigid lens fit is first assessed in white light according to the following criteria:

1. Diameter. The lens should appear to be an appropriate size for the eye. A relatively small lens may fail to cover the cornea through sitting high or resting on the bottom lid. It may also be less comfortable because of greater interaction between the upper lid margin and the lens edge. Alternatively, the lens may irritate the bottom lid by dropping between blinks. Lenses that are larger than the palpebral aperture can result in problems through interacting with the bottom lid as well as the top lid. In some cases the lens will be pushed into a high riding position by occasional interaction with the bottom lid, while in other cases the lens may rest on the bottom lid.
2. Centration. Some decentration may be acceptable if the optic zone maintains pupil coverage, but this may also indicate poor central or peripheral fit. Flat fitting lenses can show decentration in any direction, depending on factors such as lid tightness.
3. Movement. Sluggish, limited post-blink movement may indicate a relatively steep-fitting lens. Fast movement sometimes indicates a flat-fitting lens, but may also be due to strong interaction with the top lid, perhaps due to excessive edge clearance.

Fluorescein is instilled into the eye and the lens fit is assessed in cobalt blue light according to the following criteria:

1. Central fit. If the lens is half covered by the top lid, or the lens is decentred, it may not be possible to observe the central fit without retracting the lid and repositioning the lens. This is achieved by gently holding the top and bottom lids with the index finger and thumb respectively. The lids can be used to manoeuvre the lens into a central position, and can also be used to pump extra fluorescein beneath the lens. The fluorescein pattern for well-fitting lenses will vary according to corneal asphericity and astigmatism. Spherical corneas show the simplest fluorescein patterns. The optimum fit is one that

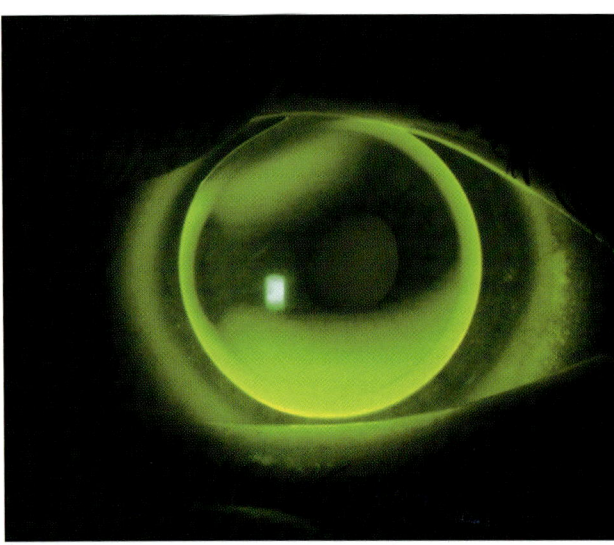

Figure F.6 • Assessing central fluorescein fit having centred the lens and retracted the top lid.

shows central alignment or just a trace of fluorescein indicating minimal central clearance. With astigmatic corneas, in the steeper meridian the central fluorescein pattern will show increasing thickness towards the edge. The most recognizable fluorescein pattern is the 'dumb-bell' pattern seen with spherical lenses on astigmatic corneas (Figure F.6). With steep-fitting lenses, fluorescein assessment will show a central pool of fluorescein, and this pool will appear brighter the steeper the fit. In extreme cases an air bubble may be present. With flat-fitting lenses, a central touch will be visible as an area of dark blue or black. The area of touch will be smaller, the flatter the fit. Fluorescein will be present in the periphery, and may be continuous with the peripheral band of fluorescein.

2. Mid-peripheral fit. Spherical lenses, particularly on astigmatic eyes, make contact with the cornea at the edge of the optic zone. If the lens is poorly blended or makes contact at a sharp angle, it may be uncomfortable and cause epithelial disruption. If a narrow line of contact between optic zones can be seen upon lens inspection, it is likely that there is a sharp junction from poor blending. A band of contact corresponding to the first peripheral zone may indicate relatively steep peripheral curves and the need for peripheral lens flattening. In the case of a flat-fitting lens, the mid-peripheral band of fluorescein may merge with that of the central zone even in the flattest meridian.

3. Edge lift. The width and the brightness of the peripheral band of fluorescein gives an indication of the extent of edge clearance. Where the edge clearance is small, the tear-film thickness may be less than the critical thickness above which the fluorescein appears a saturated yellow colour. This is generally less than the desired clearance of 80μm or more. A less-than-bright yellow peripheral ring, therefore, indicates sub-optimal edge clearance. This will be confirmed by an apparent break in the peripheral band of fluorescein when the lens decentres toward the limbus. In the case of excessive edge clearance, bubbles may be seen forming under the lens periphery. The peripheral band may also be wider than expected, and show the saturated yellow appearance over much of the peripheral band.

Once a correct-fitting lens is identified, an over-refraction is performed to determine the correct lens power and lenses can be ordered for the patient.

Fitting scleral contact lenses

Scleral lenses can be fitted by taking an eye impression or by assessing pre-formed lenses of known specifications. The objective in either case is to achieve best possible alignment over the sclera with corneal clearance. Different approaches are required for fitting polymethyl methacrylate (PMMA) versus gas-permeable scleral lenses.

A means of ventilation, most often a fenestration, is a prerequisite for PMMA scleral lenses, to give oxygenated tear flow. Fenestrations also admit air bubbles behind the lens and cause settling back by relieving the positive pressure in the pre-corneal fluid reservoir. These factors are problematic and contribute significantly to the unpredictable nature of scleral lens fitting. The relationship between the corneal curvature and the lens back optic zone radius (BOZR) is relatively unimportant with scleral lenses, where the critical feature is corneal clearance. Air bubbles greater than 0.1mm in diameter can cause visual disturbance, while small bubbles may lead to intolerable corneal contact.

Pre-formed scleral lenses are lathe cut, which results in the optic and scleral zones being co-axial. The sclera is not symmetrical about the geometric axis, but a successful result can still be achieved in most cases. A series of lenses, each with a known back scleral radius (BSR), is tried until the optimum scleral zone appearance is achieved. If the BSR is too steep, the lens vaults from the periphery, adding to the apical clearance. If it is too flat, the periphery of the lens stands off the sclera but the apical clearance is not affected.

Having established the BSR, fenestrated lenses for optic measurement (FLOMs) are used to determine the optimum optic zone clearance by variation of the BOZR and back optic zone diameter (BOZD). A steeper BOZR with an unchanged BOZD, or a larger BOZD with an unchanged BOZR, increases the optic zone sagittal depth and hence the apical clearance. The BSR, BOZR and BOZD must all be varied to obtain the optimum fit. Because the typical nasal sclera is much flatter than the temporal sclera, co-axial scleral lenses tend to decentre temporally and downwards to a position of approximate symmetry, increasing the variation in the depth of the pre-corneal fluid reservoir. This may cause intractable bubbles and contact zones even when the cornea is reasonably regular. The spherical back surface of a pre-formed lens never matches the asymmetric corneal surface, so there can be large variations in the depth of the pre-corneal fluid reservoir. If bubbles form in the deeper areas, reducing the clearance may be the only way to reduce their size, but this may lead to compressive corneal contact.

With the impression method of scleral lens fitting, a mould of the anterior eye is made using dental alginate.

This is allowed to set and plaster is then poured into the mould, giving rise to a stone cast of the eye. A PMMA sheet is thermally moulded over the stone cast, excess PMMA is cut off to the desired lens shape, the edge is polished, and substance is removed from the optic zone to give appropriate clearance between the lens and cornea. This gives a near glove-fit over the sclera irrespective of scleral topography, and enables the closest possible match to the corneal contour. Large air bubbles are therefore less likely to form beneath the lens and interfere with vision.

The great majority of eyes can be fitted, using pre-formed fitting methods, with sealed (rather than fenestrated) lenses made from gas-permeable materials. There is some disagreement as to whether sealed gas-permeable scleral lenses transmit sufficient oxygen to maintain normal corneal physiology, or whether they need to be fenestrated. The depth of the pre-corneal fluid reservoir and the quality of corneal contact zones are the key features to evaluate, as they have a bearing on both tolerance to lenses and visual performance.

The reduced 'settling back' with sealed gas-permeable scleral lenses enables precise control of corneal clearance. Assessment of corneal clearance is effected by simple observation with a thin optical section on a slit lamp; a slit width of 0.25mm – i.e. approximately half the thickness of a normal cornea – is optimal. The extent of clearance is estimated with respect to the thickness of the cornea. The optimum corneal clearance is achieved by using combinations of the BOZR and BOZD to vary the sagittal depth, or by changing the optic zone projection (OZP) in progressive increments.

The main limitation of sealed gas-permeable scleral lens fitting is an insufficiently regular scleral zone, which leads to intrusion of bubbles into the pre-corneal fluid reservoir. This can occur immediately following lens insertion, or after a period of wear. The apical clearance can be reduced so that bubbles are displaced to the periphery of the optic zone, but the lens may be less comfortable as a result. If intrusion of bubbles is intractable, an impression is necessary. Gas-permeable scleral lenses can be produced from impressions, but the process is cumbersome compared to the pre-formed approach.

Fitting soft contact lenses

The behaviour of a soft lens on the eye is determined by trial lens fitting. The selection of the first trial lens for a patient can take into account the horizontal visible iris diameter, particularly if the cornea appears to be unusually large or small (there should be a 1.0–1.5mm overlap of the lens on to the white sclera; Figure F.7). The selection of back optic zone radius is a process of trial and error unless there is useful information from experience of the patient with previous lenses. For example, if the patient previously required a relatively steep lens in order to achieve a successful fit, this will suggest the need for a similarly steep lens to obtain a good fit. The lens material and wearing regimen are also key factors in the selection of the initial trial lens. While compromises occasionally have to be made, the appropriate lens should be selected based on an assessment of the requirements of the patient rather than prescribing habits or practice policy.

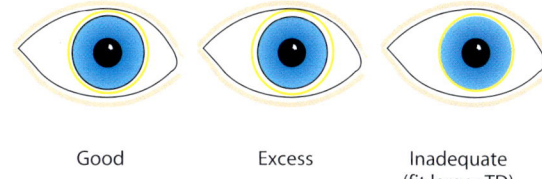

Good   Excess   Inadequate (fit larger TD)

Figure F.7 • Diameter selection of a soft lens.

The selected lens is placed on the eye, allowed to settle (see *Settling time*), and the following assessment techniques (although not necessarily all of them) can be applied:

1. Initial lens comfort. The reaction of the patient to the lens in terms of comfort is the first clue to the lens fit. A well-fitting soft lens is a comfortable lens. Tight-fitting lenses are also usually comfortable initially, but some discomfort or lens awareness may indicate a loose-fitting lens. Due to the overlapping distribution of corneal nerves, it is difficult for patients precisely to locate the source of any discomfort; however, it is worth asking the patient roughly to describe the discomfort. Also, the severity of any discomfort can be gauged by observing the patient. Clearly, excessive lacrimation, blepharospam and other forms of aversion response would tend to suggest a more severe reaction.

2. Vision. An over-refraction is usually unnecessary as part of the fitting procedure. Current spherical soft lenses, because of their thinness and flexibility, rarely support a tear lens between the lens and cornea. Where an over-refraction yields an unexpected result, the labelled lens power may be incorrect; this can be checked by measuring the lens power with a focimeter. Unstable vision may indicate a loose, relatively mobile fit.

3. Lens centration. Some lens decentration is acceptable, provided the lens shows full corneal coverage at all times (the entire limbus is overlapped by at least 0.5mm) and does not appear to compromise comfort. It is important to ensure that the pupil is fully covered by the optic zone of the lens. Loose-fitting lenses tend to show greater decentration, typically greater than 0.3mm. Tight lenses show similar centration characteristics to those of well-fitting lenses.

4. Lens movement. Some lens movement (at least 0.2mm) is necessary with each blink to maintain post-lens lubrication and, in turn, ensure a complete post-lens tear film. Excessive movement can cause unnecessary discomfort and disrupt vision. The absence of post-blink movement is a key indicator of lens tightness, as virtually all tight-fitting lenses show little or no movement. Loose-fitting lenses do not necessarily show excessive movement, so the assessment of lens movement on its own is an inadequate measure of lens fit. In a normal fit, the lens usually remains stationary when the lid moves downward during the first part of the blink (lid closure) but then moves upwards by a small amount during the second part of the blink (lid opening), returning to its original position immediately after the

blink – hence the description 'post-blink movement'.

5. Lag on upgaze and version. The lens should decentre about 0.3mm upon upgaze or lateral version.

6. Push-up test. This test is undertaken by digitally moving the lens upwards by pushing the lower lid against the lens edge. The test consists of an assessment of the amount of force necessary to dislodge the lens upwards (which should be minimal), and the speed of recentration of the lens from its dislodged position (which should not be sluggish).

7. Peripheral fit. A slight, barely visible edge stand-off can cause discomfort due to interaction with the lids. Excessive peripheral tightness is rarely seen with modern lenses due to their relatively thin edges; when seen, tight peripheral fits show some indentation of the bulbar conjunctiva, which may be visible on lens removal by instillation of fluorescein and observation of tear pooling in the indentation.

8. Keratometry mire assessment. The keratometry mires tend to distort when the lens is not aligned with the lens surface. Mire distortion tends to clear immediately after a blink with tight-fitting lenses, and between blinks with loose-fitting lenses.

9. Videokeratoscopy. This gives a more detailed picture than keratometry. The final contour map, however, unlike keratometry, is a static assessment.

10. Retinoscopy. This can be useful in confirming that the optic zone gives proper coverage of the pupil, and may be particularly useful with some bifocal designs.

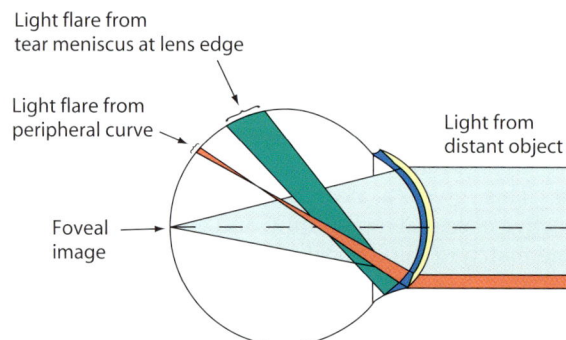

Figure F.8 • Causes of rigid lens flare.

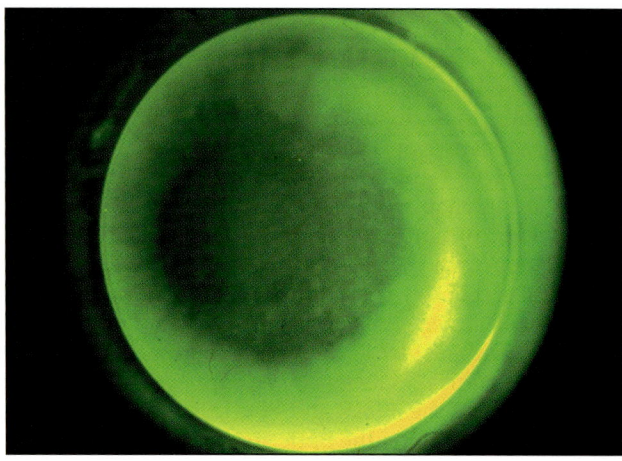

Figure F.9 • Flat-fitting rigid lens revealed by fluorescein.

Once a correct-fitting lens is identified, an over-refraction is performed to determine the correct lens power, and lenses can then be ordered for the patient.

Fixation disparity

Confirmation of the cover test results and assessment of the level of decompensation (if any) is useful in any binocular vision assessment. This can be done by utilizing any of the recognized methods of heterophoria measurement. The aligning prism, often called the fixation disparity (or associated heterophoria), can be measured using the Mallett unit. The unit is extremely helpful as an aid to the management of decompensation, particularly for prescribing prism and monitoring the effect of exercises.

Flare associated with contact lens wear

Because the overall diameter of a rigid lens is less than that of the cornea, discontinuities and flare effects may arise in the peripheral field. Flare refers to the formation of transient defocused secondary arcuate or annular images, which are observed at variable locations in the mid-periphery. This phenomenon is encountered more frequently when the pupils are enlarged, such as at night, and is due to refractive effects of the tear meniscus at the lens edge and/or the peripheral curve (Figure F.8). Patients seem to become less troubled by this phenomenon over time.

Flat contact lens fit

A lens that has a curvature which is less than that of the anterior eye (especially the cornea) is deemed to be fitting flat. The degree of flatness cannot be simply predicted by comparing the back central optic radius of the lens with central corneal curvature, because the curvature of both the lens and cornea can change dramatically towards the periphery. In general, a flat-fitting lens will appear to be loose. A flat rigid lens fit, when examined using fluorescein, will display a broad region of central touch and substantial peripheral and edge lift off (Figure F.9).

Flexure, contact lens
- See *Dimensional stability, rigid lens.*

FLOMs
- See *Fitting scleral contact lenses.*

Fluid lens
- See *Tear lens beneath a contact lens.*

Fluorescein sodium

Fluorescein sodium is a water-soluble dye. It absorbs most light in the blue part of the spectrum but the majority of its emitted light is in the yellow part of the

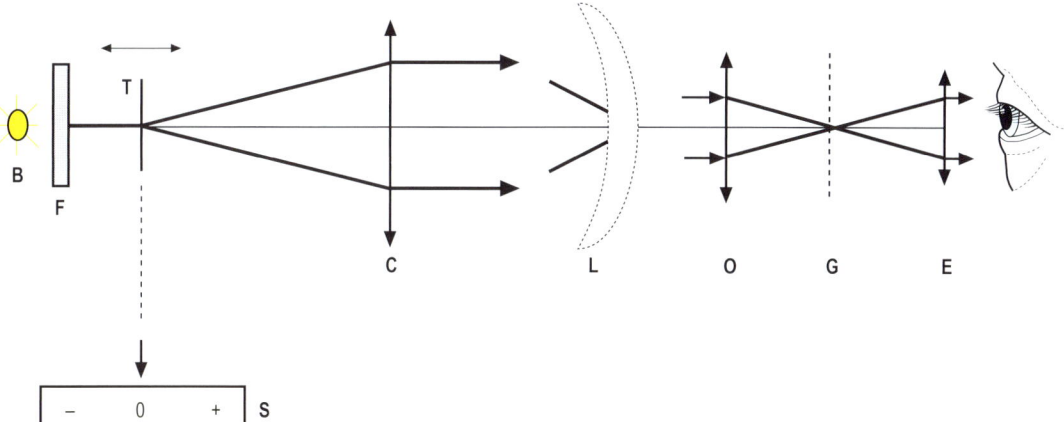

Figure F.10 • Ray diagram of eyepiece focimeter.

spectrum, with some in the green. The intensity of light emitted is governed by the concentration and pH of the solution and, critically in rigid lens fitting, the thickness of the fluorescein sample. Fluorescein is not visible until a critical thickness of about 15μm is reached. The intensity of fluorescence increases with increasing thickness until another critical thickness of about 60μm is reached, beyond which the fluorescein is seen as a uniform bright yellow colour.

This dye has three main uses in contact lens practice:

1. Assessing the adequacy of fit of a rigid lens
2. Assessing the ocular surface for evidence of trauma or physiological decompensation
3. Highlighting the tear film for the purpose of measuring tear break-up time.

In rigid lens fitting, the fluorescein pattern is a simple two-dimensional representation of a complex three-dimensional shape. This provides useful information about the relationship of the lens with the shape of the eye. Areas of tear pooling appear bright yellow. Where the tear layer is absent or extremely thin, there is no visible fluorescence and the area appears dark blue or black. Between these extremes, varying thicknesses of post-lens tear film are seen as varying intensities of yellow/green. Fluorescein therefore provides a contour map of the thickness of the tear film.

Fluorescein will fill spaces on the corneal surface where tissue is missing. It will also enter and stain the cytoplasm of dead or devitalized epithelial cells. Therefore, bright areas of fluorescence on the corneal surface observed following instillation of fluorescein indicate either cell damage or cell loss. A dull glow around a bright area of fluorescence indicates that fluorescein has diffused into surrounding epithelial and/or stromal tissue.

If fluorescein is instilled into an eye and the eye is held open for a few seconds, dark areas will begin to appear among the normal even fluorescent glow across the cornea; these dark areas indicate tear thinning or break-up. This phenomenon forms the basis of the tear break-up time test.

Fluorescein sodium, instillation of

The preferred method of instilling fluorescein sodium into the eye is to use a filter strip impregnated with this dye (i.e. a 'fluorescein strip'). A drop of non-preserved saline is placed on the orange (impregnated) tip of the fluorescein strip. The patient is instructed to look down and the strip is lightly touched on the superior conjunctiva for less than one second. The patient is instructed to execute a couple of blinks in order to spread the fluorescein. Placing a drop of fluorescein on the superior sclera will maximize the length of time the dye remains in the eye.

In rigid contact lens wearers, the process can be simplified by touching the fluorescein strip against the front of the lens. A thick fluorescein-stained pre-lens tear film may confound interpretation of the true post-lens fluorescein pattern (the object of interest), so it may be necessary to wait until this has dissipated before assessing the pattern.

Fluoro-silicone-acrylates

- See *Rigid contact lens*.

Fluting of contact lenses

Lifting off of the edge of the lens from the surface of the eyeball. This phenomenon can occur with lenses of relatively high modulus (stiffness), such as thick, low water content soft lenses, silicone elastomer lenses, and silicone hydrogel lenses. Lens fluting should be avoided; if it is observed, a different lens base curve should be chosen (typically steeper).

Focimeter

The focimeter (also known as a lensometer or vertometer) is an instrument used for the measurement of lens power. A ray diagram of a typical arrangement of an eyepiece focusing focimeter is shown in Figure F.10. An illuminated target (T) moves longitudinally along the optic axis of the instrument, and is connected to a power scale (S) reading vertex lens power in dioptres. The unknown spectacle lens is placed on a holder (L) at the second principal focus of the positive collimating lens (C). The purpose of this design feature, which is an example of a Badal lens system, is to ensure that the magnification of the focimeter image remains constant regardless of the power of the unknown spectacle lens: the spectacle lens is said to be in the 'unit magnification' position. The astronomical telescope, consisting of an objective (O) and

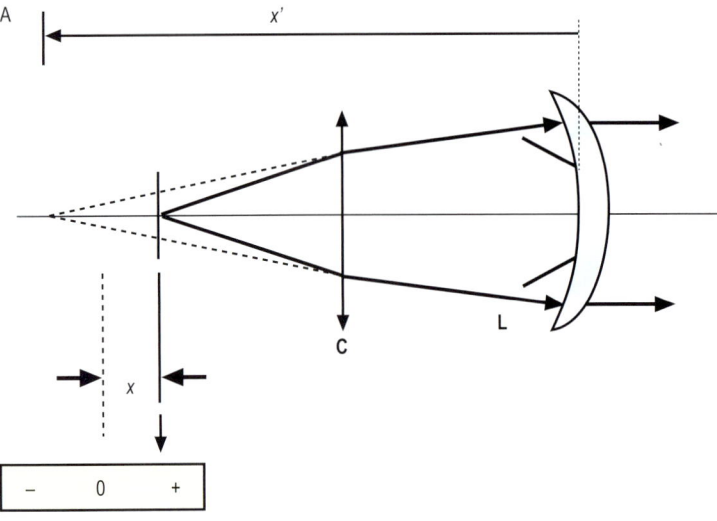

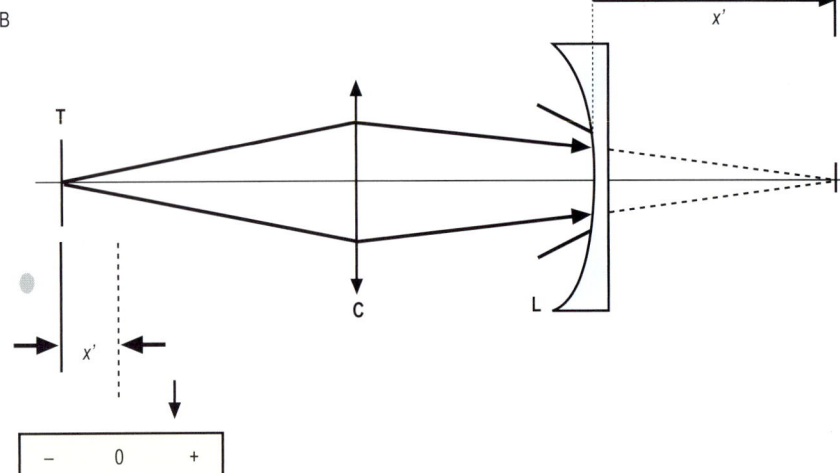

Figure F.11 • (A) Focimeter with positive lens. (B) Focimeter with negative lens.

an eyepiece (E) is adjusted so that it is focused on infinity, and therefore only parallel light will be seen in focus. The graticule (G) in the eyepiece of the telescope contains axis and prism scales. Note that a narrow band-pass filter (F) is used to provide a peak illumination at either 546.07nm or 587.56nm.

In Figure F.10, the instrument is shown at zero adjustment with no spectacle lens in place. Light emerges from the collimating lens system in parallel, and the image seen through the telescope is sharp with the target positioned at zero on the power scale, where the target is coincident with the first principle focus of the collimating lens. In the top diagram in Figure F.11, a positive power spectacle lens has been introduced at the lens holder (L). The target has been moved closer to the collimating lens by a distance x in order that parallel light leaves the front of the spectacle lens and is seen in focus by the telescope. The image of the target is situated at a distance x' from the rear surface of the unknown spectacle lens. In the bottom diagram in Figure F.11 the alternative situation with a negative power spectacle lens is shown. In this case, the target has been moved further away from the unknown lens, by a distance x, in order to be seen in focus by the telescope. The distance x' again gives the distance from the rear lens surface to the image focus.

The relationship of target movement to the power of the unknown lens can be deduced from Newton's relationship:

$$f^2 = x.x'$$

As x' is the back vertex focal length of the lens being measured, this means that the target movement per dioptre (x) is proportional to the back vertex power of the lens, and that the focimeter power scale is linear. The term f is the focal length of the collimating lens, sometimes known as the 'standard' lens of a focimeter.

The selection of collimating lens power is a compromise between the range, accuracy, and dimensions of the instrument. The equation can be re-arranged to give the target movement (in mm) per dioptre of unknown lens power:

$$x = 1000/F^2$$

where F is the power of the collimating lens in dioptres. For a collimating lens power of +25.00D, the target movement is 1.6mm/D. This demands a very precise calibration and control of target movement in order to obtain accurate results, but on the other hand, in order to measure over a range of +10.00D to –10.00D, a target movement of only 32mm is required. If as an alternative design a collimating lens power of +10.00D were to be used, this would give a target movement of 10mm/D, and a total target movement of 200mm, requiring a very large instrument, but theoretically more accurate.

In order to obtain accurate results from a visually focusing eyepiece instrument, the eyepiece must first be adjusted to minimize any proximal accommodation. If the target and graticule cannot be made to appear jointly in focus at zero indicated power, then a more fundamental adjustment is required by an instrument mechanic. In order to overcome some of the above potential problems when using eyepiece focimeters, instruments known as projection focimeters have been developed. In these cases the image is projected on to a translucent screen, which is optically coincident with the plane of the graticule. It is also claimed that projection instruments are less tiring to use over a long period of time than those with eyepieces.

Folds
- See *Oedema*.

Follow-up consultation, low vision

A patient who has received a low vision aid (LVA) must be seen again by the clinician in 2 or 3 weeks to assess progress. It is important to ensure that the patient can actually carry out the task for which the aid was intended. A shorter time interval may not give the patient the opportunity to fully try out the aids, but if the return appointment is delayed beyond this the patient may be disillusioned and have already become convinced that LVAs are unsuccessful. On return the patient should be asked about experiences with the aid, and then asked to demonstrate how the aid is being used.

If the strategy has not been successful, there are three possible reasons:

1. Vision has deteriorated; a check of distance and near acuities under the same conditions as at the previous visit would confirm this. A different (presumably higher powered) aid would need to be selected and the trial period repeated.
2. The aid is being used suboptimally, perhaps positioned too far from the eye, or at the wrong distance from the task, with inadequate lighting, using the eye with poorer acuity, or with the wrong spectacles. The patient should be given the instructions again, perhaps considering ways in which the misunderstanding could be avoided. This might involve a change to a magnifier with internal illumination if the patient cannot arrange task lighting, or the placement of an occluder over one lens of the spectacles to ensure that the best eye is used.
3. The patient is trying to use the aid for a different task than that for which it was intended, e.g. trying to read the newspaper whereas large print books had been the designated goal, or trying to read with a telescope designed for knitting. The use of the magnifier should be explained again, checking with the patient that the task for which the magnifier is intended is still a priority. If it is not, a different magnifier may be needed, and the trial period repeated.

In the case of (2) or (3) above, the possibility of a more formalized instruction or training in the use of the aid should be considered for this patient. See *Low vision training*.

If the aid has proved successful, the patient can be questioned to determine if he/she has any requirements not dealt with previously. If all requirements have been met, the patient can be discharged until there is either an alteration in the visual or personal circumstances such that the aid is no longer effective, or the requirements of the patient have changed. This may be dealt with in a number of ways, such as providing the patient with clear written (large print) instructions on how to request an appointment on demand, or instituting a rigorous pre-planned system of reviews, in which the patient returns at 6-monthly (or appropriate) intervals. It is also important that the patient knows how to obtain a replacement magnifier in the case of loss or breakage, so that unnecessary appointments do not need to be made.

Food and Drug Administration

In the United States of America, the control of contact lenses and contact lens care products is governed by the Food and Drug Administration (FDA). The FDA has classified contact lenses as a drug, and therefore demands rigorous testing and evaluation before contact lenses can be released onto the market. This process is controlled by the Centre for Devices and Radiological Health, which has the following mission: 'Protecting the public health by providing reasonable assurance of the safety and effectiveness of medical devices and by eliminating unnecessary human exposure to radiation emitted from electronic products.'

Forces acting on a rigid contact lens

A number of forces that act on a rigid lens have to be suitably balanced in order to achieve a satisfactory fit (Figure F.12). The gravitational force of the lens and pre-lens tear film causes the lens to drop. The effect will be greater, and the lens less stable, the further forward the centre of gravity lies. The centre of gravity is further forward in plus lenses compared with minus lenses. It is shifted posteriorly by increasing the diameter, steepening the back optic zone radius, or decreasing the thickness of the lens. With both plus and minus lenses, the greatest shift and most effective stabilization is achieved through changing the lens diameter.

The lens is held in place by the capillary forces in the post-lens tear film and the surface tensional force in the tear meniscus at the lens edge. The capillary force increases with increasingly closer alignment of the lens and the cornea. The force is therefore greater with spherical corneas compared with astigmatic corneas.

Surface tension forces act at the lens edge where the edge meniscus is not covered by the lid. There will be no surface tension where a meniscus is absent due to excessive edge clearance. This force can be increased by reducing edge clearance and edge thickness.

Eyelid forces (primarily the upper lid) act to move the lens in a vertical direction during the blink. Between blinks these forces help to stabilize the lens in the case of an extra-palpebral fit, but have no effect in the case of an intra-palpebral fit.

Forces acting on a soft contact lens

A range of forces act on a soft lens, which keeps the lens in place on the eye but allows it to move a small amount

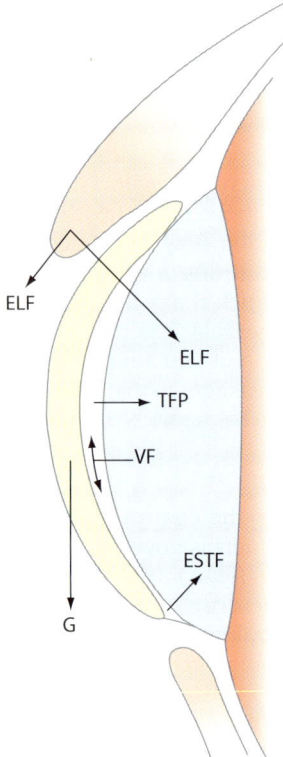

Figure F.12 • Forces acting on a lid-attached rigid lens. ELF = eyelid forces; ESTF = edge surface tension force; G = gravity; TPF = tear fluid pressure; VF = viscous forces.

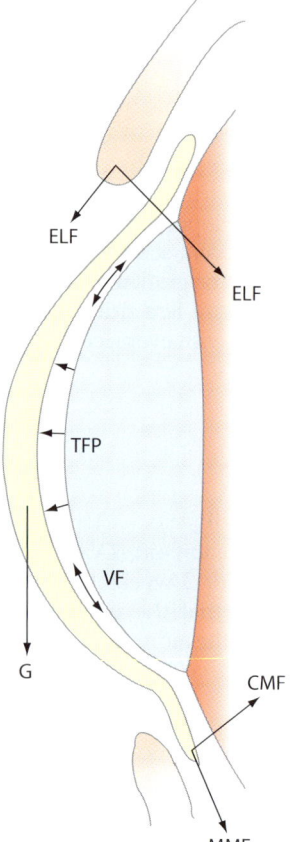

Figure F.13 • Forces acting on a soft lens. CMF = circumferential membrane force; ELF = eyelid force; G = gravity; MMF = meridional membrane force; TFP = tear fluid pressure; VF = viscous forces.

between blinks (Figure F.13). Soft lenses are usually required to flex in two directions in order to align to the shape of the cornea and sclera. Since soft lenses are generally flatter than the central corneal curvature they steepen in order to align with the cornea, but at the periphery they are required to flatten so as to align with the sclera. The stresses formed in the lens are proportional to the mechanical properties of the material as well as the dimensions of the lens. Due to the viscous nature of the tear fluid, this deformation of the lens to match the shape of the eye results in a 'squeeze pressure' being developed in the post-lens tear film. This squeeze pressure is related to the amount of force required to move the lens across the eye, and will therefore influence lens fit. The amount of force required to move the lens is also related to the viscosity of the post-lens tear film. This helps to explain why the movement of a soft lens can vary markedly during a given wearing period. Soft lens retaining forces are relatively large compared with those of rigid lenses, and therefore gravitational force has less of an effect.

Foreign bodies

Foreign bodies (FBs) account for about half of all types of ocular injuries. They generally result from a person not realizing the hazard of the task; for instance, when using a hammer and chisel, cutting wire, or using a grinding wheel. The natural defence mechanisms of the eye may be penetrated and FBs may become embedded in the globe, or they may pass through the cornea or sclera to become lodged within the globe. The symptoms can vary from little or no discomfort to severe pain. Figure F.14 shows the common sites of foreign bodies.

Many small FBs will be washed out of the eye by the tears. Sometimes, however, the FB will become embedded in the subtarsal conjunctiva of the upper lid, which will cause pain on blinking and a vertical corneal abrasion. The area of abraded cornea, where the epithelium has been removed, will be seen as a disturbance of the corneal reflection. This can be viewed by instilling fluorescein and viewing the eye under ultraviolet light. The upper lid must be everted if these FBs are to be located and removed. The healing of the epithelium may sometimes be incomplete, resulting in recurrent corneal erosions.

An eye with a corneal FB usually shows marked vascular injection closest to its position. Ocular pain will be experienced but it will be difficult to localize. If the corneal FB has been present for a couple of days, a grey ring of infiltration may occur around it and, on removal, a small, pitted ulcer will remain. It may leave a permanent scar, although this will generally only affect vision if it is over the centre of the cornea. An FB embedded in the conjunctiva or sclera is often surrounded by haemorrhages.

Many FBs are metallic, with iron particles being the most common, followed by copper and aluminium. The softer metals (e.g. magnesium) are a less frequent cause of FBs, as they tend to fragment less during drilling, sawing, grinding, or cutting. Metallic FBs left embedded in the eye will rapidly oxidize under the influence of the enzymes of the cornea and tears. This may set up a severe inflammation of the cornea or iris. The oxidation of steel is much faster than that of aluminium or magnesium, and a rust ring may be apparent within a couple of hours. A rust deposit left in the cornea will partially dissolve and an iron stain will diffuse into stromal or subepithelial layers.

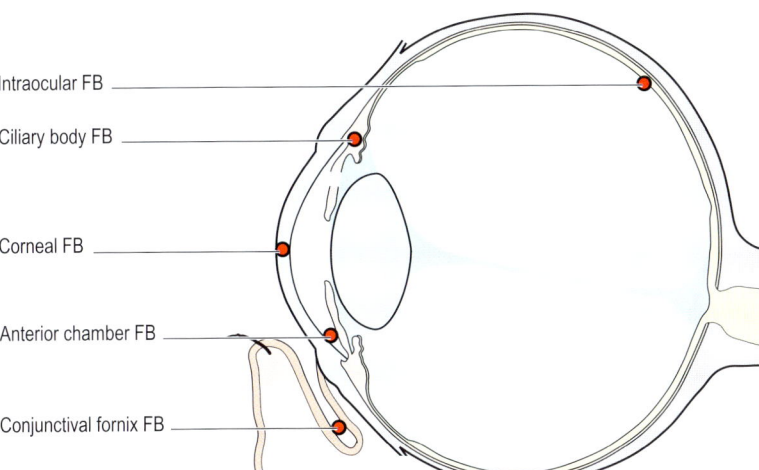

Figure F.14 • Sites of ocular foreign bodies.

The possible presence of an intra-ocular foreign body (IOFB) should always be investigated, especially when the symptoms are a gush of fluid from the eye with blurring of vision. Small, hot FBs hitting the eye at great speed may penetrate the globe and actually seal their route of entry. As only a slight pain is experienced, it is essential not to miss an IOFB, as it may eventually lead to loss of vision. Ideally when an eye is perforated, an X-ray should be taken to exclude the presence of a metallic IOFB. The classic signs of a perforating injury are a shallow anterior chamber, eccentricity of the pupil, and prolapse of the iris. However, care must be taken in the following two cases:

- A small conjunctival haemorrhage, while being the only clue, may obscure deeper scleral laceration.
- The eye appears normal but there is a history suggestive of an IOFB.

The IOFB may have been stopped by the iris and fallen into the anterior chamber angle to be hidden from view. If an IOFB has penetrated through the vitreous, fibrous tissue will form along its path. The fibrous tissue may impair vision if it crosses over the visual axis and a vitrectomy may then be required to restore vision and/or to prevent tractional retinal detachment.

Vegetable FBs may cause infections so severe that a purulent panophthalmitis may occur in only a few hours. Other FBs may be retained without noticeable reaction, e.g. gold, silver, platinum, glass, and many plastics. Less well tolerated by the eye are lead, zinc, nickel, and aluminium particles. These are often coated in an inert salt and later encapsulated by a fibrous tissue coating, rendering them less toxic. The most dangerous IOFBs are iron and copper, which cause siderosis and chalcosis, respectively. In siderosis the iron oxidizes and causes a slow, insidious intra-ocular reaction as it permeates most of the ocular tissues; this can lead to complete blindness. It is a late-occurring syndrome and the ferrous pigmentation causes a rusty coloration of the cornea, iris, or lens. In addition, a series of chronic degenerative changes occur, which lead to pupil dilation because of atrophy of the sphincter pupillae, cataract, and then retinal detachment and open angle glaucoma. These complications usually occur between 2 months and 2 years after injury. Surgery is therefore urgently required after injury to remove the iron IOFB.

Pure copper will cause a rapid inflammation of the eye (chalcosis) and the eye may be lost if endophthalmitis occurs. Copper alloys (bronze and brass) may induce chronic degenerative processes by slow diffusion of the copper, which tends to be taken up by the limiting membranes of the eye. A green ring may develop in the peripheral cornea in Descemet's membrane (Kayser-Fleisher ring) and a sunflower cataract in the anterior capsule of the lens can form.

Four prism dioptre base out test

The four prism dioptre base-out test is advocated for use with patients suspected of having a small angle squint or other motor or sensory disturbances that are not readily detected and may result in suppression. An advantage of this method is that it does not rely on the patient's subjective response. The test is performed with the patient fixing at a distance target. As stable fixation is important the test may not work very well in young children or uncooperative patients. A four base-out prism dioptre prism is quickly inserted then removed before each eye in turn. The examiner observes the eye without the prism. In the case of a patient with suspected small angle squint, the prism is usually inserted in front of the fixing eye. Where there is no central suppression of either eye (i.e. a normal response), the eye being observed should make a version then a vergence eye movement. These movements are in accordance with Hering's law of equal innervation. Insertion of the prism in front of the first eye results in a version eye movement due to the retinal disparity produced by the prism. The fellow eye also moves in the same direction and by the same amount in order to satisfy Hering's law. Finally, when bifoveal fixation is re-established, the fellow eye makes a vergence movement.

In the case of suppression of the observed eye, the eye will make a version eye movement but not a vergence eye movement. In this case the suppression scotoma in the observed eye is just large enough so that the stimulus to initiate the vergence movement is not perceived. Where suppression exists in the eye where the prism is inserted, the expected version eye movement does not occur as the retinal disparity induced by the prism is within the suppression scotoma of that eye and therefore not perceived.

The four base-out prism test should be used with caution as responses may vary considerably between

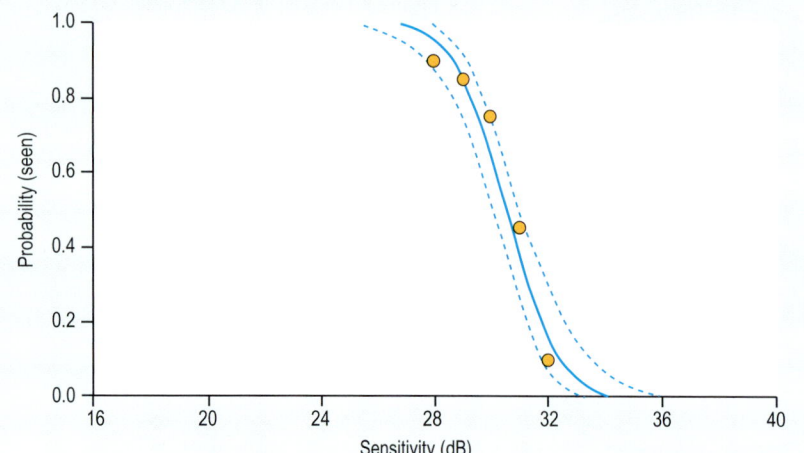

Figure F.15 • Frequency-of-seeing curve.

patients even in the absence of suppression. It is important to use an isolated fixation target, or peripheral fusion might be used to give a normal response in a patient with central suppression. In any event, confirmation of the presence of suppression should be made in combination with at least one other test.

FOZD
- See *Front optic zone diameter, contact lens.*

FOZR
- See *Front optic zone radius, contact lens.*

Frequency of seeing curve
One of the best ways of measuring the sensitivity of the eye is to plot what is known as a frequency-of-seeing curve. To do this, a range of intensities is found that straddles the patient's sensitivity, i.e. the bright ones are above the patient's threshold and the dim ones are below it. Several different intensity levels (normally 5 to 9 levels) between these two values are chosen and stimuli are presented over and over again, in a random manner, at all the chosen intensity levels. The percentage of time that the stimulus was seen at each of the intensity levels is plotted. At the high intensity levels the percent seen will be close to 100% while at the dim levels it will be close to 0%. When all the values are joined together they should form an 's' shaped curve like that shown in Figure F.15. This type of curve is known as an ogive.

The gradient of the frequency-of-seeing curve is a measure of variability. The steeper it is, the less variability there is. There are 3 important factors that affect the gradient of the frequency-of-seeing curve:

- The patient – Some patients are more variable than others and there is not a lot that the perimetrist can do about it.
- The amount of experience – More experienced patients generally have steeper gradients. This is one reason why many of the psychophysical papers report data on very small highly trained groups of subjects.
- The sensitivity of the eye – The gradient of the frequency-of-seeing curve reduces and variability increases when the sensitivity is low. Figure F.16 shows two frequency-of-seeing curves recorded during the same session on an eye with glaucomatous visual field loss. At one location, where the sensitivity is normal, the gradient of the frequency-of-seeing curve is steep while at the other, where the sensitivity is depressed, the gradient is shallow.

Fresnel lenses and prisms
A Fresnel lens is a thin plastic vinyl sheet; one side is perfectly flat, and the other side has a series of fine hemispherical lens forms etched into the surface. These lens forms are arranged in a concentric pattern to create what is effectively a flat plus or minus power lens. A series of prism forms can be arranged in parallel lines to create what is effectively a large flat prism. Because one side of the Fresnel lens/prism is perfectly flat, it can adhere to an existing conventional glass or plastic lens. The advantage of a Fresnel lens/prism is that it has a flat form irrespective of the lens or prism power, is extremely light weight and relatively inexpensive. The main disadvantage is that image quality is slightly degraded as a result of the fine striations that are required to create the lens or prim power. Fresnel lenses/prisms are generally used in the eyecare field as a temporary measure for prismatic correction as part of a course of orthoptic treatment, or for temporary refractive correction, e.g. for a patient who has been rendered aphakic because it has not been possible to insert an intraocular lens following cataract removal for medical reasons.

Front optic zone diameter (FOZD), contact lens
This is the diameter of the optic zone of the front surface of the lens as measured through the lens centre. The front optic zone diameter (FOZD) of a rigid lens should be at least 0.5mm larger than the back optic zone diameter (BOZD). Except in low powers, most rigid lenses are lenticulated to reduce thickness and weight. Lenses occasionally incorporate a negative carrier in order to encourage lid attachment and centre the lens. A negative carrier is a peripheral zone that is thinner at the optic zone junction than the lens periphery. A positive carrier or tapered edge design – where the peripheral zone is thicker at the optic zone junction than the lens periphery – is occasionally used to discourage lid attachment in a high riding lens. See *High plus power contact lens design.*

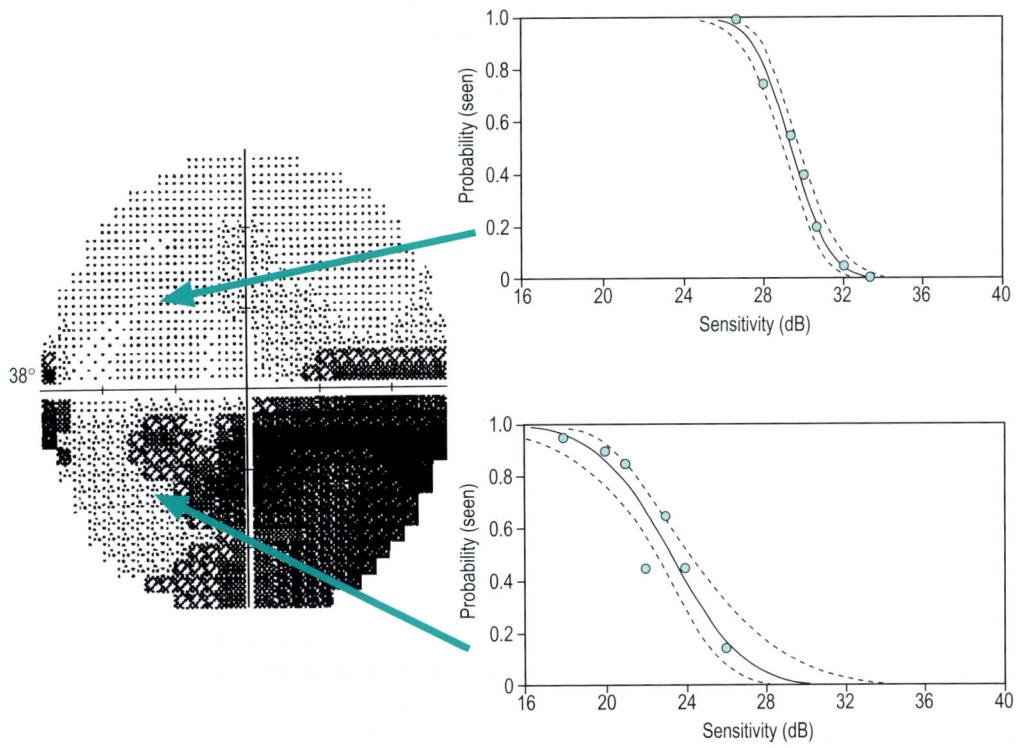

Figure F.16 • Two frequency-of-seeing curves: one from a part of the visual field where the sensitivity is normal and one from a region where the sensitivity is depressed.

Front optic zone radius (FOZR), contact lens

The front optic zone radius (FOZR) is the radius of curvature of the front surface of a contact lens (see Figure B.1). This parameter is varied to achieve the desired optical correction once the BOZR has been determined to achieve an optimum fit.

Front surface rigid toric contact lenses

- See *Cylindrical power equivalent rigid toric lenses*.

Fuchs's dystrophy

- See *Corneal dystrophies, degenerations and depositions*.

Fundus camera

An image of the ocular fundus can be captured using a camera system especially designed for this purpose. In essence, a fundus camera is an indirect ophthalmoscope. A flip mirror within the optical path allows the fundus to be viewed and the instrument to be positioned to capture the area of the fundus of interest, the mirror flips out of the optical path when the camera shutter is pressed. The field of view of such instruments extend up to 45°. Fundus cameras are available in table-mounted or hand-held portable configurations. Some instruments are claimed to require no mydriatic; however, mydriatics are often used to ensure a larger pupil, which will typically afford superior image quality, increased brightness and a greater field of view.

Table F.3 • Typical values of fusional ranges at near.

Base Out	Base In
Blur point 15 to 17$^\Delta$	Blur point 12 to 13$^\Delta$
Break 30 to 40$^\Delta$	Break point 20 to 21$^\Delta$
Recovery point 8 to 11$^\Delta$	Recovery point 11 to 13$^\Delta$

Fusional reserves

This is a measure of the ability of a patient to react to increasing demands on vergence by having to adjust the fusional vergence. Fusional reserves are measured either by use of a prism bar, in which case a stepped vergence response is being tested, or by use of Risley rotary prisms which induces smooth increasing demands. The test can also be performed using a synoptophore, vectograms and tranaglyphs. It is normal to use a speed of $4^\Delta/s$. The fusional range is tested at distance and at the patient's usual reading distance. Prisms are introduced, and slowly increased, with the patient fixing a target that is appropriate to ensure good accommodative interest.

It is customary to measure the point when the patient reports diplopia or the clinician notices misalignment of the eyes. This is called the *break point*. The value of prism when binocular function is restored is also recorded. This is known as the *recovery point*. The normative values expected are different depending on whether step or smooth vergence testing is performed. Typical values are indicated in Table F.3.

Table F.4 • General approaches, with examples, of methods used in fusional reserve exercises.

Method	Example	Advantages/disadvantages
Haploscopic instruments	Aperture Rule Trainer	can be used for home or 'in-practice' exercises can be used to treat most horizontal deviations, including eso-deviations instructions included; easy to use
Tranaglyphic methods	Computer orthoptics (LCD or red/green goggles)	comprehensive range of exercises good for child motivation since transforms exercises into a 'computer game' particularly well-suited to practices with optometric assistants home computer-assisted regimens are available
Polarized vectograms	Bernell vectograms	more naturalistic than tranaglyphs stereoscopic relief can be employed which increases patient interest inexpensive and well-suited to use by optometric assistants
Free-space techniques	Institute free-space stereograms (IFS) Dinosaur exercise	suitable for home or practice training inexpensive IFS employs stereoscopic relief, increasing patient interest and allowing checks to ensure proper use natural, so improvement may better translate into everyday life
Facility training	Flip prisms or loose prisms	suitable for home or practice training inexpensive probably best combined with ramp exercises

Additional valuable information may be gleaned by asking the patient to report when the object of regard becomes blurred. This will be the point at which the patient can no longer maintain accommodation on the target and begins to lose comfortable binocular function. This value may be more significant from a functional point of view than the break point since it is unlikely that any patient will continue to be able to function efficiently after this *blur point* has been reached.

When a patient reports that the target seems to be moving, suppression is present. Good observers will also notice that for base out demand, the target will appear to be reducing in size. Understanding the information gleaned in measuring fusional ranges will aid the practitioner in deciding the significance of the binocular problems and will help in re-evaluation during progress checks whilst treatment progresses.

Fusional reserve exercises

When patient (and parent) motivation is good, fusional reserve exercises are the treatment of choice for exo-deviations of up to about 15 to 20$^\Delta$. In exo-deviations, the ability to converge at the relevant distance(s) is trained (positive fusional reserves). Training divergent (negative) fusional reserves in eso-deviations is harder, but can be successful in well-motivated cases. The general approaches are listed, together with examples, in Table F.4. It should be noted that some exercises treat the positive or negative relative accommodation instead of the fusional reserves. Vertical fusional reserves do not respond well to treatment, but increasing horizontal fusional reserves may help a hyperphoria that is combined with a horizontal heterophoria.

Gap junctions
- See *Corneal epithelium*.

Gas discharge lamps
Gas discharge lamps can be grouped according to:
- pressure – high or low
- gas – sodium or mercury.

These lamps utilize the ionization of a gas to produce light. As electrons pass through the gas between the electrodes they accelerate and collide with the atoms of the gas (usually sodium or mercury). The collisions may cause:
- ionization of the atoms, i.e. the release of an increasing number of free electrons, which themselves cause collisions, resulting in a cumulative ionization; or
- absorption by the gas atoms of most of the energy of the electrons, which raises the energy state of the electrons to higher levels. Subsequently, when the electron falls back to a lower energy level it emits radiation (Figure G.1).

The spectral emissions from discharge lamps tend to be discontinuous (line spectra), unlike those of incandescent lamps. At low gas pressure the emission is concentrated in narrow spectral lines, but these broaden as the pressure is raised. The envelope of the lamp is filled with a mixture of gases and vapours. The main gas is the one responsible for the emission of light, i.e. mercury or sodium. Other gases are included to aid the starting of the electron discharge, such as argon, neon, xenon, or argon mixed with nitrogen.

Control gear is necessary, first to be able to provide a high voltage for starting the lamp, and second to be a current limiter/controller once the arc has been established. This is achieved by either a large resistor or an inductive resistor, which is known as a choke or ballast. Virtually all discharge lamps require control gear of some sort and it will vary in size and weight in proportion to the lamp wattage and lamp complexity.

Gas-permeable scleral contact lenses
- See *Fitting scleral contact lenses*.

General directive on the mutual recognition of higher education diplomas
The general directive on the mutual recognition of higher education diplomas (89/48/EEC) is intended to harmonize professional groups within

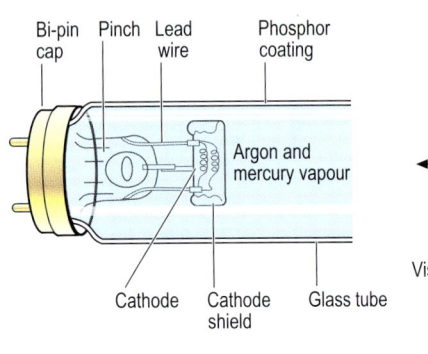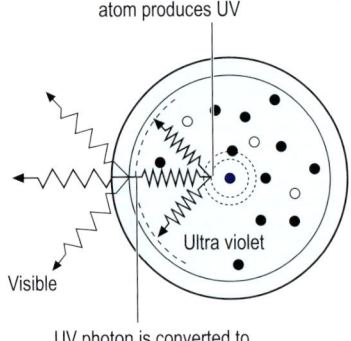

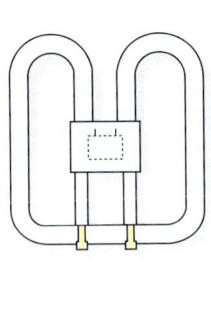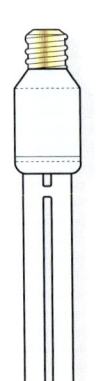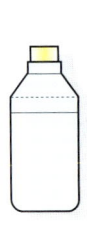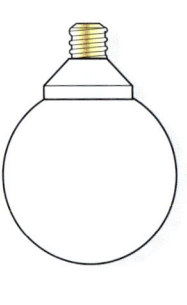

Figure G.1 • (A) Simplified mechanism of a low pressure mercury vapour fluorescent lamp. (B) Range of lamp designs (adapted from the Thorn Lighting Technical Handbook, courtesy of Thorn Lighting Ltd).

the member countries of the EC, has laid down the basis for optometric interchange within Europe. The Directive is extremely general in its coverage and does not require prior harmonization of education and training. In order to produce equivalence it is understood that the optometrist in each state covered by the proposal will complete a full course of upper secondary education followed by successful completion of a 3-year full-time course leading to a higher education diploma. The Directive also covers those who take an equivalent 3-year full-time course on a part-time basis.

Because of the differing national legislation throughout the European Community, experience and knowledge of varying areas of clinical optometry may be restricted in certain individuals. The legislation, again by its general nature, does not interfere with this but provides for optometrists intending to migrate to a member state to have their training and qualification assessed to identify any significant shortfalls. Once identified it is for the migrating optometrist to overcome these differences by further training, supervised practice or examination as determined by the accepting country. The optometrist will always be allowed to return to the home country however and would carry the extended qualification.

The introduction of this Directive encouraged many European countries to develop a new 3-year full-time university course in optometry. This enables member states to participate in the movement of qualified personnel. In addition there have been discussions to develop a syllabus and examination structure for the introduction of a European Diploma in Optometry. This, combined with a slow but steady movement of individuals between countries, could see the expansion of optometry and harmonization of the profession in Europe.

General Optical Council (UK)

Part 1 of the Opticians Act 1958 set out the basis for the General Optical Council (GOC). There are currently 28 GOC members and the Council is constituted as shown below. This body has the role of promoting high standards of professional education and professional conduct among optometrists and dispensing opticians and such additional functions as defined within the 1989 Opticians Act (amended 2005).

In addition to a Registrar, the Council is comprised as follows:

- nine persons nominated by the Privy Council;
- six persons chosen to represent registered optometrists;
- five persons chosen to represent registered dispensing opticians;
- four persons nominated by the assessing bodies;
- four registered medical practitioners.

Members of Council are appointed or elected for a period of five years and election by registered optometrists is on a regional basis.

The Council is required to establish seven main committees, as follows:

- Education Committee – for the purpose of giving advice and assistance to the Council on matters relating to optical training, education and assessment.

- Companies Committee – for the purpose of giving advice and assistance to the Council on matters relating to business registrants, other than matters required by the Act to be considered by the Investigation Committee, the Registration Appeals Committee or the Fitness to Practice Committee.
- Investigating Committee – for the purpose of investigating any allegation that: (a) a registered optometrist's or a registered dispensing optician's fitness to practice is impaired; (b) a business registrant's fitness to carry on business as an optometrist or a dispensing optician or both is impaired; or (c) a student registrant's fitness to undertake training as an optometrist or dispensing optician is impaired.
- Registration Committee – for the purpose of giving advice and assistance to the Council on matters relating to registration, other than matters required by the Act to be considered by the Registration Appeals Committee.
- Registration Appeals Committee – for the purpose of hearing and determining appeals against any decision of the registrar refusing to enter the name of an individual or body corporate in, or restore it to, the appropriate register.
- Standards Committee – for the purpose of giving advice and assistance to the Council on matters relating to the standards of conduct and performance expected of registrants or those seeking admission to the register.
- Fitness to Practice Committee – for the purpose of inquiring into and determining allegations relating to: (a) the fitness of registered optometrists or registered dispensing opticians to practice; (b) the fitness of business registrants to carry on business as an optometrist or a dispensing optician or both; and (c) the fitness of student registrants to undertake training as an optometrist or dispensing optician.

The Council has the power to make rules governing the practice of optometry and dispensing optics. The rules currently in force are as follows:
- 2005 – 2006 Registration Fees Rules
- 2005 Registration Rules
- 2005 Registration Appeals Rules
- 2005 Fitness to Practice Rules
- 2005 Continuing Education and Training Rules
- 2005 Committee Constitution Rules
- 1999 Rules Relating to Injury or Disease of the Eye
- 1993 Testing of Sight by Persons Training as Optometrists Rules
- 1989 Sight Testing (Examination and Prescription)(No. 2) Regulations
- 1989 The Contact Lens (Specification) Rules
- 1988 The Contact Lens (Qualifications etc.) Rules
- 1985 Rules on Publicity
- 1985 Rules on the Fitting of Contact Lenses
- 1985 The Disciplinary Committee (Procedure) Rules
- 1984 Sale of Optical Appliances Order of Council

Details of these rules, and of any other matters relating to the General Optical Council, can be found at: www.optical.org

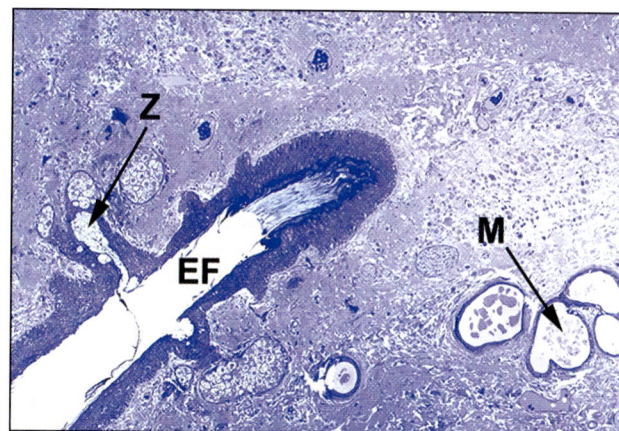

Figure G.2 • Histological section through the ciliary zone of the eyelid. Glands of Zeis (Z) discharge their contents into an eyelash follicle (EF), which contains the remnants of an eyelash. M= gland of Moll.

Ghost vessels
- See *Neovascularization, contact lens-induced*.

Glands of Krause
- See *Accessory lacrimal glands*.

Glands of Moll
These are ciliary glands found in association with eyelash follicles (Figure G.2). Glands of Moll are modified sweat glands consisting of an unbranched spiral tubule. The exact function of these glands is unclear.

Glands of Wolfring
- See *Accessory lacrimal glands*.

Glands of Zeis
These are ciliary glands found in association with eyelash follicles (see Figure G.2). The glands of Zeis are unilobular sebaceous glands that open directly into the follicle. The function of their oily secretion is to lubricate the lashes to prevent them from drying out and becoming brittle.

Glare
Discomfort glare occurs physiologically (and transiently) in normal vision when an individual is suddenly subjected to a much higher level of luminance than that to which he or she has adapted. The discomfort can be long-lasting if the visual environment requires a difference in adaptation level between adjacent areas of the visual field. The amount of discomfort glare created by a discrete light source within the visual field is proportional to the brightness of the source and its angular subtence at the eye, and inversely proportional to its distance from the visual axis and the brightness of the background. Discomfort glare can be a symptom of many ocular diseases, when the eye is subjected to levels of illumination which are higher than those to which it can adapt, although the precise mechanism of the visual symptoms is unknown. This phenomenon cannot be

measured objectively in the clinical setting, although its severity is sometimes assessed in symptom surveys by subjective grading.

Disability glare may occur at the same time as discomfort glare, but is distinguished by the change in retinal image contrast, and hence reduction in acuity, which it creates. In the presence of high ambient illumination (an extremely bright white background, or a separate glare source), there may be scattering of light, especially within an eye which has optical irregularities in the ocular media (e.g. cataract or corneal oedema), or it may have its origin outside the eye, such as from particles on otherwise transparent surfaces (e.g. car windscreens, spectacle lenses or contact lenses). Disability glare can also be of retinal origin, when strong stimulation of one large region of the retina affects the sensitivity of other regions of the retina. As might be expected, the glare source has a greater effect as its luminance increases, and as it moves closer to the line of sight. In fact, in a normally sighted individual, the effect is negligible once the glare source has moved more than 10° from the visual axis.

Scattering of light creates a 'veiling luminance' which is present across the whole retinal image. There is thus an equal increase in the luminance of the retinal image in both the light and the dark areas, which has the effect of reducing image contrast, which will impair vision. Many different tests have been devised to measure this phenomenon (see *Disability glare, tests for*) which has particular clinical significance in the assessment of cataract sufferers, contact lens wearers, and those who have undergone refractive surgery. It can often provide useful corroboration and quantification of patient complaints when high-contrast visual acuity is normal.

Adaptation to glare expresses the ability of an eye to function optimally with as short a delay as possible, when tested under different lighting conditions than those to which it is adapted. The relatively lengthy period required for dark adaptation is well known, and any extension of this time is indicative of rod photoreceptor disease, such as in retinitis pigmentosa. More common, and of greater functional significance, is the ability of an eye to recover acuity in normal lighting conditions, after brief fixation of a bright light. There is no universally accepted method of conducting this 'macular dazzling' or 'photostress' test, which is measuring a successive glare phenomenon. During the test the photoreceptor pigments are bleached by the intense light, leading to a scotomatous after-image overlying the letters to be read. Recovery occurs by the re-synthesis of visual pigment and this depends on the proper relationship between photoreceptor outer segments and the retinal pigment epithelium. Such tests have therefore been suggested to be useful in the early detection of diseases which affect this relationship (such as age-related maculopathy or diabetic retinopathy) when recovery is slowed.

Effective alleviation of the symptoms of glare is based on avoidance (but see *Tints for low vision*) and whenever possible, illumination levels should be uniform. It is therefore recommended that the ratio between the task illuminance and the illuminance of the surrounding region should not be greater than 3:1. Other advice that may be given to reduce glare includes:

- adjacent rooms and corridors should have equivalent illuminance
- the patient should wear a tinted overspectacle in the bright outdoor environment which can be removed on coming indoors
- a visor, eyeshade or hat with a brim should be used to shield the eye from light from a discrete glare source.

Glass, ophthalmic
- See *Spectacle lens materials*.

Glasses
- See *Spectacles*.

Glaucoma

Glaucoma is a term that encompasses a group of conditions, which have in common the development of a potentially blinding optic neuropathy. The optic neuropathy is a result of a progressive loss of ganglion cell axons, the cause of which remains controversial. Ganglion cell loss may be brought on by factors such as ganglion cell apoptosis, reduced blood flow to the nerve head or the physical effects of elevated intraocular pressure. Glaucoma is assessed from possible changes in intraocular pressure (IOP), optic nerve head morphology, visual field (VF) integrity, or the anterior chamber angle, as well as other secondary signs.

Most glaucoma syndromes are asymptomatic, because the central visual field is not affected until late in the disease process. The patient history may reveal risk factors for glaucoma, such as a family history of glaucoma in siblings or parents. In *acute* angle closure, the patient often presents in the evening or over night with a severe dull ocular ache, reduced vision, haloes around lights and even nausea and vomiting. Despite the usually dramatic nature of the presentation some patients have remarkably few symptoms.

Ocular hypertension is defined in the Ocular Hypertension Treatment Study (OHTS) as an IOP in the range of 24 to 32mmHg, with normal optic nerve appearance, normal VF findings, open anterior chamber angles and no other related ocular pathology. However, care is needed with applanation tonometry (e.g. Goldmann), as it is subject to false positives due to a number of patient factors including blepharospasm, above average corneal thickness (over 555µm with ultrasound) and even tight neckties in males.

The various types of glaucoma can be classified as follows:

Primary open-angle glaucoma (POAG). Usually has the following triad: glaucomatous optic neuropathy (GON), VF loss and raised IOP (as above). Anterior chamber angles are open and there are no other pathological changes or signs of inflammation. VF loss with static threshold perimetry can be defined as significant loss at the 5% level in more than 3 contiguous points. The field loss should be repeatable. Field loss is most often in an arcuate zone between 10 and 20 degrees of fixation and characteristically respects (i.e. does not cross) the horizontal midline.

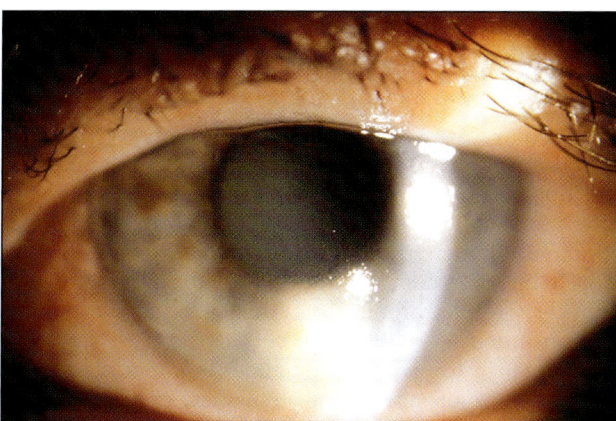

Figure G.3 • Acute angle closure glaucoma with conjunctival injection, corneal oedema and dilated pupil.

GON features include: (a) notching of the neuroretinal rim; (b) thinner rim margin superiorly or inferiorly than the nasal or the temporal margins; (c) increased cup-disc ratio over time or inter-ocular asymmetry more than 0.2; (d) blacked-out areas of the radiating nerve fibre layer; and (e) nerve fibre layer (Drance) haemorrhage crossing the disc margin. An enlarged vertical cup–disc ratio (>0.6) is suspicious but less specific.

Normal tension glaucoma. IOP is less than 21mmHg, in the presence of GON or VF defect or both. Neurological causes including causes of optic atrophy, where the disk pallor is greater than the cupping, need to be excluded. May be related to a thin cornea.

Angle closure glaucoma. The eye is injected, the cornea oedematous (Figure G.3) and the IOP raised, usually to between 50 and 80mmHg. The anterior chamber is shallow and the iris bowed forward, the pupil is totally non-reactive, often oval and in mid-dilation. Gonioscopy is difficult due to corneal oedema but if possible reveals the angle to be fully occluded. If the optic nerve head is visible it is usually swollen and vascular flow non-existent. Risk factors are an anterior chamber central depth of less than 2mm, or gonioscopy failing to show the trabeculum angle structures. Creeping angle closure glaucoma may show no acute signs or symptoms.

Secondary glaucomas include:
- Pseudoexfoliative (P×F), with white pseudoexfoliative material deposited on the anterior crystalline lens;
- Pigmentary, as evidenced by iris transillumination, trabecular pigmentation and Kruckenberg spindle;
- Neovascular, characterized by abnormal blood vessels or fibrovascular membrane occluding anterior angle;
- Inflammatory, due to uveitis or phacolysis;
- Steroid-induced, which can be caused by more than 2 to 4 weeks of topical corticosteroids;
- Post-traumatic or post-operative.

Congenital glaucoma. Glaucoma in infants is usually bilateral, with hazy and enlarged corneas due to increased IOP.

The glaucomas are most often managed by a therapeutic reduction in IOP. If IOP is over 40mmHg or VA is hand movements or worse, then IOP reduction is urgent and all topical glaucoma medications should be used, subject to the medication contraindications and precautions. IOP should be checked every 10 to 20 minutes and both eyes should be treated. In acute angle closure, with IOP over 45 to 50mmHg, oral or intravenous (IV) agents may be helpful in treatment, such as carbonic anhydrase inhibitors (e.g. acetazolamide 500mg) and hyperosmotics such as mannitol. Systemic contraindications and precautions must be observed.

Ocular hypertension with IOP <24mmHg, or exfoliation syndrome without glaucoma, may only require close observation. Treatment of ocular hypertension may be started with IOP in the range of 24 to 30mmHg, although the more recent OHTS guidelines favour the lower end of the range, particularly when other risk factors are present, including positive family history, increased optic disc cupping, systemic risk factors, or a thinner cornea.

Medical treatment delays glaucomatous progression. First line medical treatment in recent years has become the prostaglandin-analogues such as Latanoprost (Xalatan). Prior to this, beta-blockers such as Timolol 0.5% were the mainstay of treatment, although caution was required in patients with certain systemic conditions. Secondary glaucomas are usually treated according to the underlying cause.

Argon laser trabeculoplasty (ALT) is considered equally effective as medical therapy for POAG. Furthermore, ALT has a higher initial success rate than medical therapy in PXF glaucoma. Selective laser trabeculoplasty (SLT) is a newer technique than ALT, but with less data available. A YAG laser peripheral iridotomy is a definitive treatment for angle closure glaucoma. Trabeculectomy filtration surgery is beneficial in lowering IOP when medical treatment fails.

In cases of advanced glaucoma, consideration should be given to low vision referral. Fundus photos or scanning laser ophthalmoscopy can help identify change in GON. Glaucoma and glaucoma suspect patients are usually reviewed at 6 or 12 month intervals, the aim being to identify any change in the VF or GON.

Glaucoma, drugs for the treatment of

In primary open-angle glaucoma and ocular hypertension, topical agents having different pharmacological modes of action can be used to reduce intraocular pressure, either by reducing the formation of aqueous humour or by facilitating its outflow. The different categories of drugs used in the treatment of glaucoma are outlined below.

Beta-adrenoreceptor antagonists (β-blockers). Beta blockers have been regarded as ideal drugs for the treatment of open angle glaucoma since they are well tolerated and cause few adverse reactions. They act by blocking β_2 receptors in the ciliary epithelium so that the secretion of aqueous humour is reduced. Although only relatively minor adverse ocular effects are caused by β-blockers, they can be responsible for an important range of systemic side effects.

Timolol is a non-cardio selective β adrenergic antagonist that blocks both β_1 and β_2 adrenoreceptors and is particularly effective in lowering intraocular pressure. Since β_1-receptors are present in cardiac tissue, a lowered heart rate could occur as a systemic side effect. Also, as the lung contains β_2-receptors, their blockade can result in bronchoconstriction. The use of timolol is, therefore, contraindicated in patients with asthma, obstructive pulmonary disease and those with sinus bradycardia, uncompensated cardiac failure and a number of other conditions.

Betaxol is an adrenergic antagonist that is selective for β_1-receptors. Since it is cardioselective, it less likely to cause bronchoconstriction. Other β-blockers are carteolol, levobunolol and metipranolol.

Beta blockers have represented the first line in the treatment of open angle glaucoma in patients without pulmonary disease or conditions such as congestive heart failure.

Miotics or cholinergics. The cholinergic or parasympathomimetic agent, pilocarpine, has been used in the treatment of glaucoma since the late 19th century. Miotics stimulate the muscarinic receptors on the longitudinal muscle fibres of the ciliary muscle with the result that the trabecular meshwork opens and increases the outflow of aqueous. The consequent spasm of accommodation constitutes a significant disadvantage in patients under the age of about 50 years. Vision in lower levels of lighting is also handicapped by the miosis. The use of pilocarpine in glaucoma treatment has declined due to its disadvantages and side effects and also due to the advent of alternative drugs. It is available in unpreserved single dose form which might be useful on rare occasions for the emergency treatment of glaucoma.

Since carbachol is especially resistant to hydrolysis by the cholinestersases that inactivate acetylcholine, its effects are more sustained than those of pilocarpine and fewer instillations are necessary. However, it is absorbed poorly by the cornea.

Carbonic anhydrase inhibitors (CAIs). These drugs are isoenzyme II inhibitors and block the enzyme carbonic anhydrase in the ciliary epithelium resulting in decreased production of aqueous. The CAI, acetazolamide, has low ocular penetration that necessitate its oral administration as tablets and it is associated with a number of side effects that include thirst, headache, flushes, and drowsiness. In acute angle-closure glaucoma, acetazolamide can either be administered orally or by intravenous injection, the latter providing a more rapid reduction in intraocular pressure.

Two topical CAIs are available, dorzolamide and brinzolamide. Although these drugs can be used as a monotherapy, they are often used as adjunctive agents when beta-blocker monotherapy has proved inadequate. Carbonic anhydrase is present in the endothelium, so these drugs affect its pump mechanism and their use is inappropriate in patients in whom this corneal structure is compromised.

Non-selective sympathomimetics. Adrenaline is a non-selective sympathomimetic and acts as an agonist at α_1-, α_2-, β_1- and β_2-receptors. The non-selective stimulation of α- and β-receptors leads to opposing effects on the production of aqueous humour. The effect of α_1 stimulation is vasoconstriction in the ciliary body, which reduces the output of aqueous, while the β stimulation in the ciliary epithelium increases it. Increased outflow of aqueous results from the effect on the β_2-receptors in the trabecular meshwork and upon the α_2-receptors controlling uveoscleral outflow. The overall effect is a reduction in intraocular pressure. Initial conjunctival vasoconstriction following instillation of adrenaline is likely to be followed by a rebound hyperaemia and prolonged use can result in problems such as corneal and conjunctival pigmentation. In order to improve its efficacy, adrenaline was combined with the adrenergic neurone blocker, guanethidine, but this product has been discontinued.

Dipivefrin (dipivalyl adrenaline) is a modified form, or prodrug, of adrenaline that has enhanced lipid solubility facilitating its penetration of the cornea. Whilst associated with fewer systemic complications than adrenaline, dipivefrin does have some side effects.

Selective sympathomimetics (α_2 agonists). Apraclonidine is a non-selective α_2-agonist that reduces the production of aqueous humour. Adverse effects restrict the use of this drug to the prevention or short-term treatment of a postoperative rise in intraocular pressure following anterior segment laser surgery.

Brimonidine is a highly selective α_2-agonist that both reduces aqueous output and promotes its uveo-scleral outflow. Allergic reactions are much less frequent than with apraclonidine and it has a significant additive effect when used as an adjunctive agent. Brimonidine has also proved to be a useful adjunctive agent when added, for example, to latanoprost.

Prostaglandin $F_{2\alpha}$ analogues. The $F_{2\alpha}$ class of prostaglandin lowers intraocular pressure by increasing both the uveo-scleral and the trabecular outflow, but does not decrease the production of aqueous humour. Analogues of $F_{2\alpha}$ have a potent hyoptensive action and can reduce intraocular pressure by 25 to 35% compared to baseline readings and can reduce the magnitude of diurnal variation. Adverse effects of their use include conjunctival hyperaemia (which can subside within two weeks), hypertrichosis and darkening of iris pigmentation.

Latanoprost and travoprost increase uveo-scleral outflow and bimatoprost, which is a prostamide analogue, also increases trabecular outflow.

Prostaglandin analogues may be used together with any ocular hypotensives with the exception of cholinergic agonists. A prostaglandin analogue is commonly the drug of first choice in glaucoma and can also be used when patients fail to respond to other drugs or become intolerant of them. It can be employed as an adjunct to a β-blocker.

Combination drugs. A combination of dorzalamide with timolol or latanoprost with timolol can be used when β-blocker monotherapy has proved to be inadequate.

Guidelines issued by the Royal College of Ophthalmologists in 2004 indicate that the drugs of first choice in the treatment of primary open-angle glaucoma and ocular hypertension are prostaglandin analogues or β-blockers with carbonic anhydrase inhibitors and agonists representing second choice. Combination drops are becoming increasingly popular.

Topical drugs used in the treatment of glaucoma in multidose and single dose forms are listed in Tables G.1 and G.2, respectively.

Table G.1 • Drugs for the treatment of glaucoma: preserved multidose preparations.

Mode of action	Non-proprietary name	Proprietary name	Formulation	Preservative
β Blocker Miotic	Betaxol hydrochloride	Betoptic®	Drops 0.5% as solution Drops 0.25% as suspension	Benzalkonium chloride 0.01%*
	Carteolol hydrochloride	Teoptic®	Drops 1%	Benzalkonium chloride 0.025%
	Levobunolol hydrochloride	Betagan®	Drops 0.5% with polyvinyl alcohol 1.4%	Benzalkonium chloride 0.004%*
	Timolol maleate	Timoptol®	Drops 0.25% and 0.5%	Benzalkonium chloride 0.01%
		Timoptol®-LA	Drops 0.25% as gel	Benzododecinium bromide 0.012%
		Nyogel®	Drops 0.1% as gel	Benzalkonium chloride 0.005%
	Pilocarpine hydrochloride	Pilogel®	Gel 4% with carbomer 940 3.5%	Benzalkonium chloride 0.008%*
Carbonic anhydrase inhibitor	Dorzolamide hydrochloride	Trusopt®	Drops 2%	Benzalkonium chloride 0.0075%
	Brinzolamide	Azopt®	Drops 1%	Benzalkonium chloride 0.02%*
Non-selective sympathomimetic	Dipivefrin hydrochloride	Propine®	Drops 0.1%	Benzalkonium chloride 0.005%*
Selective sympathomimetic	Apraclonidine hydrochloride[†]	Iopidine®	Drops 0.5%	Benzalkonium chloride 0.01%
	Brimonidine tartrate	Alphagan®	Drops 0.2%	Benzalkonium chloride 0.005%
Prostaglandin $F_{2\alpha}$ analogue	Bimatoprost	Lumigan®	Drops 0.03%	Benzalkonium chloride 0.005%
	Latanoprost	Xalatan®	Drops 0.005%	Benzalkonium chloride 0.02%
	Travoprost	Travatan®	Drops 0.004%	Benzalkonium chloride 0.015%
Combined carbonic anhydrase inhibitor and β Blocker	Dorzolamide hydrochloride Timolol maleate	Cosopt®	Drops dorzolamide 2% with timolol 0.5%	Benzalkonium chloride 0.0075%
Combined prostaglandin and β Blocker	Latanoprost Timolol maleate	Xalacom®	Drops latanoprost 0.005% with timolol 0.5%	Benzalkonium chloride 0.02%

* with disodium edetate
[†] for short-term use to prevent post-operative increase in intra-ocular pressure

Table G.2 • Drugs for the treatment of glaucoma: unpreserved single dose preparations.

Mode of action	Non-proprietary name	Proprietary name	Formulation
β Blocker	Betaxolol	Betoptic®	Drops 0.25% as suspension
	Levobunolol hydrochloride	Betagan®	Drops 0.5% with PVA 1.4%*
	Metipranolol	Minims® Metipranolol	Drops 0.1 and 0.3%
	Timolol maleate	Timoptol®	Drops 0.25 and 0.5%
Miotic	Pilocarpine nitrate	Minims® Pilocarpine Nitrate	Drops 2 and 4%
Selective sympathomimetic	Apraclonidine hydrochloride[†]	Iopidine®	Drops 1%

* with disodium edetate
[†] for short-term use to prevent post-operative increase in intra-ocular pressure

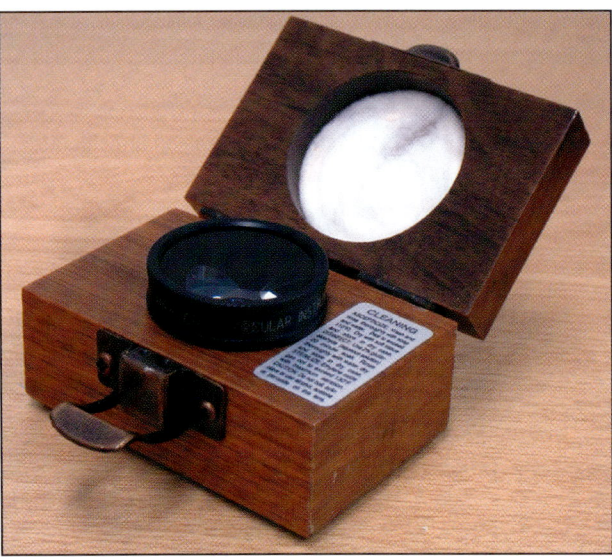

Figure G.4 • Gonioscope.

Glaucomatous visual field defects
- See *Visual field defects associated with glaucoma*.

Glycocalyx
- See *Corneal epithelium*.

GOC
- See *General Optical Council*.

Gonioscopy

Gonioscopy is a technique that allows practitioners to examine an area of the eye otherwise hidden from view. The anterior chamber wall cannot be directly observed externally because of the limbal overhang. As the observer moves parallel to the iris surface, the light rays from the chamber angle undergo internal reflection, which prevents the light from leaving the eye. The word gonioscopy, derived from Greek, means to view the angle. This procedure allows evaluation of the width of the anterior chamber angle and involves the use of a mirrored contact lens (or 'gonioscope'; Figure G.4) held against the anaesthetized cornea.

The purpose of gonioscopy is to permit visualization of the irido-corneal angle, better known as the anterior chamber angle, and often referred to simply as 'the angle'. This is the area in which the trabecular meshwork lies, and is therefore responsible for aqueous outflow. The appearance of the anterior chamber angle varies according to congenital individual differences and with acquired changes through age, injury or disease. From anterior to posterior, the gonio-anatomy consists of 10 normally visible structures:

- cornea
- Schwalbe's line
- Schlemm's canal
- trabecular meshwork
- scleral spur
- ciliary body
- iris processes (not always present)
- iris root
- iris surface
- pupil border.

Gonioscopy will indicate areas where the angle is narrow as less of these structures will be visible. Furthermore, gonioscopy should reveal the presence of any material such as pigment within the angle – a possible risk factor for secondary open angle glaucoma.

Gothenburg Study

A critically important research study, conducted in Gothenburg, Sweden, during the 1980s that revealed the long-term adverse effects of extended hydrogel contact lens wear on the cornea. Specifically, a contralateral-eye paradigm was employed by examining a cohort of contact lens patients who had worn lenses in one eye only (due to unilateral amblyopia or unilateral myopia) for an average of 62 months. Any changes observed were compared with the contralateral non-lens-wearing eye. This methodology afforded an extremely powerful and sensitive assessment of the physiological changes induced by lens wear, as it obviated variability due to intersubject differences. It was discovered that the extended wear of hydrogel lenses induces a reduction in epithelial oxygen uptake and thickness, the induction of epithelial microcysts, stromal thinning, and increased endothelial polymegethism. Although the epithelial changes recovered within 1 month, the principle of ocular compromise during lens wear was firmly established.

The Gothenburg Study also revealed four key strategies for alleviating these changes: removing lenses more frequently, regularly replacing lenses, fitting lenses of higher oxygen performance, and improving tear exchange beneath lenses. These strategies formed the blueprint for future contact lens developments, such as the development of mass production manufacturing facilities for disposable lenses and silicone hydrogel lenses. (Holden, B. A., Sweeney, D. F., Vannas, A., Nilsson, K. T. and Efron, N. (1985). Effects of long-term extended contact lens wear on the human cornea. Invest. Ophthalmol. Vis. Sci., 26(11), 1489–1501.)

Grading contact lens complications

The severity of contact lens complications can be assessed with the aid of grading scales. Grading is effected by observing the tissue change of interest directly or with the aid of a slit-lamp biomicroscope, under low and/or high magnification as required, and estimating the grading to the nearest 0.1 scale unit. For example, a tissue change that is judged to be considerably more severe than Grade 2 but not quite as severe as Grade 3 may be assigned a grade of 2.8 or 2.9. Although this procedure can sometimes be difficult, grading to the nearest 0.1 scale unit (rather than simply assigning a whole digit grade of 0, 1, 2, 3 or 4) affords much greater precision and increases the sensitivity of the grading scale for detecting real changes or differences in severity.

It is important to designate clearly the grading system used and the specific tissue change being graded. A more expedient approach would be to print or stamp the

Table G.3 • Designation and interpretation of the various levels of severity depicted in the Efron Grading Scales.

Grade	Severity	Colour band	Clinical interpretation
0	Normal	Green	Clinical action not required
1	Trace	Lime	Clinical action rarely required
2	Mild	Yellow	Clinical action possibly required
3	Moderate	Orange	Clinical action usually required
4	Severe	Red	Clinical action certainly required

names of the various complications onto a record card, each with an accompanying box for entering the assigned grade. It may be necessary to make additional annotations to describe the condition more fully – e.g. to indicate the location of the pathology.

The five-stage 0 to 4 grading scale is based on a universally accepted concept whereby a higher numeric grade denotes greater clinical severity. This schema can be applied to any tissue change. The designation and general interpretation of each grading step is shown in Table G.3. It must be recognized that these are only very general guidelines, and are not intended to replace sound professional judgement.

When using grading scales for the first time, a confidence range of about 1.2 is to be expected; however, with experience this confidence range may reduce to 0.7 grading scale units. In general, a change or difference of more than about 1.0 grading scale unit, or a level of severity of more than Grade 2, is considered to be clinically significant.

Grading scales

As an aid to accurate record keeping, health care practitioners of all disciplines often resort to the use of standardized grading scales of various conditions.

A number of grading scales have been developed for use in the field of optometry. Appendix B displays the Optometric Grading Scales developed by Richard Pearson, which are used for quantifying the following ocular features:

- Limbal anterior chamber depth
- Age-related cataract
- Vertical cup/disc ratio
- Retinal vessels.

Two grading systems for complications of contact lens wear, each containing a wide range of grading scales, are readily available to practitioners:

1. Efron Grading Scales for Contact Lens Complications (shown in Appendix C)
2. CCLRU Grading Scales (supplied by Vistakon; Johnson & Johnson).

These grading scales provide a simple, convenient and accurate means by which clinicians can record and communicate the severity of complications of contact lens wear. The Efron Grading Scales were painted by an ophthalmic artist, and the CCLRU Grading Scales are a mosaic of clinical photographs. The advantage of using painted (versus photographic) grading scales is that greater clarity can be achieved because the precise level of severity can be depicted, all other factors can be kept constant, potentially confounding artefacts can be avoided, and artistic license can be adopted. The grading assigned to a particular condition can serve as a reference against which any future tissue change may be assessed, and can therefore influence clinical decision-making. These grading scales may act as a standard clinical reference for describing the severity of contact lens complications.

The primary design criteria upon which the Efron Grading Scales are based are simplicity, convenience, and ease of use by clinicians. Sixteen sets of grading images are depicted in two panels, each comprising eight complications. These 16 grading scales show the key anterior ocular complications of contact lens wear. Each complication is illustrated in five stages of increasing severity, from 0 to 4, with 'traffic-light' colour banding from green (normal, Grade 0) to red (severe, Grade 4). The severity of the complications is based on an appraisal of accumulated evidence in the literature and clinical experience.

Each complication in the Efron Grading Scales has been painted to an equivalent level of magnification that addresses the compromise between being large enough to depict the key features of the tissue changes, and being low enough to relate to what practitioners can observe with available clinical techniques. The magnification of the complications varies from ×1 (i.e. the whole cornea) to ×600. A consequence of these magnification levels is that, although epithelial microcysts and endothelial blebs can be detected and graded at ×40 magnification on a slit-lamp biomicroscope, they will not be viewed at the resolution depicted. Furthermore, endothelial polymegethism can only be assessed with the aid of a specular microscope. All other complications can be viewed at the resolution depicted and are capable of being graded by direct observation and/or using a slit-lamp biomicroscope up to ×40 magnification. See *Grading contact lens complications*.

Gravimetry, soft contact lens

The water content of a soft lens can be estimated by weighing the sample in air (W_1), completely dehydrating the lens in a suitable oven, and then re-weighing the dried sample (W_2). The water content is defined by $(W_1-W_2)/W_1 \times 100\%$. Alternatively, dehydration can be achieved by placing the lens above an active desiccant such as anhydrous $CaSO_4$. Although the above techniques constitute a useful approach in a research environment, they are destructive and therefore of no value to the clinician.

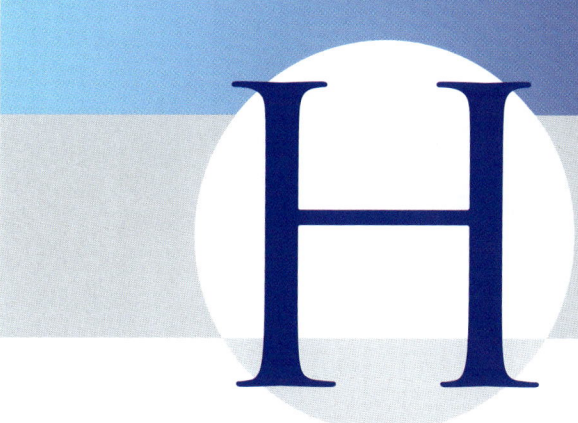

Halberg clip
This is a device that clips on to the spectacle frame that a patient is wearing. It contains two slots for inserting trial lens frames. The Halberg clip is especially useful for performing a refraction over the top of a patient's own spectacles (i.e. an 'over-refraction'), in cases where vertex distance control is important (e.g. with high refractions).

Halos associated with contact lens wear
If the optic zone of a rigid lens is small and the eye pupil is large, the outer zones of the pupil will be imperfectly corrected, leading to the formation of bright rings or 'halos' when viewing bright light sources under dim lighting conditions (e.g. oncoming headlamps when driving at night). Similar effects may occur with smaller pupils if the lenses are badly decentred.

Hand grooming with contact lenses
- See *Hygiene with contact lenses, practitioner and patient*.

Hand held plus lens magnifier
With any plus lens magnifier, the magnification remains constant regardless of the eye-to-magnifier distance, providing that the object is placed at the anterior focal point of the plus lens. This gives the option of taking the plus lens and placing it in a mounting, perhaps with a handle, and holding it away from the eye. The distance of the user from the task will be increased, even if the magnifier still needs to be held in close proximity. This can be useful when it would not be safe to approach the task too closely (perhaps setting dials and gauges on an oven), or if the patient rejects the unusual close working distance associated with spectacle-mounted lenses. The field of view through the magnifier is inversely proportional to the eye-to-magnifier distance, however, so positioning the magnifier away from the eye limits the field of view: this means that these devices are most suitable for short-term 'spot' or 'survival' reading such as price tags whilst shopping, or looking up a telephone number, rather than a longer duration task such as reading a novel. See *Reading requirements, low vision*. In these circumstances, the patient may select a magnifier based on size, weight and portability. Some designs have internal illumination, which is useful if it is to be used out of the home where lighting is unpredictable; having the light source below the lens also limits annoying reflections from the lens surfaces.

Hand magnifiers are often the most psychologically acceptable to the patient because they are freely available devices, often being sold for hobbies such as stamp-collecting or needlework, rather than for the visually impaired. They are often very familiar to the patient who has obtained and used one of these aids before reaching the stage of seeking professional advice.

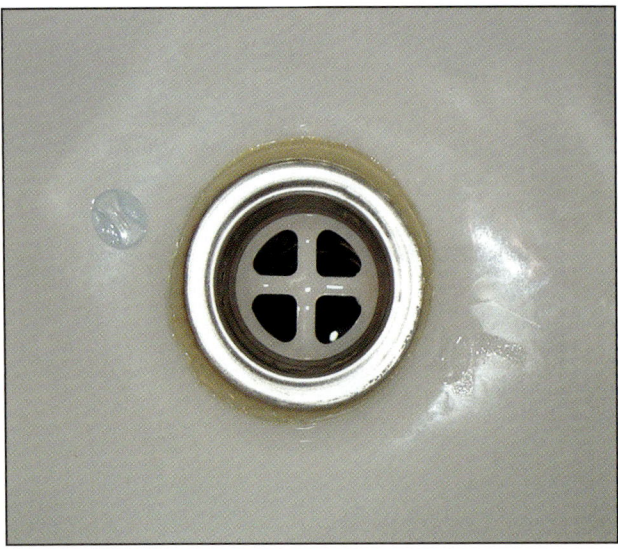

Figure H.1 • Lenses 'dropped' in a bathroom sink. The lens with the handling tint can be seen at the half-past 9 o'clock position (relative to the drain hole), whereas the untinted lens is barely visible at the 4 o'clock position.

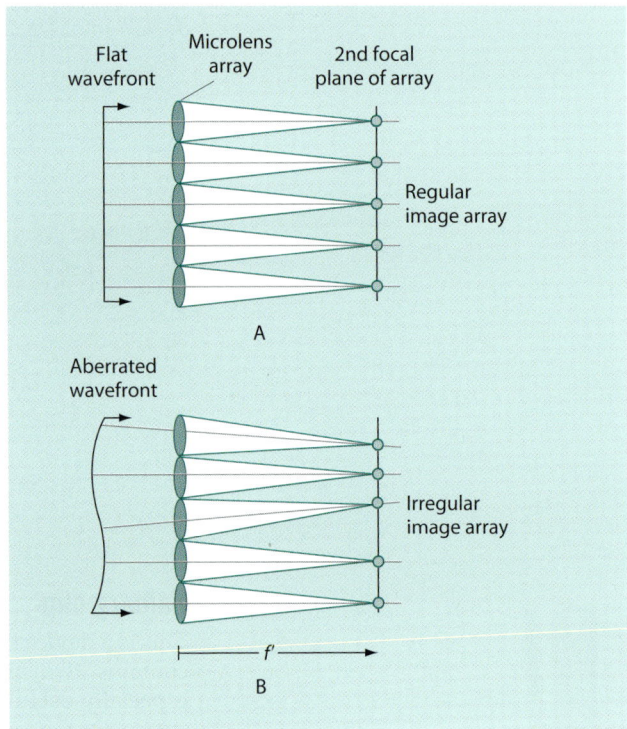

Figure H.2 • Principle of the Hartmann–Shack technique. (A) Effects with a perfect emmetropic eye, where the images are formed on the axis of each lens and hence are regularly spaced. (B) Effects with an aberrated eye, where the image ray is irregular since the images are no longer formed on the axes of the lenses.

There are literally hundreds of different designs of hand magnifier to choose from. To be used comfortably, the magnifier must have a suitable handle, and should preferably be designed for right- or left-handed use. Although glass lenses, which have greater surface hardness, are available, plastic lenses are preferred to reduce the weight: the rim around the lens forms a flange which stops the curved lens surface from being scratched when placed down on a table. The lens should be used with the most convex surface towards the eye and there must be some way for the patient to distinguish which is the correct orientation. The magnifier is placed against the object, and then it is raised up until maximum magnification is reached (when the object is at the focal point of the lens). The presbyopic user should therefore wear distance spectacles.

See *Spectacle correction, plus lens magnifiers*.

Handling tints for contact lenses

These are also known as 'visibility tints' or 'locator tints', and are incorporated into soft lenses so that these lenses can be easily seen in the lens case or on a domestic surface if accidentally dropped (Figure H.1). Such tints are very light and do not alter iris colour; however, they make the lens slightly more visible on the eye by virtue of the handling tint being visible where the lens edge impinges over the sclera. Handling tints do not affect vision or colour perception. See *Tinted contact lenses*.

Hardness, rigid contact lens

The hardness of a rigid lens material can be defined as its resistance to penetration. In a hardness test, an indentation device (e.g. a 'nail-like' probe) is pressed on the surface of the material under test, and the extent to which it sinks into the material for a given pressure and time is an inverse measure of the hardness. There are many hardness testing instruments available commercially that are suitable for plastics and rubbers, including the Vickers indenter, the Rockwell hardness tester and the Shore durometer. Other types of hardness testing include resistance to scratching and recovery efficiency (resilience). There is no common method of measurement in these tests; each uses an arbitrary scale and, although the scales can be approximately compared, precise correlation is not possible. The only true form of hardness evaluation is to consider relative data generated using the same instrument at the same time under identical test conditions.

Hartmann–Shack aberrometry

A variety of subjective and objective techniques are available for measuring the wavefront aberration of the eye. Probably the most elegant, which is beginning to be commercially available, involves the use of a Hartmann–Shack wavefront. A hexagonal array of identical microlenses allows the slope of the wavefront across a lattice of points in the pupil to be determined. The principle can be understood with reference to Figure H.2. Suppose there is a point source on the retina of a perfect emmetropic eye. The light leaving the eye can either be envisaged as a bundle of parallel rays or as a series of plane wavefronts. The array of microlenses is now placed in the path of the emerging light. Each lens will converge the parallel rays to its second focal point, so that an absolutely regular array of image points will form in the common focal plane. If now the eye suffers from aberration, the emergent rays are no longer parallel and the associated wavefronts are no longer flat. Thus the rays no longer come to a focus on the axes of the lenses: the lateral displacement from the focal point of each lens is directly proportional to the local inclination of the ray or the slope of the wavefront. It is, then, easy to calculate the form of the emergent wavefronts and the wavefront aberration from the distorted pattern of image points.

Departures from a reference sphere of more than a quarter of a wavelength would be expected to degrade image quality. The aberration in the central 2–3mm of the pupil is usually modest, but much larger amounts may be found in the periphery of dilated pupils. On the basis of wavefront aberration results, it is possible to calculate monochromatic point and line-spread functions, and also the ocular modulation and phase-transfer functions for any pupil diameter.

Haze
- See *Oedema*.

Head mounted video magnification device (HMVD)
A head mounted video magnification device (HMVD) is an electronic vision enhancement system intended to provide electronic magnification for a visually impaired user for all viewing distances and in a fully portable form. It consists of a head-mounted miniature camera, a video display mounted in front of each eye, and a power source and control panel, usually on a belt pack.

The first such device was the Low Vision Enhancement System (LVES, although often known as 'Elvis') which was developed in a joint research project between the Johns Hopkins University, NASA, and the Department of Veterans Affairs, and manufactured and marketed by a company in Minneapolis, USA, named Visionics. Despite their wearability, these devices are only intended for sedentary use, with the manufacturers warning against use in any mobility task. HMVDs share many of the advantages of closed circuit televisions (CCTVs): there is variable magnification and zoom facility which can provide an overall view at low magnification before increasing to concentrate on detail; more use is made of electronic image manipulation, with edge enhancement as well as reverse contrast often available; and they are available with colour or monochrome displays. HMVDs also offer a much wider field of view (especially for near and intermediate tasks) than telescopes (see *Telescopes, near and intermediate viewing*). Apart from the cost, HMVDs suffer a number of practical disadvantages: poor cosmetic appearance; controls cannot be viewed whilst the user is wearing the headset; and high weight which causes discomfort and is likely to increase head instability, which causes the user to observe 'image shake'. To avoid this, it is common for a stand to be provided to 'park' the headset and plug in to an external monitor, thus converting it into a CCTV for prolonged reading. HMVDs with hand-held, table-mounted or 'mouse' cameras are also available.

Health and Medicines Act 1988 (UK)
The Health and Medicines Act 1988, in addition to removing the previous right of any individual to apply for a National Health Service (NHS) examination, amended certain sections of the Opticians Act 1958. The amendments related to s.20 dealing with restrictions on the testing of sight, supply of optical appliances and the use of titles and descriptions and also s.21 which dealt with restriction on sale and supply of optical appliances.

Health and Social Security Act 1984 (UK)
The Office of Fair Trading published a report, 'Opticians and Competition' in December 1982. This report concluded that although opticians did not make undue profits there were certain measures which would, in the opinion of those producing the report, improve the service to the public. The main improvement would be the introduction of competition into supply of spectacles through the removal of the professional 'monopoly'. Coupled with this, greater freedom to advertise would offer a wider choice and greater information to the public considering spectacles.

The Government took the Office of Fair Trading report as the basis for drawing up a bill with far greater scope than had been anticipated. In fact, the Health and Social Security Act 1984 had such far-reaching consequences that many of the organizations that had campaigned so vigorously for change now campaigned against the proposed legislation. The Act as a whole was designed to amend or supplement existing legislation regarding optical services and the optical profession but also included changes to:

- The status and constitution of Family Practitioner Committees.
- Finances within the Health Service.
- Disablement allowances.
- Social Security benefits.
- Occupational pension schemes.
- Membership of Social Security appeal panels.

The sight testing service provided through the General Ophthalmic Services was left untouched by this legislation on the grounds that the screening service provided by optometrists was necessary. On the other hand, the legislation covering the supply of spectacles and the regulations governing the practice of optometry and the provisions of the Health Service were radically altered.

Heat disinfection, soft contact lens
This physical method of soft lens disinfection relies on thermal energy being imparted to micro-organisms to cause lethal cell changes. Heating was the first soft lens disinfection method approved by the USA Food and Drug Administration (in 1972). Disinfection using this approach requires a temperature of 80°C to be maintained for at least 10 minutes. A representative example of one of the heating units available at this time was the Bausch & Lomb system, which reached 96°C for a period of about 20 minutes (Figure H.3). In terms of lens disinfection, the heating systems were recognized as being highly effective, even against the protozoan Acanthamoeba. Furthermore, after the initial purchase of the heat unit, the ongoing costs of operation were minimal.

There were a number of disadvantages associated with heat disinfection. In normal circumstances the protein that

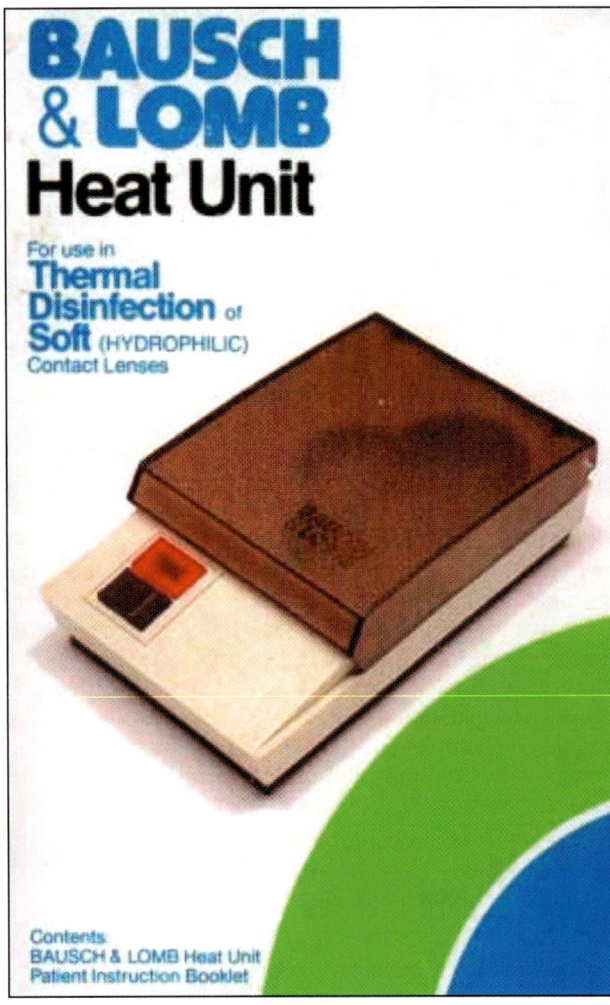

Figure H.3 • Early advertisement for the Bausch & Lomb Heat Unit.

spoils the surface of a soft contact lens does not denature, but heating the lens tends to denature protein, with adverse clinical consequences such as reduced acuity, the potential for ocular surface reactions such as papillary conjunctivitis, and altered physical lens parameters. With the popularity of low water content, non-ionic lenses in the early and mid-1970s, this was not a significant problem. However, heat disinfection is unsuitable with the higher water content materials that dominate the market today; such lenses, especially if ionic in nature, absorb much greater quantities of proteins, and turn yellow and become deformed when heated.

The heating process is also inconvenient for many wearers. Not only does this method require a nearby source of electricity, but the system also uses unpreserved saline, which does not offer any antimicrobial activity. The opportunity for microbial contamination arises if the lenses remain in the cooled saline for a prolonged period, so this disinfection system requires the process to be repeated each day with fresh solution if the lenses are not used. With the advent of planned replacement lenses, which are generally of mid-to-high water content and are often manufactured from ionic materials more prone to parameter changes, the popularity of heat disinfection has waned and this technique is rarely used today.

HEMA
- See *Poly (2-hydroxyethyl methacrylate)*.

Hemi-desmosomes
- See *Corneal epithelium*.

Hemianopia, aids for

A homonymous hemianopia is a loss of vision on the same side of the visual field in both eyes. The sufferer therefore cannot see any objects to either the left, or to the right side of fixation (Figure H.4). There are often problems with reading which can be aided with a typoscope, but more significant difficulties in navigation, with complaints of bumping into objects on the blind side. Some hemianopes become very good at scanning – systematically moving their eyes to explore the whole visual field – and this can be taught if necessary. See *Low vision training*. Alternatively, there are various optical devices which aim to allow the hemianope to view (or to be aware of) objects in the blind field more easily.

An angled mirror can be placed on the nasal side of the eye rim of a pair of spectacles, on the same side of the bridge as the hemianopic defect, and with the reflecting surface towards the eye (Figure H.5A). This would mean, for example, a mirror on the right side of the bridge for a right hemianopia. Although the mirror is small, it will obscure part of the seeing left hemi-field for the right eye, although the view of the left eye will be uninterrupted. Through the mirror, the right eye will be aware of objects in the non-seeing right (temporal) field, superimposed by the mirror onto the left field (Figure H.4C).

As an alternative, prisms can be attached to the spectacle lenses to refract the light from objects in the blind field. In order not to affect the image from the other hemifield, a prism of power $\approx 20^\Delta$ is only placed over the side of the lens closest to the defect. Because of their ease of use and replacement, good cosmesis and low weight, flexible Fresnel prisms are often used to create this partial aperture or sector prism. The aim is to find a position for the prism which is as close as possible to the pupil, but where it will not be noticed by the patient in straight ahead gaze. The prism is placed with its base towards the non-seeing area, and moves the image of objects $\approx 12°$ from the periphery of the blind area closer to the midline. When the patient scans into the blind hemifield, the amount of eye rotation required is therefore reduced, and objects are more easily detected. If the prism is fitted binocularly (Figure H.5B), in a symmetrical position on the two lenses, however, a strip of the blind hemi-field ($\approx 10°$ wide) immediately beyond the midline is 'lost' as more peripheral images appear to jump towards the prism apex (Figure H.4D). This can be avoided by fitting the prism monocularly (Figure H.5C), which creates diplopia with the 'true' image seen by the eye without the prism, and the displaced (more peripheral) image seen superimposed through the prism (Figure H.4E). This requires greater adaptation by the patient but gives potentially more useful information from the missing hemifield.

Monocular prism placement is also the principle of the Gottlieb Visual Awareness System (Rekindle, Gottlieb

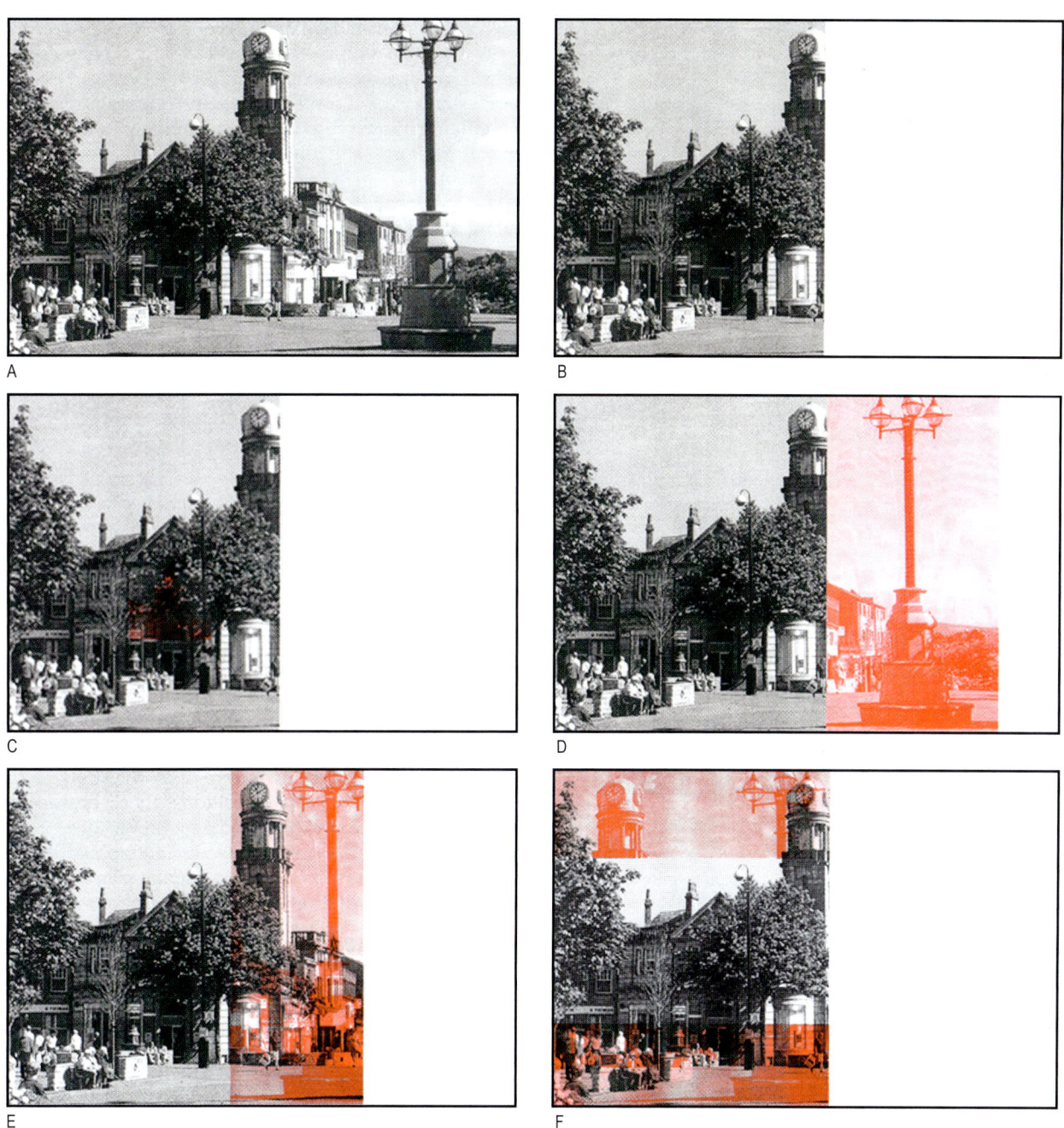

Figure H.4 • A schematic representation of a street scene as observed by (A), a normally-sighted observer and (B) an observer with right hemianopia. The view available to this individual when using various optical devices is illustrated. In each case the view through the device is seen in red. The views shown are as seen when using (C) the mirror; (D) binocular partial aperture prisms; (E) monocular partial aperture prism; (F) the prism to optically induce peripheral exotropia.

Vision Group, Stone Mountain, GA, USA). In this case the prism is a glass component mounted into the carrier prescription lens (Figure H.5D). The use of a conventional prism avoids the poor image quality and reflections apparent to the wearer of Fresnel prisms. An alternative monocular prism has been described as 'optically induced peripheral exotropia'. The prism is placed across the full width of one lens, above and/or below the line of sight, base towards the blind hemifield (Figure H.5E). A higher powered prism (≈35$^\Delta$) is used to produce ≈20° field shift. The poor image quality and diplopia are less disturbing to the wearer because gaze is never through the prism, and the diplopia is only present in peripheral vision (Figure H.5F). Nonetheless, as with any of the devices described, the patient still needs training to adapt to the 'true' location of objects (see *Low vision training*).

Herpes simplex keratitis

The herpes simplex virus is a double stranded DNA virus and is the most ubiquitous viral infection in

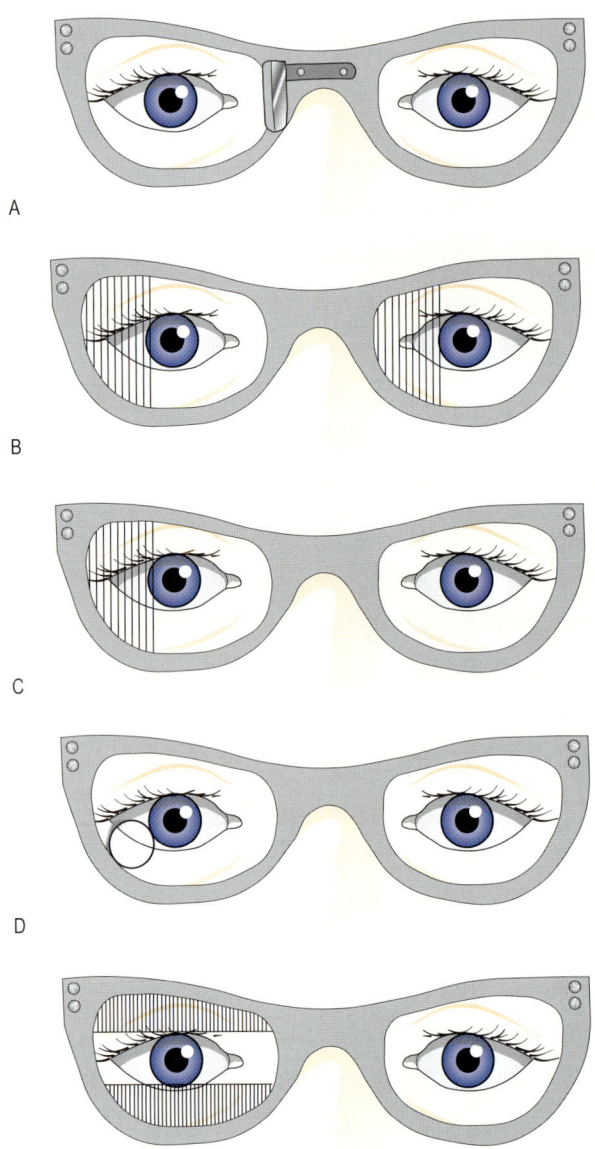

Figure H.5 • Schematic representation of the different optical systems available to aid mobility for hemianopia. The positioning shown is for a right-sided hemianopia. (A) Mirror on nasal bridge of spectacle frame, (B) binocular Fresnel partial aperture prisms, (C) monocular Fresnel partial aperture prism, (D) Gottlieb Visual Awareness system, (E) prism to optically induce peripheral exotropia.

humans. Humans are its only known host. Ocular infection is common; it is estimated that approximately 500,000 people in the USA have had herpes simplex keratitis (HSK) and that approximately 10% of these have at least one recurrence each year. The extremely protean nature of its corneal involvement is one of the distinctive features of HSK and has led to it being labelled a 'great masquerader'. The initial or primary infection typically occurs in childhood and leads to a blepharokeratoconjunctivitis, characterized by eyelid skin vesicles, follicular conjunctivitis and corneal microdendrite. Following the primary infection the virus remains in the body, resident in the trigeminal ganglion. This establishment of dormant virus within the neuronal cell bodies is termed latency. Secondary disease occurs when the virus becomes reactivated and travels down the sensory neuronal axon to infect the cornea. Several manifestations of secondary disease occur as a result of an inflammatory response to residual, often non-replicatory, viral antigen rather than from florid viral replication.

The different types of corneal involvement with secondary HSK can be classified on an anatomical basis or by the degree of viral replication and inflammation. The latter is more useful from a clinical perspective as it helps to direct the usage of topical antivirals and corticosteroids. The anatomical classification is as follows:

Epithelial:

- Dendritic ulcer
- Geographic ulcer
- Metaherpetic (indolent) ulcer.

Stromal:

- Stromal necrotic keratitis
- Disciform (herpetic keratouveitis) keratitis
- Interstitial keratitis
- Limbal vasculitis.

Endothelial:

- Linear endotheliitis.

While some viral replication within the cornea may occur at a low level in all these conditions, those caused by viral replication are dendritic and geographic ulcers.

Blurring of vision, increased lacrimation, photophobia and ocular discomfort are common with all manifestations of HSK. Significant pain is rarely a symptom of HSK, probably due to the neurotrophic nature of the virus leading to reduced corneal sensation. This is especially the case with recurrent disease. Signs of ocular inflammation and viral activity will be present. Ocular inflammation usually leads to corneal oedema, keratic precipitates, an anterior chamber reaction and an increased intraocular pressure. Viral replication is most obviously manifest by an epithelial dendritic staining pattern (Figure H.6). Herpes simplex keratitis affects approximately 1/5000 people every year. Metaherpetic ulcers, interstitial keratitis, limbal vasculitis and linear endotheliitis are all very rare.

Each condition requires specific treatment. Patients with recurrent disease should be advised to avoid known trigger factors such as UV light exposure and ocular trauma with the use of tight fitting wrap around sunglasses. They should also be especially attuned to the possibility of a recurrence around the time of a significant intercurrent illness such as influenza. Patients should also be advised of the need for prompt presentation if they feel they may have a recurrence of HSK. Culture or more commonly direct immunofluorescent staining can be undertaken from tissue swabs to identify specific viral antigen.

Topical antiviral agents are used either in a full treatment dose, i.e.: acyclovir ointment 5× daily for 7 days to treat active viral replication, or prophylactically, i.e. acyclovir b.i.d. to prevent viral reactivation during steroid usage. Topical steroids are used to suppress

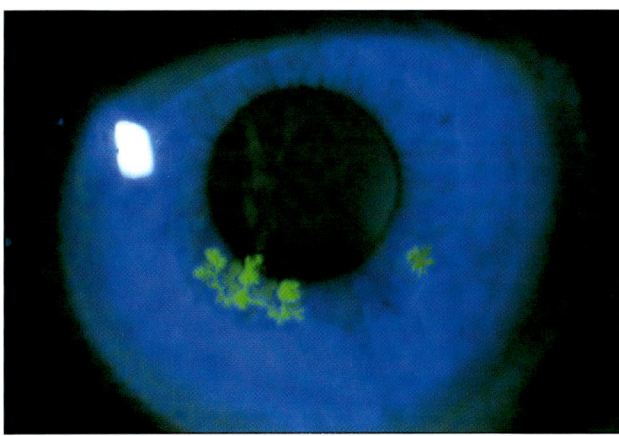

Figure H.6 • Small dendritic ulcers stained with fluorescein in herpes simplex keratitis.

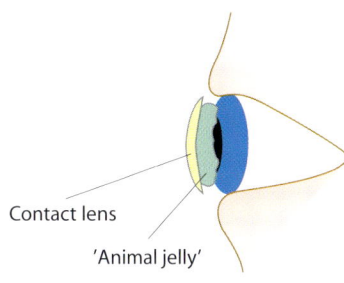

Figure H.7 • 'Animal jelly' sandwiched between a 'spherical capsule of glass' (contact lens) and cornea, as proposed by Sir John Herschel.

inflammation and are usually tapered over several months to prevent rebound inflammation from occurring. Long-term low dose oral acyclovir has been shown to be effective in reducing the number of recurrences especially in patients with recurrent disease.

Herpes zoster ophthalmicus
- See *Eyelid pathology, therapeutic contact lenses for*.

Herschel, John
In a footnote in his treatise on light in the 1845 edition of the Encyclopedia Metropolitana, Sir John Herschel suggested two possible methods of correcting 'very bad cases of irregular cornea'. These were '... applying to the cornea a spherical capsule of glass filled with animal jelly' (Figure H.7), or '... taking a mould of the cornea and impressing it on some transparent medium'. Although it seems that Herschel did not attempt to conduct such trials, his latter suggestion was ultimately adopted some 40 years later by a number of inventors, working independently and unbeknown to each other, who were all apparently unaware of the writings of Herschel.

High minus power contact lens design
A rigid contact lens of –10.00D would have an unfinished edge thickness of approximately 0.32–0.35mm if the diameter was 8.8–9.6mm. Because unfinished edge thickness for best comfort and lens stability should be approximately 0.10mm, lenticularization of high minus lenses is essential (Figure H.8). A computer-numeric controlled lathe can be used to cut a steeper anterior lenticular radius to obtain the proper edge thickness.

Typical front optic zone diameters range from 7.2mm (in a lens of 8.8mm total diameter) to 7.8mm (in a lens of 9.6mm total diameter) and are about 0.2mm larger than the back optic zone. The lenticular radius may be cut flatter for a smaller front optic zone or steeper for a larger front optic zone. The latter design will result in higher mid-peripheral thickness. The higher the power (with the same front optic zone), the thicker will be this mid-peripheral area. This may complicate the fit and cause

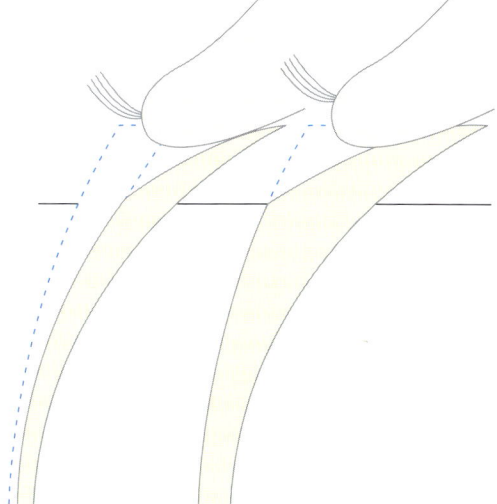

Figure H.8 • Low minus power lens (left) with same front optic zone diameter as high minus power lens (right). Junction thickness (horizontal straight line) is greater for the high minus power lens.

discomfort if the lens does not attach to the upper eyelid. Greater mid-peripheral thickness may also cause a high-riding lens to ride even higher. Mid-peripheral thickness can be reduced with proper polishing or advanced multi-curve computer-controlled anterior surface lathing.

High plus power contact lens design
Silicone lenses of high plus power are typically 11.3–12.5mm in diameter and are fitted with base curve near (or only slightly flatter than) K. Silicone hydrogel high plus lenses are fitted like soft contact lenses, and will be beneficial for these patients when they are available.

High plus rigid lenses, unless they are of very small diameter (8.5mm or less) and fit steep, must be made in regular (parallel) carrier form or minus (edge thicker than junction) carrier form (Figure H.9). Lenticular lenses are thinner, have less mass, and centre better than non-lenticular designs. Typically these lenses are 9.0–10.5mm in diameter. Regular carrier designs are better for lens positioning between the eyelids. Minus carrier lenses are better for lid-attachment fitting. The smaller the front optic zone diameter, the thinner the lens. The front optic zone diameter may be equal to, larger than or smaller than the back optic zone diameter. Typically the front optic zone diameter is 7.0–8.0mm in diameter, and the

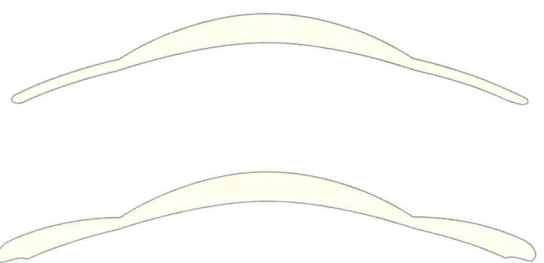

Figure H.9 • Lenticular designs for plus powered lenses. Top: regular (parallel) carrier. Bottom: minus carrier.

back optic zone is designed as needed for fitting. Junction thickness for lenticular rigid plus lenses should be thin enough to minimize lens thickness but thick enough to allow adequate lens strength (about 0.15mm). Regular carrier unfinished edge thickness is typically 0.10–0.12mm, and minus carrier unfinished edge thickness is typically approximately 0.2mm. Lenticular (front peripheral) radii range from approximately 0.2mm flatter than the posterior secondary curve (regular carrier) to 3.0mm flatter than the posterior secondary curve (minus carrier).

Hir-Cal grid
- See *Non-invasive tear break-up time.*

HMC (Oculus) anomaloscope
- See *Anomaloscope.*

Home delivery plans
- See *Contact lens supply routes.*

Hormonal changes
- See *Indications and contraindications for contact lens wear.*

Horopter
The locus of objects in space that stimulate corresponding retinal points of the two eyes when the eyes are fixating binocularly towards a central object is termed the horopter. The concept of the horopter is a useful theoretical model that enables many aspects of binocularity and space perception to be explained. Various experimental paradigms can be employed to demonstrate the location of the horopter in space, and these give rise to the different results and hence different names, such as the apparent fronto-parallel plane, the nonius horopter and the Veith-Müller circle. The essential experimental technique for plotting the location of the horopter is to have a subject view a thin vertical reference rod about 1 m away from the observer – set against a blank, amorphous background – and to instruct the observer to position a series of rods, set to each side of the central rod, so that all rods appear to be equidistant from the observer. The shape formed by the array of rods constitutes the horopter, and this shape will change as the distance of the reference rod from the observer is changed.

Horner's syndrome
Horner's syndrome is characterized by 'miosis, ptosis and anhydrosis' of the affected eye. The condition is due to interruption of sympathetic innervation to the eye. The ptosis and anhydrosis is due to the fact that the sympathetic system controls Müller's muscles of the eyelids and the facial sweat glands. The efferent lesion causing Horner's syndrome may be anywhere in the long sympathetic pathway from the cervical spine to the eye. The consition can be congenital or acquired. Trauma is the leading cause of this syndrome in those under 20 years of age. In patients over 20 years, tumours are the cause in about half the cases. The location of any pathology can be considered in relation to the superior cervical ganglion. As a general rule, postganglionic lesions are benign and preganglionic lesions are indicative of a serious problem.

Hue discrimination
- See *Wavelength discrimination.*

Hydrogel
Hydrogels are, both historically and potentially, the largest group of contact lens materials in terms of structural variety. PolyHEMA is in many ways typical of other hydrogels, and is still undoubtedly the most important single material of its class across a wide range of biomedical applications.

It is simplest to regard hydrogels as 'washing line' polymers having a long backbone (the 'washing line') from which a variety of chemical groups may be suspended (the 'washing'). The function of the chemical groups in hydrogels is primarily to attract and bind water within the structure. Greater physical stability is achieved by fastening the washing lines together at intervals by the use of cross-links. Cross-links are introduced by the use of cross-linking agents, which are simply monomers with two active carbon–carbon double bonds. Networks are never perfect, and contain entanglements, chain loops and wasted chain ends. In addition to hydroxyethyl methacrylate (HEMA), other important monomers used to achieve an attraction for water include N-vinyl pyrrolidone (used in FDA Group II materials) and methacrylic acid (used in all FDA Group IV materials). In the silicone hydrogels the same 'washing line' principle applies, but here groups that contain silicon-oxygen bonds (silicones) are attached, in order to increase oxygen permeability. This is achieved with the monomer commonly referred to as 'TRIS', which is a component of both rigid and silicone hydrogel materials.

Hydrogen peroxide disinfecting solution for contact lenses
Hydrogen peroxide has been used as an antimicrobial agent for about 200 years. It is widely used medically for disinfection and sterilization, and is generally available in concentrations ranging from 3 to 90%, depending on its purpose. Hydrogen peroxide has a broad-spectrum efficacy against bacteria, viruses and yeast by producing hydroxyl free radicals that attach essential cell components such as lipid and proteins, and is often considered

to be the 'gold standard' in terms of soft contact lens disinfection. For example, 3% hydrogen peroxide will kill trophozoites and cysts of Acanthamoeba castellanii in 3min and 9h of soaking, respectively. Hydrogen peroxide can be chemically broken down into oxygen and water, and is therefore considered to be environmentally friendly. It tends to decompose on standing, and therefore needs to be stabilized, typically with phosphates or phosphorates. The use of stannate as a stabilizer has been associated with hazing of ionic lenses due to an interaction between the stannate ions, methacrylic acid groups in the lens material and tear-derived lysozyme.

Although hydrogen peroxide has a high efficacy in terms of its antimicrobial action it is toxic to the eye, and neutralization is required before a lens that has been placed in hydrogen peroxide can be worn comfortably. Conjunctival hyperaemia is induced by levels of hydrogen peroxide greater than 200ppm, and concentrations in excess of 100ppm are associated with subjective stinging; however, concentrations of this order of magnitude do not cause corneal or conjunctival staining.

Storage in hydrogen peroxide has been reported to alter lens parameters. There is a temporary reduction in lens hydration after prolonged lens storage in hydrogen peroxide. High water ionic lenses (FDA Group IV) appear to be most susceptible to changes in diameter and base curve, although the clinical consequences of these changes are generally not significant because of their temporary nature – for example, a soaking period of 20 minutes in neutralizer returns lens parameters to their original specification within 1 hour of lens wear.

The approaches to neutralization have varied since the introduction of hydrogen peroxide as a contact lens disinfectant. The initial approach was to allow for the storage of the lenses in 3% hydrogen peroxide, with neutralization undertaken as a secondary process before lens insertion. These two-step systems are considered to provide the best antimicrobial action, especially when the lens is exposed to 3% hydrogen peroxide overnight. The two most popular approaches for neutralization in a two-step hydrogen peroxide system are the catalytic and reactive methods. In the Oxysept system (Allergan), a solution containing the enzyme catalase is added to the lens storage case after the hydrogen peroxide has been discarded. This quickly breaks down the remaining hydrogen peroxide into water and oxygen, with the production of the latter requiring a vented storage case. With this system, no hydrogen peroxide is detectable 1 minute after the introduction of the neutralizer. An example of the reactive method was the 10:10 product (CIBA Vision). Here, after the hydrogen peroxide storage solution has been discarded, the lens case is filled with a solution containing sodium pyruvate, which completely neutralizes the hydrogen peroxide in about 6 minutes. This product has now been discontinued.

Despite the antimicrobial efficacy of two-step systems, this approach is probably the most complex of all soft lens disinfection regimens and carries an unacceptably high risk of the patient suffering a severe 'peroxide burn' after accidentally placing a lens directly into the eye from the 3% hydrogen peroxide solution. This led to a reduction of the popularity of two-step systems and the subsequent development of one-step systems. The one-

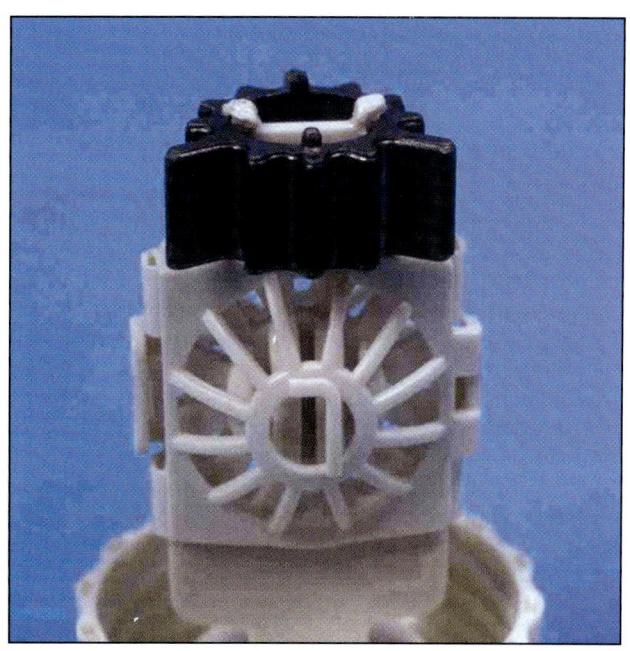

Figure H.10 • The neutralizing platinum disc in this one-step hydrogen peroxide system is attached to the lens holder. In other systems, it is fixed in the base of the case.

step systems negate the requirement for a separate neutralization process by the contact lens user. After the lens storage case is closed, the disinfection and neutralization steps take place without further intervention from the wearer. Two approaches are common. In the first, such as in the Oxysept 1-Step system (Allergan), the lens case is filled with hydrogen peroxide and a coated tablet containing catalase is added. The coating of the tablet is dissolved, releasing catalase into the solution and leading to neutralization of the hydrogen peroxide within about 2 hours. A number of products use a second method of neutralization – a platinum disc (Figure H.10). In this approach, the disc is either attached as an integral part of the lens holder or is permanently lodged in the base of the storage case. There is a rapid neutralization over the first 2 minutes – from the original 30000ppm (or 3% concentration) to about 9000ppm – followed by a slower phase to 50ppm after 3 hours and 15ppm after 6 hours.

The trade-off for the increased convenience for the user of a one-step system is two-fold. First, as the lenses are held only in neutralized solution within a few hours of entering the case, long-term storage is not advisable because the residual solution has no antimicrobial capabilities. Secondly, the reduced time in relatively high concentration hydrogen peroxide compared with the two-step systems affords a reduced antimicrobial power to the system. Furthermore, the speed of hydrogen peroxide neutralization differs between the tablet systems and the platinum disc systems. Although activity against bacteria is likely to be adequate with these systems, the storage period is unlikely to be sufficient for efficacy against Acanthamoeba. However, antimicrobial efficacy can be enhanced by appropriate lens cleaning and rinsing.

Hydroxyethyl methacrylate
- See *Poly (2-hydroxyethyl methacrylate)*.

Hygiene with contact lenses, practitioner and patient
It is imperative that the importance of hand washing prior to lens handling is reinforced in the course of contact lens patient education. The best way of achieving this without appearing to be patronizing to the patient is for the instructor to wash his or her hands prior to lens handling, in full view of the patient. A very brief explanation as to why this is so important – the prevention of lens contamination and reduction of the risks of infection – can be given to patients before inviting them to wash their hands. At all future instruction or aftercare visits, patients should be prompted to wash their hands if they forget to do this before proceeding to handle lenses.

Hand grooming is an important factor related to hygiene. The nails of all fingers that are likely to be involved in lens manipulation should be cut short and filed smooth to avoid both lens damage and the potential for corneal insult.

Hygienist, contact lens
- See *Patient education*.

Hypercapnia
This term refers to a level of carbon dioxide in excess of that normally found in a specified condition. For example, the partial pressure of carbon dioxide in the atmosphere is 0.3mmHg at sea level under conditions of standard temperature and pressure. This is considered to be the baseline reference at the anterior corneal surface, where higher levels of carbon dioxide infer hypercapnia.

Hypermetropia
Often referred to by the foreshortened term 'hyperopia', this is a refractive defect of the eye in which light from a distant object is focused behind the retina when accommodation is relaxed, resulting in blurred distance and near vision. The hypermetropic patient can make distance objects appear clear by accommodating the eye, assuming that the accommodation facility equals or exceeds the dioptric degree of the refractive defect; however, constant accommodation to clear distance objects can lead to eye strain. Plus powered lenses can be used to obviate the need for constant accommodation and afford comfortable and clear distance vision. The refractive error may be a result of an eye having a relatively short axial length or reduced dioptric power of one or more of the refractive elements.

Hyperopia can be classified in a variety of ways, as follows:
- Anatomical features of hyperopia. Axial hyperopia infers that the eye is too short for its refractive power. Refractive hyperopia infers that the refractive system is too weak for the axial length of the eye. The refractive elements that can contribute to the insufficient power are: decreased refractive index of clear media (cornea, aqueous, lens or vitreous), decreased curvature of the cornea or lens, or a decrease in anterior chamber depth.
- Degree of hyperopia. Hyperopia can be classified as being low (< +3.00D), moderate (+3.00D to +5.00D) and high (> +5.00D).
- Physiological and pathological hyperopia. Physiological hyperopia can be defined as that in which each component of refraction lies within the normal distribution for that population. Thus, hyperopia arises from a failure of correlation between the refractive components of the eye. Pathological hyperopia described hyperopia that is accompanied by pathology such as a presence of space-occupying lesions in the eye (e.g. tumor, haemorrhage, oedema) or a pathologically flattened cornea (cornea plana). Aphakia and lens dislocation are also causes of hyperopia.
- Action of accommodation. Since hyperopia is due to the eye being 'underpowered', an increase in accommodation may serve to alleviate at least some of the hyperopia. However, constant accommodation to correct for hyperopia can lead to symptoms of asthenopia, and problems of convergence excess (esotropia or esophoria). Hyperopia can be further sub-classified with regard to the action of accommodation as follows: latent hyperopia – that which is masked by accommodation and can not be revealed by noncycloplegic refraction (a cycloplegic agent is required to reveal the full amount); manifest hyperopia – that which is indicated by the maximum plus lens that provides optimum visual acuity; total hyperopia – the sum of latent and manifest hyperopia. Total hyperopia can also be classified as facultative (that which is masked by accommodation and can be revealed by noncycloplegic refraction) and absolute (that which can not be compensated for by accommodation).

Hyperopia
- See *Hypermetropia*.

Hyperphoria and hypophoria
Hyper/hypophoria occurs where both visual axes are directed towards the fixation point but deviate on dissociation. The cover–uncover test reveals vertical movement when the eyes are dissociated. For hyperphoria the eye behind the cover moves up, for hypophoria the eye behind the cover moves down. When the cover is removed the eye moves in a compensatory movement in the opposite direction. Anatomical causes of vertical heterophorias include displaced globes, abnormal extraocular muscles or ptosis. Refractive causes are high myopia, also known as 'heavy eye syndrome'. Weak vertical fusional reserves also play a role.

Hyperthyroidism
- See *Systemic disease, contact lens wear in*.

Hypertropia and hypotropia
Small comitant vertical deviations may occur as isolated conditions or associated with moderate or large angle horizontal deviations. Onset is typically between birth and about three years. Angles are small, between 1 and 10°. The magnitude of the deviation and the fusional status determine whether the deviation is constant or intermittent. Treatment is the prescription of vertical prism for deviations of 10° or less. Vision training is a second choice as a treatment option to increase vertical fusional ranges, but can be difficult. Hypertropia and hypotropia greater than 10° often requires surgical management, principally for cosmetic reasons.

Hypophoria
- See *Hyperphoria and hypophoria*.

Hypotropia
- See *Hypertropia and hypotropia*.

Hypoxia
This term refers to a finite level of oxygen less than that normally found in the atmosphere, which is 155mmHg at sea level under conditions of standard temperature and pressure, and allowing for a water vapour pressure of 4mmHg. Adj: hypoxic.

IACLE
- *See International Association of Contact Lens Educators.*

Identification tint for contact lenses
Polymer buttons used for rigid lens manufacture are often colour-coded with light tints by some manufacturers who supply a wide range of products, so as to facilitate correct product identification at the lens fabrication stage. Such tints are barely visible in the finished lens, and do not affect vision or colour perception. See *Tinted contact lenses*.

Illuminance
When a ray of light reaches a surface it is referred to as illumination. The quantity of illumination or illuminance (E) is defined as the luminous flux (F) that is incident on a given surface area (A), i.e. the luminous flux per unit area. This is expressed in SI units of lumens per square metre, or lux, where:

$E = F/A$

For example, if an area of 0.1 square metre receives a luminous flux of 40 lumens, the illuminance, E, will equal 40/0.1 = 400 lux.

One of the basic laws to enable the calculation of illuminance is the 'inverse square law', which states that the illuminance (E) equals the intensity of the light source (I) divided by the square of the distance (d); that is:

$E = I/d^2$

In principle this applies only to a single point source of light in a completely dark room. However, for most practical applications a luminaire can be considered to be a point source if its largest dimension is less than one-fifth of the distance from itself to the point of illumination. Therefore, the inverse square law can be applied to a 1m fluorescent tube at a distance greater 5m. For example, light from a small point source with a luminous flux of 1lm, strikes a surface 1m away, illuminating an area of $1m^2$. Hence, the illuminance is 1 lux (because E=F/A). If the surface is moved to 2m from the light source, the luminous flux will remain the same but the illuminated area will increase in size to $4m^2$, i.e. the area has increased in proportion to the square of the distance of the light source. The illuminance will be reduced to 0.25 lux, i.e. the illuminance has changed inversely with the square of the distance.

Illumination recommendations, low vision
It is recognized in the standards which govern the design of interior lighting that higher levels of illuminance are required in areas where the users are elderly, or where more visually demanding tasks are carried out. It is

therefore almost invariably the case that visually impaired individuals require high levels of illuminance to achieve optimal performance since they are inevitably working closer to their threshold, and are often elderly.

Four aspects of optimizing illumination can be considered:

1. Increasing the general ambient level of illuminance. It will usually be impossible to change the entire lighting installation in the home, but a great deal can be achieved with relatively simple measures. For example:

- Draw curtains well back, clean windows regularly and only use net curtains if essential. Privacy can be retained by restricting the net curtains to the lower half of the window.
- Use fluorescent fittings where possible. If an incandescent bulb is to be used, a large pale-coloured lampshade with white reflective interior should be selected. This size will obstruct less light and allow safe use of a higher wattage bulb without overheating. If a pendant fitting is used, this should be open at the top to allow light to be reflected from the ceiling.
- Choose pale matt decorative finishes to give diffuse reflection and increase the illuminance falling on the surface under the luminaire. Judicious use of dark borders (dado rails, door surrounds, window frames, skirting boards) can aid orientation, without significantly reducing the total reflected light.
- Aim for near-uniform light levels throughout the area, making sure that corridors and stairs have no less than one-third to one-quarter of the illuminance of the rooms opening onto them. Adapting to changing light levels is likely to be slowed in a significant percentage of visually impaired patients.

2. Providing adequate enhanced illumination for detailed tasks in a discrete localized area (task lighting). To find out how the individual patient responds to different levels of task illuminance will require a test to be made in the consulting room. This should begin using dim room lighting (approximately 5 to 20 lux), then normal room illumination augmented by a task lamp positioned about 1m from the patient (approximately 100 to 300 lux), then the reading lamp should be brought to 20cm or less to produce high illumination (approximately 2000 to 5000 lux).

The effect of the use of localized task lighting must be demonstrated to the patient, along with the types of lamp which are available: the patient often already has a lamp with tungsten bulb, and this may be adequate if it can be positioned close to the task, but not so close to the patient that it becomes uncomfortably hot with prolonged use. A lamp with a compact fluorescent tube is preferred because it will not get hot, and it will have a higher efficacy and thus be more economical to use (an 11W fluorescent tube gives approximately the same task illuminance as a 60W tungsten bulb from the same distance). For the patient requiring the highest levels of illuminance (≈ 10000 lux), a lamp with halogen bulb will be required. The following measures should be considered in order to produce optimum localized task lighting:

- Localized lighting is not just used when reading, but might be necessary over the telephone, under wall-mounted kitchen cupboards to illuminate work-surfaces, over the dining table, or over a tool shed work-bench. It may be needed during the day to supplement natural daylight.
- The traditional position for a reading lamp is behind the patient so that light comes over the shoulder onto the task. This can be very effective for 'normal' reading distances, but is difficult to combine with the use of a magnifier and/or a very short working distance, when it is almost inevitable that the patient's body will shadow the task, and the light will create annoying reflections from the magnifier surface. A better arrangement in this instance is to place the light in front of the face, with the shade arranged so that there is no light shining directly into the eyes. This inevitably places the lamp housing very close to the face, which can be uncomfortably warm unless a fluorescent lamp is used. If the lamp is to be adjusted to different angles, it must have a flexible or jointed arm with sufficient reach and have a heavy base or table clamp so that it will be stable, even when the arm is fully extended.

3. Incorporating illumination in magnifiers.

Hand held and stand-mounted plus lens magnifiers are commonly available with built in illumination, and if well designed then this ensures that the illumination falls exactly on the task area from a close distance. As the light is under the magnifier there is no possibility of annoying reflections from the surfaces. It means that the magnifier can still be used optimally outside the home where illumination is unpredictable. There are however a number of practical difficulties: if battery powered there is additional bulk and weight; the patient must be able to change bulbs and batteries; batteries can prove costly if not rechargeable; and if mains-powered the device cannot be used outdoors, and trailing wires may pose a safety hazard. Fluorescent lamps may be available in a variable focus stand magnifier, but tungsten, halogen, or light-emitting diode (LED) light sources are more common. Halogen bulbs are the brightest (but can prove uncomfortable for some users), although these usually have to be mains-powered. LED sources have the advantage of very long device and battery life.

4. Supplying additional light outdoors, for mobility.

Difficulty with vision at night is a common complaint of visually impaired patients with severe visual field restriction. As the peripheral retina contains a preponderance of rod receptors, they will be preferentially lost as the visual field reduces. There are a number of mobility lights which are commercially available, either in the form of a headlamp, or attached to a waist-belt. Requirements are for a beam with wide, even illumination; a simple torch is often adequate for this purpose if the patient is able to carry it in the hand.

Impression fitting, scleral lens

- See *Fitting scleral contact lenses*.

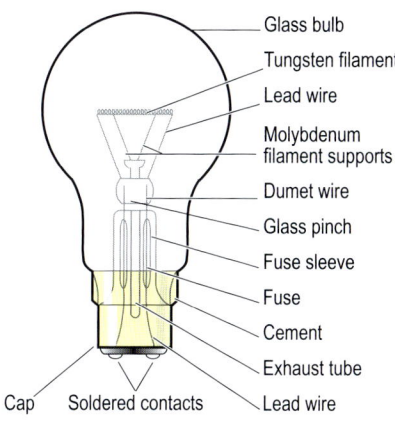

Figure I.1 • A tungsten filament lamp (adapted from Thorn Lighting Technical Handbook, courtesy of Thorn Lighting Ltd.).

Incandescent lamps

Tungsten lamps operate by heating a tungsten filament to incandescence in a glass envelope filled with an inert gas, usually argon or krypton (Figure I.1). The passage of electricity through the filament raises the temperature of the tungsten molecules to the point where they emit light or incandesce. The resulting spectral emission is a function of the temperature of the filament. The main characteristic of the incandescent lamp is that the spectral emission forms a continuum. As the temperature of the filament increases, the peak of its emission moves from the red to the blue end of the spectrum. Although the melting point of tungsten is 3600 K, the rate of evaporation increases markedly above 2800 K. This can be reduced by raising the vapour pressure in the lamp with an inert gas such as argon.

The advantages of tungsten lamps are as follows:

- immediate full light output
- operate in all positions
- easy to control lamp output by varying applied voltage.

The disadvantages of tungsten lamps are as follows:

- short life (1000 to 2000h); frequent replacement necessary
- high running cost due to poor luminous efficiency (11 to 19lm/W)
- emphasize red strongly and yellows and greens to a lesser extent; blue is strongly subdued
- should not be used for colour matching
- light output and life sensitive to small voltage variation
- sensitive to vibrations
- at too high a temperature the tungsten evaporates from the filament, leaving black deposits on the inside of the bulb, which reduce the light output.

Tungsten halide lamps are filament lamps. The filament is contained in a tube of fused silica or quartz, which is filled with a halogen compound gas. Whereas conventional tungsten filament lamps must not be run at too high a temperature, a tungsten halide lamp can be run at much higher temperatures because, although the tungsten is evaporated off the filament, it combines with the halogen, e.g. iodine vapour, to form a reusable compound – a halide. This compound is carried on the convection currents within the bulb; when it passes the filament, it dissociates into tungsten, which is deposited on the filament while the halogen is released to repeat the cycle (Figure I.2). This increases lamp efficacy and life.

The advantages of tungsten halide lamps are as follows:

- higher luminous efficacy than tungsten (17–25lm/W)
- longer life of lamp (2000–4000h)
- no decline in light output with time (there is no blackening of the inner surface of the glass)
- higher colour temperature
- lamps can be made small and compact, and therefore ideal for optometric instruments.

The disadvantage of a tungsten halide lamp is that the surface of the bulb is liable to deteriorate if touched with the fingers; fats from the skin migrate into the quartz envelope, causing it to blister.

Extra low voltage lamps are used for projectors and car headlamps. Low voltage dichroic reflector lamps, which are frequently used for display lighting, are designed to reflect light forward and transmit the heat (infrared radiation) through the back of the lamp.

Incomitant deviations

These are strabismic deviations that vary in size according to the direction of gaze and depending on the eye that is fixing. Recognition and interpretation of incomitant strabismus often pose a problem to optometrists, who rarely encounter such deviations.

Familiarity with the primary and secondary actions of the extraocular muscles is fundamental to the inter-

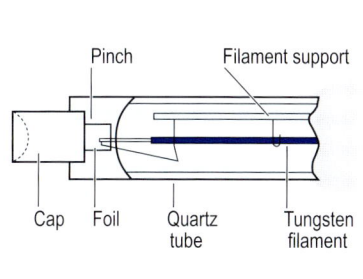

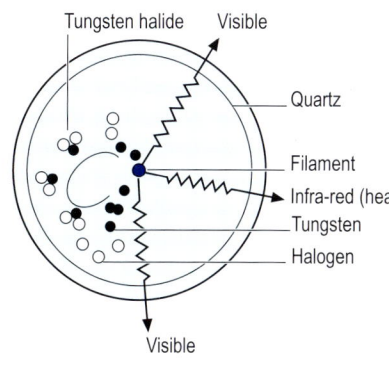

Figure I.2 • Simplified mechanism of the tungsten halogen lamp (adapted from Thorn Lighting Technical Handbook, courtesy of Thorn Lighting Ltd.).

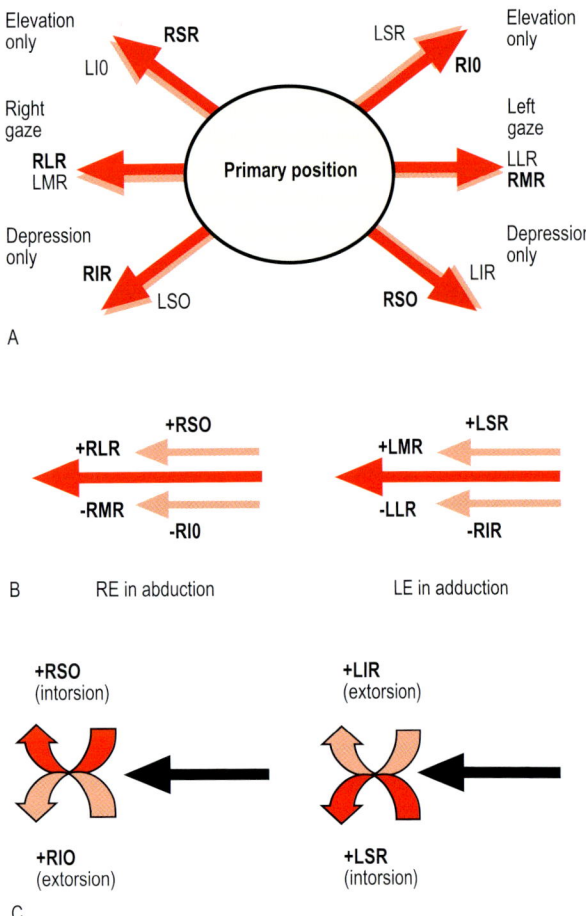

Figure I.3 (A)–(C) • Extraocular muscle actions.

A neurogenic paralysis reduces ocular rotation in the field of action of the affected muscle under binocular viewing conditions. Unless the nerve is severed, full ocular rotation is achieved monocularly when excess innervation is provided. Thus, the incomplete movement seen binocularly becomes complete on monocular testing with a cover and is referred to as an under-action. In some longstanding neurogenic pareses the weak muscle becomes fibrotic with time, resulting in incomplete rotation even on monocular testing.

In mechanical deviations such as those due to muscle fibrosis or entrapment, the muscle defect prevents rotation of the globe. Thus, the reduced rotation seen under binocular viewing conditions is still evident on monocular testing. This type of motility defect is referred to as a restriction or limitation. In addition, since the muscle can neither contract nor relax, both its agonist and antagonist functions are prohibited which may result in restriction of movement in more than one direction of gaze. For example, a restricted right medial rectus muscle may result in limitation of movement in both right and left gaze on the affected side. Finally, since the defect is not neurogenic in origin, the full sequelae do not develop. Only over-action of the contralateral synergist occurs. If the defect is present in opposite directions as described, the corresponding over-actions to both restrictions are seen in the fellow eye. A simple alternate cover test in the direction of gaze of the defect will differentiate these abnormalities.

Formation of muscle sequelae follows the onset of muscle weakness (palsy) to some extent depends on the nature of the initial defect. This pattern of events also results in the primary and secondary deviations that can be used to identify the involved eye. The pattern of events are:

- Under-action of the primarily affected muscle.
- Over-action of the contralateral synergist. Always present, this over-action occurs when the affected eye is fixing. It results from the increased innervation required to rotate the affected muscle into its field of action. As a result of Hering's law, an over stimulation of the contralateral synergist follows. This is always the largest over-action in the sequelae. Under-action of the primarily affected muscle and over-action of the contralateral synergist together result in the primary deviation.
- Over-action of the direct antagonist. If the patient fixes with the non-involved eye, within days to weeks a contracture will develop in the direct antagonist muscle. This occurs because the normal contracture of the direct antagonist is unopposed by the weak muscle.
- Inhibitional palsy of the contralateral antagonist. With the involved eye fixing, the movement of the involved eye into the field of action of the antagonist of the weak muscle requires less innervation than would ordinarily be necessary due to the contracture. Thus, by Hering's law, less innervation is supplied to the contralateral antagonist which under-acts. This process is sometimes called 'spread of comitance' and results in gradual uniformity of the deviation across the binocular visual field with time.

pretation of abnormality. Figure I.3A shows the primary actions of the extraocular muscles. The primary action of each muscle is achieved when the line of action of the muscle is located over the centre of rotation of the eye. For example the primary action of the superior rectus muscle is elevation, which occurs in abduction. That is not to suggest that the superior rectus muscle is a primary abductor, but that when the eye is relatively abducted (such as following lateral rectus contraction) the superior rectus is most effective as an elevator. In this position there are no secondary muscle actions.

When the eye is rotated 90° away from the position of primary action of the muscle, the primary action is reduced and the secondary actions of that muscle become more effective. In the case of the superior rectus muscle, for example, the elevation is diminished and adduction and intorsion increase, reaching a peak when the eye is relatively adducted (such as following medial rectus contraction). At this time there is no residual elevation. An easy way to remember the secondary actions is *RAdSIn* (recti adduct; superiors intort) from which all secondary actions can be determined. These rotations are summarized for binocular right gaze in Figures I.3B and I.3C. Note that horizontal secondary actions are additive, while cyclo-rotations cancel out.

Reductions in ocular rotation may be caused by neurogenic paralysis or muscular (mechanical) defects. These behave differently and can be easily differentiated by examination of a Hess chart plot or on motility testing.

In incomitant strabismus the angle of deviation varies according to the eye used for fixation. The primary deviation arises with the non-involved eye fixing. The secondary deviation occurs with the involved eye fixing and is larger than the primary deviation. This is because the innervation to the weak muscle that is required for that eye to fixate in the primary position is greater than when the healthy eye is used. The over-action of the contralateral synergist is correspondingly larger. As the sequelae develop, spread of comitance results in a reduction in the differential angle between the primary and secondary deviations, and greater uniformity of the angle of deviation throughout the binocular field of view.

Incomitant defects may be congenital or acquired. Aetiology can often be ascertained from a careful history. In the case of neurogenic palsies this should be supplemented with a working knowledge of the cranial nerve pathways to determine the site of a lesion. This has important implications for the referral process.

Congenital palsies may be familial, although the specific cause is often unknown. Neurogenic palsies are often associated with hydrocephalus and cerebral palsy. Palsies of this nature may be multiple, bilateral, and asymmetric. Most mechanical defects are congenital and Duane's syndrome in particular is often familial.

The main aetiological factors in neurogenic paralysis are trauma, inflammation, vascular abnormalities, metabolic disease or raised intracranial pressure such as following space occupying brain lesions. Acquired mechanical defects may also be traumatic, or following other diseases with muscular effects such as thyrotoxicosis, myasthenia gravis or spondylitis.

In acquired cases, removal of the cause of the defect is often followed by spontaneous partial or complete recovery. Surgical management is usually delayed until consecutive Hess plots are stable for at least six months.

A basic awareness of neuro-anatomy will help to identify the probable site, or even the cause, of a neurological defect. The minimum essential knowledge relates to the three cranial nerves supplying ocular motor function. These are the third (oculomotor), fourth (trochlear) and sixth (abducens) cranial nerves. The three nerve nuclei are vertically aligned within the brainstem from where the nerves diverge. The third and sixth nerves diverge laterally and forward from either side of the brainstem. The fourth nerve decussates on the dorsal side of the brainstem at the level of the foramen magnum, before passing temporally and forwards via the middle cranial fossa. The sixth nerve passes over the petrous temporal bone making a 90° bend as it does so. The three nerves converge again, together with the trigeminal nerve, passing through the cavernous sinus lateral to the pituitary gland before entering the orbit via the optic canal. Within the orbit the nerves diverge, and the superior and inferior divisions of the third nerve separate. In this respect, the most vulnerable sites for damage are:

- The foramen magnum, resulting in unilateral or bilateral trochlear nerve damage such as following whiplash injury.
- The petrous temporal bone, resulting in compressive lesions from above following raised intracranial pressure, or from below such as following otitis media infection, each resulting commonly in abducens palsy.
- The cavernous sinus, resulting in multiple palsies, although these are much less common.
- Orbital lesions, resulting in single or multiple muscle palsies.

Indications and contraindications for contact lens wear

As part of an initial assessment as to the suitability of a patient for contact lens wear, any specific indications or contraindications for lens wear must be established. These are best considered in the following categories:

1. Ocular anatomy. In elective fitting (i.e. non-therapeutic use) there are few anatomical features that influence the suitability for contact lenses. However, extremely steep or flat corneas or extremes of corneal astigmatism may present particular fitting difficulties that could increase the time spent on fitting. With bifocal contact lens fitting, lower lid tension and position may be critical to the visual outcome and pupil size may also influence fitting success. In such cases, the implications for likely success and the increased fitting time and expense should be explained carefully to the patient.

2. Ocular health. Since a contact lens will come into intimate contact with the ocular surfaces, it is essential that there are no presenting ocular conditions that might be aggravated by lens wear. Disorders such as recurrent infection, irregular corneal surface, recurrent erosions, dry eye or meibomian gland dysfunction may be partial contraindications for elective contact lens wear, depending on severity.

3. General health. There are numerous health problems that may influence the suitability for contact lenses, including those that have a direct effect on the ocular tissues and those that may cause secondary problems. In addition, several systemic medications may influence the tear film and thus the ability to wear lenses comfortably.

4. Allergies. Those who are susceptible to allergies may experience problems from two sources. Wearers with atopy may be more intolerant to contact lens wear by a factor of five times compared to non-atopic wearers. Wearing time should be limited during the allergy season. Those with other more specific allergies may be at risk from reactions to the chemicals within preservative-based lens care systems. These chemicals can interact with deposits on the lens surface, creating an allergic-type response. In such cases, preservative-free systems or daily disposable lenses are indicated.

5. Chronic infection. Those with chronic sinusitis or catarrh may be more at risk of developing infection secondary to corneal abrasion. The associated mucus in the tears may cause visual problems from lens surface wetting anomalies, as well as blocking the nasolacrimal ducts and causing epiphora.

6. Metabolic disorders. Disorders of metabolism may have varying effects on the eye and its physiology. Hyperthyroidism, with its associated exophthalmos, may create problems in tear film distribution, while diabetes may influence the stability of refractive error, corneal deturgescence and epithelial wound healing.

7. Pregnancy, lactation and hormonal changes. Owing to hormonal changes during pregnancy and lactation, female patients may be prone to corneal oedema and mucus build-up. Comfort and overall tolerance can be reduced, although the response of a previously-adapted lens wearer during pregnancy may often be good. It is less desirable to commence fitting lenses during pregnancy and lactation. Disruption to the tear film can occur during puberty and the menopause, and while taking oral contraceptives or hormone replacement therapy, giving rise to chronic or transient problems of intolerance and dryness.

8. Systemic medication. As well as the systemic conditions that can affect tolerance to lenses, medication used in the treatment or control of those conditions can also have undesirable side effects. These generally affect the tear film, either causing symptoms of dryness or in some cases leading to soft lens discoloration.

9. Psychological factors, including motivation. In addition to anatomical and health-related issues, it is important to judge the motivation to wear contact lenses and the personality type of the potential wearer. Contact lenses are considered to give a more normal cosmetic appearance and may significantly enhance overall appearance, particularly when the refractive error is high. In addition, there are cases where lenses can be used specifically to conceal significant cosmetic defects such as iris anomalies, corneal opacities, inoperable squint or microphthalmos. A particularly exacting personality type may find the adaptation period and the initial learning of handling techniques too intrusive to outweigh the overall benefits of lens wear.

10. Lifestyle/occupational issues. In addition to motivational and psychological factors, consideration should be given to lifestyle and occupational issues. Often contact lenses are believed to be inappropriate for certain occupations, and while this may be true for particularly contaminated atmospheres, contact lenses may provide some protection from both foreign bodies and chemicals. In certain vocations, contact lenses may offer no obvious disadvantages and therefore employees should not necessarily be precluded from wearing lenses (e.g. in the fire service). Whatever the situation, hygiene is important, and attention to this factor must be of the highest order. Additionally, lens handling requires some degree of dexterity, and particularly rough or calloused hands may render lens handling and cleaning process difficult, leading to frustration and inadvertent lens damage.

11. Financial considerations. It is important that the patient understands the financial implications of the fitting and, perhaps more importantly, the ongoing costs relating to continuing clinical care, lens care solutions and lens replacements. Fitting lenses to a patient without the financial means to care for them will inevitably lead to non-compliance and an increased potential for adverse events to occur.

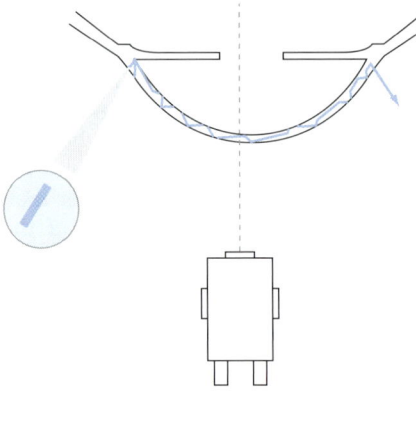

Figure I.4 • Sclerotic scatter slit-lamp technique. Adapted from L.W. Jones, D.A. Jones (2001) Slit lamp biomicroscopy. In: N. Efron (ed.) The Cornea: its Examination in Contact Lens Practice, pp.1–49. Butterworth-Heinemann, Oxford.

Indirect illumination, slit-lamp technique of

This refers to any technique with the slit-lamp biomicroscope where the focus of the illuminating beam does not coincide with the focal point of the observation system. Indirect illumination can be achieved by 'uncoupling' the instrument and manually displacing the slit beam to the side. However, it is possible to effect indirect illumination without uncoupling the instrument; this is simply achieved by directing a slit beam on to a section of the cornea adjacent to that of interest.

The following two specific types of indirect illumination are possible:

1. Sclerotic scatter. This technique is used to investigate any subtle changes in corneal clarity occurring over a large area, such as central corneal oedema. The slit lamp is set up for a wide-angle parallelepiped (45–60°) and the viewing system is focused centrally. The beam is manually offset ('uncoupled') and focused on the limbus (Figure I.4). The slit beam is totally internally reflected across the cornea, and a bright limbal glow is seen around the entire cornea. Any specific area of abnormality, such as a corneal scar, will interrupt the beam in its passage and produce a light reflection in the otherwise dark cornea.

2. Retro-illumination. This refers to any technique in which light is reflected from the iris, anterior crystalline lens surface or retina, and is used to back-illuminate an area more anteriorly positioned. The area may be seen against a light background (direct retro-illumination, Figure I.5) or a dark background (indirect retro-illumination, Figure I.6), depending whether or not the illumination and viewing systems are coincident. Direct retro-illumination is used most often, and here corneal opacities will appear black against a bright field. Retro-illumination is particularly useful for examining epithelial microcysts, neovascularization, scars, degenerations and dystrophies.

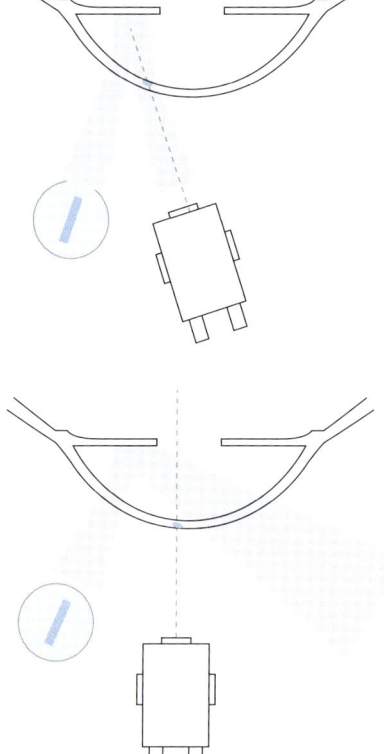

Figure I.5 • Direct retro-illumination slit-lamp technique. Adapted from L.W. Jones, D.A. Jones (2001) Slit lamp biomicroscopy. In: N. Efron (ed.) The Cornea: its Examination in Contact Lens Practice, pp.1–49. Butterworth-Heinemann, Oxford.

Figure I.6 • Indirect retro-illumination slit-lamp technique. Adapted from L.W. Jones, D.A. Jones (2001) Slit lamp biomicroscopy. In: N. Efron (ed.) The Cornea: its Examination in Contact Lens Practice, pp.1–49. Butterworth-Heinemann, Oxford.

Induced astigmatism with rigid toric contact lenses

This is the astigmatic effect created in the contact lens/tear lens system by the toroidal back optic zone bounding two surfaces of different refractive index - namely the lens (refractive index 1.432 to 1.490 depending on the material) and the tears (refractive index 1.336). See *Compensated rigid bitoric lenses; Cylindrical power equivalent rigid toric lenses; Residual astigmatism with rigid toric lenses; Stabilization of rigid toric lenses; Toric lens design, rigid; Toric lens, rigid.*

Infants and contact lenses

- See *Paediatric contact lenses; Paediatric contact lens examination; Paediatric contact lens fitting.*

Informed consent, contact lens

Informed consent means that a patient embarking on contact lens wear should be made aware of both the risks and benefits of contact lens wear, as well as having the opportunity to ask questions. The information provided verbally should be reinforced with written material. As well as providing the patient with information about the recommended lenses and/or solution system of choice, the practitioner must also have discussed the possible alternatives.

A comprehensive list of every possible contact lens complication does not need to be discussed, but a practitioner is required to discuss those that any reasonable member of the profession would expect to be told. A practitioner would be expected to mention the more common non-serious aspects of lens wear, such as the normal adaptation symptoms, in addition to the less common risks that could lead to a serious complication such as visual loss from corneal infection.

Prospective wearers should also be made aware of the consequences of not following the recommended instructions. This may be perceived by some practitioners as a negative approach, as it does not present contact lenses in a positive light. However, discussing such possible scenarios will preclude patients from claiming lack of informed consent should they be non-compliant with advice.

A standard form can be used, which patients sign to acknowledge that they have been given the necessary advice and instructions. They should be given a copy of this, with the other copy retained in their records. In the case of minors, the form should be signed by both the child (where possible) and the parent or guardian.

Insertion and removal, rigid contact lens

Before inserting a rigid lens in a new wearer, it is helpful to prepare the patient for some initial discomfort, to advise that this will recede, and to suggest that any discomfort will be minimized by raising the chin and looking downwards (this posture causes the upper lid to stabilize the lens). Anxiety may also be reduced by explaining that any irritation will be to the eyelid rather than the eye itself, which will be unaffected. Applying wetting solution to the lens prior to insertion will tend to make the lens more comfortable and transfer more readily to the eye, but care should be taken to avoid applying more than a small drop as too much can make fluorescein assessment more difficult. For reasons of hygiene, the hands of the practitioner (and the patient, if handling lenses) should be washed and dried immediately prior to lens handling.

The standard technique that a practitioner will use to insert a rigid lens into the eye of a patient is as follows:

1. If you intend inserting the lens with your right hand, stand on the right-hand side of the patient. Lenses can be inserted into both eyes of the patient from the same side using the same hand. The opposite arrangement applies if you intend inserting the lens with your left hand. The following description assumes insertion with the right hand.
2. Ask the patient to fixate a distant object, straight ahead, so as to steady the eyes.
3. Place the lens on the forefinger of your right hand.
4. Hold the top lid using the forefinger or thumb of the left hand. If this proves difficult, have the patient first look down until the lid is securely held.
5. Hold the bottom lid using the middle finger of the right hand, and place the lens directly on to the cornea. Instruct the patient to blink (Figure I.7).
6. Release the bottom lid but continue to hold the top lid, and ask the patient to look down.
7. At this point, the lens is often quite comfortable. Warn the patient that once you let go of the lid, he or she will be more aware of the lens.

If the lens locates onto the sclera, the lens will probably not be uncomfortable. Have the patient look in the opposite direction to where the lens is located, e.g.

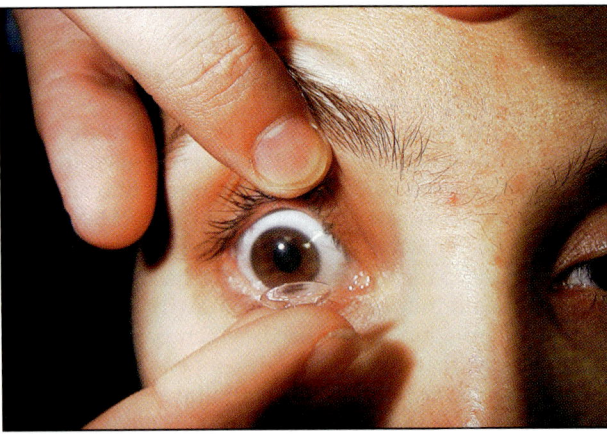

Figure I.7 • Lids retracted and rigid lens in position ready for insertion.

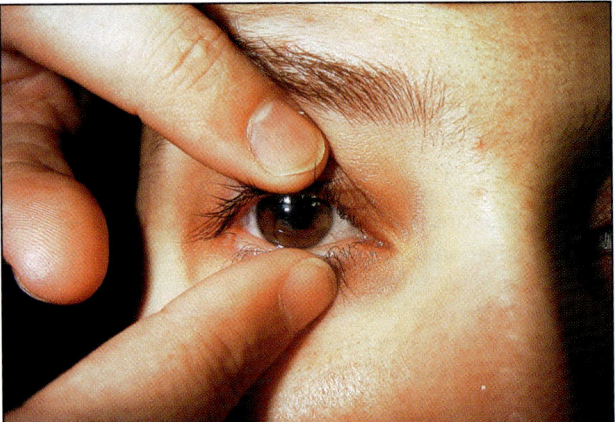

Figure I.8 • Preparing to remove a rigid lens by 'flicking' it from the eye.

4. With the forefinger of the left hand (approaching from above the head) hold open the top lid, while with the middle finger of the right hand hold open the bottom lid.
5. Place the lens directly on to the cornea and slowly remove your finger.
6. Release your lids, raise your chin and look down. This will initially stabilize the lens and decrease any discomfort.
7. Let go of the lid and start blinking normally. You will now be more aware of the lens. If the lens locates onto the sclera, the lens will probably not be uncomfortable. Look in the opposite direction to where the lens is located, e.g. upwards if located on the lower sclera. With two fingers, manipulate the lids to push the lens so that it is manoeuvred back onto the cornea. If this proves difficult, remove the lens by lid squeezing.

A patient can remove a rigid lens from his/her eye as follows:

1. To remove a lens from the right eye, place the forefinger of the right hand towards the outer canthus of the upper lid and place the middle of the right hand towards the outer canthus of the lower lid.
2. Open the eyes wide so that the upper and lower lid margins are above and below the top and bottom lens edge, respectively.
3. Cup the left hand beneath the right eye, resting the edge of the cupped hand against the cheek.
4. Tilt the head slightly downwards, pull the lids taut (away from the nose) and execute a firm blink.
5. The lens will be flipped out of the eye into the cupped hand (or it may end up resting on the lower lid). If the lens remains in the eye, try again.
6. Use the opposite hands to remove a lens from the left eye.

Insertion and removal, scleral contact lens

To insert a scleral lens into the eye of a patient, the following procedure is followed:

1. If you intend inserting the lens with your right hand, stand on the right-hand side of the patient. Lenses can be inserted into both eyes of the patient from the same side using the same hand. The opposite arrangement applies if you intend inserting the lens with your left hand. The following description assumes insertion with the right hand.
2. Hold the lens between the thumb and either the index or the middle finger of the right hand.
3. Retract the upper lid and lift it away from the globe, using the thumb and forefinger of the left hand to pull on the lashes.
4. Place the upper edge of the lens under the upper lid and hold it firmly in place with the left hand.
5. Evert the lower lid over the lower lens edge, using the right hand.

Sealed gas-permeable scleral lenses must be inserted filled with saline, so it is necessary to have the patient bend forward and look down to the floor so that the lens

upwards if located on the lower sclera. With two fingers, manipulate the lids to push the lens so that it is manoeuvred back onto the cornea. If this proves difficult, remove the lens by lid manipulation or by using a suction holder (miniature suctions holders are available for in-office lens removal by practitioners only; such devices should not be given to patients).

A practitioner can remove a rigid lens from the eye of a patient as follows:

1. Place the forefinger of one hand on the middle of the bottom lid and the forefinger of the other hand on the middle of the top lid.
2. Gently pull the lids apart, away from the nose and then together so that the tightened lids flick the lens from the cornea (Figure I.8).

The standard technique that a patient can be advised in order to insert a rigid lens into his or her eye is as follows:

1. Use the same hand for inserting lenses into either eye. The following description assumes insertion and removal with the right hand.
2. Fixate a distant object, straight ahead, so as to steady the eyes.
3. Place the lens on the forefinger of the right hand.

is horizontal. This can be difficult to do without letting in bubbles. Manually closing the upper lid over the lens before everting the lower lid often helps.

A scleral lens can be removed from the eye of a patient as follows:

1. Retract the upper lid with the thumb of the left hand and press the lid margin behind the upper edge of the lens.
2. A small movement of the lid over the globe towards the temporal side is usually enough to ease the suction between the lens and eye.
3. Instruct the patient to make a small upwards eye movement to release the lens from the surface of the eye.

A sealed gas-permeable scleral lens may be more difficult to release, in which case a small solid suction holder applied to the front of the lens, as the lid is pressed behind the lens, will help ease the lens off the eye.

The standard technique that a patient can be advised in order to insert a scleral lens into his or her eye is as follows:

1. Use the same hand for inserting lenses into either eye. The following description assumes insertion and removal with the right hand.
2. Hold the lens between the thumb and either the index or the middle finger of the right hand.
3. Retract the upper lid and lift it away from the globe using the thumb and forefinger of the left hand to pull on the lashes.
4. Place the upper edge of the lens under the upper lid and hold it firmly in place with the left hand.
5. Evert the lower lid over the lower lens edge with the right hand.

When instructing patients how to handle lenses, it is often necessary repeatedly to remind them not to let go until the lower lid is fully over the lower edge of the lens. Sealed gas-permeable scleral lenses must be inserted filled with saline, so it is necessary for the patient to bend forward and look downwards so that the lens is horizontal. This can be difficult to do without letting in bubbles. Manually closing the upper lid over the lens before everting the lower lid often helps.

The standard technique that a patient can be advised in order to remove a scleral lens from his or her eye is as follows:

1. Retract the upper lid with the forefinger of the left hand and press the lid margin behind the upper edge of the lens.
2. Move the lid a small amount over the globe towards the temporal side; this is usually enough to ease the suction between the lens and eye.
3. Look upwards slightly; this will release the lens from the surface of the eye.

Insertion and removal, soft contact lens

For reasons of hygiene, the hands of the practitioner (and the patient, if handling lenses) should be washed and dried immediately prior to lens handling.

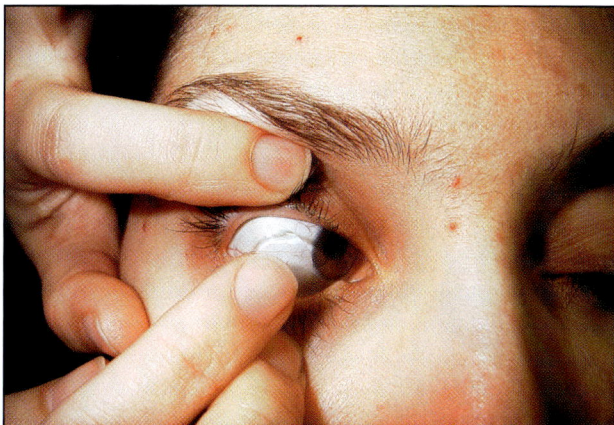

Figure I.9 • Insertion of a soft lens.

The standard technique that a practitioner will use to insert a soft lens into the eye of a patient is as follows:

1. If you intend inserting the lens with your right hand, stand on the right-hand side of the patient. Lenses can be inserted into both eyes of the patient from the same side using the same hand. The opposite arrangement applies if you intend inserting the lens with your left hand. The following description assumes insertion with the right hand.
2. Prior to inserting a soft lens, place it between the forefinger and middle finger of the right hand and rinse with saline to remove any debris.
3. Allow the excess saline to drain before placing the lens on the dry forefinger of the right hand.
4. Use the forefinger or thumb of the left hand to hold the top lid open while, with the middle finger of the right hand, holding the bottom lid open.
5. With the patient looking superiorly and nasally, apply the lens to the exposed bulbar conjunctiva. Then press the lens firmly to expel any air bubbles from under it.
6. Slide the lens onto the cornea (Figure I.9). Once the soft lens is centred on the cornea, and without air bubbles beneath it, your finger can be removed. Instruct the patient to look straight ahead. Hold the lids open for a few seconds to allow the lens to settle, and then ask the patient to look down. With thin soft lenses, the lens can be easily folded or dislodged if it has not settled properly.

If the patient finds the lens uncomfortable, debris may have inadvertently become trapped beneath the lens. In such a case, temporarily dislodge the lens onto the sclera and then re-centre the lens.

A practitioner can remove a soft lens from the eye of a patient as follows:

1. Ask the patient to look up or away.
2. Hold open the top lid with the forefinger or thumb of one hand.
3. Hold down the bottom lid with the middle finger of the same hand.
4. Pinch and remove the lens with the thumb and forefinger of the other hand (Figure I.10).

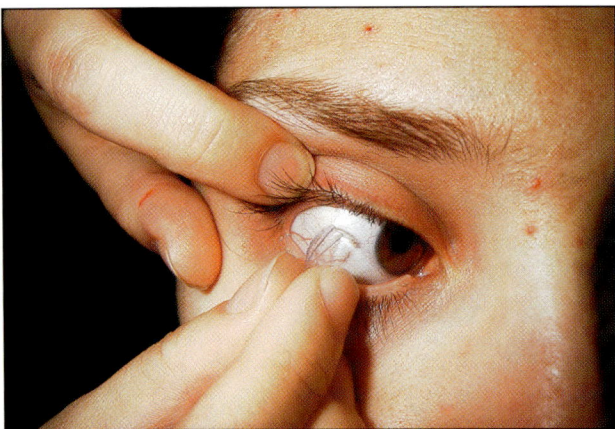

Figure I.10 • Removal of a soft lens.

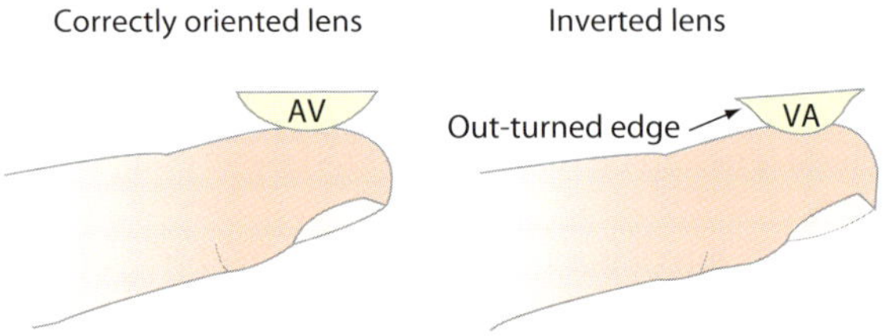

Figure I.11 • A lens can be checked for inversion by examining the lens rim at eye level.

The standard technique that a patient can be advised in order to insert a soft lens into his or her eye is as follows:

1. Use the same hand for inserting and removing lenses into either eye. The following description assumes insertion and removal with the right hand.
2. Prior to inserting a soft lens, place it between the forefinger and middle finger of the right hand and rinse with saline to remove any debris.
3. Allow the excess saline to drain before placing the lens on the dry forefinger of the right hand.
4. With the forefinger of the left hand (approaching from above the head), hold open the top lid while, with the middle finger of the right hand, hold open the bottom lid.
5. Look slightly upwards and apply the lens to the inferior bulbar conjunctiva. Then press the lens firmly to expel any air bubbles from under it.
6. Slide the lens up onto the cornea. Once the soft lens is centred on the cornea, and without air bubbles beneath it, your finger can be removed. Look straight ahead. Hold the lids open for a few seconds to allow the lens to settle and then look down. With thin soft lenses, the lens can be easily folded or dislodged if the lens has not properly settled.
7. The lens will sometimes be uncomfortable immediately after insertion because debris may have inadvertently become trapped beneath it. In such a case, temporarily dislodge the lens onto the sclera and then re-centre the lens.

A patient can remove a soft lens from his or her eye as follows:

1. Look up.
2. Hold open the top lid with the forefinger of the left hand (approaching from above the head).
3. Hold down the bottom lid with the middle finger of the right hand.
4. Place your finger on the bottom of the lens and slide it downwards. Pinch and remove the lens with the thumb and forefinger of the right hand.

Inside-out check, soft contact lens

Before inserting a soft lens into the eye, it is necessary to perform an 'inside-out' check. The lens is balanced on the forefinger and the lens profile is examined. If the lens is inside out, its edge will be slightly turned out. The profile will resemble that of a 'dish' rather than a 'bowl' (Figure I.11). A lens that is placed on the eye 'inside-out' may display excessive movement and be slightly uncomfortable.

Instructing patients
- See *Patient education with contact lenses*.

Integrated approach, low vision
- See *Multidisciplinary team, low vision*.

Interdisciplinary team, low vision
- See *Multidisciplinary team, low vision*.

Interferometric measurement of contact lens back optic zone radius (BOZR)

There are two types of interferometry, optical and geometric. Optical interferometry is one of the most precise methods for estimating the shape of a reflecting surface relative to a test surface of known parameters. Using Newton's rings, or a similar optical arrangement, the resolution of the technique is of the order $\lambda/2$. A Newton's rings arrangement is cumbersome, time consuming and difficult to use with unstable devices such as soft lenses. This has limited its popularity. The technique is eminently suitable for checking non-spherical surfaces, and for any minute imperfections on either the front or back surface of a contact lens.

'Moiré fringes' are geometric interference patterns produced when two gratings overlap. An example of this enigmatic pattern is shown in Figure I.12, where two gratings consisting of parallel dark and clear lines are inclined by an angle θ relative to each other. The angular direction of the resultant pattern (φ) depends on the ratio of the frequency of one grating relative to the other and the angular separation of the two gratings (θ). The ratio of frequencies is the same as the ratio of the apparent sizes of the gratings. If the apparent size of one grating is known for a particular Moiré pattern, as well as the values of θ and φ, then the apparent size of the other grating can be calculated as follows:

$$B/A = \{\sin \theta / \tan \varphi\} + \cos \theta$$

where A is the apparent size of the lines in grating 1, and B is the apparent size of the lines in grating 2 at the viewing plane. In Figure I.12, A = B. However, keeping θ constant and separating the gratings along the viewing axis (i.e. out of the plane of the paper), the direction of

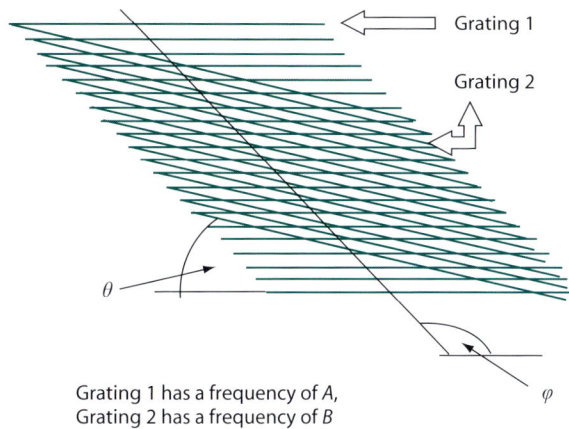

Figure I.12 • Moiré pattern resulting from an overlap of two gratings.

the Moiré pattern φ would change because A would no longer equal B at the plane of observation. A curved reflecting surface has magnifying properties, depending on its radius. If the image of a grating of known frequency is formed by reflection from the back surface of a soft lens, and this image is analyzed in a Moiré pattern arrangement, it is possible to create an optical system whereby the radius of the unknown surface is a relatively simple function of φ. Soft lens measuring devices are commercially available which contain a built-in programme that analyses the resulting Moiré pattern and allows an assessment of the form and regularity of aspheric lens surfaces and lens power distribution over a central 5-mm aperture. Moiré pattern systems are valuable for checking non-spherical surfaces in multifocal lenses.

International Association of Contact Lens Educators (IACLE)

This is a global educational organization dedicated to raising the standard of contact lens education worldwide and promoting the widespread, safe use of contact lenses. This is accomplished by: helping to improve the quality of contact lens teaching; providing educational infrastructure; increasing the number of skilled contact lens practitioners throughout the world; and increasing the number of qualified contact lens educators.

The association presently has 462 members in 60 countries; their members include optometrists, ophthalmologists, opticians and 'contactologists'. Membership is open to persons who are significantly involved either full-time or part-time in contact lens education and are members of staff of a recognized teaching institution. Membership applications are approved by the Executive Board.

IACLE operates an accreditation system, publishes a contact lens curriculum, distributes educational resources, sponsors a teacher exchange programme, and hosts numerous courses and workshops around the world. Website: www.iacle.org

International Society for Contact Lens Research (ISCLR)

The ISCLR is a group committed to international communication in the field of contact lens research and related sciences. Established in 1978 by an international group of leading researchers, ISCLR has become a crucial way in which researchers and industry in the field of contact lenses may be brought rapidly up to date with important developments and directions.

The ISCLR is a 'closed' society in that its membership is limited to only about 100 active workers in the contact lens field. There are strict requirements for admission to, and for retaining, membership; members must demonstrate that they are actively engaged in ongoing research in the contact lens field, and are required to attend all biennial meetings. The society is heavily supported by the contact lens industry, whose representatives participate in its meetings. Website: www.isclr.org

Internet supply

- See *Contact lens supply routes.*

Interpupillary distance

This is the distance between the pupils of the two eyes. The interpupillary distance is often simply referred to as the 'PD'. The typical PD when the eyes are directed to a distance fixation target is 64mm for men and 62mm for women. The PD reduces when the eyes fixate at near; the shorter the fixation distance, the smaller the PD. In certain circumstances – such as the fitting of progressive addition ophthalmic lenses – the positioning of ophthalmic lenses is critical. In such cases, the distance of the pupil of each eye to the facial mid-line is measured separately; these are known as monocular PD measurements. The PD can be measured by an instrument that is (incorrectly) called a 'pupillometer' (the strict definition of a pupillometer is a device that measures the diameter of an individual pupil); some instruments operate by determining the pupil centres, and others rely on determining the location of corneal reflexes. Some models of videokeratoscopes, aberrometers and autorefractors will give a readout of interpupillary distance after both eyes have been measured.

Intraocular pressure

This is the positive pressure within the eyeball. It is a function of the balance between the rate of production or aqueous humour in the eye and the rate of drainage of aqueous humour from the eye. Intraocular pressure (IOP) can theoretically be measured directly using a manometer. However, this is not viable in humans as it would involve placing a small puncture in the eyeball. Therefore, intraocular pressure is measured indirectly using one of a variety of techniques known as tonometry. Normal IOP falls within the range 10 to 22mmHg. If aqueous outflow is blocked, IOP can become elevated and lead to glaucoma. There is a small increase in IOP (of about 2mmHg) with age. Intraocular pressure is generally about 4mmHg higher in the morning than in the evening, and is higher when lying down. During accommodation, IOP decreases by about 4mmHg.

Inventory, contact lens

- See *Practice logistics*, *contact lens.*

Ionizing radiation

Ionizing radiation consists of very short wavelengths (< 0.01 nm) and is caused by the disintegration of atoms. This occurs naturally as cosmic radiation from radioactive isotopes, such as radium. Artificial sources can produce X-ray and gamma radiation, as well as corpuscular radiation, which include alpha- and beta-particles, electrons, positrons, protons, and neutrons. Those employed in occupations such as radiology, nuclear physics, and uranium mining and engineering, can be at risk from ionizing radiations.

Most of the ionizing radiation passes through the eye, but a small amount is absorbed and, depending upon the exposure time and concentration, can cause damage to nearly all of the ocular tissues. In general, low penetrating forms of radiation, such as beta-particles, require excessive and repeated exposure for damage to occur, whereas high penetrating forms of radiations, such as X-ray and gamma-radiation and neutrons, require relatively small doses.

The sensitivity of the various ocular tissues will depend upon the miotic activity of the cells, i.e. division and growth, and the ability to repair radiation-induced damage. The foetal eye is far more sensitive to radiation exposure than the adult eye. Of the ocular tissues, the conjunctiva, cornea, and lens are most susceptible, as they undergo constant replication and, in the case of the lens, growth throughout life.

Ionizing radiation may have a direct or an indirect effect upon the ocular tissues. Direct action upon the cells can result in the development of abnormalities, or in cell death. Indirect effects can occur as a result of damage of the blood vessels, leading to a reduced blood supply to the tissues.

The most common effect of radiation exposure is the formation of cataracts, because the lens contains the ocular tissues that are most sensitive to this type of radiation. The lenticular changes are similar regardless of the type of radiation; fine dot-like subcapsular opacities in the anterior cortex and granular and vacuolar subcapsular opacities at the posterior pole of the lens. These may progress to involve the peripheral portions of the posterior cortex. It may take several years for the cataracts to develop after exposure to the radiation. The latent period and the severity of lens damage depends on:
- Radiation dose – duration and concentration; single or multiple exposures.
- Type of radiation – low or high penetration.
- Age of person – the younger the person the shorter the latent period and the greater the lens damage.

Iris

The iris is a thin muscular diaphragm, continuous with the ciliary body and separating the anterior and posterior chambers of the eye (Figure I.13). The central aperture, the pupil, can vary in diameter from about 2 to 8mm under natural conditions, governed by the actions of two smooth muscles, the sphincter and dilator pupillae. Iris colour is determined by melanin pigment within melanocytes (principally within the anterior border layer). Cells containing sparse pigment granules (melanosomes) will produce a grey colour and with increasing concentration, the colour produced is mid-brown, then

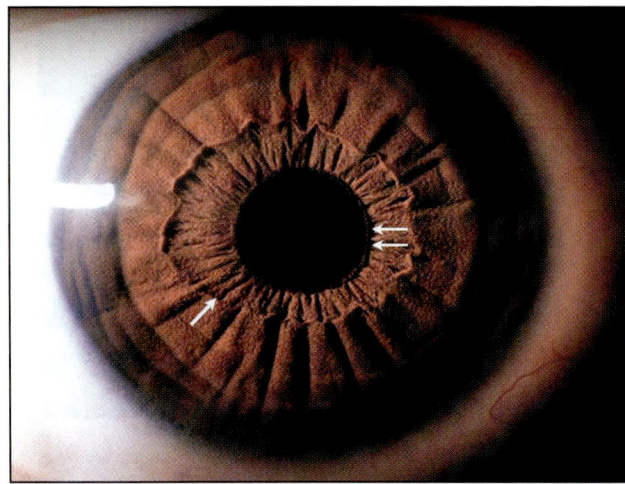

Figure I.13 • Gross appearance of the iris. The pigment ruff (double arrow) is visible at the pupil margin. The collarette (single arrow) marks the border between pupillary and ciliary zones. Radial folds and circumferential contraction furrows can be seen within the ciliary zone.

dark brown. When the iris is sparsely pigmented, shorter wavelengths are selectively scattered back to the observer and the longer wavelengths penetrate to the pigmented posterior epithelial layers and are absorbed. Consequently the iris appears blue.

From the posterior surface forward, four tissue layers of the iris are resolved:
- posterior pigment epithelium
- anterior epithelium and dilator pupillae muscle
- substantia propria (stroma) including the sphincter pupillae muscle
- anterior border layer.

The posterior pigment epithelium consists of melanin-rich columnar cells mounted on a thin basement membrane. The anterior epithelium forms a thinner, rather less heavily pigmented layer. The anterior epithelium has two morphologically distinct portions: an apical 'epithelial' portion and a basal 'muscular' portion. The muscular portion forms the specialized dilator pupillae. Activation of its sympathetic nerve supply induces contraction of the muscle, dilating the pupil.

The sphincter pupillae is located in the posterior stroma encircling the pupillary margin. Its constituent smooth muscle fibres are spindle-shaped with their axes disposed circumferentially, forming a 1mm band in the plane of the iris. The sphincter is innervated by myelinated parasympathetic nerve fibres from the oculomotor nerve.

The stroma is composed of a loose network of connective tissue containing a number of cellular elements including: fibroblasts, melanocytes, clump cells and mast cells.

The anterior border layer represents a modification of the stroma. It is composed of two types of cell: a discontinuous layer of fibrobasts overlying a dense aggregation of pigmented melanocytes. The anterior border layer is the principal determinant of iris colour; it is thin in a blue iris and thick and densely pigmented in brown irises.

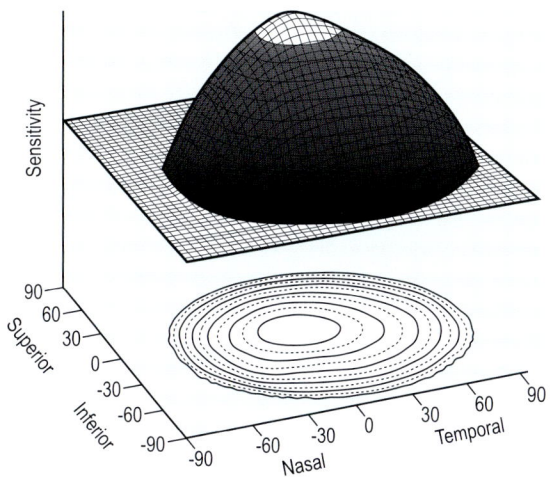

Figure 1.14 • The island of vision.

Iron deposition
- See *Deposits, contact lens.*

ISCLR
- See *International Society for Contact Lens Research.*

Ishihara test
- See *Pseudoisochromatic plates.*

Island of vision

The sensitivity of the eye is not constant across the whole of the visual field but varies in a rather complicated way with eccentricity, adaptation level and the nature of the test stimulus. As a means of representing the different sensitivities at different regions, the visual field is often described as an island, a concept attributed to Traquair who described the visual field as an 'island of vision in a sea of darkness'.

The height, or elevation, of the island represents the sensitivity of the eye. Stimuli whose parameters place them above the island are too dim to be seen. Those that fall outside of the island (over the sea) are outside of the field of view (e.g. behind your head) and cannot be seen no matter how bright they are made. Only stimuli whose parameters place them within the island of vision can be seen.

Just as geographers use contour lines to represent the height of an island on a map, so perimetrists use isopters to represent the sensitivity of the eye on a field chart. A contour line is a line joining points of equal height above sea level. An isopter is a line joining points of equal sensitivity (Figure I.14).

The island of vision changes with the state of adaptation. When the eye is light-adapted it will appear as a relatively low-lying island with a peak at its centre, the fovea. When the eye is dark-adapted the island will be much higher (more sensitive) and because of the distribution of rods and cones will have a crater at its centre.

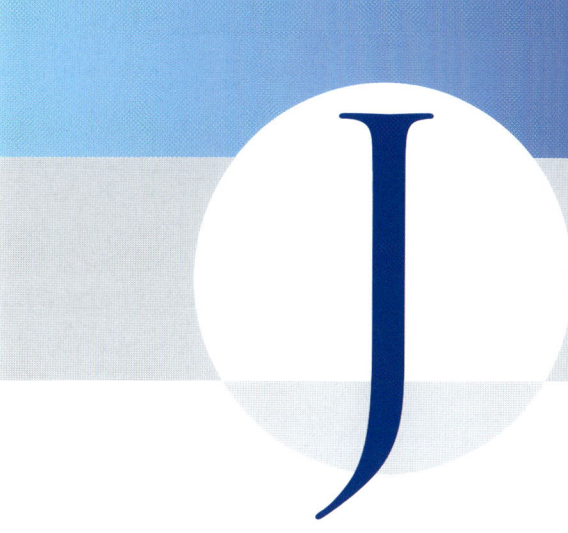

Jackson cross-cylinder technique
- See *Cross-cylinder technique*

Jelly bumps
- See *Deposits, contact lens.*

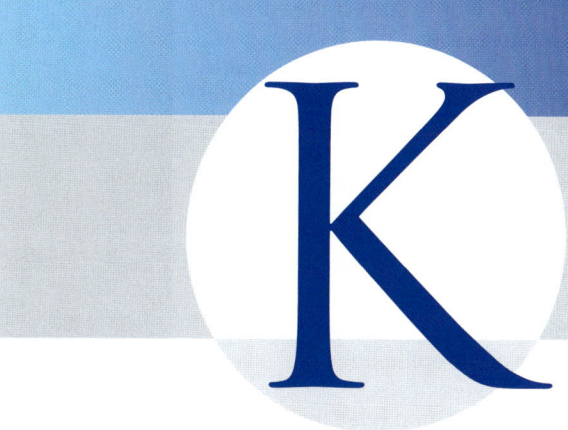

Keratitis
- See *Bacterial keratitis.*

Keratoconus

Keratoconus is a progressive, asymmetric, non-inflammatory disease of the cornea characterized by steepening and distortion, apical thinning, and central scarring of the cornea (see Figure D.11). These corneal changes lead to a mild to marked decrease in vision secondary to high irregular astigmatism and, frequently, central corneal scarring. There are several characteristic biomicroscopic corneal signs that become more prevalent as the disease progresses, including:

- an inferiorly displaced, thinned protrusion of the cornea
- corneal thinning over the apex of the cone
- scars in Bowman's layer
- Vogt's striae in the posterior stroma
- Fleischer's ring, consisting of iron in the corneal epithelium at the base of the cone.

Although the aetiology of keratoconus is unknown, this condition has been putatively associated with atopic disease, eye rubbing, inheritance, and contact lens wear. Estimates of the prevalence of keratoconus vary from 4–108 per 100 000 population.

Management varies with disease severity. Non-surgical alternatives are the primary method of patient management in keratoconus. Although the visual disturbances in keratoconus may be managed with spectacles or soft lenses early in the disease process, rigid lenses are the treatment of choice for the irregular astigmatism associated with the condition. Occasionally, in later stages soft lenses are used in conjunction with rigid lenses in a 'piggyback' combination, or scleral lenses are prescribed.

Patients are generally referred for penetrating keratoplasty when they can no longer tolerate contact lenses or when contact lenses provide inadequate vision. Poor vision with contact lenses is often accompanied by apical corneal scarring, but vision can be compromised even with optimal contact lens correction and no corneal scarring. With concerted effort, the vast majority of patients initially referred for corneal transplants can be successfully refitted with contact lenses without surgery, yielding improved visual acuity and contact lens wearing time.

Keratoconus, contact lens correction of

The use of rigid contact lenses is the mainstay of the optical management of keratoconus. These lenses, which are manufactured in a large variety of unique designs, effectively resurface the irregular cornea and allow the intervening fluid lens to correct the corneal astigmatism adequately in most cases.

Certainly, a rigid contact lens allows for a far more uniform refracting surface than the irregular astigmatic surface of the keratoconic cornea. The local irregularities of the (often) stained and (sometimes) raised epithelial lesion are filled in by the tears behind the rigid lens. However, the lacrimal lens only eliminates about 90% of the astigmatic error of the cornea due to the index difference between the tears and cornea. Corneal scarring and epithelial staining diffuse light and result in worse low contrast visual acuity. The rigid lens may also further distort the cornea. A flat or steep fit may cause wrinkling of the epithelium, and a very flat fit may decrease axial length.

Although rigid lenses often position over the apex of the displaced ectatic area, they eliminate the difficulties associated with this displacement by also superimposing the visual axis. Rigid lens fitting in keratoconus is, however, by no means simple. Numerous lenses are often required, even for an initial fitting, and achieving an adequate cornea-lens fitting relationship with reasonable vision becomes more difficult as the disease progresses. Although most practitioners who fit a large variety of keratoconus patients have their preferences for lens design, most practicing clinicians still find each keratoconus patient a trial-and-error experience.

The major rigid lens fitting techniques are:

- apical bearing, with primary lens support on the apex of the cornea, where the central optic zone of the lens actually touches or bears on the central corneal epithelium
- apical clearance, with lens support and bearing directed off the apex and onto the paracentral cornea, with clearance of the apex of the cornea
- divided support or 'three-point touch', with lens support and bearing shared between the corneal apex and the paracentral cornea.

Typically, an apical bearing fit is the easiest to achieve in keratoconus. Almost all rigid contact lenses touch the apex of the cone unless steps are taken to alleviate the bearing or to clear the corneal apex. In three-point touch – although possibly viewed as a variant of apical touch – the objective is to minimize the touch on the corneal apex by steepening the lens centrally and allowing the peripheral cornea to show areas of light touch, thereby minimizing trauma to all areas of the cornea (Figure K.1). The major disadvantage of apical touch is the possibility of epithelial trauma and the inducement of corneal scarring. The advantages of apical touch include the possibility of superior acuity. In lenses fitted with an apical clearance technique, trauma to the central cornea and epithelium is presumably minimized. Lens wearing time may be lessened relative to lenses supported more by the central cornea. See *Fitting scleral lenses*.

Keratocytes
- See *Corneal stroma*.

Keratoglobus
- See *Distorted corneal shape, therapeutic lenses for*.

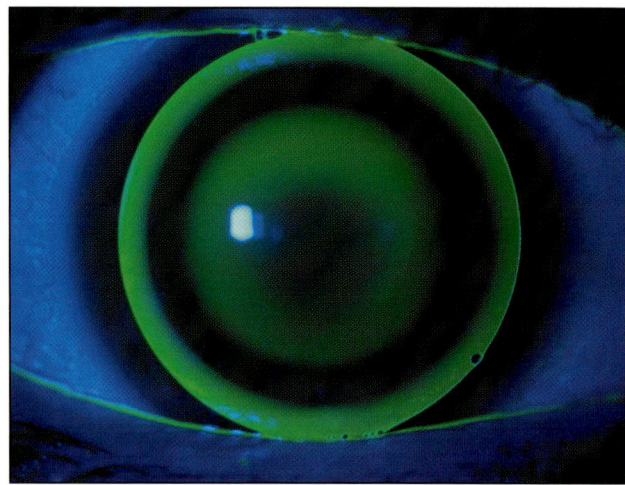

Figure K.1 • Three-point-touch technique of fitting a rigid lens to a keratoconic eye.

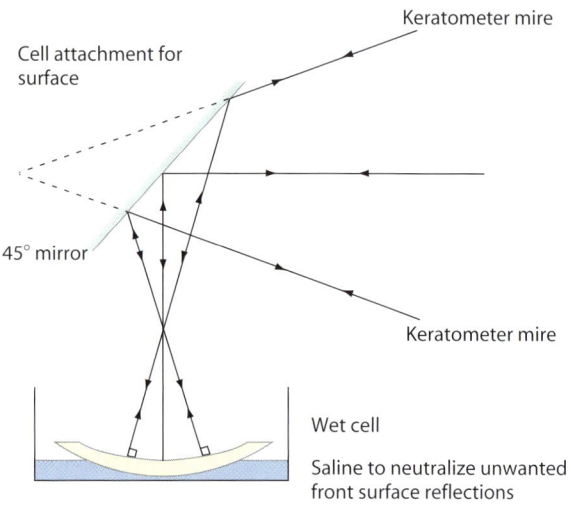

Figure K.2 • Optics of measuring the BOZR of a rigid lens using a keratometer.

Keratometer, for contact lens curvature measurement

With slight modification, a keratometer can be adapted for measuring any reflective curved surface. In conjunction with a mirror and wet cell, this is a precise although cumbersome method for measuring the back optic zone radius (BOZR) (Figure K.2) or front optic zone radius (FOZR) of soft or rigid lenses. Keratometer scales are calibrated for corneal radius and/or corneal surface power, and thus the keratometer scale needs to be re-calibrated when using it for estimating the BOZR of a soft lens. Re-calibration can be achieved using rigid contact lenses of known BOZR.

Keratometer, for corneal curvature measurement

Knowledge of corneal curvature is primarily of interest as an aid in determining the initial contact lens to be placed on the eye in cases of rigid contact lens fitting. The amount of keratometric astigmatism can be compared to the ocular astigmatism. This identifies lenticular astigmatism, which may be the cause of residual astigmatism

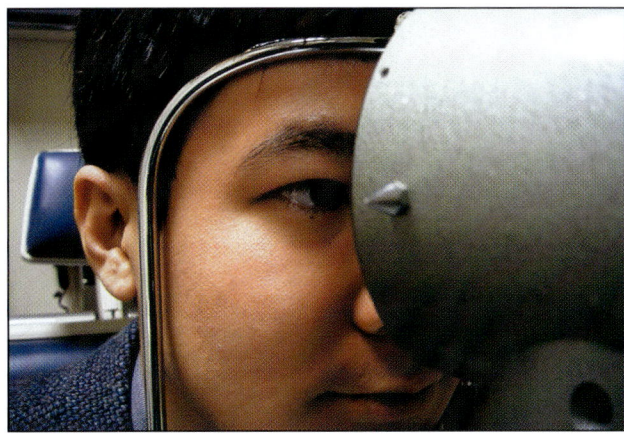

Figure K.3 • Alignment of the keratometer with the eye of a patient.

in rigid lens wear. For soft lens fitting, particularly disposable lenses, which might, for example, be available in only two back optic zone radii (BOZR), keratometry may be used simply to identify steeper corneas, which require the lens with the smaller BOZR.

For all lens wearers (and indeed non-lens-wearers), keratometry can provide an indication of progressive or rapid changes in curvature, which can be indicative of a compromised cornea. Keratometric assessment can also aid in the diagnosis of keratoconus.

Keratometric measurement of the radius of curvature of the cornea is based on the fact that the front surface of the cornea acts as a convex mirror. The reflection of an object (or mire, from the French for 'target') of known size at a known distance is viewed using a short focus telescope, and a relatively simple equation allows the corneal front surface radius of curvature to be determined directly from the instrument. The corneal power that results from a given radius is often also indicated on the keratometer; alternatively, this can be calculated or determined from tables (Appendix F).

Keratometry is a simple, rapid and non-invasive test (Figure K.3), but it does have some limitations. The actual region over which the standard keratometer measures corneal radius is that of two small areas approximately 1.5mm on either side of the central fixation point. Different types of keratometers use differing sized mires at differing separations. It is thus of no surprise that different keratometers may give differing radius values on the same eye. The keratometer only measures at one corneal radius, it assumes regular astigmatism (i.e. that the principle axes are orthogonal), and it has a limited range of powers (36.00–53.00D). The latter problem can be overcome by interposing a –1.00D lens (for low corneal powers, i.e. very flat corneas) or a +1.25D lens (for high corneal powers, i.e. very steep corneas) in front of the entrance aperture of the keratometer (on the patient side of the instrument). The doubled mires are aligned in the usual way, and the keratometer reading is converted to the actual corneal power using tables such as those given in Appendix E.

The latest development in automated keratometry involves the use of infrared devices that rapidly and automatically determine central keratometry and refractive error simultaneously.

In addition to determining central radius of curvature, it is useful to measure peripheral radius values, particularly in complicated conditions such as post-penetrating keratoplasty and post-refractive surgery. Conventional keratometers have been traditionally adapted by using peripheral fixation points. However, in reality keratometers cannot be used to determine corneal curvature accurately if the surface being measured does not have a constant radius of curvature or is not radially symmetric. For this reason, dedicated instruments using other technologies, such as computer-assisted corneal topographic analysis, have been developed to measure the overall corneal topography.

Keratopathy, superficial punctate
- See *Corneal staining*.

Keratoplasty, contact lens fitting following
- See *Post-keratoplasty, contact lens fitting*.

Keratoscopy
- See *Corneal topographic analysis*.

Kollner's rule
A classification of acquired colour deficiency was suggested by Kollner in 1912. Kollner's rule is often incorrectly abbreviated as stating that acquired 'blue-yellow' colour deficiency is caused by retinal disease and acquired red-green colour deficiency is caused by optic nerve disease. This distinction is no longer tenable.

Krause gland
- See *Accessory lacrimal glands*.

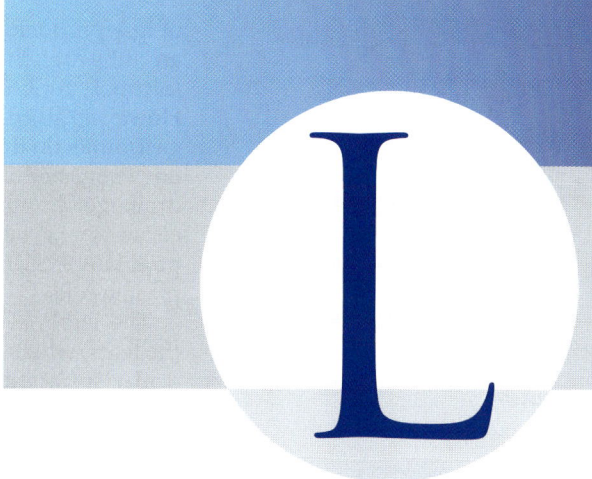

Lacrimal drainage system

Tears collect at the medial canthal angle, where they drain into the puncta of the upper and lower lids (Figure L.1). Each punctum is a small oval opening, approximately 0.3mm in diameter, which is located at the summit of an elevated papilla. From each punctum the canaliculus passes first vertically for about 2mm and then it turns sharply to run medially for about 8mm. At the angle, a slight dilation, the ampulla, can be seen. The canaliculi converge towards the lacrimal sac, usually forming a common canaliculus before entry. The lacrimal sac occupies a fossa formed by the maxillary and lacrimal bones. It measures 1.5–2.5mm in diameter and approximately 12–15mm in vertical length. From the lacrimal sac tears drain into the nasolacrimal duct, which extends for about 15mm, passing through a bony canal in the maxillary bone to an opening in the nose beneath the inferior nasal turbinate. A fold of mucosa is often observed at the termination of the duct, which has been termed the 'valve of Hasner', although there is no strong evidence that it functions as a valve.

Tear drainage is an active process mediated by the contraction of the orbicularis during blinking. Tears enter the canaliculi principally by capillary action. During the early part of the blink, the puncta are occluded as the orbicularis further contracts. The canaliculi and lacrimal sac are also compressed, forcing fluid into the nose. An alternative hypothesis has been proposed, whereby orbicularis contraction dilates the sac, thus creating a negative pressure that draws in the tears from the canaliculi. A vascular plexus is embedded in the wall of the lacrimal sac and duct, and this may influence tear outflow. It is postulated that opening and closing of the lumen of the lacrimal passages can be achieved by regulating blood flow within this plexus.

Lacrimal gland

The main lacrimal gland is the key provider of the aqueous component of the tears. The gland is located in a shallow depression of the frontal bone behind the superolateral orbital rim. It is partially split by the aponeurosis of the levator palpebrae into an upper larger orbital lobe and a lower palpebral lobe, which can often be visualized through the conjunctiva upon lid eversion. The gland is pinkish in colour, with a lobulated surface. Between 6 and 12 ducts leave the gland through the palpebral lobe and discharge into the conjunctival sac at the upper lateral fornix.

At a microscopic level, the lacrimal gland is tubulo-acinar in form (Figure L.2). Its secretory units (acini) contain secretory cells surrounded by myoepithelial cells. Acinar secretory cells show extensive folding of their plasma membrane and apical microvilli. Adjacent cells are linked by tight junctions, which restrict diffusion between cells. The most prominent feature of these cells is the presence of abundant secretory granules. Two principal secretory cell

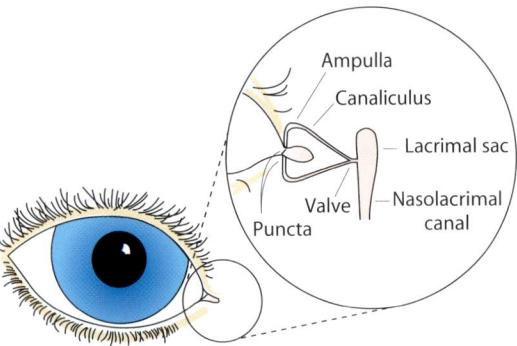

Figure L.1 • Lacrimal drainage system.

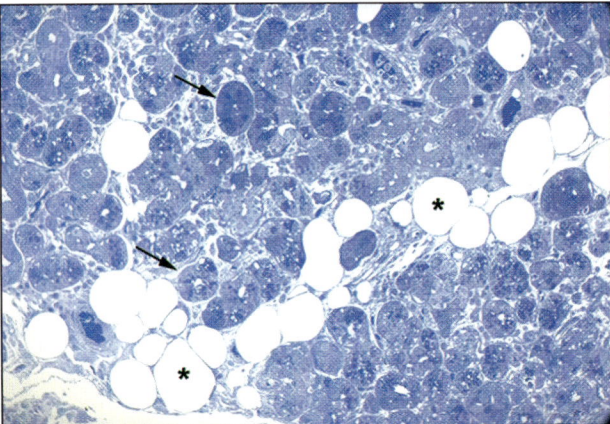

Figure L.2 • Low-power light micrograph of the lacrimal gland. Acini are arrowed. Adipose connective tissue (asterisks) extends across the gland.

sub-types have been identified on the basis of their granule content. The majority of cells contain dark granules (dark cells) with a smaller number of cells containing light granules (light cells). The functional significance of this heterogeneity is uncertain at present. Ducts consist of a single layer of cuboidal cells, which lack secretory granules. Myoepithelial cells are dendritic cells that are closely associated with the perimeter of acini and ducts. It is likely that these contractile cells play a role in the expulsion of tears from the gland. The interstices of the gland contain numerous blood vessels and nerves. A large population of immune cells (particularly IgA-secreting plasma cells) are also found between acini.

The arterial supply to the lacrimal gland is provided by the lacrimal artery, which enters the posterior border of the gland. Venous drainage occurs via the lacrimal vein. A rich autonomic innervation includes secretomotor (para-sympathetic) fibres, which issue from the pterygopalatine ganglion, and sympathetic (vasomotor) fibres from the carotid plexus. The lacrimal nerve traverses the gland to provide a sensory innervation to the conjunctiva and lateral aspect of the eyelid.

In addition to its role as the principal provider of the aqueous phase of the tear film, the lacrimal gland is also a major component of the ocular sensory immune system, which acts as the first line of defence against microbial infection. The secretory immune system is mediated through secretory IgA. The lacrimal gland is the main source of tear IgA, and the gland contains a large number of IgA-producing plasma cells. The mechanism by which an antigenic challenge of the ocular surface induces a lacrimal antibody response is not fully understood. However, since the administration of an antigen by a gastrointestinal route raises specific IgA levels in tears, one suggested mechanism is that ocular antigens – after drainage through the nasolacrimal duct – stimulate B cells in gut Peyer's patches. These sensitized B cells then populate the lacrimal gland, where they transform into plasma cells.

The lacrimal gland also secretes growth factors into the tears, which are important for the maintenance of the ocular surface and epithelial wound healing. Prominent amongst these growth factors are epidermal growth factor (EGF) and transforming growth factor beta (TGFb).

Lacrimal lens
- See *Tear lens beneath a contact lens.*

Lacrimal puncta
- See *Lacrimal drainage system.*

Lacrimal sac
- See *Lacrimal drainage system.*

Lacrimal system
The lacrimal apparatus provides for the production and maintenance of the pre-ocular tear film. The normal function of this system is essential for the integrity of the ocular surface and the provision of a smooth refractive surface. The lacrimal apparatus comprises a secretory system, which includes the main and accessory lacrimal glands, and a drainage system, which consists of the paired puncta and canaliculi, the lacrimal sac and the naso-lacrimal duct. See *Lacrimal drainage system; Lacrimal gland.*

Lactate
- See *Oedema.*

Lactation
- See *Indications and contraindications for contact lens wear.*

Laminate tint constructions for contact lenses
An opaque tinted iris pattern can be incorporated within a contact lens using a laminate construction. An iris pattern is painted, using opaque dyes and tints, onto the surface of an unhydrated HEMA button that has been lathed to the curvature of the intended finished lens. A second pouring of HEMA over the top of this pattern is effected. Once set, the laminate button is lathed to create the finished lens form, which is then hydrated in the usual way. The advantage of this process is that the painted features are encapsulated, and therefore protected, within the lens. The disadvantages are that the lens is thicker, thus reducing oxygen transmissibility, and the tensile properties of the lens are altered, which can affect fitting characteristics.

A variation of laminate construction, known as sandwich technology, has been developed. The top and bottom layers of clear HEMA are co-polymerized with a thin middle layer of coloured non-toxic pigments, allowing the composite button to be lathed and then hydrated into an ultra-thin lens design. An alternative approach is to use non-coloured opaquing agents to create an iris pattern in the centre of the two HEMA buttons, and then tinting the top HEMA section to create the desired cosmetic colouration. See *Tinted contact lenses*.

Lamp life

The term 'life' of an electric lamp can have two different meanings:
- The time after which the lamp ceases to operate, e.g. filament lamps fail due to filament breakage.
- The time after which the light output is so reduced that it is more economical to replace the lamp, e.g. discharge lamps.

Lantern colour vision tests

Colour vision lanterns originated in the 19th century and are intended to select people for employment in transport. A lantern test aims to demonstrate that recruits are able to identify coloured light signals by name. Different lanterns are used in different countries. Most lanterns show paired red, green and white lights which are equivalent to navigation signal lights. The x, y chromaticity coordinates of these lights and their spectral content are specified by the CIE. Colour naming does not fulfill the ideal criteria for a colour vision test but it is assumed that people with severe colour deficiency will name the colours incorrectly and fail the test whereas people with slight colour deficiency will pass. The latter are deemed to be 'colour deficient safe'. This grading function is not always realized either because the lantern is inappropriately designed, poorly operated or because the examination is too short. Permitted colour names are explained before the examination and this helps candidates to guess the correct response particularly when the examination is short. Prolonged testing is needed to demonstrate inconsistent colour naming. This method of occupational selection is currently under review especially since different approved lanterns have been shown to pass different cohorts of colour deficient people. An additional problem is that most transport services seek to exclude protans and some people with this type of colour deficiency are able to pass a lantern test.

There are 2 Holmes-Wright lanterns containing paired red, green and white signal lights. The Type A lantern is intended to select personnel for occupations in rail transport, the UK armed services and in civil aviation. The Type B lantern is used to select people for occupations in civilian merchant marine transport. These lanterns have an acknowledged provenance and a fixed examination protocol. A full examination, consisting of 3 runs of the 9 colour pairs, with the Type A lantern in either photopic or scotopic viewing at high brightness is an excellent screening test for red-green colour deficiency. A proportion of normal trichromats fail examinations with the Type A lantern in scotopic viewing at low brightness and also fail examinations with the Type B lantern. An examination with the Type B lantern is only given to recruits on appeal following identification of colour deficiency with the Ishihara plates.

The Beyne lantern was developed in France. The construction of this lantern is very complex. The exposure time and angular subtends of the spectral colours varies over a wide range. Test protocols use a limited selection of these options. Some people with normal colour vision make mistakes and a final decision on recruitment is made on the results of a test battery which includes achieving an acceptable error score on the F-M 100 hue test.

The Spectrolux lantern (Switzerland) includes blue and yellow as well as red, green and white lights. The examination protocol is not clearly defined but is generally not rigorous. The colours are displayed singly and in pairs. Pass/fail of the initial test with single colours depends on the order of presentation. The colours are not signal light colours and some normal trichromats fail by interchanging blue and green colour names.

The Farnsworth lantern (Falant lantern) was developed in the USA and is designed as a grading test which aims to fail people with severe colour deficiency and pass people with slight colour deficiency. The red, green and white lights shown are within isochromatic zones and are not specified signal colours. The lantern is easy to use and has a set examination protocol. Pass/fail is determined by an error score.

There are 2 simple versions of the UK-designed Giles-Archer lantern ('Standard' and 'Aviation'). Only single colours are shown. The colours are obtained with gelatine filters and are not signal light colours. There is no fixed examination protocol and pass/fail results vary in different examination locations. More colour deficient people are able to pass if the examination is short. A dark red is included specifically to identify protans. Protans should respond 'no light' but are frequently able to guess the correct response. These lanterns are not approved by the CIE for occupational selection.

Lanthony colour vision tests

Phillipe Lanthony designed 3 colour vision tests in the 1970s which utilize Munsell colour samples and are intended to evaluate acquired colour deficiency.

The Lanthony desaturated D15 test has the same hues as the Farnsworth D15 test but has Munsell value 8 and chroma 2. The colours are therefore very desaturated and it is difficult for normal trichromats to arrange the hues correctly at standard light levels (350–500lux). Specificity is therefore low. Lanthony recommends at least 1000lux for this test.

The New Colour test is primarily designed to demonstrate the range of neutral colours in acquired colour deficiency. There are 70 caps with Munsell samples. The hues are divided into a series of 4 D15 tests with Munsell value 6 and chromas of 2, 4, 6, and 8 respectively. There are 10 grey samples representing an achromatic lightness scale. The test is time consuming and is performed in 2 steps for each chroma series. In the first step the samples perceived to be coloured are separated from those perceived to be achromatic. In the second step the colour caps and the perceived achromatic caps are arranged in sequence of hue and lightness, respectively.

The Tritan Album has 5 pseudoisochromatic plates intended to identify and grade the severity of congenital tritan and acquired Type 3 colour deficiency. This is not achieved. Congenital tritanopes fail only the most desaturated plate. Each plate consists of a square matrix of grey dots. The dots in one corner are violet. The visual task is to identify this corner.

LASEK

- See *Laser refractive surgery, contact lenses following; Laser-assisted epithelial keratomileusis (LASEK).*

Laser-assisted epithelial keratomileusis (LASEK)

LASEK is one of a number of laser-based surgical techniques to correct refractive error. In LASEK, the epithelium is cut not with a microkeratome cutting tool as used in laser-assisted in situ keratomileusis (LASIK), but with a finer blade called a trephine. Then the surgeon covers the eye with an alcohol solution (typically one part alcohol and four parts sterile water) for around 30 seconds. The solution loosens the attachment of the epithelium to the underlying stroma. After sponging the alcohol solution from the eye, the surgeon uses a small hoe to lift the edge of the epithelial flap and gently fold it back out of the way. An excimer laser, as in LASIK or photorefractive keratectomy (PRK), is used to sculpt the stromal bed. The epithelial flap is then put back in place. The technique can be used to correct myopia, hypermetropia and astigmatism. See *Laser refractive surgery, contact lenses following; Laser-assisted in situ keratomileusis; Photorefractive keratectomy.*

Laser-assisted in situ keratomileusis (LASIK)

LASIK is one of a number of laser-based surgical techniques to correct refractive error. In LASIK, a special cutting tool called a microkeratome is used to create a circular flap of cornea, leaving part of the flap connected to the remainder of the cornea (via a 'hinge'). Then the surgeon uses a small hoe to lift the edge of the corneal flap and gently fold it back out of the way. An excimer laser is used to sculpt the stromal bed. The corneal flap is then put back in place. The technique can be used to correct myopia, hypermetropia and astigmatism. See *Laser refractive surgery, contact lenses following; Laser epithelial keratomileusis; Photorefractive keratectomy.*

Laser refractive surgery, contact lenses following

The contact lens management of patients following laser refractive surgery poses far fewer problems than those encountered after radial keratotomy (RK), the latter being rarely performed today. Patients may present for contact lens fitting after having various forms of laser-based refractive surgery, including photorefractive keratectomy (PRK), laser-assisted in situ keratomileusis (LASIK) or laser epithelial keratomileusis (LASEK) surgery performed on both eyes simultaneously.

The LASIK flap presents few, if any, problems in the fitting or wearing of contact lenses. In fact, there has been no discernable difference with respect to contact lens fitting or physiologic response between post-PRK and post-LASIK/LASEK patients.

The amount of corneal tissue removed in a myopic laser procedure will play an important role in the post-surgical management of the patient with contact lenses. Irregular astigmatism is a rare finding in both PRK and LASIK/LASEK, and therefore it is not a significant issue for the contact lens practitioner.

Three contact lens options are used for post-PRK and post-LASIK/LASEK patients:

1. Conventional rigid lens designs. Many patients who have undergone PRK or LASIK/LASEK can be successfully fitted with traditional spherical or aspheric rigid lenses. With myopic ablations, the mid-peripheral cornea (beyond the central 6.0–7.0mm) remains unchanged. Therefore, the major concern in fitting rigid or soft contact lenses is the relative difference between the flatter central cornea and the steeper (normal) mid-peripheral cornea. This difference creates few problems for patients who were low-to-moderate myopes prior to surgery. In such cases, the small amount of tissue ablated does not noticeably affect the contact lens fit or the on-eye lens dynamics. These individuals are often best fitted with a BOZR designed to align the mid-peripheral corneal topography 4.0mm from the centre of the cornea.

2. Reverse geometry rigid lens designs. A patient with high pre-operative refractive error (i.e. greater than –10.00D) might end up with a large difference in thickness between the central and mid-peripheral cornea, such that a traditional rigid lens (designed to align with the mid-peripheral cornea) may exhibit excessive apical clearance. The subsequent large volume of tears centrally can result in unstable optics, and trapped bubbles can form beneath the centre of the lens. In situations such as this, patients may be best managed with reverse geometry lens designs. A standard rigid design mimics the prolate shape of the normal, un-operated cornea, which is steeper in the centre than the periphery. The reverse geometry design more closely parallels the post-refractive surgery topography by incorporating a flat central radius of curvature with a steeper mid-peripheral design. This creates a 'plateau' configuration on the posterior lens surface, which dramatically decreases the volume of tear fluid present beneath the central portion of the lens.

3. Soft lenses. Most of the currently available daily disposable or frequent replacement soft lenses are viable options for the post-laser correction. However, after surgery a complex relationship exists between visual acuity, defocus (refractive error), diffraction and optical aberrations. The loss of post-operative central corneal asphericity can result in a form of spherical aberration that will be symptomatic, especially in patients with large pupils. Improved optical correction can be achieved with soft lens designs that incorporate aberration-correcting anterior aspheric optics.

With both PRK and LASIK/LASEK, rigid lens fitting is best delayed until approximately 8–12 weeks after surgery. At this point, the refraction and topography have stabilized. At 3 months post-surgery, the integrity of the flap interface is usually sufficient to withstand the minor trauma associated with lens insertion and removal, as well as the normal on-eye movement that occurs with blinking.

Practitioners need to be aware of the level of corneal sensitivity following laser refractive surgery if contact lenses are to be fitted. Following PRK, the decrease in central corneal sensitivity will last for about 1 month. Following both LASIK and LASEK, there is a decrease in central corneal sensitivity that takes about 6 months to recover.

Patients frequently experience dry eye symptoms after LASIK; however, the mechanisms that lead to these changes are not well understood. Tear film dysfunction has obvious implications if contact lenses are required after surgery.

LASIK
- See *Laser refractive surgery, contact lenses following; Laser-assisted in situ keratomileusis (LASIK)*.

Lathe cutting for contact lens manufacture

This technique is used to manufacture both soft and rigid contact lenses. It essentially involves the use of a special contact lens lathe to cut a solid piece of plastic into the required shape. In the case of a soft lens, a block of anhydrous plastic material (xerogel) is lathed and then hydrated to form the finished product. In the case of a rigid lens, the material is simply cut to the desired final form.

Lathe cutting is labour intensive, which means that the cost of manufacturing soft lenses using lathe-cutting technology is necessarily more expensive than that using spin casting or cast moulding. Therefore, lathe cutting is generally reserved for the production of rigid lenses and for custom-ordered soft lenses which contain design features that are not amenable to mass production – such as lenses of high spherical power and/or high toric power.

The lens material is supplied to the lens manufacturer in the form of 'rods' or 'buttons'. A rod is a solid cylindrical piece of plastic, about 16mm in diameter and 40cm long. The rod is then sliced, tangentially to the long axis, into buttons of about 1cm thick. More commonly, the materials are fabricated and supplied in button form.

The button is first secured to a back surface lathe in a clamp or 'collet', and this assembly is set spinning at a high rate about its central axis. A diamond-tipped tool cuts the posterior surface lens shape into the button. A second diamond tool advances from the side to reduce the diameter to the required size. The surface is rendered smooth by either fine machining or polishing. The dimensions of these cuts are calculated to allow for eventual expansion when the xerogel is later hydrated.

The button is removed from the collet and the cut posterior surface of the button is mounted onto a support tool of a front surface lathe, using low melting point wax. A diamond-tipped tool cuts the anterior surface down to the required thickness (Figure L.3) and the surface is smoothed. Polishing tools may be used to smooth the lens edge, although some advanced lathes obviate this step. Finally, all relevant lens parameters are inspected and measured.

In the case of soft lenses, the xerogel lens form is hydrated in normal, unpreserved saline, re-inspected,

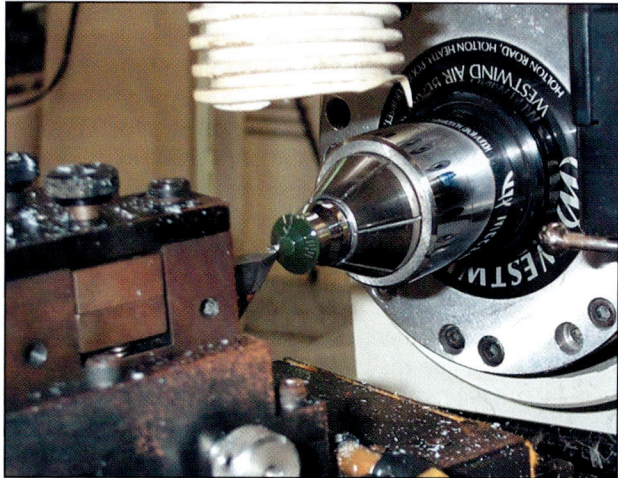

Figure L.3 • Front surface curve being lathed onto a rigid lens.

sealed in small glass vials, and autoclaved at 120°C for 15 minutes to effect sterilization. Advances in lathing technology and computer-controlled processing have led to the development of semi-automatic systems whereby stacks of buttons are automatically fed into lathes; however, even this technology cannot match the mass-production capabilities of cast moulding.

Lattice dystrophy
- See *Dystrophies of the corneal epithelium, therapeutic contact lenses for*.

Laws of motility and muscle pairs

Binocular eye movements are governed principally by two basic laws of motility concerned with the ocular rotation of each eye separately and for the eyes as a pair.

- Sherrington's law of reciprocal innervation – this law is concerned with the co-ordination of muscle pairs of one eye. It dictates that when an agonist muscle contracts, there is inhibition of the innervation to its direct antagonist, which relaxes. The relaxation of the direct antagonist is in proportion to the contraction of the agonist.
- Hering's law of equal innervation – this law is concerned with the co-ordination of muscle pairs for the two eyes together. When an impulse to perform an eye movement is received by one eye, muscles of the other eye, which rotate the eyes into the same direction of gaze, receive equal innervation. The muscles involved are 'yoke muscles'.

There are three types of muscle pairs that are governed by these laws.

- Agonist/antagonist pairs – these are those muscle pairs, within one eye, which move the eye in opposite directions. Sherrington's Law therefore governs them. A simple example of such a pair is the medial and lateral rectus muscles of one eye, which rotate the eye into adduction and abduction respectively. Muscle pairs may be antagonistic for some rotations and not for others. For example the inferior and superior rectus muscles are antagonists for vertical and torsional rotations but not for horizontal rotations, as shown in Figure I.3B.

- Synergists – these are muscles of one eye that move the eye in the same direction. For example the superior rectus and inferior oblique muscles are synergistic for elevation, both rotating the eye upwards. They are also antagonistic for torsional and horizontal rotation, as shown in Figure I.3C.
- Yoke muscles – these are pairs of muscles, consisting of one muscle from each eye, that produce simultaneous rotations of the eyes in either the same direction (conjugate movement) or opposite direction (disjugate movement). Hering's law of equal innervation governs these rotations. Examples are the right medial rectus and left lateral rectus for laevo-version; the right medial rectus and left medial rectus for convergence; and the right superior rectus and left inferior oblique for dextro-elevation. Understanding the yoke muscle pairings for primary muscle actions are essential for the clinical interpretation of incomitant strabismus.

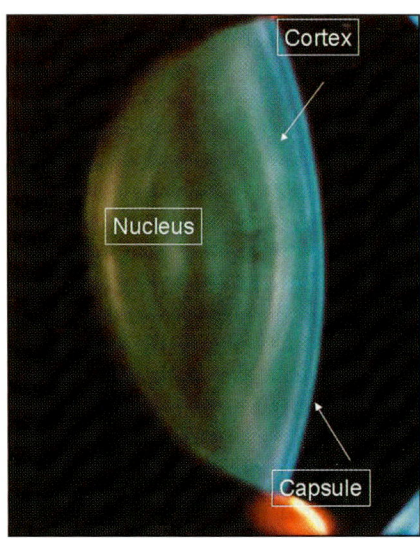

Figure L.4 • Optical section through the crystalline lens.

Layout, optometry practice

The layout of an optometry practice will be governed by the physical limitations of the site and the sequence and order of activities that the patient undergoes during a visit to the practice. The key features are as follows:

1. Reception area and front desk. This is the first personal contact position for the visiting patient, and should be a welcoming point as well as a help desk. The reception area will often be the last point of contact before the patient leaves the practice.
2. Waiting area. The waiting area needs to be comfortable, with sufficient seating to accommodate potential patients and customers. A 'rule of thumb' worth considering is that this area should be furnished and decorated to a standard similar to that of the sitting rooms of the patients and customers attending the practice.
3. Consulting room. Depending on the patient workload of the practice, more than one room may be dedicated to the consultation and examination activity. Increasingly, delegation of data collection tasks (e.g. non-contact tonometry, visual field analysis, auto-refraction etc.) to support staff means that an area or room will be utilized for this pre-examination screening or adjunct data collection. The consulting room will have all the equipment found in a modern optometry practice. In addition to this, it will be necessary to have some contact lens verification equipment. If the practice specializes in contact lens fitting, the need for specialist diagnostic fitting sets and materials (e.g. pre-formed rigid scleral lenses, bifocal lenses, eye impression materials etc.) will be dictated by the profile of patients attending the practice.
4. Spectacle dispensary. The spectacle dispensary should be able to provide for the functional and aesthetic needs of the patient. In the case of a highly specialized contact lens practice that does not have a spectacle dispensary, there should be the facility to refer patients to a convenient dispensing practice nearby.
5. Contact lens dispensary. The contact lens dispensing area is where patients will attend for instruction and for practising insertion and removal of contact lenses. See *Patient education*. It is also here that patients will receive their (starter) contact lens care systems, obtain advice on wear, care and hygiene with respect to their contact lenses, and complete the paperwork etc. This area should therefore have the furniture, facilities, materials and equipment to allow this to happen effectively. Employing videos and CD-ROMs in this area to support the education process, along with written materials, is now a common practice.

Lens, crystalline

The primary function of the crystalline lens is to transmit visible light and to sharply focus it on the retina. It contributes one third of the total dioptric power of the eye and by changing its shape it is able to fulfill the requirements of the accommodative process (Figure L.4). The lens is a relatively simple structure, comprising of regularly arranged concentric layers of elongated lens fibres that are continually formed at the equatorial germinative zone. The inner part of the lens, that contains those fibres that were laid down in early life, is termed the nucleus and the outer part containing younger fibres is known as the cortex. This unique aspect of lens growth means that old cells are not replaced by new, and so the lens has developed strategies to minimize damage from the cumulative effects of ultraviolet radiation and other oxidative insults. An elastic capsule that is synthesized by the lens epithelium, which postnatally is found only on the anterior surface and equatorial zone, encloses the lens. In keeping with its optical properties, the lens is highly transparent in the visible region of the spectrum. This is surprising for a structure containing a high concentration of protein (33%). Nevertheless, a young lens transmits most light between 450 and 1400nm. The basis of lens transparency is a series of special anatomical and physiological features that keep light scatter to a minimum; these are:

- Lens fibres contain a high concentration of a unique series of proteins, termed crystallins (α, β and γ; hence the term 'crystalline lens') that are tightly packed and demonstrate short-range order
- Lens fibres possess narrow cell membranes and are grouped in regular hexagonal arrays with minimal extracellular space
- Lens fibres do not possess nuclei or cytoplasmic organelles that could act as potential scatter sources
- Changes in refractive index within the lens occur over distances less than the wavelength of light
- The electrolyte balance of the lens is tightly regulated to maintain the constant hydration level that is critical for lens transparency.

The lens continues to grow throughout life through the regular addition of new lens fibres. Adult lens dimensions change in a complex manner, and from the end of the second decade, the sagittal thickness shows a greater percentage increase than the equatorial diameter. This would be associated with an increased dioptric power, were it not for a compensatory change in refractive index. Increased growth also results in changes in the mechanical properties of the lens, which is a major contributor to presbyopia. The young human lens transmits approximately 100% of incident light. With age, light transmission is reduced, with an associated increase in light scatter. Increased scatter occurs in all regions, although it is maximal in the deep cortex and nucleus. The intensity of back-scattered light from the lens continues to increase until physiological scatter gradually merges into the pathological scatter of nuclear cataract. The newborn lens is faintly yellow. With age, the post-natal accumulation of yellow chromophores leads to an increased yellow colouration. These molecules also contribute to the increased 'blue fluorescence' that is a feature of the ageing lens. The increased light absorption of the lens is greatest at the blue end of the spectrum (460–470nm). This is thought to be an adaptive process to protect the retina from potentially damaging wavelengths.

Lens edge fluting
- See *Fluting of contact lenses*.

Lens flippers
Lens flippers are used for the training of accommodative facility, whereby a determination is made of the ability of the patient to maintain a visual target in focus when the lens powers are rapidly alternated. They consist of two pairs of lenses mounted on either side of a central bar that is continuous with a finger grip. By rolling the finger grip between the thumb and forefinger by 180°, the position of the lenses can be reversed. A lens flipper is usually comprised of two pairs of lenses of the same numeric power but opposite sign e.g. a pair of +1.00D lenses on one side of the flipper bar and a pair of –1.00D lenses on the other side; such a configuration would be used to test the facility of the patient to alter accom-

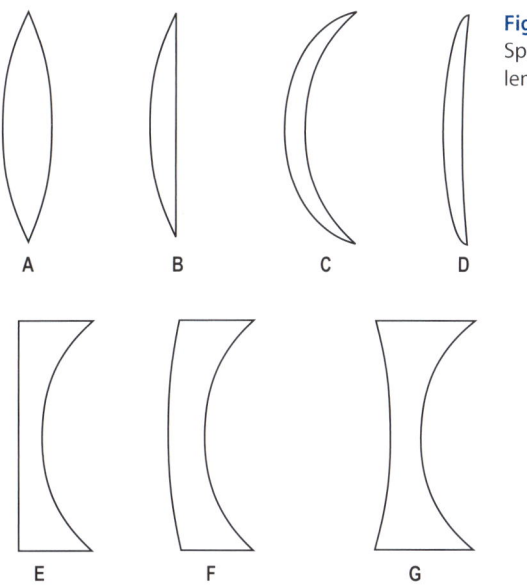

Figure L.5 • Spherical lens forms.

modation by 2.00D. Lens flippers are also available with lens powers of 1.50D and 2.00D).

Lens form, ophthalmic
Ophthalmic lenses with the same back vertex power can be manufactured in a wide variety of different forms. Early lenses were made in what is now known as flat form, whereas now the majority are produced as curved. The differences between these forms are defined in BS 3521 part 1,1991 as follows:

- Curved lens – a lens having one surface convex in all meridians, and one surface concave in all meridians.
- Flat lens – any other type of lens.

Thus, it is important to remember that a flat lens does not have to have a plane surface. The comment concerning 'in all meridians' in the definition is to cover the case where a cylindrical correction is incorporated into the lens. Spherical curved form lenses are known as *meniscus* lenses. In Figure L.5, lenses are shown in the position that they would be normally fitted, with incident light coming from the left, and the more negative curve next to the eye. Lens C is a steep meniscus form, whereas D would be classified as a shallow meniscus. Lens A is equi bi-convex, both surfaces having identical curvature. Lens G is bi-concave, but with a steeper rear surface compared to the front.

There are several reasons for using different forms of lens. Changing the form from flat to meniscus will usually improve the vision through the edge of the lens. However, flat form lenses are generally thinner and lighter than curved forms. The cosmetic appearance in medium to high plus prescriptions is also better in flatter form lenses, because the front surface curvature is reduced compared with meniscus forms.

Lens inventory, contact lens
- See *Practice logistics, contact lens*.

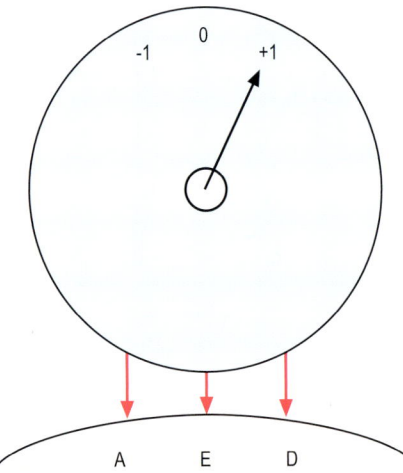

Figure L.6 • Lens measure with fixed outer 'legs' A and D, and central moveable sensor at D connected to the dial indicator.

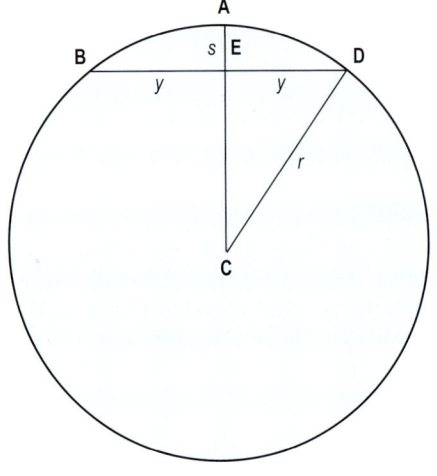

Figure L.7 • Calculation of sag of a surface.

Lens measure

Sometimes known as the Geneva lens measure, this instrument is used to measure the curvature of an ophthalmic lens surface. As shown schematically in Figure L.6, the instrument consists of two fixed supports at A and D, separated by a distance $2y$.

Pointer E is movable vertically and measures sag s, relative to chord AD, displayed by pointer on the dial.

Instruments usually assume a lens refractive index of 1.523, so that a direct conversion to surface power can be made, with the scale in dioptres. Note that A, E and D are all in a straight line so that the instrument can be used to measure the surface curvature along the different principal meridians of a toroidal surface.

In Figure L.7, AD (=$2y$) is a chord of surface radius r. EB is the sag of the chord (s)

Hence in triangle BDC:

$$r^2 = y^2 + (r-s)^2$$
$$r^2 - y^2 = (r-s)^2$$
$$\sqrt{(r^2 - y^2)} = r - s$$
$$s = r - \sqrt{(r^2 - y^2)}$$
$$\text{or } r = (y^2 + s^2)/2s$$

Thus there is a direct relationship between the sag s of the chord AD and the radius of curvature of the surface being measured.

Before using a lens measure it is important to check the zero reading on an optically flat piece of glass, e.g. the surface of a trial case prism. This is because the central pointer (E) is spring loaded in order that negative surface powers can be measured. So when a lens measure is held with the pointers not in contact with a lens surface, the scale reads the most negative power of which the instrument is capable of reading. When measuring the surface curvature of an ophthalmic lens made from a material with a refractive index which differ from 1.523, a correction factor must be used in order to give the true surface power.

Lensometer

- See *Focimeter*.

Lens power

Three lens powers are used to describe spectacle lenses:

Back vertex power – this is the standard value quoted as the 'power' of a spectacle lens, and is designated as F'_v and often quoted as the BVP.

$$F'_v = \frac{F_1}{\left\{1 - \left[\left(\frac{t}{n'}\right)F_1\right]\right\}} + F_2$$

where F_1 is the front surface power (D)
F_2 the back surface power in (D)
t is the lens thickness (m)
n' is the refractive index of the lens material

The BVP is the dioptric distance from the rear surface of the lens to the second principal focal point, F'. In other words, it is the reciprocal of the back vertex focal length. In the case of a spectacle lens, it represents the power of the lens from the perspective of the person wearing the lens, i.e. viewing from the rear side of the lens.

Front vertex power – light from an object placed at the first principal focus, F, of a lens will emerge in parallel from the rear surface of the lens. In this special case the front vertex power, F_v or FVP, is calculated from:

$$F_v = \frac{F_2}{\left\{1 - \left[\left(\frac{t}{n'}\right)F_2\right]\right\}} + F_1$$

The FVP of the lens is of less immediate importance to the spectacle lens wearer, since it represents the power of the lens when viewed from the front surface. Front vertex power is only measured when assessing the addition of front surface multifocals. Looking at the equations for F_v and F'_v however, it should be apparent that the two values will be similar unless t, the thickness of the lens, is substantial.

Equivalent power – the equivalent power (F_e) is the power of the single thin lens which could be used to replace a thick lens or lens system. It can be calculated from:

$$F_e = F_1 + F_2 - \frac{t}{n'}F_1 \cdot F_2$$

Although equivalent power is commonly used for describing the lens characteristics of optical instruments, it is mainly used in spectacle lenses when calculating magnification effects.

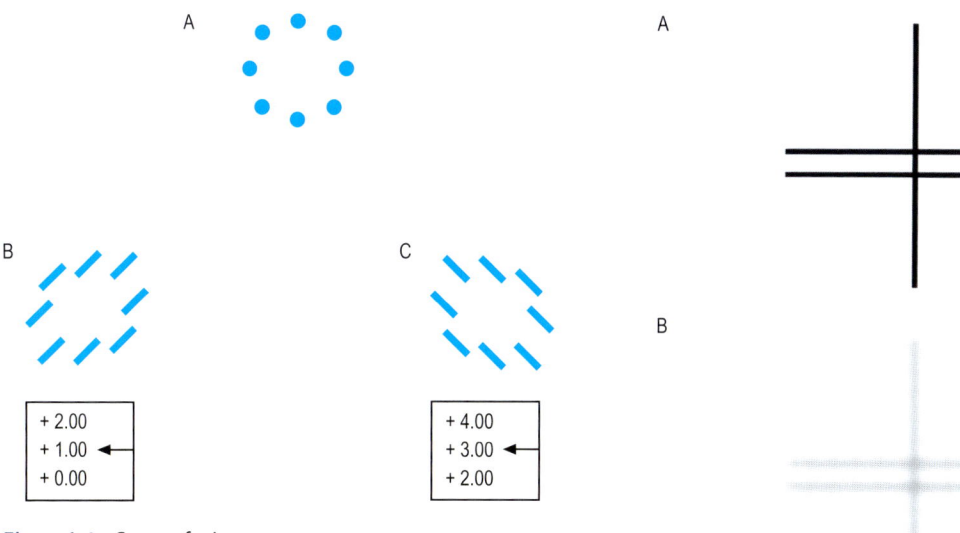

Figure L.8 • Corona focimeter target.

Lens power measurement

The commonest instrument for measuring ophthalmic lens power is the focimeter. Most instruments of this type use an eyepiece, and before measuring a lens, this must be focused correctly according to the following procedure:

- Before inserting an unknown lens into the focimeter, set the target position at zero by means of the power drum control.
- Unscrew the eyepiece adjustment control until the target goes completely out of focus.
- Screw in the eyepiece control until the target just comes into focus. The graticule should also be in focus at the same time.
- Check by setting the power control drum to a random value and then visually refocusing the target: the value on the power control should read zero.

If the target and graticule cannot be made to appear jointly in focus at zero indicated power, then a more fundamental adjustment is required by an instrument mechanic.

Several different designs of illuminated target are used in focimeters. The simplest of these is the circle of dots or corona target (Figure L.8). The spectacles or lens to be measured should be placed, rear surface down, on the aperture of the focimeter so as to measure back vertex power as opposed to front vertex power. The lens should be positioned so that the boxed centre or other appropriate reference point is over the centre of the aperture, and the lens is supported by the frame table.

The frame table is an adjustable support that enables a horizontal reference to be found for a pair of spectacles. The height is adjustable so that the optical axis can be positioned vertically at the required height. It is important for finding the cylinder axis accurately that both lens rims of a pair of spectacles being measured rest on the frame table.

A lens-marking device is normally provided which marks three ink dots on the front surface of the lens. The central dot is coincident with the optical axis of the instrument, and a line through all three dots is coincident with the 0–180 line on the axis scale of the protractor.

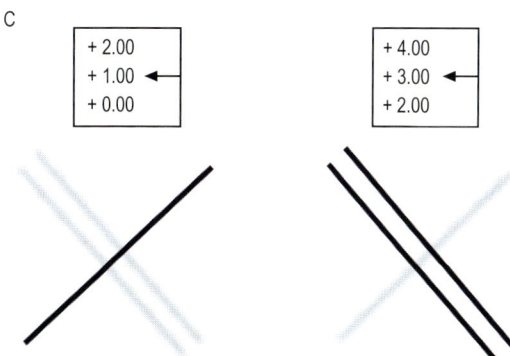

Figure L.9 • (A) Line focimeter target. (B) Blurred image due to target not being orientated parallel to the principal meridians of the lens. (C) Target correctly orientated, viewing the principal lens powers of +1.00/ +2.00 x 135.

This line should also be parallel to the frame table. A spherical lens will give an image the same as the object. That is, the power wheel should be adjusted until the corona is again sharp, and the lens power read off from the scale.

In the case of an astigmatic lens, the image will be distorted into a series of lines, rather than appearing as a ring of dots. Since all astigmatic lenses form two images with mutually perpendicular orientations, two positions of focus can be found (Figure L.8). In order to determine the cylindrical axis, a marker on the graticule is generally made rotatable so that it can be made parallel with the clearest image line, and the axis can be read off the graticule protractor. The length of the line images in a corona target focimeter depends on the difference in power between the two meridians: the greater the power of the cylinder, the longer the line images that are formed.

In order to make a focimeter more accurate at determining the power of low power cylindrical lenses targets are sometimes used which contain a line or series of lines (Figure L.9). The lines can be used at any orientation with a spherical lens, but in order to obtain a clear focus with an astigmatic lens the target must first be orientated parallel to the relevant principal meridian.

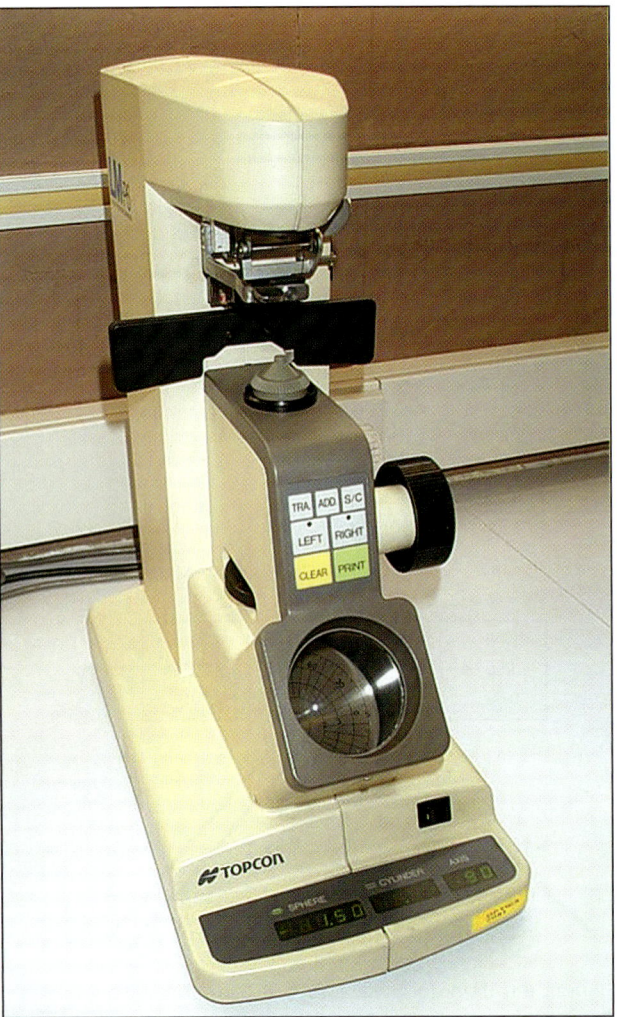

Figure L.10 • Focimeter with a reduced aperture stop suitable for measuring the power of contact lenses

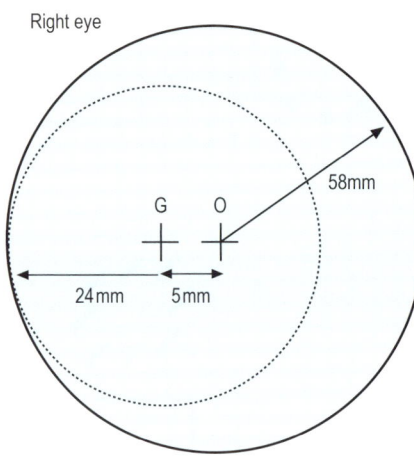

Figure L.11 • Calculation of minimum blank size or minimum uncut size.

The standard focimeter is calibrated for spectacle lenses placed at a specific location on the instrument measuring stop. The physical limitations of the focimeter combined with the highly curved back surface of the lens cause the lens to rest in a position away from this location. This will result in a systematic error when reading off lens power, and this error is significant especially when checking high-powered lenses. The particular focimeter should be recalibrated for contact lens checking, and ideally a dedicated focimeter should be set aside for the exclusive purpose of checking the powers of contact lenses. The focimeter is also used to measure the magnitude and direction of prismatic power in prism ballast and scleral lenses. In addition to the quantitative data obtained using this technique, the clarity of the viewed image formed by transmission through the contact lens can provide an indication of lens optical quality.

The optical configuration of most focimeters is such that lens power is checked by sampling over an aperture of approximately 4mm diameter. In many advanced rigid lens designs (e.g. bifocal, multifocal and aspheric) there can be significant power variations within such a small range, and this will not be detected by standard focimetry. Reducing the aperture can help; however, in advanced optical designs lens power variations are best checked using optical interferometric techniques such as the Twyman-Green interferometer.

The target orientation control is often calibrated in standard notation, and can be used as a cross-check to the axis finder in the graticule for determining the axis of the cylinder. The target orientation control is particularly useful when it is impractical to position the focimeter image in the centre of the graticule, e.g. when measuring the near addition in multifocals.

A standard optical focimeter also can be used to measure the back vertex power (BVP) of a contact lens (Figure L.10). Care must be taken to prevent flexure and damage to the lens. A flat plastic disc with a range of circular apertures is often used to support the lens during focimetry. An automatic focimeter can also be used. Any surface droplets, distortions or lens surface depositions (even fingerprints) will decrease the quality of the viewed image, especially with soft lenses, and this increases the likelihood of an error in assessing BVP. The recommended technique, therefore, is to surfactant-clean the lens, dab it dry with a lint-free tissue, and place the lens on the focimeter support using rubber-tipped tweezers. It is important to measure the BVP of a soft lens as soon as possible following removal from its storage medium to avoid possible effects of lens dehydration. A graduated rotating device is useful for checking toric lenses.

Lens size, minimum uncut

When glazing a lens into a frame it is obviously vital that the uncut lens is large enough to occupy the whole of the lens shape. The minimum uncut size necessary depends on the size and shape of the finished lens. If the finished lens is also to be decentred, then this will also affect the smallest uncut, or blank size, from which the finished lens can be cut. This is particularly important in positive power lenses, where it is always desirable to use the minimum sized uncut so that the thinnest and lightest lens is produced.

The method for determining the minimum uncut lens size is given in the following example. A prescription of +6.00DS with 3D base-in prism is required. The patient has chosen a frame that requires the finished lens to be circular with a diameter of 48mm. The prescription must be correct at the centre of this lens. A determination needs to be made of the minimum diameter of a circular uncut lens that is required if the prism were to be produced by decentration (Figure L.11).

First, a calculation is made of the decentration required to give the desired prism:

$P = cF$ (Prentice's rule)

thus

$c = P / F$
$c = -3 / +6 = -0.5 = 5$mm In

To calculate the size of uncut required, consider Figure L.11. In the diagram, the reference point G is the point the patient will look through and is at the centre of the finished lens, which has a radius of 24mm. The optical centre O is decentred 5mm in from G, as calculated above. Thus the optical centre is the centre of a circle of radius 29mm. Therefore, the minimum uncut diameter required is 58mm. In practice, another 2mm or so will be allowed for edging the lens.

In summary, the formula for calculating the minimum uncut lens size is as follows:

Minimum size uncut = maximum visible lens aperture + (2 × decentration) + wastage

Calculation of blank size in this way is often required for exaggerated lens shapes, and in cases where the distance between centres of the frame and the interpupillary distance of the patient differ.

Lens stock
- See *Practice logistics, contact lens*.

Lens supply
- See *Delivery systems, contact lens; Contact lens supply routes*.

Lenticular ophthalmic lenses

A lenticular lens is one in which the aperture containing the prescribed power is smaller than the frame aperture in which it is glazed. They are used for high power positive or negative prescriptions where a full aperture lens would be too thick or heavy. Originally, lenticular lenses were made in cemented form, where the prescription aperture was cemented to a carrier lens. The development of lenticular manufacturing technology closely followed that of bifocals, so that solid and fused glass versions are now available. Currently, the majority of mass-produced products are moulded in plastics material.

The majority of positive powered lenticular lenses are now manufactured in solid form with a circular aperture in plastic materials. The front surface of the aperture is commonly aspheric and has a typical diameter of 40 to 42mm. Spherical surface lenticular lenses commonly have an aperture diameter of 34mm. Blended lenticular lenses are also available where a good cosmetic appearance is required with a large diameter. In this type of lens, the central powered zone is smoothly blended

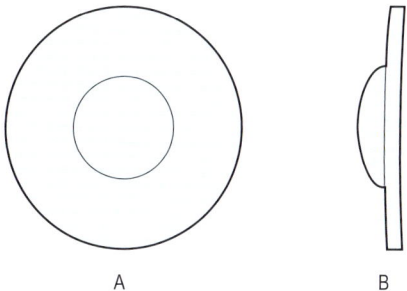

Figure L.12 • Plus lenticular lens form. (A) Plan view of round aperture lenticular. (B) Cross-section cement positive power lenticular.

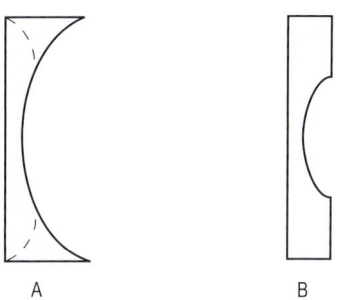

Figure L.13 • Minus lenticular lens form. (A) A flattened lenticular. Edge thickness reduced (to dotted line) by applying convex rear curve. (B) Plano margin lenticular.

into the carrier portion of the lens. Unfortunately the optical properties in the blending zone are very poor (Figure L.12). Positive power lenticulars will have a restricted field of view, unless the wearer makes a head movement.

There is a greater variety in design of negative lenticular lenses, since some of these lenses can be manufactured on conventional lens prescription generators, unlike solid positive power lenticular lenses. The simplest design is the flattened lenticular lens, where a positive power is applied to the periphery of the rear surface in order to reduce the edge thickness. This process can be applied manually to give an aperture similar to the frame aperture (hand flattened) or applied on a generator (machine flattened) where a circular aperture is produced. Lenticular lenses are also produced for negative prescriptions by grinding a negative curve into a nominally plano lens (plano margin lenticular). Blended negative lenticulars are also available where the edge of the powered aperture is smoothed off to improve the cosmetic appearance (Figure L.13). As with the positive blended lenticulars, this gives poor optical quality in the blending zone.

Lenticulation, contact lens

The process of altering lens design to minimize edge thickness in a negative-powered lens, or to minimize centre thickness in a positive-powered lens, is referred to as 'lenticulation'. The general strategy is to reduce the optic zone diameter as much as possible without compromising visual function, and form a thin lenticular supporting rim outside the optic zone. See *High minus power contact lens design; High plus power contact lens design*.

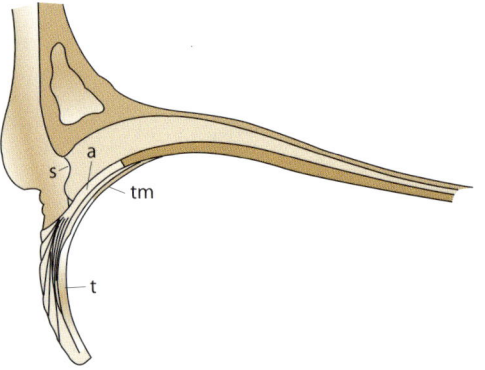

Figure L.14 • Relations of the levator palpebrae superioris. a = levator aponeurosis; tm = superior tarsal muscle (of Müller); t = tarsal plate; s = orbital septum. (Adapted from Gray H, Bannister LH, Berry MM, Williams PJ. In Gray's Anatomy: The Anatomical Basis of Medicine and Surgery, 38th edn. Churchill Livingstone, Edinburgh, 1995.)

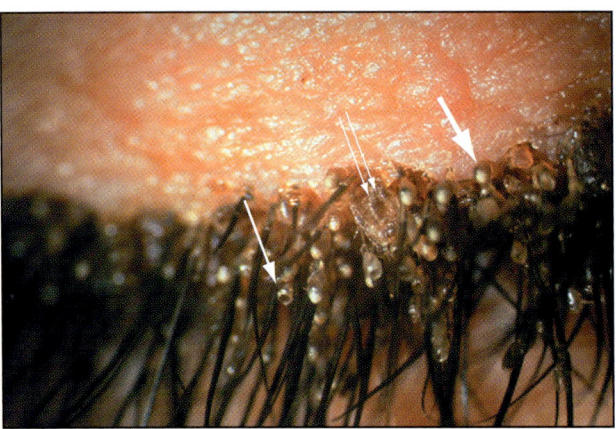

Figure L.15 • Lice infestation of the upper eyelashes. A single louse (double arrow) sits at the base of the lashes surrounded by full (thick arrow) and empty (thin arrow) nit shells.

Levator palpebrae superioris

This muscle is primarily responsible for elevating the upper lid during blinking, and for maintaining an open palpebral aperture. The levator palpebrae arises from the lesser wing of the sphenoid, above and anterior to the optic canal, and runs forward along the roof of the orbit above the superior rectus before terminating anteriorly in a fan-shaped tendon known as the aponeurosis. Some fibres are attached to the anterior surface of the tarsal plate, whilst the remainder pass between fascicles of the orbicularis. The superior palpebral sulcus forms at the upper border of the attachment to the orbicularis (Figure L.14).

Lice

The louse (Phthirus pubis) has two pairs of strong grasping claws on its central and hind legs, allowing it to hold on to eyelashes with considerable tenacity (Figure L.15). Crab louse infestation (phthiriasis) is considered to be a venereal disease because it is passed on by sexual contact, although infestation from contaminated bedding, towels, etc. is another possible mode of transfer.

Signs of phthiriasis include:
- pruritis of the lid margins
- blepharitis
- marked conjunctival injection
- madarosis
- presence of lice
- presence of oval, greyish-white nit shells attached to the base of lashes.

Additional signs include preauricular lymphadenopathy and secondary infection along the lid margins at the site of lice bites. The most predominant symptom is intense itching. The initial course of action is to attempt physically to remove as many mites and mite eggs as possible. Patients should be advised to engage in vigorous lid scrubbing twice daily, using commercially available preparations. In general, contact lens wearers presenting with parasitic infestation of the eyelids should be treated in the same way as similarly infested non-lens-wearers.

Syns. Pubic louse; crab louse.

Lid eversion
- See *Eyelid eversion*.

Lids
- See *Eyelids*.

Life expectancy, contact lens

The life expectancy of high water content soft lenses is 6 months. In the case of rigid lenses, life expectancy is related to material oxygen permeability (Dk). The mean life expectancy of rigid lenses is 20 months for low Dk materials, 16 months for mid-Dk materials, and 9 months for high Dk materials.

Lifestyle
- See *Indications and contraindications for contact lens wear*.

Light levels

Colour vision is present when retinal cone receptors are stimulated in daylight (photopic vision) and in twilight (mesopic vision). Colour vision is absent in the dark when only rod receptors are stimulated (scotopic vision). Photopic vision occurs at luminance levels greater than 3 candelas per square metre and scotopic vision occurs at luminance levels less than 0.001 candelas per square metre. Intermediate levels are described as mesopic and both cones and rods are stimulated. See *Luminance*.

Light meters

There are two types of light meters: those that measure the illumination and those that assess the luminance level.
- An illuminance meter usually consists of a light-sensitive cell, which is connected by an amplifier to a display; the display may be analogue or digital. The light-sensitive cell may consist of a selenium or silicon

Table L.1 • Classification of light sources.

Lamp group	Lamp type	Old code*	New code*
Incandescent	Filament – tungsten, – tungsten halogen	GLS/TH	I/HS
Discharge – Low pressure	Fluorescent (tubular and compact)	MCF	FD/FS
	Low pressure sodium	SOX	LS
Discharge – High pressure	High pressure sodium	SON	S-
	High pressure mercury	MBF	QE
	High pressure metal halide	MBI	M-

*International Lamp Coding System

photo-voltaic cell, although neither of these have a spectral response similar to that of the human visual system. One method of matching the spectral sensitivity of the cell to spectral sensitivity of the eye is to superimpose a coloured filter. This is known as a 'colour-corrected' illuminance meter. The other method is to use correction factors, which are provided by the manufacturer for various light sources. It is also desirable to use a light meter that is 'cosine-corrected'. Ideally, all the light falling on the photocell should be measured, but light falling on the cell at an oblique angle may be reflected and not measured. To reduce these reflections, a transparent hemisphere or diffusing cover is placed over the cell. Illuminance metres measuring illuminances from 0.1 to 100 000lux, i.e. from moonlight to daylight, are available.

- A luminance meter usually consists of an imaging system (some form of small telescope), a photoreceptor, and a display. The imaging system is adjusted so that it forms an image of the object of regard on the photocell. Like the illuminance meter, the photocell must be colour-corrected. Luminance meters that can operate over the range of 10^{-4} to $10^8 cd/m^2$ are available. They can be used for areas varying in size from a few seconds of arc up to a few degrees.

Light sources

There are two basic sources of light – natural daylight and electric (artificial) light. Although daylight appears to have a great advantage over electric light in being free of charge, it does have a major disadvantage in that it is a continually varying source. An electric light source is constant and, provided there is a supply of electricity, it is always available. Daylight, unfortunately, varies in quantity, colour, and direction depending upon the time of day, season, and weather conditions. For example, the range of illuminances can vary from 100,000lux on a bright, sunny day, to 5000lux on an overcast day, to 0.5lux from moonlight. To utilize the available daylight efficiently, large windows are required. When selecting the type of window consideration should be given to:

- the thermal barrier
- the noise barrier
- routine maintenance.

The spectral composition of daylight varies, as do the correlated colour temperatures (CCT) which can vary from 4000K on an overcast day to 40 000K on a clear, bright day; the most common value is about 6000K. Five phases of CCT have therefore been agreed, which represent the typical spectral distribution of irradiances produced by the sun. As the CCT increases, i.e. with clear sky conditions, the blue end of the spectrum becomes more dominant. Correlated colour temperature is the temperature of a full radiator, which emits radiation having a chromaticity nearest to that of the light source being considered; it is measured in degrees Kelvin.

There are 2 main types of artificial light sources, incandescent and discharge (Table L.1). To enable a comparison to be made between the different light sources the following factors can be assessed:

- Luminous efficacy
- Colour properties – colour appearance and colour rendering
- Lamp life.

Lighting levels

The illuminance required for a particular task will depend on many factors, including the size of the detail, the contrast of the detail with its background, the accuracy and speed with which the task must be performed, the age of the worker, etc. Recommendations that take these factors into account are given in the CIBSE Code for Lighting, which provides levels of illuminance for a variety of tasks and occupations. The Code gives a scale of maintained illuminance, which increases as the visual task becomes more difficult (Table L.2). This is the value below which the average illumination on the task should not fall. However, it can be modified if the visual conditions differ from normal.

Modifying factors include visual difficulty, duration of the work, the visual abilities of the worker being below normal, and the consequence of any mistakes. The illumination should be modified by at least one step on the scale of illuminances if the visual conditions are not considered to be normal.

The recommended scale of illuminances is: 20 – 30 – 50 – 75 – 100 – 150 – 200 – 300 – 500 – 750 – 1000 – 1500 – 2000 – 3000 – 5000 lux.

Table L.2 • Example of activities/interiors appropriate for each standard maintained illuminance (CIBSE (1994), reproduced courtesy of the Chartered Institution of Building Services Engineers).

Standard maintained illuminance (lux)	Characteristics of activity/interior	Representative activities/interiors
50	Interiors used rarely with visual tasks confined to movement and casual seeing without perception of detail	Cable tunnels, indoor storage tanks, walkways
100	Interiors used occasionally with visual tasks confined to movement and casual seeing calling for only limited perception of detail	Corridors, changing rooms, bulk stores, auditoria
150	Interiors used occasionally or with visual tasks not requiring perception of detail but involving some risk to people, plant or product	Loading bays, medical stores, plant rooms
200	Interiors occupied for long periods, or for visual tasks requiring some perception of detail	Foyers and entrances, monitoring automatic processes, casting concrete, turbine halls, dining rooms
300†	Interiors occupied for long periods, or when visual tasks are moderately easy, i.e. large details >10min arc and/or high contrast	Libraries, sports and assembly halls, teaching spaces, lecture theatres, packing
500†	Visual tasks moderately difficult, i.e. details to be seen are of moderate size (5–10min arc) and/or high contrast; also colour judgement may be required	General offices, engine assembly, painting and spraying, kitchens, laboratories, retail shops
750†	Visual tasks difficult, i.e. details to be seen are small (3–5min arc) and of low contrast; also good colour judgements or the creation of a well lit, inviting interior may be required	Drawing offices, ceramic decoration, meat inspection, chain stores
1000†	Visual tasks very difficult, i.e. details to be seen are very small (2–3min arc) and can be of very low contrast; also accurate colour judgements or the creation of a well lit, inviting interior may be required	General inspection, electronic assembly, gauge and tool rooms, retouching paintwork, cabinet making, supermarkets
1500†	Visual tasks extremely difficult, i.e. details to be seen extremely small (1–2min arc) and of low contrast; optical aids and local lighting may be an advantage	Fine work and inspection, hand tailoring, precision assembly
2000†	Visual tasks exceptionally difficult, i.e. detail to be seen exceptionally small (<1min arc) with very low contrasts; optical aids and local lighting will be of advantage	Assembly of minute mechanisms, finished fabric inspection

†1 minute of arc (min arc) is 1/60 of a degree. This is the angle of which the tangent is given by the dimension of the task detail to be seen divided by the viewing distance.

A good lighting system must provide suitable lighting for all employees, whatever their task and whatever their age. The recommendations provided are for 40–50 year olds. Older employees require higher levels of illuminance to achieve the same levels of visual efficiency. Therefore, the level of illumination may need to be increased; this is most easily achieved by the use of local lighting. Care must be taken to ensure that this additional lighting does not become a glare source to other employees working in the surrounding area. Older individuals are more sensitive to glare than the young, due to increased light scattering within the eye, and also take longer to adapt from one lighting level to another.

Lighting systems

There are several methods by which a task may be illuminated. The three most common in use are shown in Figure L.17; these are generalized lighting, localized lighting and local lighting.

Generalized lighting systems are designed to provide an approximate average illuminance over the entire working area. This has the advantage of allowing flexibility of work stations, as there is even illumination over the working area. However, energy is wasted because the whole area is illuminated to a level needed for the most critical task. It is therefore more costly than it need be. The luminaires are generally arranged in a regular layout, which is easy to plan using the lumen method of lighting

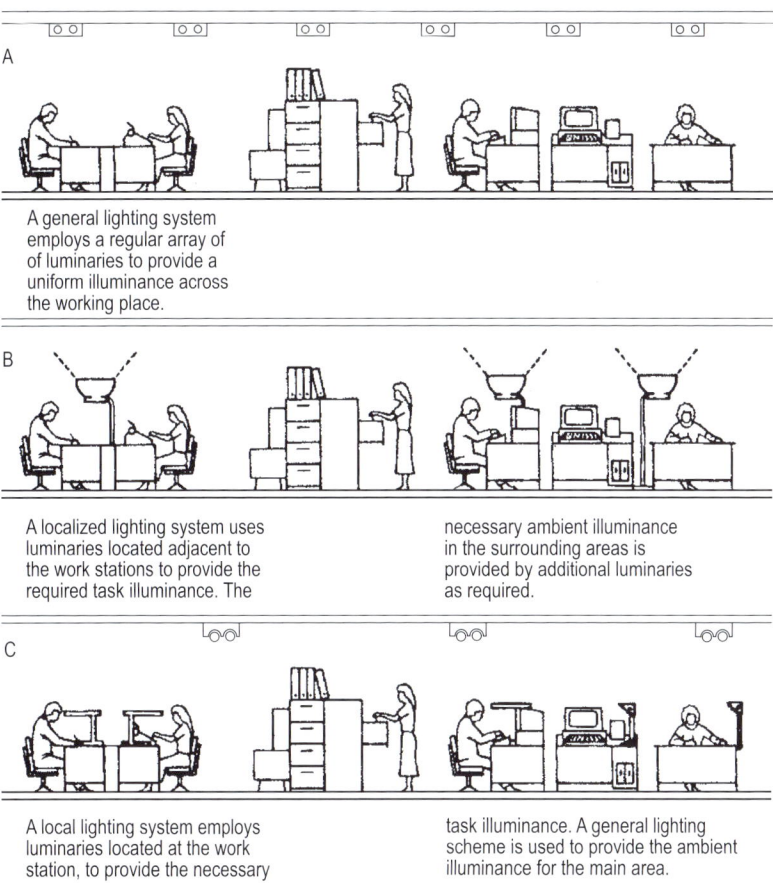

Figure L.16 • Lighting system: (A) general, (B) localized; and (C) local. (Adapted from CIBSE (1994), reproduced courtesy of the Chartered Institution of Building Service Engineers).

A general lighting system employs a regular array of of luminaries to provide a uniform illuminance across the working place.

A localized lighting system uses luminaries located adjacent to the work stations to provide the required task illuminance. The necessary ambient illuminance in the surrounding areas is provided by additional luminaries as required.

A local lighting system employs luminaries located at the work station, to provide the necessary task illuminance. A general lighting scheme is used to provide the ambient illuminance for the main area.

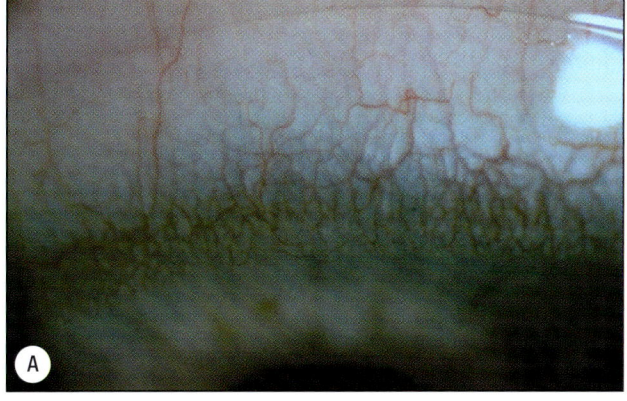
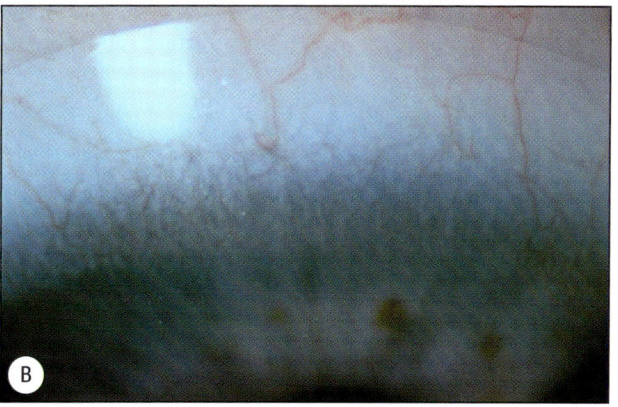

Figure L.17 • (A) Hyperaemia is evident at the superior limbus of a patient wearing a low Dk/t hydrogel lens in one eye, whereas (B) less hyperaemia is evident at the superior limbus of the contralateral eye wearing a high Dk/t silicone hydrogel lens.

design (see below). It is recommended that the uniformity of illuminance over the task area should be not less than 0.7 (ratio of minimum illuminance to average illuminance).

Localized lighting systems are designed to provide the required illuminance on the working surface, together with a lower level of illuminance for other general areas. The difference in illuminance between the task and general areas should be in the ratio of 3:1 or less. Great care must be taken at the design stage of this system to match the lighting to the work stations. If at a later date, the work stations are relocated, there may be a problem with fixed luminaires. This can be overcome if uplighters (stand or desk-mounted) are used, as they can easily be moved to a new location. Localized lighting will generally use less energy but may require more maintenance than generalized systems.

Local lighting systems are comprised of two separate lighting arrangements: one to provide the ambient background lighting and the other to provide supplementary lighting at the task. Local lighting is a very efficient method of providing high task illuminance that can be flexible, directional lighting for detailed tasks. It is also a method whereby additional lighting can be provided at the task, the luminaire usually being mounted at the work station. Care must be taken when positioning the luminaire at the work station so that it does not create veiling reflectances or shadows, or become a glare source for the surrounding workers. Local light should not be placed directly in front of the worker as it will reduce the visibility. The best position is to the left of the work station or desk if the worker is right-handed, so that the reflections will mainly go across the line of sight. For left-handed workers, the local light should be positioned to the right. The task to background illuminance ratio should not be less than 3:1. This system has the advantage of providing the necessary level of lighting; however, the luminaires may be inefficient, rather expensive, and have higher maintenance costs due to increased wear and tear.

The lumen method of lighting design provides for uniform illumination of an area when the luminaires are arranged in a regular layout. If the lighting is to vary over the working area, then the point-by-point method should be used. The lumen method can be used to calculate the average illumination produced by a lighting installation, or the number of luminaires required to achieve the desired illuminance. The light received on a work surface will depend on the direct light and the reflected light. Therefore, when calculating the lighting to be installed to give a certain level of illuminance on the work surface, factors such as room size, reflectance of the surfaces, and type of lamp have to be taken into account. The number of luminaires (N) may be calculated from the equation:

$$N = \frac{E \times A}{F \times n \times MF \times UF}$$

where A is the area of the work surface (m^2), E is the average illuminance on the working surface (lux), F is the lamp luminous flux (lumens), MF is the maintenance factor, n is the number of lamps per luminaire, and UF is the utilization factor.

Limbal redness associated with contact lens wear

Assuming that a given case of eye redness is lens related, it is necessary to determine whether the source of the problem is the cornea or the conjunctiva. Conjunctival redness associated with a quiet limbus and the absence of pain indicates a primary conjunctival problem. Conjunctival redness associated with an injected limbus and corneal pain indicates corneal involvement, or indeed a problem that is related exclusively to the cornea. Careful slit-lamp examination of the anterior ocular structures, and inspection of the lens at high magnification, will generally reveal the cause of the problem. It may also be necessary to prescribe different care systems and differentially diagnose the effects of various solutions over time.

In the absence of any clinically observable ocular pathology, corneal hypoxia is the likely cause of excessive limbal redness (Figure L.18). Hypoxia stimulates the release of inflammatory mediators from the limbal vessel walls, leading to vasodilatation; this is an automatic reaction designed to facilitate a greater flow of oxygenated blood to the distressed tissue. This mechanism fails in the case of the limbus because limbal

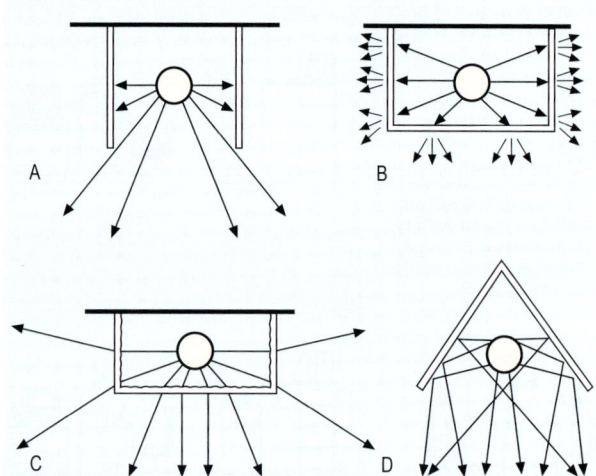

Figure L.18 • Four methods of light control: (A) obstruction, (B) diffusion; (C) refraction; (D) reflection. (Courtesy of the Electricity Association Services Ltd 1990, previously The Electricity Council.)

blood flow contributes little to corneal oxygenation; the cornea derives virtually all of its oxygen supply from the atmosphere. The result, therefore, is contact lens induced hypoxia maintaining chronic limbal vessel engorgement in a vain attempt to re-oxygenate the cornea.

There is a significant relationship between the oxygen transmissibility of the peripheral region of a soft lens and limbal redness. Indeed, one of the key benefits of high-permeability silicone hydrogel lenses is that they induce low levels of limbal redness. Although hypoxia is presumed to be the key determinant of limbal redness, practitioners should be alert to the possibility of other causes, such as poor lens edge design or pathology of the anterior ocular structures – especially the cornea. Recovery from chronic contact lens induced limbal redness after removal of lenses and cessation of wear takes about 7 days.

Syn. limbal hyperaemia, limbal injection.

Lipid deposition on contact lenses

- See *Deposits, contact lens*.

Lipids in tears

- See *Tear lipids*.

Liquid lens

- See *Tear lens beneath a contact lens*.

Lissamine green stain

This is a green dye that can reveal the presence of ocular surface damage in patients with keratoconjunctivitis sicca. It is said to be tolerated better than rose bengal by patients.

Local Optical Committees

Local Optical Committees (LOCs) are local representative committees formed where a primary care trust (PCT) or group of PCTs are satisfied that a committee is representative of the optometrists in their area. The role of the LOC

Table L.3 • The WHO definitions of visual impairment (WHO, 1979).

Category of visual loss	Description	Maximum visual acuity	Minimum visual acuity	Maximum visual field*	Minimum visual field*
0	Normal	6/6	6/18		
1	Low vision – visual impairment	<6/18	6/60		
2	Low vision – severe visual impairment	<6/60	3/60		
3	Blind	<3/60	1/60	≤ 10° around central fixation	>5° around central fixation
4	Blind	<1/60	Light perception	≤ 5° around central fixation	
5	Blind	No light perception	No light perception		
9	Undetermined	Cannot be measured	Cannot be measured		

*Even if central acuity normal

is to provide a local perspective on eye care to the PCT. The administrative costs of the LOC are funded through a statutory levy made on each GOS sight test claim processed.

Representatives of optometrists and dispensing opticians providing ophthalmic services in an area were formally recognized for the first time in the NHS Act 1949. As the General Ophthalmic Services changed and the supply of spectacles was partially deregulated, representation of dispensing opticians by right was excluded from the LOC.

Locator tints
- See *Handling tints for contact lenses*.

Loose contact lens fit
A lens that moves or lags excessively is deemed to be fitting loosely. Loose-fitting lenses can cause peripheral corneal staining, symptoms of discomfort, and variable vision. Patients may also complain of lenses being displaced from the cornea during wear. The first possibility to consider is whether the lens is inside out. Switching to a similar lens of steeper back optic zone radius may not always overcome the problem, particularly with thin lens designs. It may therefore be necessary to change to a lens with a tendency towards tight fitting.

Loveridge grid
- See *Non-invasive tear break-up time*.

Low vision
Low vision is reduced visual acuity, which even with the best refractive correction provided by spectacle or contact lenses still results in a visual performance on a standardized clinical test which is less than that expected for an individual of that age. The definition does not include those who are monocular: these patients have different problems and are rarely considered in this category. The term also implies that some form of vision remains (that is, the ability to recognize shapes, no matter how close they must be placed), and that vision is not simply confined to light perception. Refractive correction in this context includes reading additions up to +4.00DS (an arbitrary threshold of historical origin). The individual with low vision requires various vision enhancement strategies (such as magnification, illumination, or contrast) in order to make the best use of their remaining vision for carrying out practical activities of daily living.

If the visual loss is so severe that the individual can no longer use vision to recognize objects, to read or write, or to navigate or orientate in the environment, then they are functionally blind: such an individual must use sensory substitution in which visual stimuli are replaced by auditory or tactile information (such as books recorded on audiotape, or CD, or transcribed into Braille). To the layperson, blindness is often equated to 'no perception of light', but in reality the dividing line between low vision and blindness is not so precise: many individuals will use both vision enhancement and sensory substitution strategies in their everyday life. The World Health Organization publishes guidelines as to the levels of acuity and visual field which equate to these definitions, and these have become widely accepted in epidemiological surveys (Table L.3). See *Registered visual impairment, visual disability*.

Low vision aids
A low vision aid is any piece of equipment used by a person with low vision in order to enhance their vision. Such aids may be:
- Optical: including hand held, stand mounted and spectacle mounted plus lens magnifiers; and telescopes for distance and intermediate/near viewing.

- Electronic: including closed circuit television systems (CCTVs) (see *Electronic vision enhancement systems*) and specialized computer adaptations (e.g. image enlargement software)
- Non-optical: such as optimization of illumination and contrast; and tints and typoscopes.

Low vision aids, monocular versus binocular use

If the acuities of the two eyes are similar (difference ≤ 2×), it is visually beneficial in most cases to use binocular viewing. If the acuities are unequal, there is unlikely to be any visual advantage in binocular correction, and monocular correction of the better eye will usually be more appropriate. Even if no visual advantage will accrue, the patient may feel a psychological benefit from binocular viewing.

Other advantages of binocular correction are:

- If the low vision aid is spectacle mounted (see *Spectacle-mounted plus lens magnifiers*; *Telescopes, near and intermediate viewing*) binocular mounting can equalize the weight and cosmetic appearance, although may increase cost.
- An occluder can be provided to change to monocular viewing with either eye if binocular viewing later becomes tiring or difficult.
- For a patient with patchy vision loss, the functional field in one eye could theoretically compensate for the missing areas in the other eye: clinical experience suggests that this rarely occurs.

Binocular correction would however be contraindicated if there was:

- very distorted vision in a previously dominant eye which appeared to interfere with the vision of the better fellow eye of the patient. If this eye cannot be suppressed, occlusion must be provided. Sometimes a blurring lens, or a frosted occluder, will suffice, but it may prove necessary to use an opaque black cover.
- too large a convergence demand created by the close working distance, causing discomfort or diplopia.

The design of the magnifying device, or the limitation on viewing conditions which it imposes, may also dictate that viewing must be monocular. The reasons for this must be fully explained to the patient, who must be reassured that ignoring one eye will not cause it to deteriorate, nor will using the fellow eye exclusively cause it to be put under excessive strain.

Hand-held and stand-mounted plus lens magnifiers can rarely be used binocularly, since the (typically) small diameter lenses must be used close to one eye in order to optimize the field of view. They could only be considered for binocular viewing if the lens is of large aperture (and therefore of low power and low magnification) and held at a long eye-to-magnifier distance. If the monocular fields are to overlap, it is also necessary that the lens be placed on the user's midline. This means that each eye views obliquely through the lens and thus experiences greater aberrations than if the lens is directly in front of one eye, whose visual axis coincides with the optical axis of the lens.

Binocular viewing through a magnifying plus lens can be achieved by spectacle mounting the lenses. See *Spectacle mounted plus lens magnifiers*. With the object positioned at the focal point of the lens, the working distance is inevitably short and the convergence demand is great: 1^Δ for every mm of interpupillary distance is required to view an object at a distance of 10cm from the centre of rotation of the eye. Since the lenses are high-powered positive lenses, the amount of base-out prism to be overcome will be increased still further if the lenses are not sufficiently decentred inwards.

It has therefore been suggested that the optical centres of the lenses be decentred further in for near than the visual axes, to create a base-in prismatic effect to help in near viewing. If the decentration is too large to be practical, introducing 1^Δ base-in prism per dioptre of reading add is a possible solution. Despite this, the convergence demand remains high, and it is suggested that +10.00DS (2.5×) is the highest binocular magnification usable by most patients.

Fixed focus telescopes (for both distance and near) are available in binocular and monocular versions. In order to overlap the fields of view of the two eyes, the telescope tubes must have an adjustable interpupillary distance, and be angled (converged) appropriately for the required viewing distance (the tubes of a distance telescope will be parallel to each other). Near telescopes can be used binocularly with higher magnification (≈5×) than spectacle mounted plus lens magnifiers (≈2.5×), because of the increased working space. See *Telescopes, near and intermediate viewing*.

If a telescope has variable focus, it should also have variable angling of the tubes, but this is rarely available in practice. Instead, for Galilean telescopes where the focusing range is more limited, a compromise convergence angle is chosen; whereas for astronomical binoculars the focusing range is artificially restricted (infinity to ≈2m, compared to infinity to ≈20cm with an astronomical monocular).

Low vision assessment

This is a rehabilitative or habilitative process which provides a range of services for people with low vision (and their carers), in timely and easily accessible fashion, in order to enable them to make optimum use of their eyesight to achieve maximum potential. The patient and his/her family should receive:

- advice and information about available services and how to obtain them, and about the eye condition
- psychological and emotional support
- support in understanding the limitations of rehabilitation
- an assessment of visual function, including provision of appropriate low vision aids and training (see *Prescribing magnification*)
- appropriate modification to the home, school, and work environments

The consequences of visual impairment affect many aspects of the patient's life, and it can be seen that care of the patient requires a wide range of expertise in a number of different areas. Such assistance is unlikely to be available from a single professional group, and an interdisciplinary, or multidisciplinary team approach has been implemented in many developed countries. See *Multidisciplinary team, low vision*.

Low vision assessment, paediatric

A major concern for the visually impaired child and their parents is their access to education, and this will be a major consideration when a child attends for assessment. The Children's Act 1989 provides for each child 'in need' to be assessed for any services required. It is not necessary for the child to be registered as visually impaired in order for this to be done. Local Education Authorities (LEAs) identify all children from 2 years of age (up to the age of 19 if they are still in full-time education) who are likely to have 'special educational needs (SEN)'. Regardless of the degree of visual impairment, most children will be educated in mainstream schools (unless they have additional disabilities), although there may be some special arrangements made for them. Examples might include the use of special equipment, a non-teaching classroom assistant with them for part or all of the time, or withdrawal from classes for a few hours each week in order to have special tuition from a peripatetic specialist teacher. If the resources required are beyond the SEN budget of the mainstream school, a statutory assessment involving consultation with medical and educational professionals and parents will take place, following which a 'statement' of the requirements of the child will be drawn up by the LEA. Several professionals are called on to produce reports on the child, and this may include a report by the optometrist on visual performance and the use of low vision aids (LVAs).

The assessment of a child involves several important components:

- Refraction, and determining optimal spectacle correction

The full refractive correction should be determined, and the required wearing time agreed with the child and parents, and communicated to teachers. If there are problems with the spectacles being mislaid, a separate pair may be required to be kept in school. Dispensing multifocals to make close work more comfortable should be considered. To determine the reading add, print of the required size should be held at the preferred distance, ensuring that the print can be read clearly. Plus lenses are then introduced in +0.50DS steps until blurring of the print occurs, and the patient has to bring the reading material closer in order to get it clear. The addition to be prescribed is the highest value that gives clear vision at the preferred working distance.

- Assessment of visual performance

This will allow common-sense guidance to be offered to parents and teachers on the tasks which may cause problems, and any ways in which they may need to be modified. Tests may include: binocular and monocular distance acuity, reading acuity and speed, contrast sensitivity, colour vision, binocular visual field, oculo-motor status, and ocular motility (for investigation of nystagmus).

- Assessment for low vision aids

It has been traditional to expect children to only begin to use LVAs at around 5 to 7 years of age, when they begin to read print: even then, early reading primers are often printed in very large type. Children as young as 2 years of age can, however, benefit, providing they are encouraged to use the aid by their parents. The aid must be introduced in conjunction with meaningful tasks, such as the examination and identification of small objects and pictures. The greatest benefit is often for distance tasks, since these involve objects which the child cannot get close to: very young children may lack the manual dexterity required for efficient telescope use, but a fixed-focus type may be a useful introduction. The benefit of using an LVA at this age is that the child is much less self-conscious and less likely to reject an aid because of the cosmetic appearance, or because it makes them different to their peers; it can therefore become established as part of their life which they will be reluctant to abandon later. At the opposite end of the age range, it is also customary to believe that the secondary school pupil needs to read a blackboard, to access normal print textbooks, and to make handwritten notes. This may be the case, but the use of a classroom assistant to read the board, large print textbooks and a laptop computer are adaptations that may have been made for the child. It is therefore important to know exactly what school activities are to be carried out, with what existing help and equipment, any particular causes for concern, and any plans that the teaching staff have to change the methods of support. This is best achieved by the specialist teacher being encouraged to attend the assessment, along with the parents. If they cannot attend in person it may be possible to request completion of a questionnaire. Alternatively, within a multi-disciplinary clinic, members of the team (such as a rehabilitation officer or orthoptist) may visit the child at school to assess the situation, and have discussions with the teaching staff.

- Follow up and monitoring

If aids appear appropriate, they will only be used successfully if the child is supported in their use. Parents might be asked to spend some time with the child each day using their magnifier: for example, spotting street signs with a telescope as the child is driven to school. A report should be written for the teaching staff explaining what aids have been given and when they should be used, since many different staff may be involved with the child. Awareness training may need to be provided for some mainstream teachers, and for other pupils in the class, to avoid any negative responses to the aids. Aids may well need to be introduced gradually, as in the initial stages the child may work more slowly with normal print and a magnifier than they did with enlarged print. Training in the use of aids is important, and this may be carried out by a suitably trained teacher or classroom assistant, or by a member of the clinic team. See *Low vision training*. This person may be able to return to see the child in school after the assessment to make sure that aids are appropriate, and being used effectively. Information on progress can be fed back to the clinic. It is essential that follow-up can be arranged on demand, since the child's requirements are constantly changing, and aids which are well used often need adjustment or repair. Low vision assessments should remain accessible for children who have rejected aids initially, since new tasks may arise which would require their use.

Low vision, causes and prevalence

On the basis of the definition adopted by the World Health Organization (WHO) (see *Low vision*) it is estimated that there are approximately 45 million blind and 135 million with low vision worldwide. Around 90% of the world's blind live in the developing countries, with 60% in sub-Saharan Africa, China and India. Up to 80% of global blindness is avoidable, however, resulting from conditions that could have been prevented or can be successfully treated. Five conditions have been identified as immediate priorities within the framework of the WHO campaign to tackle preventable blindness called VISION 2020. These are cataract, trachoma, onchocerciasis (river blindness), childhood blindness, refractive errors and low vision. It is recognized that the lack of general and ophthalmological health services, particularly in rural areas, needs to be tackled. In both the developed and developing countries, the prevalence of childhood blindness is only one-tenth of that in the corresponding adult population; however, it is estimated that at least 50% of the children who become blind from causes related to infections (e.g. measles), malnutrition (e.g. Vitamin A deficiency) and neglect, will die within the following 12 months.

In the UK, registration of the visually impaired provides data on the number of such people within the general population. See *Low vision*. Registration is, however, voluntary, and it is likely that only about 25% of over 1 million eligible individuals are actually registered. The visually impaired population is predominantly elderly, with approximately 70% of those registered being over 75 years of age. In the general population, 10% of this age group have low vision and 2% are blind (as defined by the WHO guidelines). Age-related macular degeneration is responsible for over 50% of all registrations: cataract does not feature heavily because although it is very common in the elderly population, treatment will usually be rapid and successful and no permanent impairment will result. In younger adults, major causes are diabetic retinopathy and genetic conditions such as retinitis pigmentosa. For children, prenatal factors (including genetic causes) are involved in the majority of cases, and in only about 10–20% does the cause appear to arise later than the perinatal period: just over 50% of visually impaired children have additional disabilities.

Low vision devices
- See *Low vision aids*.

Low vision service
- See *Low vision assessment*.

Low vision services committees

In 1999 in the UK, a framework document was produced by the Low Vision Services Consensus Group, which represented professional bodies, patient organizations and charities working with the visually impaired. The document described the basic elements of a good quality low vision service and suggested how the service might be delivered. It recognized that a multidisciplinary team approach would offer the best service, but did not offer precise guidelines on how the service would operate, believing that this should be arranged individually in each locality, so that the most appropriate use could be made of existing expertise and facilities. The report recommended establishing a Low Vision Services Committee (LVSC) in each area which could ensure the delivery of a service which matched the specifications laid down in the document, and could monitor the effectiveness of that service. See *Outcome measures, low vision*. In England the LVSC have been formed under the auspices of Primary Care Trusts and/or Health Authorities, in partnership with Social Services. In addition, members are drawn from professionals working in the field, hospital trusts, voluntary organizations, and, perhaps most importantly, the users of the service. Once the document had been published, the Consensus Group became an Implementation Group and appointed an Implementation Officer whose role has been to advise on, and encourage, the setting up of the network of LVSC needed to cover the whole of the UK.

Low vision training

Low vision training is any individually tailored tuition in the use of vision or low vision aids. Such training may include:

- Training in the use of vision such as using discernible visual landmarks for orientation, or adopting different eye movement techniques for locating objects or reading (see *Eccentric viewing and steady eye strategy*)
- Training in the adaptation of the environment such as optimizing illumination and avoiding glare, or using contrast
- Training in the use of low vision aids such as how to position a magnifier and optimize field of view. This is probably the most significant aspect of training for the majority of patients.

The professional responsible for training (see *Multidisciplinary team, low vision*) has a pivotal role in extending the ability demonstrated in the clinic into the patient's home, work or school environment. It is clear that satisfying acuity requirements does not necessarily guarantee effective and sustained use of an aid. The optimum method of use of an aid is rarely obvious, and the patient needs to practise applying the aid to the particular task in which they are interested. It is probably the failure to appreciate this which has contributed to significant numbers of patients never using the magnifier they were given.

If full task-related training in the use of the aid is not available or appropriate, complete verbal instructions should be given to the patient, and to any carer accompanying the patient, perhaps backed up by written instructions in large print. Note which spectacles to use with the magnifier (see *Spectacle correction, telescopes; Spectacle correction, plus lens magnifier*), the working distance required, which eye to use, and what the magnifier can and cannot be used for. Emphasize how the illumination should be arranged, how to clean and care for the magnifier, how to change bulbs and batteries (if appropriate), and how to contact the clinician if any difficulties are experienced. The patient must then have the opportunity to attend for a follow-up visit within a short period of time, so that any difficulties can be resolved.

Lubricants

- See *Re-wetting solutions, soft contact lens; Wetting solutions, rigid contact lens*.

Lumen method of lighting design

- See *Lighting design*.

Luminaires

Most light sources emit light in all directions, but this can be wasteful and cause visual discomfort. The function of most luminaires is to:

- redistribute the light from the lamp in preferred directions with the minimum of loss
- reduce glare from the source
- be acceptable in appearance and, in some cases, make a definite contribution to the decor
- provide support, protection, and electrical connection to the lamp.

Four methods of light control commonly used are: obstruction, diffusion, refraction and reflection (Figure L.18):

- Obstruction: The lamp is surrounded by an opaque enclosure with a limited size aperture. An example of this type is a downlighter in a refined metal tube with an open bottom.
- Diffusion: The lamp is enclosed by a translucent material, which increases the apparent size of the light source. This will reduce the brightness of the source. Most diffusers also absorb light, with as much as 60% being lost. The diffusion is achieved by: (a) ribbing or stippling a specular reflector; (b) providing a glass cover of diffusing material, such as acid-etched or sand-blasted glass; or (c) translucent glass or a plastic filter.
- Refraction: This technique uses numerous prisms to deviate the rays of light and redirect them in the direction required. The luminaire is generally made of glass or plastics and is highly suitable for general office lighting as it combines good glare control with reasonable efficiency.
- Reflection: This technique makes use of reflecting surfaces, which may vary from a matt finish to a highly polished one. This type of luminaire is very efficient, as all the light can be directed where required. This is one of the oldest methods of controlling light and is seen in vehicle headlights, which have highly specular reflectors.

The methods described above are often combined in one luminaire. For example, a reflecting plate may be used above a lamp whilst prismatic controllers are used at the sides and below. The Standard that covers most of the luminaires in the UK is BSEN60 598.

Luminance

Luminance is the intensity of light emitted or reflected in a given direction per projected area of a luminous or reflecting surface. Luminance is expressed in candelas per square metre. For a matt surface the relationship is:

Luminance = Illuminance x reflectance

It should be noted that the terms 'luminance' and 'brightness' have similar meanings; however, the objectively measured photometric quantity should be referred to as luminance. For physiological purposes, the following approximate luminance ranges are recognized:

- scotopic conditions: 10^{-6} to 10^{-3} cd/m^2
- mesopic conditions: 10^{-3} to 3 cd/m^2
- photopic conditions: >3 cd/m^2.

Luminous efficacy

The amount of light given by a lamp for each watt of power consumed. It is measured in lumens/watt. It is important to note that a discharge lamp cannot normally be operated directly from a mains electricity supply unless it has control gear to stabilize the lamp current. This control gear also consumes energy and, therefore, the efficiency of the discharge lamp circuit depends on the power taken by both lamp and control gear.

Luminous flux

The quantity of light emitted from a light source or received by a surface is expressed in units of lumens (lm). This is a measurement of the rate of flow of luminous energy, which is more commonly called the luminous flux (F).

Luminous intensity

This is a measure of the capacity of a source or illuminated surface to emit light in a given direction. It is the luminous flux emitted in a very narrow cone containing the given direction divided by the solid angle of the cone. Luminous intensity (I) is expressed in candelas (cd). One candela is equal to one lumen per steradian:

$I = lm/sr$ (Figure L.19)

If a source emits the same luminous flux in all directions, its luminous intensity is uniform in all directions. However, for most sources the flux is not the same in all directions. A spotlight, for example, may have a luminous intensity of 2000cd at the centre of the beam but, if it were angled, the intensity directed downwards may be reduced to only 200cd. Applying the inverse square law to the spotlight when directed downwards on to a surface 2m below, the illuminance will be:

$E = I/d^2 = 2000/2^2 = 500$ lux

where I is intensity (cd) and d = distance (m). This law applies to light striking a surface at right angles. However, if the surface is tilted or turned so that the rays hit it at an angle, the illuminated surface will increase in size and the illuminance will decrease. The ratio of the

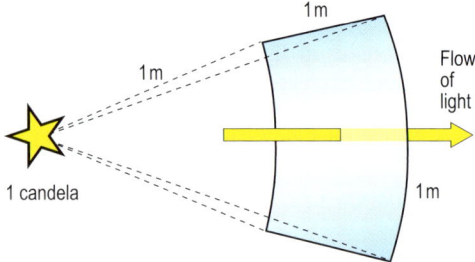

Figure L.19 • Luminous intensity. One lumen is the flow of light through an area of one square meter on a surface of a sphere of one metre radius with a point source of one candela at its centre (Courtesy of the Electricity Association Services Ltd and the Lighting Industry Federation Ltd 1986).

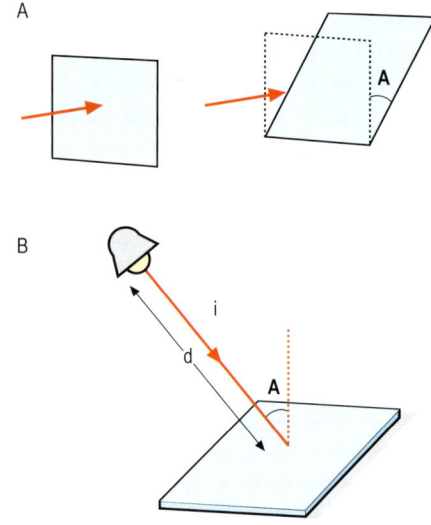

Figure L.20 • (A) the effect upon the illuminance of tilting a surface. (B) Inverse Square Law and the Cosine Law (adapted from the Thorn Lighting Technical Handbook, courtesy of Thorn Lighting Ltd.).

originally illuminated area to the new area is equal to the cosine of the angle through which the surface has been tilted. The illuminance will decrease by the factor of the cosine of the angle. This is known as the Cosine Law of Illuminance. For example, if a surface originally illuminated to 200 lux is tilted through an angle of 60 degrees, the illuminance will be reduced by half, to 100 lux, because the cosine of 60 degrees is 0.5 (Figure L.20A).

The Cosine Law can be combined with the Inverse Square Law (Figure L.20B), thus:

$$E = \frac{I \cos A}{d^2}$$

This equation can be used for one or more light sources provided the total illuminance at a point is the sum of the illuminance by the individual sources; this is known as the point-by-point method.

MacAdam ellipses
- See *CIE chromaticity diagram 1931*.

MacBeth easel lamp
- See *Standard illuminants*.

Macular degeneration, age-related

Age-related macular degeneration (AMD) is the most common cause of irreversible vision loss in people over 50 years of age in western countries. Loss of central vision in AMD occurs following the deposition of material in Bruch's membrane, beneath the retinal pigment epithelium (RPE). The material is manifest clinically as drusen, which is a sub-retinal pale yellow deposition located mainly in the posterior pole area (Figure M.1). Vision is not affected unless there is an associated loss of pigment and atrophy of the RPE, degeneration of the choriocapillaris and photoreceptor atrophy. Ultimately a geographic atrophy may develop. Less commonly, (in only 10–15% of patients), choroidal neovascularization (CNV) may develop and grow through defects in Bruch's membrane into the sub-RPE or sub-retinal spaces. CNV carries the likelihood of leakage leading to RPE detachment, sub-retinal haemorrhage or lipid, and ultimately disciform scarring and central blindness. A vascular basis for AMD has been suggested in several studies, with associations having been documented between AMD and systemic conditions such as hypertension, cerebrovascular disease, atherosclerosis and serum cholesterol level. AMD may reflect systemic conditions as well as local processes, as evidenced by a higher mortality rate in patients with age related maculopathy (ARM; see below). Underlying mechanisms proposed for these associations have included effects on the choroidal circulation and lipid deposition within Bruch's membrane.

In the early stages of AMD patients may note slight distortion in their vision (metamorphopsia), or blurring in their vision. The hallmark of AMD is the presence of drusen. The small hard drusen are usually considered innocuous and a normal part of aging. Their size is comparable to the width of the smaller retinal blood vessels.

AMD can be classified as follows:

1. Normal: minimal or no drusen

2. Mild: multiple small hard drusen (< 63µm), non-extensive intermediate drusen (63–124µm) or pigmentary changes. If vision is unaffected, this form of the condition may be termed Age Related Maculopathy (ARM).

3. Moderate: extreme intermediate drusen, any large drusen (= 125µm) or non-central geographic atrophy without advanced AMD. The intermediate and large drusen are often termed soft drusen.

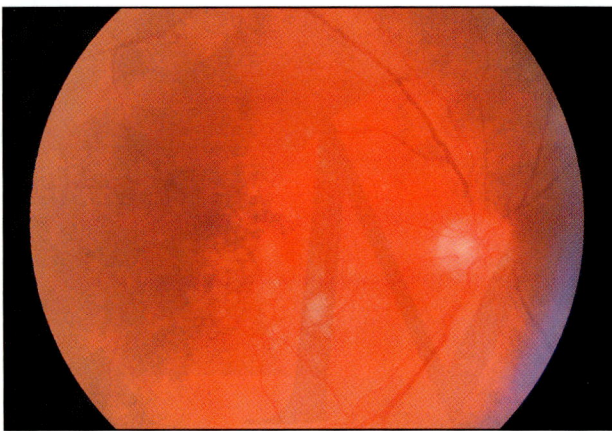

Figure M.1 • Drusen in moderate age-related macular degeneration.

4. Advanced: choroidal neovascularization, other exudative maculopathy, or geographic atrophic maculopathy in one eye but not the other eye. These forms of AMD carry a high risk of sudden, severe central vision loss.

5. The most severe form of AMD is bilateral advanced AMD. Only 10 to 15 per cent of affected patients progress to exudative AMD; however, this form of the condition is responsible for up to 90 per cent of the associated severe vision loss. In more than 40 per cent of patients with exudative AMD, the condition becomes bilateral within five years.

AMD is the leading cause of vision loss in the developed world. The Blue Mountains Eye Study showed the prevalence of AMD in an Australian population to be about 2 per cent, with a significant increase in prevalence over 65 years of age. There is a similar incidence in males and females.

Currently, there are no available therapies for AMD that are proven to restore the visual acuity of the patient. However some strategies are designed to reduce the risk of progression. Patients should be encouraged to consume fruit on a daily basis (3 or more servings per day) and to give up smoking. Smoking is thought to be a risk factor for the development of AMD due to oxidative stress, the promotion of atherosclerosis or some other mechanism. The antioxidants vitamins C (500mg), E (400IU), and beta carotene (15mg) as well as zinc oxide (80mg) afford some reduction in the risk of progressing to advanced AMD in patients with intermediate AMD. Cholesterol lowering medication may also be beneficial, but the effect is not considered proven.

Fluorescein angiography is used to diagnose CNV and to direct treatment. The composition of a CNV lesion is classified on the fluorescein angiography appearance as either classic (showing a well-demarcated hyperfluorescence in the early phase) or occult (poorly demarcated boundaries with late progressive hyperfluorescence). Indocyanine green (ICG) angiography is a technique that displays the choroidal rather than the retinal circulation and may further assist the retinal specialist to localize the lesion.

The two established treatments that stabilize vision and limit severe vision loss in patients with CNV are argon laser photocoagulation, and more recently, verteporfin photodynamic treatment. Argon laser treatment is mainly used for extra-foveal CNV, as treatment of foveal lesions adversely affects vision. Argon laser treatment may be beneficial for extrafoveal lesions, particularly in eyes with poorer initial visual acuity and smaller lesions. Verteporfin photodynamic treatment (PDT) allows treatment at the fovea, increasing the proportion of patients eligible for treatment to between 25 and 40 per cent. PDT has been shown to significantly decrease visual loss in patients with predominantly classic CNV in the macular area. However, even with laser treatment, there is a high risk of the recurrence of membrane growth and the need for re-treatments.

Macular pigment

Macular pigment permeates the neural layers of the macular area of the retina and is a mixture of two carotenoids, zeathanin and lutein. These pigments have similar absorption spectra with peaks near 460nm. Pigment concentration varies individually by more than a factor of 10 (1 log unit) and is a major source of normal variation in threshold short wavelength ('blue') sensitivity. Macular pigment is thought to provide some protection against the development of age-related macular degeneration which is a major cause of blindness in the elderly. Macular pigment does not normally change with age but research is progressing towards enhancing pigment density in older people through lutein-rich dietary supplements. Macular pigment subtends 5–10 degrees horizontally and 3–5 degrees vertically and can be demonstrated as a subjective entoptic phenomenon known as 'Maxwell's spot'.

Maddox rod

Despite the name, the Maddox rod is a flat, red transparent optical element into which a series of parallel grooves are engraved. This is placed in front of one eye while the gaze of both eyes is directed toward a distant bright spot of light. The Maddox rod causes a long red streak of light to be imaged on the retina, with the red streak being parallel to the cylindrical striations. Since the eye behind the Maddox rod cannot see any of the surroundings apart from the red streak, the eyes are effectively dissociated and will adopt their passive position. If the optical axes are perfectly aligned, the red streak will appear to run through the spot of light. If the patient has a distance phoria, the red streak will appear to one side of the red streak. The necessary amount of horizontal prism can be introduced in front of the Maddox rod to cause the red streak and spot of light to be coincident; the amount of prism used is a measure of the degree of heterophoria. The Maddox rod can also be used to measure the degree of vertical phoria or cyclophoria.

Maddox wing

The Maddox wing is a hand-held device that is used to measure the degree of heterophoria at near. The device consists of a septum to dissociate the two eyes and a separate slit aperture for each eye. One eye sees a graduated vertical and horizontal scale, calibrated to

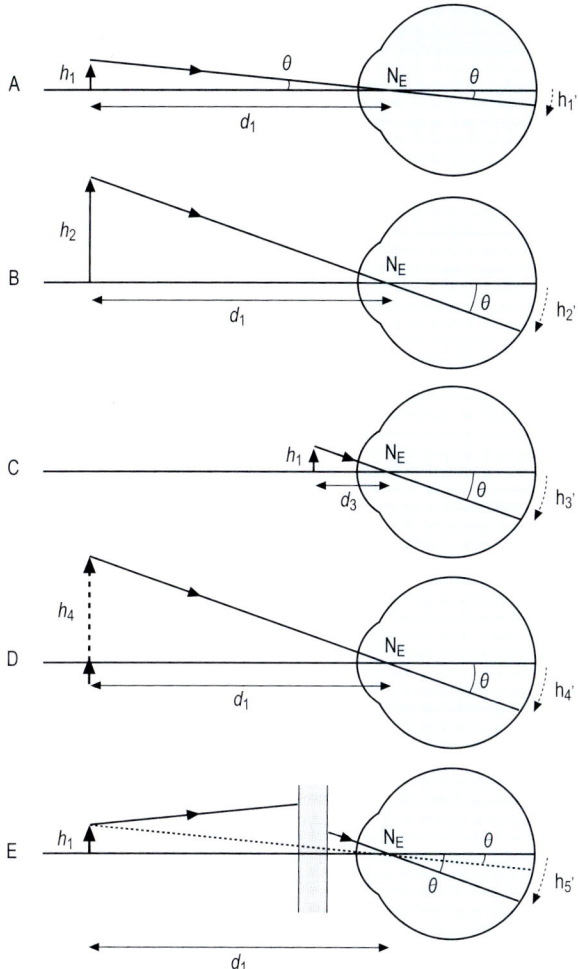

Figure M.2 • A schematic representation of the retinal image size created by (A) an unmagnified object, in comparison to (B) to (E) which illustrate the four alternative ways to magnify the retinal image: (B) increasing the object size, (C) decreasing the viewing distance, (D) real image or transverse magnification; (E) telescopic magnification.

read in prism dioptres, and the other eye sees a white arrow pointing upward and a red arrow pointing horizontally. Fusion is avoided because the eyes are viewing very different images; the eyes therefore adopt the passive position. The patient reports the numbers at which the arrows are pointing, giving a direct measure of the degree of vertical and horizontal phoria. The name Maddox wing derives from the wing-like appearance of the device.

Magnification for low vision

If a low-vision patient cannot resolve the retinal image, despite the fact that it is optimally focused onto the retina by refractive correction, then it is necessary for it to be made larger. From Figure M.2 it can be seen that the angles subtended at the nodal point of the eye by rays of light from the object and the image are always the same: that is, the ray of light from the top of the object passes straight through the nodal point without deviation, and forms the top of the image. Figure M.2A represents the situation before any magnifying device is introduced. It can be seen that the retinal image size is proportional to the angle subtended at the nodal point, and if there is to be an increase in the retinal image size then this ray of light must form a larger angle at the nodal point of the eye.

The most important point to be made concerning magnification is that it is relative: it is the ratio comparing the situation before and after some change in the viewing environment, or perhaps with and without some optical appliance. In mathematical terms:

Magnification (M) = 'new' retinal image size/'old' retinal image size

Figure M.2A shows the situation 'before' magnification, with the retinal image size proportional to θ, the angle subtended by the object at the nodal point of the eye (N_E). Figures M.2B to M.2E show the situation 'after' the different forms of magnification have been used, with the magnified retinal image size proportional to the new angle θ' subtended at the nodal point of the eye.

There are four ways in which magnification can be achieved:
1. Increase object size (Figure M.2B)

M = new object size/old object size = h_2/h_1

The most common example of the use of this type of magnification is in large print books, and the magnification available can be determined very simply by a direct measurement of the size of a letter in the large print sample compared to one in a sample of normal print.

2. Decrease viewing distance (Figure M.2C)

M = old object distance/new object distance = d_1/d_3

One of the simplest ways to magnify is by decreasing the viewing distance. This is also sometimes called 'approach magnification' or 'relative distance magnification'. A change in the viewing distance for watching television from 3m to 1m would give 3× magnification, for example. The method is equally applicable to near vision, where moving the reading task from the typical 30cm to 5cm, for example, would give 6× magnification. The disadvantage now is that such a viewing distance will make too great an accommodative demand. A simple plus lens can allow the viewer to bring the object closer without any accommodative demand, since if the object is placed at the focal point of the plus lens, a virtual image is created at optical infinity. This is the principle of all plus-lens magnifiers.

3. Real image or transverse magnification (Figure M.2D)

In contrast to the virtual image above, this method creates a real image in approximately the same location as the original object, and its size can actually be measured directly (with a millimetre scale) from the face of the magnifying device. This is typical of the situation with a closed-circuit television (CCTV) system where an image of the object is created on a television screen. This is then compared to the size of the original object to determine the magnification. So,

Table M.1 • Characteristics of the four available forms of magnification.

Type of magnification	Characteristics		
	Field of view	Working space	Distance of task
Increase size	No change	No change	N, and some I
Decrease distance	No change	Decreased	D, I or N
(created by plus-lens magnifier)	Decreased	Decreased	N only
Real image	Decreased	No change	D, I or N
Telescopic	Decreased	No change	D, I or N

D, distance; I, intermediate; N, near

M = size of real image/size of object = h_4/h_1

4. Telescopic magnification (Figure M.2E)

In this case

M = angle subtended at eye by telescope image/angle subtended at eye by object

This is potentially the most versatile of any of the methods of magnification, since it does not involve any change in the object or the viewing distance. Unfortunately, the optical system of the telescope presents considerable practical difficulties, which make it not so widely used as might be expected from a simple consideration of this magnification formula. Of the many different types of magnification and magnifying devices which are available, each falls into one of these four different categories and their characteristics are summarized in Table M.1.

Different types of magnification can be used in combination with each other, and the total magnification created is the product of the two individual values. Consider the example of a patient trying to read print with a letter size of 5mm directly from the page, without magnification, at a distance of 40cm. The patient then views the same print magnified to a size of 50mm on the screen of a CCTV monitor, at a distance of 20cm. This patient is combining 'real image' magnification (M_1) with 'relative distance' magnification (M_2), so taking each in turn:

M_1 = size of real image/size of object
= 50mm/5mm = 10x
M_2 = old object distance/new object distance
= 40cm/20cm = 2x

The combined magnification is:

$M_{TOTAL} = M_1 \times M_2 = 10 \times 2 = 20x$

so the retinal image of the letters viewed on the screen from the closer distance is 20× the size of the original image of the letters viewed direct from further away.

Mail order
- See *Contact lens supply routes*.

Manufacturing tolerances, contact lens
- See *Appendix G; Contact lens manufacturing tolerances*.

Map-dot-fingerprint dystrophy
- See *Recurrent erosion syndrome, therapeutic contact lenses for*.

Mast cell stabilizers

Mast cells are large and abundant and present in many body tissues, including the conjunctiva. They play a crucial role in the pathogenesis of allergic conjunctivitis, a condition that affects approximately 25% of the US population. When an airborne allergen such as pollen or dust contacts the eye of an allergic individual, it crosses the conjunctival epithelium and initiates a chain of events that leads to degranulation of mast cells and the release of chemical mediators including histamine, eosinophil chemotactic factor and tryptase.

Mast cell stabilizers are agents that stop the influx of calcium ions across the cell membrane inhibiting degranulation and reducing the release of histamine, which is the primary mediator of early-phase symptoms of itching and conjunctival hyperaemia. They may also be effective against other cells involved in the inflammatory process such as macrophages and eosinophils; these mediators are responsible for the late phase of an allergic response, which occurs from 2 to 24 hours after exposure to an antigen.

Mast cell stabilizers act prophylactically and their level needs to accumulate over several days or weeks before they become effective. Patients with seasonal allergic conjunctivitis should, therefore, institute use of a mast cell stabilizer several weeks prior to expected exposure to an allergen – for example, in the spring season. In the treatment of this condition, mast cell stabilizers need to be continued as a course of treatment until the autumn even if the symptoms have abated.

Mast cell stabilizers are less effective than antihistamines in alleviating the symptom of itching so the simultaneous use of both types of drug may be necessary. If treatment commences with both an antihistamine and a mast cell stabilizer, the former can be discontinued after one or two weeks as the latter becomes effective.

Examples of mast cell stabilizers are:
- Sodium cromoglicate (formerly 'glycate') – this drug was originally used in the treatment of asthmatic patients who required bronchodilation but in whom

Table M.2 • Mast cell stabilizers: preserved multidose preparations.			
Non-proprietary name	**Proprietary name**	**Formulation**	**Preservative**
Lodoxamide trometamol	Alomide®	Drops 0.1% as solution	Benzalkonium chloride 0.07%
Nedocromil sodium	Rapitil®	Drops 2%	Benzalkonium chloride*
Sodium cromoglicate	Opticrom™ Aqueous Eye Drops	Drops 2%	Benzalkonium chloride*

* with disodium edetate

steroid therapy was considered to be inappropriate. Sodium cromoglicate eye drops for treatment of acute seasonal and perennial allergic conjunctivitis are available under several proprietary names and can be purchased over-the-counter from a pharmacy. These can be used at a low dose on a 'long-term' basis throughout the season of high pollen count.
- Lodoxamide – this drug may have an additional anti-allergic benefit by acting as an eosinophil inhibitor. It may also be used on a 'long-term' basis. Lodoxamide has a faster onset of action than sodium cromoglicate and is licensed for the treatment of allergic conjunctivitis only.
- Nedocromil sodium – like sodium cromoglicate, this drug is also used in the treatment of asthma. In addition to stabilizing mast cells, nedocromil sodium is also effective against other cells involved in the inflammatory process, macrophages and eosinophils. It is approved for use in the treatment of seasonal and perennial allergic conjunctivitis and vernal keratoconjunctivitis.

Examples of mast cell stabilizer preparations are shown in Table M.2.

Although it is unlikely that patients would wish to wear hydrogel contact lenses while suffering from vernal conjunctivitis, seasonal allergic rhinoconjunctivitis or allergic conjunctivitis, they should be cautioned that mast cell stabilizer eye drops are preserved with benzalkonium chloride. The lenses could be inserted 15min after each instillation of the drops. Transient burning and stinging can occur as side effects of the use of each of these mast cell stabilizers. Patients using nedocromil may experience a distinctive taste.

Ketotifen and olopatadine are antihistamine agents (see *Antihistamine drugs*) that have the additional capability of stabilizing mast cells.

Materials, soft contact lens
- See *Hydrogel polymers*.

McMonnies dry eye questionnaire
- See *Dry eye questionnaire*.

Mechanical properties, soft contact lens

In its dehydrated state, polyHEMA is hard and brittle (as are most other hydrogel-forming polymers). In this way it resembles PMMA. When swollen in water, however, it becomes soft and rubber-like, with a very low tear and tensile strength. This lack of mechanical strength has a profound effect on the life expectancy of the lens, which caused significant problems before the advent of disposability and planned replacement. Although water content has a marked effect on mechanical strength within a given family of materials, the chemical structure of the polymer also plays a large part. This point is illustrated by comparing the strength of synthetic hydrogels such as polyHEMA with that of natural composite hydrophilic gels, such as articular cartilage, intervertebral discs and the cornea. Cartilage has a tensile strength more than 10 times greater than that of polyHEMA, despite having double the water content (around 80%).

The elastic behaviour and rigidity of hydrogels is closely governed by monomer structure and effective cross-link density, which includes not only covalent cross-link forces but also ionic, polar and steric interchain forces. By use of modified monomer combinations and cross-linking agents, high water content polymers with good stability and elasticity can be prepared. The currently available commercial high water content lenses are vastly superior in strength to the first generation of fragile gels of similar water content based on HEMA-NVP co-polymers. As a general rule, increasing water content reduces durability, particularly resistance to tearing; however, these considerations are of little significance when lenses made from such materials are only intended to last a matter of days or weeks. See *Young's modulus*.

Medical Devices Directive

In Europe, the control of contact lenses and contact lens care products is regulated by the European Medical Devices Directive (EMDD). This directive sets out requirements to which each device must conform. There are thousands of medical devices covered by the directive. The associated trade must devise appropriate management mechanisms to ensure the conformity of its products. Devices conforming to the directive should carry the European standard CE mark ('CE' stands for the French expression 'Commission Européenne'). Since June 1998, it has been illegal to either sell or buy a contact lens in Europe if it does not have the CE mark affixed to it.

The CE marks are dispensed through what are called Notified Bodies. Companies wishing to affix the CE mark to their products must be registered as an approved manufacturer with a Notified Body, which will provide them with authority to use the mark. In order to get on the approved list of a Notified Body, manufacturers of contact lenses are generally required to have implemented a quality system, typically ISO 9002, and then applied the medical device-specific CE requirements in the form of a further layer of bureaucratic controls set out in EN 46002. This procedure has become the de facto approach used by UK contact lens manufacturers who have obtained the CE mark for their products, and looks set to be the normal pathway to complying with the regulations. A principal activity of the Notified Bodies is to audit the device manufacturer to make sure that the procedures in use are such that devices made in the system comply with the directive.

Medication with contact lenses

Unpreserved unit-dose eye drops are indicated for concurrent use with soft lenses. Preserved eye drops are rarely used in this situation because of concerns that preservatives such as benzalkonium chloride can accumulate in the lens and be toxic to the corneal epithelium. This effect is usually of no clinical importance when disposable lenses are used for short periods. All topical drugs may be used with rigid lenses – both corneal and scleral. It is not known whether drugs achieve suitable concentrations in the ocular tissues when sealed scleral lenses are being worn. Ointment preparations should not be used concurrently with contact lenses.

Medicines Act 1968 (UK)

In January 1978, the Government published the long-awaited statutory instruments bringing into force Part III of the Medicines Act 1968, and announced that the regulations would become effective from 1 February 1978. Such was the extent of the change made in these orders, however, that a further Order was made later, postponing certain of the provisions for 6 months to give the pharmaceutical industry and the pharmacy profession sufficient time to come to terms with the new regulations. The new regulations provided the optometrist with a legal right to supply, as well as use, an even greater range of drugs than before.

The Medicines Act 1968 is divided into eight parts, containing in all 136 sections and eight schedules. Part I of the Act deals with administration; s.2 sets up the Medicines Commission, consisting of not fewer than eight members, representing medicine, veterinary medicine, pharmacy, pharmaceutical industry and chemistry.

The 45 sections of Part II deal with the licensing of the manufacture, import, export and wholesale of medicinal products. No person may manufacture or assemble or wholesale any product unless he has a licence to do so. Such a blanket law is, of course, subject to many exemptions.

The most important sections as far as the optometrist is concerned are included in Part III, which deals with the sale or supply of medicinal products.

Section 51 allows the Minister to set up a General Sale List of drugs which can be reasonably sold without the supervision of a pharmacist. All drugs not on this list may be sold only by a person lawfully conducting a retail pharmacy business or on premises registered as a pharmacy and under the supervision of a pharmacist (s.52). This restriction had been applied previously by including a substance in Part I of the Poisons List, when a sale could be made only by an authorized seller of poisons. Now, paradoxically, it is the non-inclusion of a substance in a list that brings this restriction into force. A very important rider which begins s.52 is 'subject to any exemption conferred by or under this part of the Act', since it allows certain substances to be sold other than at a pharmacy, even if they are not included on a General Sale List.

Further restrictions are imposed under s.58, which allows for the setting up of another list of medicinal substances called the Prescription Only List. Under subs. (2) medicines on the Prescription Only List can be supplied only in accordance with a prescription issued by an appropriate practitioner (a term defined in subs. (1) as being doctors, dentists or veterinarians).

Nowhere in the Act are specific medicinal substances listed. The inclusion of substances in the General Sale List or in the Prescription Only List is the subject of the various Orders brought into effect on 1 February 1978 and subsequently revised. Principal among these are the General Sale List and the Prescription Only List.

The main features of the three lists included in the Medicines Act are as follows:

- General Sale List – this is a list of human and veterinary drugs defined by section 51 of the Medicines Act, and contains the common (and some not so common) medicinal substances which can be sold other than at a pharmacy. Provided that s.53 is complied with, an optometrist may sell any substance on the General Sale List. Schedule 6 of the Order (SI 1977/2129) however, lists medicinal products which are not on the General Sale List and includes products marketed as eye drops or eye ointments. Thus, all eye drops, whether for human or for animal use, are not on general sale even though the active principle is included in the list.
- Prescription Only List – many of the drugs commonly in use by optometrists are included in Schedule 1 of the Prescription Only List. Even though the schedule exempts many of these drugs from the class of prescription only when they are applied externally, local ophthalmic use is often excluded from the exemption. For example, atropine is prescription only unless applied externally by a route other than to the eye. It can be seen that eye drops and eye ointment have been singled out for special attention both in their exclusion from the General Sale List and in the external application exemption from the Prescription Only List.
- Pharmacy List – this is a catch all list and any preparation that does not appear on the General Sale List or the Prescription Only List lists is automatically covered by the Pharmacy list as defined by section 52 of the Medicines Act. All drugs included on this list would normally be sold or supplied from a registered pharmacy under the supervision of a registered pharmacist. In the case of a Pharmacy List medicine that is an eye drop or ointment, it can be used and supplied by an optometrist – supply being by way of a signed order for presentation to a pharmacist.

It can be seen that the effect of the legislation was to increase the range of drugs that the optometrist may use and supply. Apart from an emergency, the use or supply of drugs must be in line with the practice of the profession of optometry as defined in the Opticians Act

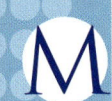

1989 (amended 2005) or laid down by the General Optical Council. Nothing in the 1968 Act has changed the restrictions concerning treatment of adverse ocular conditions.

This Act established the legislative framework for the sale and supply of medicinal products. The detail of supply was determined by a series of Statutory Instruments that were required for operation of the Act and came into force in 1978. Optometrists have rights to use and supply a variety of medicinal products by virtue of exemptions to the provisions in the Act.

Medicines and Healthcare Products Regulatory Agency (MHRA)

The Medicines and Healthcare Products Regulatory Agency (MHRA) was formed from the merger of the Medical Devices Agency and the Medicines Control Agency in 2003. The Agency has responsibility for ensuring the protection of the public health and safeguarding the interests of patients and users by ensuring that medicines, healthcare products and medical equipment meet appropriate standards of safety, quality, effectiveness and performance and that they comply with relevant Directives of the European Union.

Contact lenses fall within this regulatory framework as do Optometrists and glazing facilities assembling spectacles from CE marked lenses and frames. Under the Medical Devices Directive on spectacle frames, an optometrist or dispensing optician is not allowed to sell a non CE- marked frame that could subsequently be sent to a glazing premises to have lenses fitted to a customer.

Meesmann's dystrophy

- See *Dystrophies of the corneal epithelium, therapeutic contact lenses for.*

Meibomian gland

The tarsal plates contain the acini and ducts of the meibomian (tarsal) glands. Ducts are vertically orientated with respect to the lid margins, with multiple secretory acini that open laterally onto each duct. The glands occupy nearly the full length and width of each tarsus, and are fewer and shorter in the lower lid. Histologically, acini are lined by a layer of undifferentiated basal cells that divide, and cells are displaced from the basement membrane. As they progress towards the duct they gradually enlarge and develop lipid droplets in their cytoplasm. Ultimately, cell membranes rupture and cellular debris, together with the lipid product, is discharged into the duct.

The stimulus for meibomian gland secretion is unclear. Although a modest autonomic innervation of the meibomian glands has been demonstrated, there is still some doubt regarding a neuromodulation of glandular secretion, and it is likely that the principal control of the glands is hormonal. Androgens are known to regulate the development, differentiation and secretion of sebaceous glands throughout the body, and are thought also to influence meibomian gland secretion.

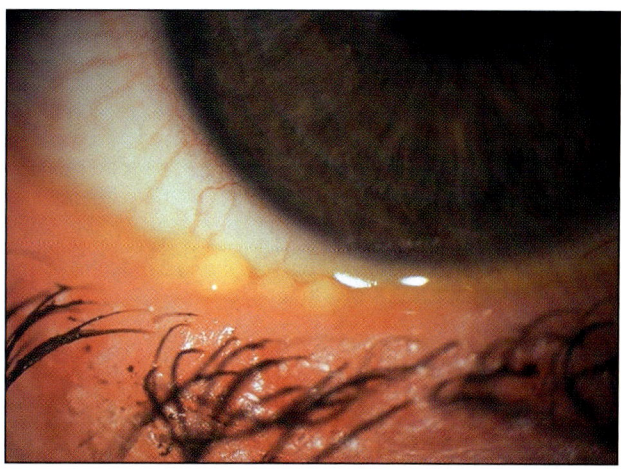

Figure M.3 • Inspissated meibomian gland secretion in the lower lid of a female patient wearing rigid lenses.

Meibomian gland dysfunction, contact lens associated

The oily secretion from the normal meibomian gland is generally clear. The key diagnostic feature of contact lens associated meibomian gland dysfunction (CL-MGD) is a change in the appearance of the clear oil expressed from healthy meibomian glands to a cloudy, creamy-yellow appearance (Figure M.3). Frothing or foaming of the lower tear meniscus is sometimes observed in CL-MGD, especially towards the outer canthus. This appearance is accompanied by symptoms of smeary vision, greasy lenses, dry eyes, and reduced tolerance to lens wear. In severe cases where the meibomian orifices are blocked, there may be an absence of gland secretion. Longstanding cases of MGD may be associated with additional signs such as irregularity, distortion and thickening of eyelid margins, slight distension of glands, mild-to-moderate papillary hypertrophy, vascular changes and chronic chalazia. The prevalence of CL-MGD is unrelated to gender but increases with age.

Associated signs of CL-MGD include all those that arise from clinical diagnostic procedures that are designed to indicate the integrity or otherwise of the lipid layer. Specifically, patients suffering from CL-MGD may display a reduced tear break-up time (measured either with fluorescein or non-invasively). Examination of the tear layer in specular reflection using a tearscope may reveal a contaminated lipid pattern, which is exacerbated by the use of cosmetic eye make-up. Symptoms of blurred or greasy vision can probably be attributed to adhesion of waxy dysfunctional meibomian oils to the surface of the contact lens; this can lead to lens surface drying, lens dehydration and sensations of dryness.

Theories for the aetiology of CL-MGD include the following:

1. It is due to excessive eye rubbing causing chronic damage to the meibomian glands
2. It occurs secondary to papillary conjunctivitis.

From a tissue pathology standpoint, MGD is characterized by increased keratinization of the epithelial walls of the

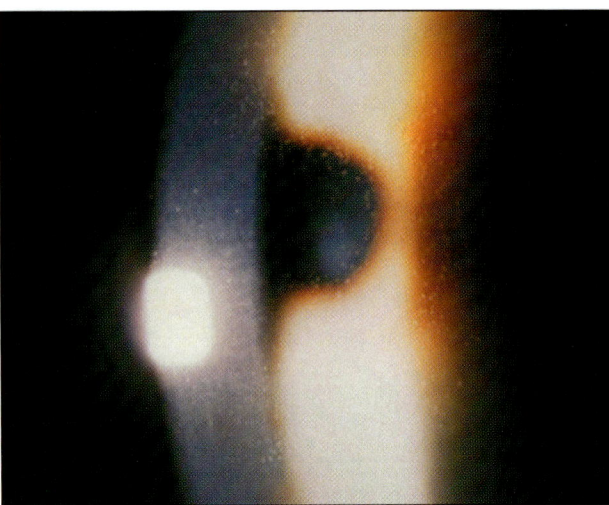

Figure M.4 • Extensive microcyst formation in the epithelium of a soft lens wearer.

meibomian gland ducts. As might be expected, therefore, this condition is often observed in combination with seborrhoeic dermatitis and acne rosacea. This leads to the formation of keratinized epithelial plugs that create a physical blockage in meibomian ducts, which in turn restricts or prevents the outflow of meibomian oils.

Although the underlying cause of meibomian gland dysfunction cannot be treated, it is possible to provide symptomatic relief by adopting one or more of the following procedures, all of which should be undertaken with the contact lenses removed:

- application of warm compresses
- lid scrubs
- mechanical expression
- prescription of antibiotics
- use of artificial tears and of surfactant lens cleaners.

By adopting these procedures, CL-MGD can be kept under good control and adverse symptoms minimized.

Mengher grid
- See *Non-invasive tear break-up time*.

Metabolic disorders
- See *Systemic disease, contact lens wear in*.

Microcysts, contact lens associated

Microcysts appear in the corneal epithelium as minute, scattered, opaque grey dots when viewed with the slit-lamp biomicroscope using low magnification and focal illumination (Figure M.4), and as transparent refractile inclusions with indirect retro-illumination. They are generally of a uniform spherical or ovoid shape and are in the order of 20μm in diameter. At high magnification (×40) using the observation technique of marginal retro-illumination, microcysts can be observed to display a characteristic optical phenomenon known as 'reversed illumination'; that is, the distribution of light within the microcyst is opposite to the light distribution of the background. This indicates that the microcyst is acting as a converging refractor, and therefore it must consist of material that is of a higher refractive index than the surrounding epithelium. Microcysts probably represent apoptotic (dead) cells which either become phagocytosed (ingested) by living neighbouring cells, or remain involuted in the intercellular spaces. In a process similar to that occurring in Cogan's microcystic dystrophy, the epithelial basement membrane duplicates and folds, forming intraepithelial sheets that eventually detach from the basement membrane and encapsulate the cellular material.

Microcysts primarily represent visible evidence of chronic tissue metabolic stress and altered cellular growth patterns. These changes are presumed to be caused by a combination of the direct effects of hypoxia, and tissue acidosis created by the indirect effects of hypoxia (producing lactic acid) and hypercapnia (producing carbonic acid). They may also have a mechanical aetiology, whereby lens-induced mechanical trauma can induce microcysts.

Whilst the actual presence of microcysts is not thought to be dangerous, their existence in large numbers is worrying, as this is representative of epithelial metabolic distress. Based on the working hypothesis that the severity of the microcyst response is related to the level of hypoxia/hypercapnia induced by lens wear, a variety of strategies can be employed in an attempt to minimize the number of microcysts. Strategies that are likely to be successful include:

- increasing lens oxygen transmissibility
- decreasing the frequency of overnight wear
- changing from extended-wear to daily-wear lenses
- changing from soft to rigid lenses
- avoiding defective lenses.

The prognosis for eliminating microcysts is good, but the time course is peculiar. Following cessation of lens wear there is an initial increase in the number of microcysts over a 7-day period, followed by a subsequent decrease. The initial increase in microcysts is thought to be due to an initial resurgence in epithelial metabolism and growth, resulting in an accelerated removal of cellular debris (formation of microcysts) and a rapid movement of microcysts towards the surface, where they are more readily observed. This is followed by a gradual decrease as the existing microcysts are completely eliminated from the cornea over a period of 3–5 months.

Microdots, contact lens associated

Examination of the living human cornea at very high magnification (×680) using a confocal microscope will reveal the presence of highly reflective 'microdot deposits' throughout the corneal stroma (Figure M.5). Microdots are small, discrete, brightly reflective spots or dots scattered throughout the stroma; they are generally round or oval in shape, and vary in diameter from about 1 to 4μm. Microdot deposits are observed in all persons, whether contact lenses have been worn or not; however, more microdots are seen in lens wearers, which indicates that contact lens wear is exacerbating otherwise normal corneal morphological features. It should also be recognized that it is not possible at present to determine

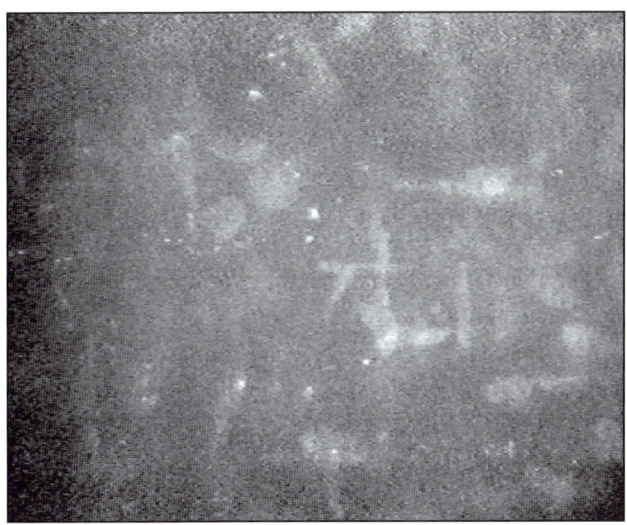

Figure M.5 • Microdots in the human corneal stroma of a soft lens wearer.

whether the appearance of microdots is related to the contact lenses, or to solutions used in conjunction with lens wear.

Microplicae
- See *Corneal epithelium*.

Microspherometer
- See *Radiuscope*.

Microtropia

Microtropia may be found as an apparently primary condition, or it may be present as a residual deviation after the treatment of a larger strabismus. It has also been suggested that it has inherited characteristics.

Anisometropia is often a major factor, and a foveal scotoma is thought to result from confusion of the blurred image with the sharp image in the more emmetropic eye. Typically, microtropia develops before the age of 3 years, but it may (rarely) break down into a larger angle strabismus and give the impression that a strabismus has developed in later childhood. It is usually an eso-deviation with a form of binocular single vision, but there are exceptional cases of micro-hypertropia that usually result from surgical intervention of a large angle hypertropia. Micro-exotropia may also exist.

Microtropia may be classified as either primary (with or without identity), primary decompensating, or secondary (as a result of reduction by optical means or surgery). Secondary microtropia is much more prevalent than primary microtropia. Microtropia is recognized as having certain characteristics that are common in many cases. They are:

Small angle. The microtropia is between 1 and 10^Δ in size. The deviation may not show on the cover test (microtropia with identity); not because it is too small, but because it is a fully adapted strabismus. There is often a heterophoric component. Microtropia is usually constant in all positions of gaze and fixation distances.

Anisometropia. There is often a difference between the refractive errors in the two eyes of more than 1.50D of hyperopia. Micro-exotropia is often associated with mixed astigmatic anisometropia, and micro-esotropia tends to be associated with spherical anisometropia. However, microtropia can occur in patients with equal refractive errors.

Amblyopia. There is reduced acuity in one eye, and as the deviation may not be apparent on the cover test, the amblyopia may be the first indication of the microtropia. Usually the visual acuity is reduced one or two lines to 6/9 or 6/12.

Eccentric fixation. Central fixation is lost in microtropia and there is likely to be a suppression scotoma in the foveal area of the amblyopic eye. The angle of the eccentricity of the fixation is usually the same as the angle of the strabismus (hence the terminology 'with identity'). This is the reason why the eye does not move on the cover test: the area of the retina on which the image falls in binocular vision is the same as the eccentrically fixing area (the area used for fixation when the other eye is covered). Occasionally in microtropia, the degree of eccentric fixation is less than the angle of the strabismus, and in these cases a very small cover test movement may be seen (microtropia without identity).

Abnormal retinal correspondence. Harmonious anomalous retinal correspondence is present in microtropia. Therefore, in most cases there will be identity of the retinal area on which the image falls in the patient's habitual vision with both the area used for fixation and the anomalously corresponding area. This leads to microtropia with identity (no movement on unilateral cover test), and most microtropia is of this type; that is, the strabismus is fully adapted. Microtropia without identity (movement on unilateral cover test) may have central or non-absolute eccentric fixation and the retinal correspondence may be either abnormal, or normal with central suppression and peripheral fusion.

Peripheral fusion. The eyes seem to be held in the nearly straight position of the small angle by the fusional impulses provided by peripheral vision. A form of 'pseudo-fusional reserves' can be measured. During the cover test it is therefore important to position the cover close to the eye in order to ensure complete dissociation; otherwise peripheral fusion may reduce the magnitude of any ocular movement and confound an accurate diagnosis.

Monofixational syndrome. In many cases of microtropia, the angle of the deviation may increase on the alternating cover test or even if one eye is covered for a slightly longer time than normal during the unilateral cover test. When the cover is removed from both eyes, the eye that was last covered will be seen to return to the microtropia position. There is the appearance of phoria in spite of the microtropia. It is as if a heterophoric movement is superimposed on the strabismus. The apparent heterophoria may be larger and more obvious than the microtropia, which as discussed above may not show at all on the cover test. This cover test recovery movement can be described as an anomalous fusional movement. A microtropia showing the superimposed phoria movement is known as 'Park's monofixational syndrome' or 'monofixational heterophoria'. These cases may not have a strabismus but in fact have a heterophoria with normal retinal correspondence and a gross fixation disparity. This is much larger than that normally found in heterophoria, but does not cause diplopia because of a large foveal suppression area in the strabismic eye. A sequence of events, which links these features and could explain the development of at least some cases of microtropia, is as follows: a decompensating heterophoria leads to an increasing fixation disparity that in time becomes associated with an enlargement of Panum's area and an increase in the deviation, resulting in a microtropia with identity and monofixational syndrome.

Stereopsis. Low-grade stereopsis has been reported in microtropia although it is not always detected with standard clinical tests. It has been argued that all cases of strabismus, including microtropia, perform subnormally at random dot stereopsis tests.

Microtropia is a fully adapted strabismus and does not usually give rise to symptoms unless other conditions have been superimposed. Patients tend to present late when reduced vision is detected at a school check. Management consists, initially, of correcting the refractive error. This is particularly important if the patient is under 5 years of age and has anisometropia. Orthoptic exercises for microtropia are very seldom successful, although it is possible to treat the amblyopia and eccentric fixation in the usual way. Full refractive correction and total full time occlusion of the fixing eye is indicated for children under 5 years old, which may result in total resolution of the deviation and complete restoration of normal visual acuity and gross stereopsis. For patients older than eight, the hyperoptic prescription can be reduced and deep anomalous correspondence will maintain a small angle. Aggressive treatment with patching of patients with microtropia under the age of 10 has been recommended as this has been found to be effective without inducing intractable diplopia.

Ill-health in older children (5 to 10 years) may cause the microtropia to break down into a larger deviation. If monofixational heterophoria is decompensated and giving rise to symptoms, orthoptic treatment for these conditions may be appropriate to restore the microtropia to its compensated and fully adapted state. Microtropic patients can also have inadequate vergence and accommodative skills for their visual requirements at school or work. Prisms and added lenses do not seem to help for these symptomatic patients, possibly due to prism adaptation. Orthoptic exercises in these cases can be successful.

Microvilli
- See *Corneal epithelium.*

Microwave disinfection, soft contact lens
Microwave irradiation has been proposed as a potentially cheap and effective method for soft lens disinfection. Although there are some parameter changes when lenses are repeatedly irradiated with a standard 650-W microwave oven, none of these changes are clinically significant. However, repeated heating (as essentially occurs with microwave radiation) is known rapidly to degrade certain polymers and to distort lenses that have absorbed high levels of protein. As patients often need to care for their lenses in locations remote from a microwave oven, this approach is often impractical or inconvenient.

Minimum recommended disinfection time (MRDT) of contact lenses
- See *Antimicrobial efficacy of contact lenses.*

Minus contact lens carrier
- See *High plus power contact lens design.*

Miotics
Miotics are drugs that reduce the diameter of the pupil either by inhibiting the dilator with a sympatholytic, or alpha blocking, agent or by stimulating the sphincter with a parasympathomimetic, or cholinergic, agent.

Sympatholytics. Sympatholytics are also known as mydriolytic or as α_1 antagonists. One drug in this category, thymoxamine, can be used to reverse the mydriasis caused by sympathomimetic agents and a 0.1% solution can overcome the effect of 2.5% phenylephrine in about two hours compared to five hours without its use. It appears to have little effect upon the ciliary muscle or upon accommodation. Dapiprazole is effective in reversing the mydriatic action of 1% tropicamide and facilitates the return of accommodation, but it does induce some conjunctival hyperaemia. Despite their clinical advantages, neither thymoxamine nor dapiprazole are available as proprietary preparations in the UK.

Directly acting parasympathomimetics. Carbachol, bethanechol, and pilocarpine act directly to contract the pupil sphincter, but suffer from the disadvantage that they cause a simultaneous spasm of accommodation resulting in pseudomyopia. The sustained action of carbachol (doryl; carcholin), a synthetic choline ester, makes it suitable for use in the treatment of glaucoma, especially where resistance or intolerance to pilocarpine is encountered. It is poorly absorbed through the cornea and the drops incorporate hypromellose as a wetting agent. Bethanecol (urecholine) is another synthetic choline ester and like carbachol it is also used in the treatment of post-operative urinary retention. As a 1% solution it can be employed as a miotic and similarly requires a wetting agent to encourage corneal penetration, but it is not available as a proprietary product.

Pilocarpine, a cholinomimetic alkaloid, can overcome the mydriatic effect of sympathomimetic agents such as phenylephrine, but fails to induce effective miosis in the case of the widely used antimuscarinic drug, tropicamide. Furthermore, the duration of action of the antimuscarinic can exceed that of pilocarpine so that the pupils dilate again. The advantages of pilocarpine compared to the anticholinesterase agent, physostigmine, are that a spasm of accommodation does not recur when undertaking close work and it causes less discomfort.

Indirectly acting parasympathomimetics. Drugs in this category inhibit the enzyme acetylcholinesterase so that miosis results from the accumulation of the transmitter acetylcholine.

Physostigmine (eserine) produces miosis accompanied by spasm of accommodation, conjunctival hyperaemia and some discomfort. Its mode of action can be described as reversible or short-term and at a given strength, it is twice as active as pilocarpine. At a strength of 0.25%, it

Table M.3 • Miotics: unpreserved single dose preparation.		
Non-proprietary name	Proprietary name	Formulation
Pilocarpine nitrate	Minims® Pilocarpine Nitrate	Drops 2 and 4%

can reverse the mydriaisis induced by an antimuscarinic agent such as tropicamide 0.5% within 30min. Physostigmine has been employed in the treatment of accommodative esotropia but has proved to be less satisfactory for this purpose than conventional refractive correction.

Ecothiopate iodide (phospholine iodide) is an example of an irreversible anticholinesterase because it binds to it permanently and its action is only terminated when new enzyme has been synthesized. It has ceased to be used as a miotic due to the adverse systemic and local side effects associated with its long-term use.

Miotics are no longer routinely used to reverse dilation of the pupil due to the relatively short duration of action of mydriatics such as phenylephrine or tropicamide and due to the fact that the risk of inducing angle closure glaucoma in carefully screened patients is remote. Pilocarpine, the only miotic to which British optometrists have access, could be instilled to reduce the glare associated with dilation but it induces a spasm of accommodation in patients under the age of about 50 years that can significantly impair vision.

In the unlikely event that acute angle closure glaucoma results from the use of a mydriatic, the patient must be referred immediately to an ophthalmologist and the general practitioner informed of the need for this course of action. It may be appropriate, subject to local ophthalmological opinion, for optometrists working in remote locations to institute emergency treatment with pilocarpine. For this purpose, one drop of the 2 or 4% strength, which is conveniently available as an unpreserved single dose preparation (Table M.3), should be instilled in the affected eye(s) every 15min for up to 30min.

Historically, miotics have played a major role in the treatment of glaucoma but are no longer regarded as the first line of therapy due to their side effects and the advent of alternative drugs. See *Glaucoma, drugs for the treatment of*.

Miotics have been employed as an alternative to spectacle correction in the treatment of accommodative esotropia. However, this mode of treatment has not proved to be superior to the use of a spectacle correction and has the disadvantage that its long-term use is associated with the risk of side effects.

A miotic is employed in the diagnosis of Adie's tonic pupil in which denervation of the post-ganglionic supply to the pupil and ciliary muscle results in a dilated pupil that exhibits:

- Minimal or no reaction to light
- Slow constriction with convergence
- Slow re-dilation

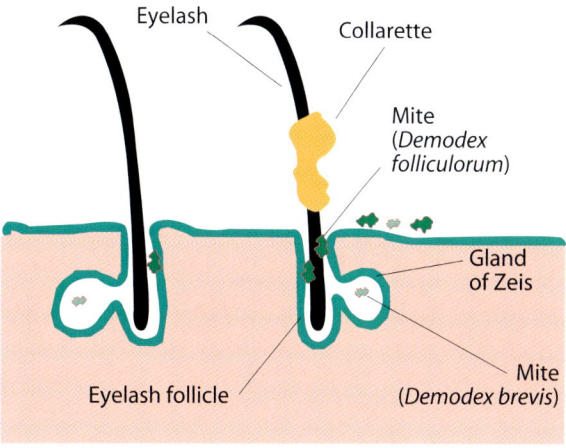

Figure M.6 • Mite habitat.

Adie's tonic pupil is unilateral in 80% of cases and is most often found in young women. A drop of 0.0625% pilocarpine is instilled into both eyes. While there is no reduction in pupil diameter in the normal eye, in Adie's tonic pupil, constriction occurs due to denervation hypersensitivity.

Mites

Mite infestation in humans is very common, and infestation of the eyelashes by mites is ubiquitous and generally sub-clinical. If present in excessive numbers, mites can lead to the following signs and symptoms:

- pruritis
- burning
- crusting
- itching
- swelling of the lid margins
- loss and easy removal of lashes.

These symptoms often parallel the 10-day mite reproductive cycle.

Two types of mite can be found in the eyelash region. *Demodex folliculorum* prefers to live in the spaces between the eyelashes and in the outermost region of the eyelash follicles. It shreds the epithelial lining of the follicle, and the shredded material mixes with lipids and sebum to form a clear sleeve around the base of the eyelashes, known as a 'cuff' or 'collarette'. *Demodex brevis* prefers an oily environment, and is found in the glands of Zeis (Figure M.6).

Although mites are very difficult to see, their presence is confirmed by the observation of epilated lashes and collarettes under the microscope. Treatment in the first instance is aimed at reducing the level of mites to subclinical levels; this can be effected by applying a topical anaesthetic and swabbing the eyelid margins and eyelashes with a cotton-tipped applicator soaked in contact lens cleaning solution. Vigorous twice-daily lid scrubbing and the application of viscous ointments at night (to suffocate the mites) over a 3-week period can cure the condition.

Modern orthokeratology

- See *Orthokeratology*.

Modification of contact lenses

A variety of procedures can be adopted to modify or adjust the form of PMMA or rigid contact lenses. These procedures usually involve the use of paraphernalia such as spinning tools, polishing pads, sponges and suction caps, and include edge and surface polishing, effecting a small change in lens power, blending peripheral curves, fenestrating, truncating and engraving. These days most practitioners prefer to return a lens to a specialist rigid lens laboratory for such modifications, although some prefer to undertake such procedures in the practice. Particular care must be exercised to avoid over-polishing (and consequent over-heating) when modifying materials of medium to high oxygen permeability, in order to avoid surface damage such as crazing and reducing lens surface wettability.

Moll gland

- See *Gland of Moll*.

Mollon-Reffin minimalist test

The Mollon-Reffin minimalist test is a test of acquired colour vision deficiency that aims to have a similar grading function as the ranked colour difference designs of the AO HRR test or paired Farnsworth and desaturated D15 tests. It also demonstrates the extent of neutral zones in acquired colour deficiency. The test is composed of three Munsell hues selected to be within typical protan, deutan and tritan isochromatic zones. These are presented in 5 Munsell value steps. The aim is to ascertain the least saturated cap, in each hue series, that can be distinguished from 5 Munsell value grey caps.

Monochromatism

A person with typical or rod monochromatism has no functioning cone receptors and is therefore achromatic. Visual acuity is about 6/60 (20/200). Photophobia and nystagmus are present. Inheritance is autosomal recessive and an equal number of males and females are affected. Consanguinity is a predisposing factor. Prevalence varies in different populations but has been estimated as about 1 in 35,000 in developed countries.

Atypical, incomplete or cone monochromatism is rare. People with this type of colour deficiency usually have short wavelength sensitive 'blue' cones only. Inheritance is x linked. The main cause is an abnormality in the locus control region which governs the expression of long and medium wavelength cone photopigments. Visual acuity is in the range 6/9 to 6/24. Photophobia and nystagmus are present if visual acuity is less than 6/18. Affected individuals have no hue (wavelength) discrimination at photopic light levels but have limited hue discrimination at mesopic levels when both rods and short wavelength cones are stimulated.

Tests for monochromatism include the Sloan Achromatopsia test and the Berson plates. These tests aim to demonstrate lack of wavelength discrimination and characteristic abnormal relative luminous efficiency. Monochromats can utilize perceived lightness differences in some designs in the Ishihara plates and the AO HRR plates and can interpret them correctly. Some monochromats are able to place the Farnsworth D15 caps in order of perceived lightness.

Monomers

- See *Polymers for contact lenses*.

Monovision contact lens correction for presbyopia

Monovision is an approach for correcting presbyopia with contact lenses whereby one eye is given the required distance refractive power and the other eye is given the required near refractive power. This approach is based upon the principle that the visual system can alternate central suppression between the two eyes when viewing is alternating between distance and near targets. The degree of interocular blur suppression, which varies between patients, may be linked to the final success of monovision. Essentially all forms of soft and rigid contact lenses can be used for monovision corrections, whether spherical or toric.

With monovision correction, there is only a slight reduction in performance in distance acuity tests when compared to spectacle correction, and no significant difference in acuity results at near. Distance and near stereopsis is compromised with monovision, but the degree of reduction is patient-specific and may or may not result in failure with this method of fitting. Contrast loss and difficulty in suppressing bright images against dark backgrounds (for example, car headlights) while wearing monovision may also contribute to poor tolerance. Despite such compromises, monovision has high patient acceptance with a success rate of around 75%. Monovision causes minimal compromise in near visual acuity performance in all illumination conditions, and thus this type of fitting option should be considered for presbyopic patients with strong near vision demands. However, when critical or sustained tasks requiring good distance binocularity predominate, it is advisable to avoid monovision or to consider supplementary correction.

No single predictive test exists to identify successful monovision patients, so systematic trial and error is the best approach. However, the initial impression of the patient can be an important indicator of likely success. The more usual fitting approach is to fit the dominant eye (see *Ocular dominance*) with the distance vision correcting lens and the non-dominant eye with the near vision correcting lens. It is important to correct any astigmatism equal to or greater than 0.75D in either or both eyes, as uncorrected astigmatism can result in reduced visual performance, asthenopic symptoms, and poor tolerance. Binocular visual acuity similar to that achieved with the spectacle correction – with no significant reduction in stereopsis or contrast sensitivity – is usually a good sign of likely success.

Some patients require spectacles to wear occasionally 'over' their monovision contact lens correction. For example, there may be a requirement for extra minus correction over the near correcting lens/eye and plano over the distance correcting lens to give full binocular vision and optimal distance acuity for night driving, especially when higher reading additions are required.

The following alternative approaches to monovision correction can improve results:

1. Partial monovision. In general, the acceptance and therefore success of monovision falls as the reading add increases. As the indicated add exceeds +2.00D, tolerance can often be improved if a reduced reading addition is given. The patient may need supplementary glasses for small print, a different pair of supplementary glasses for driving, or a secondary distance correcting contact lens. This form of monovision is ideal for social users whose near vision demands will be lower than those of full-time wearers. Partial monovision may also be a useful strategy for patients who have greater intermediate vision needs.

2. Enhanced monovision. This approach involves fitting one eye with a bifocal lens and the other with a single vision lens. A variety of options exist. The most frequent approach involves fitting the dominant eye with a single vision distance lens (spherical or toric) and the non-dominant eye with a bifocal lens. This improves binocular summation and offers some level of stereo-acuity to the monovision wearer who is experiencing increasing blur with a higher reading add. Alternatively, the same approach can be used when fitting patients who require sharper distance vision than bilateral simultaneous vision can offer with single-vision monovision lenses. The bifocal lens in the non-dominant eye usually needs more bias for near vision. This modification can be achieved effectively by increasing the distance power of the bifocal lens by +0.50D to +0.75D. Other enhanced monovision options include:

- a single-vision near lens in the dominant eye to improve near vision and a distance-bias bifocal lens in the non-dominant eye
- a single-vision lens with slightly excess plus power in the dominant eye and an intermediate-bias bifocal lens in the non-dominant eye.

3. Modified monovision. This approach involves adjusting the refractive power of the lens or selecting alternative lens designs for each eye to deliberately improve distance vision in one eye, at the expense of near performance in that eye, whilst improving near vision in the other. This can be achieved by increasing minus power/decreasing plus power on the dominant eye to enhance distance vision, while decreasing minus power/increasing plus power in the non-dominant eye. A similar bias can be obtained by using different add powers in each – the lower add power being fitted to the dominant eye to improve distance vision. Similarly, one eye may be fitted with a centre distance simultaneous design and the other with a centre near design.

Motility
- See *Ocular motility*.

Motivation for contact lens wear
- See *Indications and contraindications for contact lens wear*.

Movement, soft contact lens
- See *Fitting soft contact lenses*.

Mucin balls, contact lens induced

Approximately 50% of patients who wear silicone hydrogel lenses on an extended-wear basis display this

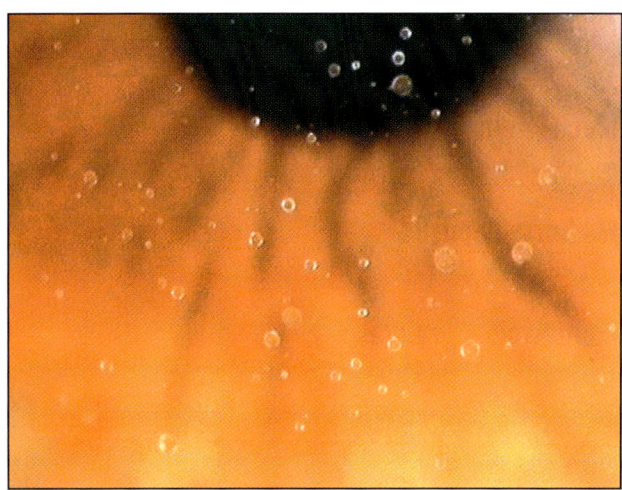

Figure M.7 • Mucin balls displaying characteristic 'doughnut' appearance.

phenomenon. Mucin balls can be observed in the post-lens tear film as small discrete particles, or 'plugs', and are similar in appearance to tear film debris. In some patients, as many as 200 mucin balls can be seen. At high magnification (×40) mucin balls appear to be of variable size and to take on a characteristic 'flattened doughnut' shape, with a thin circular annulus and broad central depression (Figure M.7). They are observed in greater numbers in patients who sleep in silicone hydrogel lenses. Mucin balls are immovable beneath the lens, and appear to be stuck to the epithelium. A higher number of mucin balls is associated with a looser lens fit. Mucin balls generally increase in number over the first months of lens wear and remain constant thereafter.

Mucin balls cause no discomfort or loss of vision, and appear to be of no immediate consequence with respect to ocular health. They are composed primarily of collapsed mucin, as well as some lipid and tear proteins. The mechanism by which mucin balls form beneath the lens may in part be related to a physicochemical phenomenon caused by the plasma-treated surface of silicone hydrogel lenses. Specifically, the lipophilic surface of these lenses establishes a complex interfacial relationship with the tear film, which creates a shearing force that has the effect of rolling up tear mucus into small spheres. The mechanical vehicles facilitating such events may be rapid eye movements during sleep and blink-induced lens movement upon awakening. The relatively high modulus of silicone hydrogel lenses may also contribute to the above mechanism. In addition, the more viscous, mucus-rich nature of the closed-eye post-lens tear film is probably of aetiological significance in the formation of mucin balls.

Following lens removal, some mucin balls remain 'stuck' to the epithelium and some are washed away with blinking but leave behind pits in the epithelial surface which fill with tear aqueous. Both the remaining mucin balls and surface fluid-filled pits stain with fluorescein. When viewed at ×40 magnification, the fluid-filled pits give rise to the optical phenomenon of unreversed illumination, which is due to the fact that they are composed of a tear aqueous which is of lower refractive index than the surrounding epithelial tissue.

Syn: Mucin plugs, lipid plugs.

Mucins in tears
- See *Tear mucins.*

Mucus in tears
- See *Tear mucins.*

Mulberry deposits
- See *Deposits, contact lens.*

Multidisciplinary team, low vision

The optimum low vision service would include a comprehensive assessment of all the needs of the individual: vocational, educational, social, psychological, financial, optometric and medical. This requires the interaction of several disciplines if the patient is to make maximal use of their vision, and live as independently as possible. Such an interdisciplinary or multidisciplinary approach is gaining acceptance, although the UK has been slower than most developed countries to realize its potential. See *Low vision services committees.* The range of professionals involved in a 'model' low-vision service can be extremely wide. An educationalist, employment specialist, physiotherapist, occupational therapist, social worker (who may offer advice on obtaining financial benefits), lighting engineer, orthoptist (whose role often extends well beyond the evaluation and treatment of oculomotor disorders), psychologist/counsellor, audiologist (since many elderly individuals also suffer a hearing impairment), and others, may be called into the 'vision team' for particular clients. It is usual, however, to have a 'core' of an ophthalmologist, an optometrist (carrying out refraction and prescribing), a low vision trainer and a rehabilitation worker. A rehabilitation worker can supply daily living and mobility aids, provide training in their use and offer advice on achieving the optimum environment for independent living. It is also becoming increasingly common to find an 'eye clinic liaison officer' as part of the team: this individual attends hospital outpatient clinics, sitting in with the ophthalmologist, and is able to form a first point of contact with individuals who are being registered, or are otherwise in need of advice about their eye condition or vision. A coordinator who can direct the patient to appropriate elements of the service, monitor their progress and help them understand what is happening, is invaluable.

The low vision trainer may be an individual with this sole responsibility, or the role may be an additional task for another member of the team. See *Low vision training.* Throughout the team, there is no absolute boundary between the roles of particular professions, and it must be accepted that the scope of services provided will vary between practitioners, depending on the experience of that individual, geographical location and local resources. The team, and the services they offer, are unlikely to be in a single physical location, and it is important that there is a clear procedure for referral between agencies, and for relevant information to be recorded and shared. If appropriate to the individual, access to any of the professionals in the team must be available at any stage: entry to the service should not be via a single professional, and should not depend on visual acuity or registration status. It is often the case that practical aids are only suggested once medical treatment has proved unsuccessful, but early intervention can have considerable benefits.

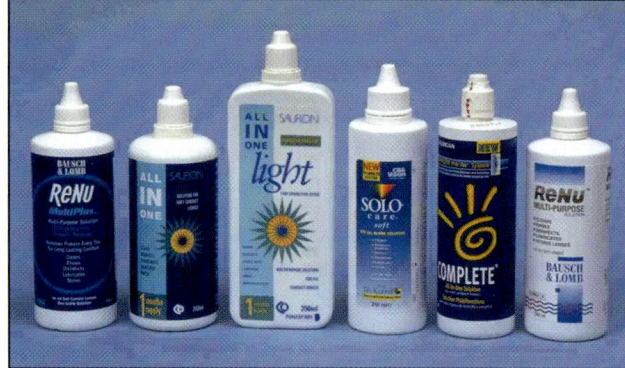

Figure M.8 • Polyhexanide-based multipurpose disinfecting solutions.

Multifocal contact lenses
- See *Bifocal and multifocal contact lenses.*

Multifocal spectacle lenses
- See *Progressive addition lenses.*

Multipurpose contact lens disinfecting solution

Multipurpose solutions (MPSs) account for about 80% of prescribed care regimens in Europe, Canada and Australia. Most of these products do not require the use of other auxiliary components in the lens care process, especially when used with lenses that are frequently replaced.

Most MPSs contain polyhexanide, which was originally developed as a pre-surgery antimicrobial scrub and then marketed for the sanitization of swimming pools and spas (Figure M.8). Polyhexanide is part of the same pharmaceutical family as chlorhexidine, and is active against a wide range of bacteria. The action of polyhexanide is thought to be due to its rapid attraction towards the negatively charged bacterial cell surface, followed by impairment of membrane activity, with the loss of potassium ions and the precipitation of intracellular constituents. Polyhexanide has a larger molecular weight than chlorhexidine, which means that it is not able to enter the matrix of soft lens materials. In turn this reduces the likelihood of the preservative reaching the ocular surface, with the consequent potential for toxic or hypersensitivity reactions.

Various MPSs contain polyhexanide at a range of concentrations from 0.6ppm to 5ppm. An increase in concentration of this active ingredient is likely to cause a general increase in its antimicrobial action. For example, a polyhexanide concentration of 5ppm provides a solution with stand-alone activity against strains of Acanthamoeba, but may increase the level of corneal staining seen in wearers of specific lens materials. Excess staining has been observed in some Group II lenses, perhaps because these materials tend to attract lipid to which polyhexanide can bind.

A surfactant component is generally included in MPSs so that they can offer a cleaning action in addition to their disinfection properties. These solutions also contain EDTA as a chelating agent to assist both cleaning and disinfecting, and a buffer to ensure a consistent pH.

More recently, 'enhanced' versions of multipurpose solutions have been introduced to the market. In the ReNu MultiPlus (Bausch & Lomb) product, hydranate has been incorporated as a sequestering agent to reduce protein deposition. This chemical forms complexes with calcium, which can act as a bridge between the lens surface and proteins. Another example of these newer products is Complete Comfort Plus (Allergan), which contains the viscosity agent hydroxypropyl methylcellulose; this ingredient is claimed to improve ocular comfort. Some products are also available in vials, which are more convenient for travelling or for the infrequent wearer.

Some MPSs have polyquaternium-1 (or polyquad) as the preservative. This compound is derived from the same pharmaceutical family as polyhexanide – the polyquats. It is a large molecule, and has a long history of use in the cosmetics industry. A number of Alcon disinfectant products have been launched which contain polyquad, such as Opti-Free. This product is usually classified as a 'multipurpose solution'; however, unlike other MPSs it does not contain a surfactant cleaner, although the inclusion of a citrate buffer (instead of the phosphate or borate generally found in polyhexanide-based MPSs) provides a cleaning effect. This negatively charged buffer is included in the polyquad products to reduce the adherence of polyquad to the surface of some ionic lens materials; this same property can reduce the protein deposition on soft lenses because positively charged proteins, such as lysozyme, can bind with the citrate rather than with the lens surface. However, citrates are not effective against lipid spoilation. Subsequent to the launch of Opti-Free, and its recommended use with a separate cleaner, the identical Opti-1™ was launched as a care product for use with frequently replaced lenses, without the recommended use of a separate cleaner.

Alcon has introduced a product which contains polyquad and another antimicrobial agent, myristamidopropyl dimethylamine (MAPD), known as Opti-Free Express. In contrast to original Opti-Free, this product contains a surfactant cleaner in addition to EDTA and a buffer. The antimicrobial performance of this new product is claimed to be similar to disinfection with a one-step hydrogen peroxide system. Many multipurpose solutions are also available in a 'no-rub' formulation in an attempt to improve patient compliance.

Traditionally, rigid lens products were preserved with benzalkonium chloride, thiomersal and chlorhexidine. However, there is some evidence that sufficient levels of chlorhexidine or benzalkonium chloride can bind to the surface of a rigid lens, leading to a toxic reaction at the ocular surface after lens insertion. More recently there has been a move away from these preservative agents or, as in the case of the Boston Advance product, a reduction in chlorhexidine concentration compared with previous care solutions. Also, polyhexanide (more traditionally part of soft lens disinfectant products) has been introduced as a second preservative in rigid lens solutions. For example, Total (Allergan) originally used benzalkonium chloride as its preservative. This was replaced by Total Care, with a new active agent – polixetonium chloride.

Munsell colour appearance system

The Munsell system was developed in 1905 and contains over 1200 colour samples in both matt and gloss finishes.

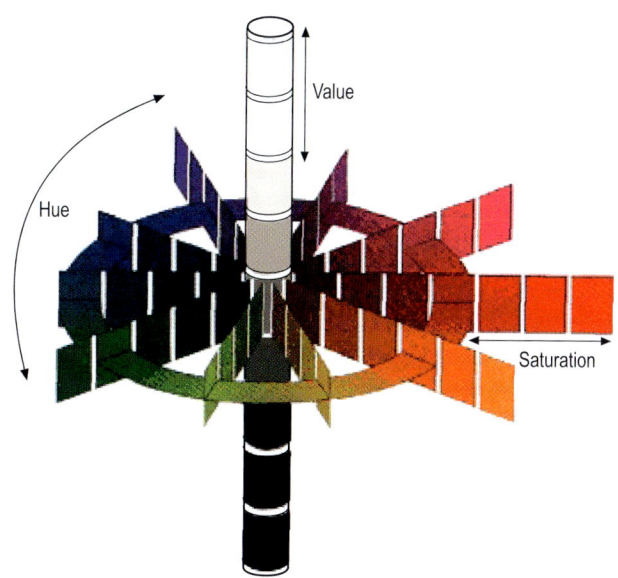

Figure M.9 • Munsell colour 'solid tree'.

The samples are arranged in uniform colour difference steps which have equal perceptual differences. Colour appearance is described in terms of hue, value and chroma. These attributes can be displayed in a 3 dimensional structure (Figure M.9) or in the pages of a book. Hue is defined as the quality expressed by colour names and is equivalent to wavelength or dominant wavelength. There are 40 standard hues derived from 5 principal hues: blue (B), green (G), yellow (Y), red (R) and purple (P) and 5 intermediate hues (BG, GY and so on). Each hue specification is divided numerically into 4 subgroups (2.5, 5, 7.5 and 10). Value is the degree of lightness or the amount of light reflected by the sample. Black has a value of zero and white has a value of 10. Chroma is similar to saturation. Saturation is defined as colourfulness in proportion to lightness and differences in saturation involve changes in both value and chroma. A white surface has a chroma of zero and a highly saturated hue has a chroma of 16 or more. Individual colours are specified using the notation 'hue value/chroma' such as '2.5 BG 5/4' or '10 RP 8/6'. The reflectance of Munsell samples have been measured in a spectrophotometer and notations can be converted to x, y chromaticity co-ordinates and vice versa. Specified Munsell hues are therefore frequently used in tests for colour vision deficiency. There are a number of other colour appearance reference systems such as the charts used by the UK Royal Horticultural Society to specify flower colours and the industrial standards developed by the National Physical Society. See *Farnsworth tests*.

Mydriatics

A mydriatic is a drug that is used to dilate the pupil in order to facilitate examination of the eye. Although cycloplegics are used as the adjunctive therapy in the treatment of anterior uveitis, they are sometimes replaced at a later stage as the condition resolves with a drug having only a mydriatic effect. Mydriasis can be achieved with a sympathomimetic (or α_1-agonist) drug, which causes the pupil dilator muscle to contract, or with

Table M.4 • Comparative performance of mydriatics.

Mydriatic	Time to maximum mydriasis after instillation of drops	Duration of mydriasis
Phenylephrine 2.5%	60 min	Up to 7h
Tropicamide 0.5%	15–30 min	Up to 6h

Table M.5 • Mydriatics: unpreserved single dose preparations.

Non-proprietary name	Proprietary name	Formulation
Phenylephrine hydrochloride	Minims® Phenylephrine Hydrochloride	Drops 2.5% & 10%*
Tropicamide	Minims® Tropicamide	Drops 0.5%

* with disodium edetate

a parasympatholytic (or antimuscarinic) drug, which paralyses the pupil sphincter muscle and also has a cycloplegic effect.

Indications for the use of a mydriatic in optometric practice include the following:

- Recent onset of vitreous opacities, especially if accompanied by the symptom of 'flashing light'
- Relatively sudden decrease in visual acuity
- Unexplained loss of visual field
- Unexplained ocular pain unaccompanied by raised intraocular pressure
- Redness of the eye which cannot be attributed to infection, allergy or raised intraocular pressure
- After contusion in order to exclude the presence of ocular damage
- Difficulty in observing the fundus due to reduced transparency of the media
- Diabetic patients
- Fundus photography.

Contraindications to the use of a mydriatic in optometric practice include:

- Patients using pilocarpine for the treatment of glaucoma
- Patients with narrow angle glaucoma
- Abnormally shallow anterior chamber (due to the risk of inducing angle closure glaucoma)
- Dislocation of the crystalline lens or of an intraocular lens
- An intraocular lens of the anterior chamber or iris-supported type.

Sympathomimetics or α_1-agonists stimulate the α_1-receptors of the pupil dilator muscle; they include hydroxyamphetamine hydrobromide (paredrine) and ephedrine hydrochloride. Cocaine is a potent anaesthetic that inhibits the re-uptake of noradrenaline into the pre-synaptic nerve terminal, increasing its duration of action so that mydriasis also occurs. The only sympathomimetic in current use is phenylephrine, which in addition to its mydriatic action, produces vasoconstriction of the conjunctiva together with some widening of the palpebral aperture. It is available in strengths of 2.5 and 1%; the weaker formulation should be used with children and the elderly due to the risk of systemic toxicity. Since the light reflex is not abolished by phenylephrine, it is unsuitable when indirect ophthalmoscopy is to be undertaken. The use of phenylephrine is contraindicated in conditions such as hypertension, coronary disease, hyperthyroidism and diabetes. Also, it may interact with β-blockers, monamine oxidase inhibitors and tricyclic antidepressants. Adverse systemic reactions to phenylephrine include cardiac arrhythmias and hypertension.

Parasympatholytic or antimuscarinic or parasympathomimetic blockers prevent acetylcholine from acting on the muscarinic receptors of the pupil sphincter muscle, resulting in mydriasis accompanied by cycloplegia. Drugs of this type include atropine, homatropine and cyclopentolate, all of which have an unnecessarily long duration of mydriatic action. Other synonyms for such drugs are anticholinergics, cholinergic antagonists, muscarinic antagonists and parasympathetic antagonists. Tropicamide is the antimuscarinic drug of choice, having a faster onset and shorter duration of onset than others. The 1% strength is customarily used as a cycloplegic for young adults and the weaker strength, 0.5%, is employed as a mydriatic for dilating the pupil by about 2mm following the instillation of one drop. Transient stinging may occur upon initial contact with the eye and, if necessary, a further drop can be instilled after an interval of five minutes. The light reflex is depressed which facilitates indirect ophthalmoscopy and retinal photography. If the patient is taking *any* medications that have an antimuscarinic effect, the action of tropicamide is likely to be augmented. Few allergic or adverse systemic reactions to tropicamide have been reported.

The comparative performance of mydriatics is shown in Table M.4, and those available as an unpreserved single dose preparation are shown in Table M.5.

Precautions for the use of mydriatics:

- Explain to the patient the reason(s) for dilating the pupil(s)
- Patients should be forewarned that photophobia is likely and that it can be alleviated by wearing sunglasses and/or a broad-brimmed hat. They should also be told that riding a motorcycle or driving a car should be avoided for several hours since vision may be blurred.

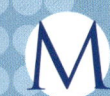

- Evaluation of anterior chamber depth.
- As with any other drug, it is wise to ask patients whether they have previously undergone mydriasis and whether there was any adverse reaction to the drug used.
- It is particularly important to establish whether the patient suffers from any illness and whether they are taking any prescribed medication or over-the-counter preparations, especially those that are antimuscarinic.
- In general, use a *single* drop. However, it may be necessary to use two or three drops with older patients and those with darkly pigmented irides.
- Measure intraocular pressure both before and upon completion of the mydriatic examination.
- Issue a note which states the mydriatic used and provides advice on what action the patient should take in the event of an adverse reaction

Myopia

Myopia can be simply defined as a refractive defect of the eye in which light from a distant object is focused in front of the retina when accommodation is relaxed, resulting in blurred distance vision. Near objects that are closer to the myopic eye than the point conjugate with the retina may appear clear without any optical correction. Minus powered lenses can be used to correct distance vision.

Myopia can be classified in a variety of ways, as follows:

- Rate of myopic progression. Stationary myopia is generally of low degree (−1.50 to −2.00) and arises during the years of physical development of the body. The level of myopia remains low with perhaps a slight regression towards emmetropia in old age. Temporarily progressive myopia arises in the early teens and progresses until the late 20s. Permanently progressive myopia increases rapidly until the age of 25 to 35 years, and advances slowly thereafter, with occasional 'spurts' of myopia progression.
- Anatomical features of myopia. Axial myopia infers that the eye is too long for its refractive power. Increases in axial length can occur in the anterior or posterior portions of the globe, or both. Refractive myopia infers that the refractive system is too powerful for the axial length of the eye. The refractive elements that can contribute to the excess power are: increased refractive index of clear media (cornea, aqueous, lens or vitreous), increased curvature of the cornea or lens, or an increase in anterior chamber depth.
- Degree of myopia. Myopia can be classified as being low (0.00D to −2.75D), moderate (−3.00D to −5.00D) and high (< −5.00D).
- Physiological and pathological myopia. Physiological myopia can be defined as that in which each component of refraction lies within the normal distribution for that population. Thus, myopia arises from a failure of correlation between the refractive components of the eye. Pathological myopia, which has also been termed malignant or degenerative myopia, describes myopia that is accompanied by degenerative changes, such as a posterior staphyloma.
- Hereditary and environmentally induced myopia. This is perhaps the most contentious approach to classifying myopia, and relates to the aetiology of the condition. Hereditary myopia infers a familial or genetic basis, whereas environmental myopia infers that prolonged and/or excessive near work is the main causative factor. Indeed, the true theory may involve a combination of both factors.
- Theory of myopic development. Three major theories of myopia development have been proposed. The 'biological-statistical theory' proposes that refractive errors form a biological continuum, ranging from high myopia to high hypermetropia. The 'use-abuse theory' suggests that myopia onset is an adaptation to use or abuse of the eyes during sustained near vision. This theory is also linked with the concept of emmetropization, which refers to the development and growth of the eye in a co-ordinated manner that tends to cause the eye to remain emmetropic.
- Age of myopia onset. This classification system relates to the age of the subject at the time of reported myopia onset. The four categories are congenital myopia (myopia is present at birth and persists through infancy); youth-onset myopia (myopia appears between age 6 and the early teens), early adult-onset myopia (myopia appears ages 20 to 40), and late adult-onset myopia (myopia appears after age 40).

Myopia, night

This refers to an increase in myopia under low luminance conditions. This occurs due to an increase in the accommodative response, typically in the order of 0.50 to 1.00D, under degraded stimulus conditions. Changes in chromatic aberration may also be involved, whereby the peak sensitivity of the eye shifts from 555nm in photopic conditions to 510nm in scotopic conditions (the 'Purkinje shift'). That is, at low luminance levels, the eye becomes more sensitive to those wavelengths undergoing a greater degree of refraction, and therefore appears to be more myopic than it is under photopic viewing conditions. Night myopia explains, for example, why stars in a dark sky may appear slightly blurred.

Myopia progression, reduction of

It has been suggested that, by prescribing rigid contact lenses (instead of soft contact lenses) to children displaying a disposition for the development of myopia, the rate of progression of myopia can be reduced. The mechanism by which this phenomenon is supposed to occur is unknown, but it is said to be unrelated to any possible lens-induced corneal moulding effects. Previous studies that purport to have demonstrated a reduction of myopia regression with rigid lenses have been flawed due to small effects, loss to follow-up, and lack of appropriate controls. Recent carefully controlled studies have failed to demonstrate such an effect, which means that the fitting of rigid lenses as a strategy to arrest myopia progression is unjustified.

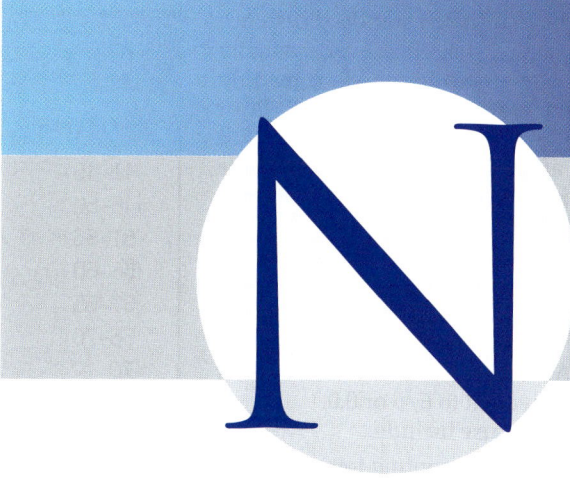

Nagel anomaloscope
- See *Anomaloscope*.

Nasolacrimal duct
- See *Lacrimal drainage system*.

National Health Service (UK)
On 6 November 1946, an Act to establish a comprehensive health service for England and Wales was passed by Parliament. This was the birth of the National Health Service (NHS). According to the Act, it was the '... duty of the Minister of Health ... to promote the establishment in England and Wales of a comprehensive health service designed to secure improvement in the physical and mental health of the people of England and Wales and the prevention, diagnosis and treatment of illness, and for that purpose to provide or secure the effective provision of services ...'.

The four basic principles underpinning the National Health Service Act were:
- Services should be financed by taxes and contributions paid when people were well rather than by charges levied on them when they were sick; and the financial burden of sickness should be spread over the whole community.
- Services should be truly national, aimed at providing the same high quality of service in every part of the country.
- Services should provide full clinical freedom to the doctors working within them.
- Services should be centred upon the family doctor team providing the essential continuity to the health care of each individual and family, and mobilizing the appropriate specialist services.

The current NHS bears little resemblance to that originally established in 1946 and now covers the whole of the UK including Northern Ireland and Scotland, although health care was one of the areas included in the recent devolution of powers to Scotland, Wales and Northern Ireland. The four over-riding principles on which the NHS was based have been 'adjusted' to take account of different political and professional developments over the last 50 years.

Near acuity
It is possible to measure near visual acuity using lines of letters on a 'reduced Snellen chart'. The chart will be analogous to that used to measure distance acuity, and lines will be labelled 6/60 to 6/6. In order for the notation to be

accurate, the chart must be placed at a standard distance (usually 38cm). Near acuity is, however, usually measured as acuity for words or sentences, since reading is the task in which the patient is interested. Print contrast, typeface, word and line spacing, word length and difficulty can each affect performance as much as letter size, especially in visually impaired patients. Nonetheless, print samples are usually calibrated on the basis of the size (and angular subtence) of the lower-case letter which has neither ascending or descending limbs (e.g. o, x, n). Providing that a standard viewing distance is specified, this angular subtence can also be converted into a Snellen or logMAR acuity. A letter with overall subtence of 5min arc is equivalent to 6/6 or 0.0.

Other notations in common use include:

- The point notation – which uses printing terminology for the size of letters, whereby 1 point is 1/72 inch. Text which is labelled as 'x-point' was set on printing blocks x/72 inches high: this is therefore the distance from the top of an ascending limb to the bottom of a descending limb. The typeface used (Times Roman) in charts produced in the UK has been standardized and text is therefore labelled as 'Nx': N to indicate 'near-vision standard test', and x to indicate the point size of the print.
- The Keeler A system – in which the letter size labelled as 'A1' has lower-case letters whose overall angular subtence at the designated standard distance of the test of 25cm is 5min arc; that is, it is equivalent to a 'normal' acuity of 6/6. From this baseline value, each successively increasing 'A' number indicates an increase in letter size by 1.25x (0.1 log units). The Keeler A series reading chart provides an excellent range of text consisting of meaningful sentences up to very large sizes (A20), with A7 being approximately equivalent to newsprint. The word separation increases dramatically, however, at the smaller letter sizes. Whilst this undoubtedly makes it easier for some visually impaired patients to read the chart, it does not resemble the real print found in books and newspapers, and results obtained should be interpreted with caution.
- The Sloan M system – whereby charts are designed to be used at a standard distance of 40cm. Each letter size bears the notation 'xM' where x is the distance in metres at which the overall height of the lower case letter subtends 5min arc. Thus 1M print size is approximately equivalent to newsprint. Patient performance could be written as, for example, '2M at 40cm', but should more accurately be designated '0.40/2' (viewing distance in metres/print size read) in a manner analogous to the Snellen distance acuity notation. The 'M' notation is the standard US terminology for print size, and its use is generally accepted in a wide variety of reading chart designs.

See *Reading tests, low vision*.

Near addition, determination of

Additional positive power, further to any dioptric power required for distance vision, is required to allow the clear focusing of tasks in those who have inadequate

Table N.1 • Suggested reading adds for increasing range.

Age in years	Initial add (D)
41–45	+0.75 – +1.00
46–50	+1.25
51–55	+1.50
56–60	+1.75
61–65	+2.00
66–70	+2.25 – +2.50
>70	+2.50 – +3.00

accommodation, typically the presbyope. There are some non-presbyopic patients where a near addition may be prescribed, such as the child with convergence excess when the addition is of a size related to the degree of over-convergence, but these are comparatively rare.

The magnitude of near addition prescribed depends on a number of factors. The age of the patient is a useful guide and typical additions for age are shown in Table N.1.

It is also useful to measure the residual accommodation present and then to maintain a fraction of this in reserve (typically a third for early presbyopes and a half for older presbyopes). It is also essential to ascertain the working distance of the near tasks for which the addition is to be used; this may vary greatly between patients irrespective of age. Finally, some knowledge of any previous correction with which the patient is content is useful as a protection against too big a change even if the previous add seems higher or lower than one might expect.

Various techniques can be used to determine the near addition. The most common method is to introduce lenses of a power chosen in consideration of the above factors and then to introduce binocularly plus or minus lenses until the target held at the appropriate working distance is best seen. Alternatively, the target may be moved closer and further away to establish the range of clear vision and ensure that the preferred position for the target is midway within this range. A near duochrome target can be used to determine the near addition. The addition which equalizes the red-green targets, or leaves the green target slightly clearer, is prescribed. A cross-cylinder technique can be adopted, whereby a cross target is placed the required distance and sufficient addition is prescribed such that a cross-cylinder presentation will render either the vertical or the horizontal lines on the target clear alternately with the flip of the cross cylinder. Whatever technique is adopted, it is important to adjust the centration of the trial lenses to the reduced interpupillary distance.

Near vision effectivity

For a series of lenses where the back vertex power (BVP) is the same in all cases, then all the images will be produced in the same position, at the second principal focus. This is irrespective of the form or material of the lens. However, when a near object at a finite distance from a lens is viewed, the situation is more complex. In such cases, the image position depends not only on the

Table N.2 • Near vision effectivity and the influence of lens form, positive power lenses.

NEAR VISION EFFECTIVITY		Trial lens A	Trial lens B	Spectacle lens C	Spectacle lens D	Spectacle lens E
Incident vergence	L_1	−4.00	−4.00	−4.00	−4.00	−4.00
Front surface power	F_1	+0.00	+5.00	+10.00	+10.00	+12.00
Lens thickness	t	+0.00	+0.01	+0.01	+0.01	+0.01
Rear surface power	F_2	+10.00	+4.92	−0.71	−0.44	−3.27
Refractive index	n	+1.50	+1.50	+1.50	+1.67	+1.50
Lens BVP	$F'_v = F_1/(1 - {}^t/_n F_1) + F_2$	+10.00	+10.00	+10.00	+10.00	+10.00
Input vergence	$V = L_1 + F_1$	−4.00	+1.00	+6.00	+6.00	+8.00
Exit vergence	$V' = V/(1 - {}^t/_n V) + F_2$	**+6.04**	**+5.92**	**+5.54**	**+5.72**	**+5.27**

LENS FORM
A: Plano-convex
B: Bi-convex
C: Shallow meniscus
D: Shallow meniscus
E: Deep meniscus
(Diagrams not to scale)

back vertex power of the lens, but also the form and material. These effects can be calculated either by using a 'step along' calculation method, or alternatively by use of a modified version of the back vertex power formula.

Table N.2 illustrates some examples of these calculations for a variety of lens forms, with the object on the lens axis at a distance of 250mm from the lens. All the lenses are of +10.00D BVP, but the form varies considerably. Lens A is a plano-convex trial case lens, manufactured so that the rear surface is curved. This lens form has the advantage that the BVP does not alter with lens thickness. It will be noted from the value of exit vergence (V′) that the value does not depart significantly from the theoretical 'thin' lens value of +6.00D. The same is true for the second type of trial case lens (B), which is bi-convex in form. However, note the situation in the three spectacle lens forms illustrated. Lens C is a shallow meniscus lens, of normal (1.50) refractive index. The exit vergence of +5.54D is approximately half a dioptre less than the trial lens value. This means that the spectacle lens will be giving an effective near power that is under-corrected by half a dioptre. The situation is improved in lens D, which is a thinner, flatter, high index meniscus design; however, the lens power is still under-corrected by a quarter of a dioptre. The final lens (E) is a steep meniscus form, and illustrates that the effect of a deeply curved front surface and appreciable centre thickness is to give a near error of three quarters of a dioptre. How much of a problem this effect causes depends on what happens to the lens power at other points on the lens.

In the case of negative power lenses, there is much less difference between the trial case lens exit vergence and that from the finished spectacle lens. This is because minus lenses have much flatter front surface curves than is the case with plus powers, and also the centre thicknesses are less.

Negative contact lens carrier
- See *High plus power contact lens design*.

Negligence
- See *Duty of care and negligence*.

Neitz anomaloscope
- See *Anomaloscope*.

Neophyte
- See *Case history, non-contact lens wearer*.

Neovascularization, contact lens-induced
Corneal neovascularization can be defined as the formation and extension of vascular capillaries within and into previously avascular regions of the cornea. Superficial neovascularization is the most common of the various forms of contact lens induced vascular response (Figure N.1). Vision loss is rare, and will only occur if vessels encroach on the pupillary axis or if there has been an extensive leakage of lipid into the stroma (Grade 4). Deep stromal neovascularization develops insidiously, usually in an already compromised cornea (e.g.

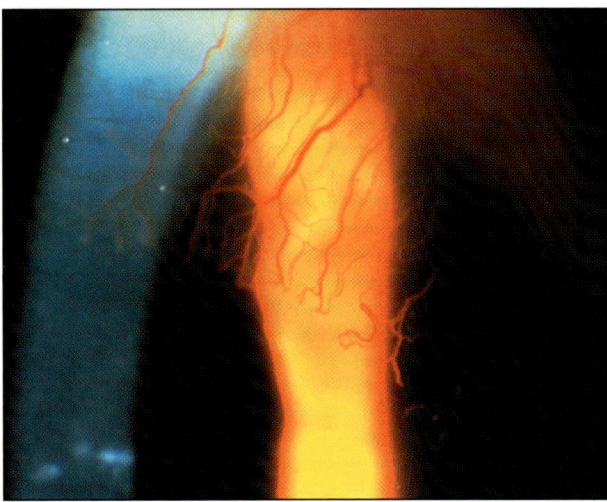

Figure N.1 • Contact lens induced corneal neovascularization.

keratoconus), and may also progress in the absence of acute symptoms.

In contact lens induced corneal neovascularization, vessel lumina are approximately 15–80μm in diameter and contain erythrocytes and sometimes leukocytes. Numerous extravascular leukocytes are observed around blood vessels, and the surrounding stromal lamellae are disorganized and separated, with lines of keratocytes lying between them. The overlying corneal epithelium is often affected, with general oedema, cell loss, and the presence of large, fluid-filled vesicles. The underlying Descemet's layer and endothelium are apparently unaffected.

Contact lens induced corneal neovascularization can be explained in terms of a dual aetiology model. Chronic hypoxia induces stromal oedema, which 'softens' the stroma and renders this tissue more susceptible to vascular penetration. Some secondary factor must act to stimulate vessel growth – for example, this could be mechanical injury to the epithelium, resulting in a release of enzymes. Inflammatory cells migrate to this site and release vasostimulating agents that cause vessels to grow in that direction.

The limits of 'normal' or 'expected' vascular ingrowth (i.e. less than Grade 1), measured from the limit of visible iris, should be 0.2, 0.4, 0.6 and 1.4mm for no-wear, daily-wear rigid, daily-wear hydrogel and extended-wear hydrogel regimes, respectively. If corneal neovascularization is a primary concern, the prescription of lenses with design features known to provide minimal interference with corneal physiology are indicated, namely those with:

- high oxygen transmissibility, to minimize oedema and metabolic acidosis
- minimal mechanical effect, as judged by patient comfort and good movement, to avoid venous stasis resulting from limbal compression in soft lenses.

Other factors to be considered include:
- avoidance of care systems likely to induce toxic or allergic responses
- changing from extended-wear to daily-wear lenses
- changing from hydrogel to rigid or silicone hydrogel lenses
- replacing lenses more frequently
- reducing wearing time
- ceasing lens wear.

Regular aftercare visits are essential. Cessation of lens wear will halt the progression of vessel infiltration into the cornea, but empty 'ghost' vessels may remain in place for months or years. Resumption of lens wear in a previously vascularized cornea will result in immediate refilling of the vessels. Thus, in advanced cases of neovascularization, long-term cessation of lens wear is indicated until ghost vessels can no longer be detected.

Neutralization of corneal astigmatism with contact lenses

A rigid lens of spherical power will neutralize virtually all corneal astigmatism. In fact the situation is a little more complex than this because of the contribution of the rear surface of the cornea to the overall corneal astigmatism, but this is generally a small effect. This neutralization effect does not depend upon the refractive index of the correcting lens. Any residual astigmatism due to the crystalline lens will remain uncorrected. Very occasionally a patient may be encountered who has a spherical refractive error but non-zero corneal astigmatism. This therefore implies that the residual (lenticular) astigmatism is of opposite sign to the corneal astigmatism and that correcting the corneal astigmatism with a spherical rigid lens will leave the residual astigmatism manifest. In such cases a spherical soft lens will result in better visual acuity, since the failure of the soft lens to correct the corneal astigmatism will allow the balance between the corneal and lenticular astigmatism to be maintained.

Irregular astigmatism and general corneal irregularity will similarly be masked by a spherical rigid lens and its accompanying tear lens. Although nominally a spherical rigid lens will neutralize any value of corneal astigmatism, the fitting relationship is likely to be unsatisfactory for corneal astigmatism greater than about 2.00DC. Thus for higher levels of astigmatism some form of toroidal correction is required.

NIBUT
- See Non-invasive tear break-up time.

Nicotine
- See Deposits, contact lens.

Non-compliance with contact lenses

'Compliance' can be defined as 'the extent to which a patient's behaviour coincides with the clinical prescription'. This definition highlights the critical importance of the practitioner–patient relationship in avoiding adverse events. Failure of the patient to comply with advice and instructions from an eye care practitioner can compromise the likelihood of success with contact lens wear. In general, non-compliance will result in:

- reduction of treatment efficacy
- secondary problems
- incorrect prescribing
- wasting of practitioner chair time
- wasting of patient time.

Clearly, health care delivery will be enhanced if the above adverse consequences of non-compliance can be minimized or eliminated.

It is not possible simply to characterize the behaviour of a patient as compliant or non-compliant, because there will be variations in the pattern of non-compliance over time, and in the extent of non-compliance at a given instance in time. Such cases are difficult to deal with, because the non-compliant behaviour may continue undetected for some time. There is a greater likelihood of detecting consistent and/or total non-compliant behaviours at an aftercare visit.

About 40–90% of contact lens wearers are non-compliant in at least some aspects of their contact lens care regimens. The types of transgressions that can occur include:

- keeping solutions too long
- failing to clean the lens case
- irregularly cleaning lenses
- failing to disinfect lenses daily
- not washing hands prior to handling lenses
- wearing lenses too long
- failing to rinse lenses after cleaning
- failing to clean lenses
- cleaning lenses in tap water.

The reasons for non-compliance are complex. In some cases patients may be deliberately non-compliant; this intentional non-compliance may be unintelligent (as in a patient adopting a dangerous procedure such as not bothering to clean his or her lenses) or intelligent (as in a patient adding an additional lens rinsing step prior to lens insertion). On the other hand, patients may be unintentionally non-compliant through forgetfulness or misunderstanding. Practitioners detecting non-compliance in a patient should seek to determine which of the reasons outlined above apply. See *Compliance enhancement*.

Non-contact aesthesiometry

Over the last 10 years a number of devices have been tested and developed to overcome the problems inherent in contact aesthesiometry. All of these devices use non-contact means of stimulating the cornea. Initially, mechanical stimulation alone was investigated, but more recently aesthesiometers have been produced that stimulate the cornea using a variety of thermal, chemical or mechanical stimuli (Figure N.2). These have included non-contact pneumatic devices, which deliver compressed air as the stimulus, the application of a carbon dioxide laser to determine the threshold for the detection of an increase in corneal temperature, and a device that measures chemical stimulation via the administration of varying concentrations of carbon dioxide.

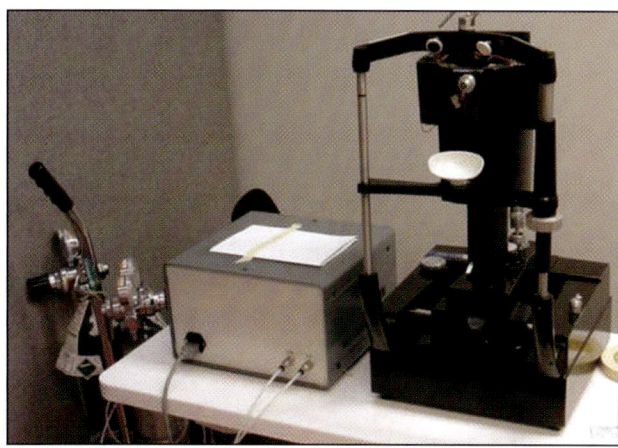

Figure N.2 • Custom-designed non-contact aesthesiometer.

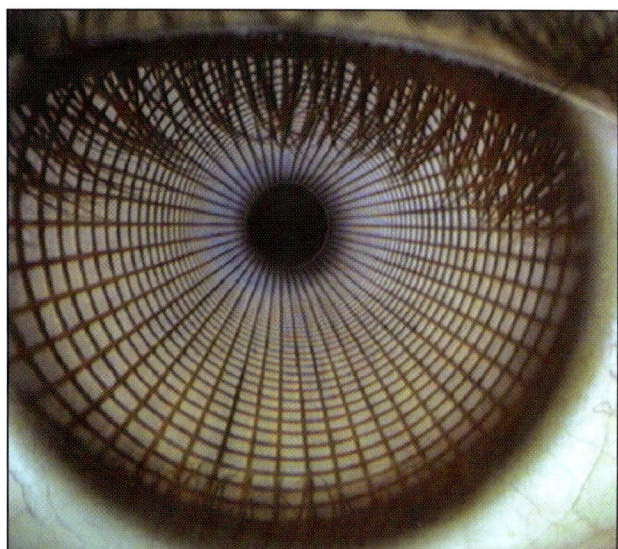

Figure N.3 • Reflection of the NIBUT grid attachment of the Tearscope-plus as seen in the pre-corneal tear film.

Non-invasive tear break-up time

The non-invasive tear film break-up time (NIBUT) can be determined by optically projecting a grid pattern onto the cornea and timing how long it takes for the grid to become disrupted. Numerous devices that employ this principle have been produced, including the instrument-stand-mounted 'NIBUT dome' or 'Mengher grid', and hand-held devices such as the keratometer-mounted Hir-Cal grid, the Loveridge grid, and the Tearscope-plus with NIBUT grid attachment (Figure N.3).

Non-ionizing radiation

Damage to the eyes occurs as a result of absorption of harmful radiation, and the severity will depend upon the wavelength of the radiation and the photon energy. Long wavelength radiation has low photon energies. Infra-red radiation has photon energies that range from 0.01 to 1eV. When it is absorbed, it will induce rotational and vibrational changes in the molecules. This increase in molecular agitation is generally referred to as a thermal effect.

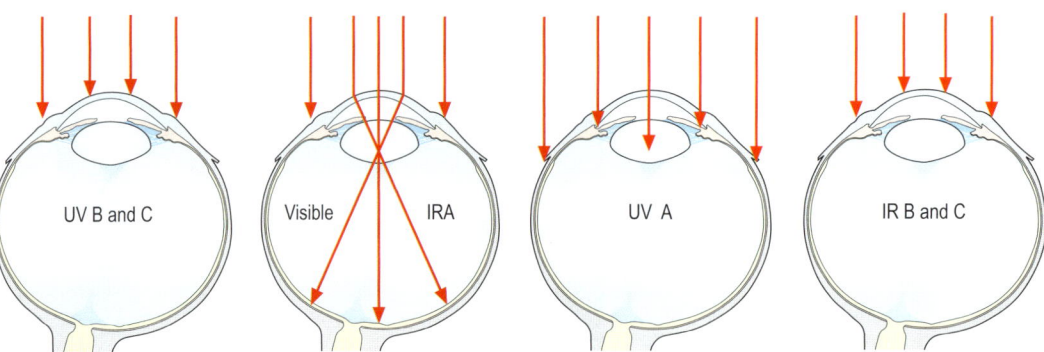

Figure N.4 • Sites of radiation absorption (reproduced by kind permission of J. Marshall and Blackwell Publishing Ltd, Oxford, 1985).

Visible and short wavelength radiations have higher photon energies. For visible and ultra-violet radiation, the photon energies range from 1 to 4eV. Absorption results in changes to the electron energies within the molecule. This excitation of the electrons may be large enough to break some of the chemical bonds and even cause ionization (usually due to absorption of photon energies > 6eV).

Figure N.4 illustrates the sites of absorption of the various wavelengths and hence the potential sites of damage, and Table N.3 summarizes some of the sources of non ionising radiation and the type of ocular damage that may occur.

Non-planned replacement of contact lenses

In certain instances contact lenses can be prescribed to be used for as long as the lenses will last; this is referred to as 'non-planned lens replacement'. Patients for whom non-planned replacement lens use might be indicated include, for example, those who require specially prepared, hand-painted cosmetic lenses; those who wear lenses infrequently and are outside the daily disposable lens prescription range; and those who previously have been demonstrated to have few problems with non-planned replacement lenses. However, the main reason for prescribing on a non-planned replacement basis probably relates to a 'traditional' approach adopted by some practitioners who are perhaps unaware of, or reluctant to embrace, the vast array of planned replacement and disposable lens systems that are available in the marketplace.

The cost of disposable lens systems has come down to such a large extent over the past decade that the current cost to a patient for a monthly lens replacement system would be about the same, or perhaps even less, than the cost of a single pair of lenses for ongoing use (i.e. non-planned replacement) that might last, say, for 12 months. If the more frequent and intensive professional care required for patients wearing lenses on a non-planned replacement basis is factored in, then the cost of this modality of lens wear is prohibitive. Thus, 'cost saving' can no longer be cited as a reason for prescribing lenses on a non-planned replacement basis.

Being outside the available prescription range is also becoming less of a reason for prescribing lenses on a non-planned replacement basis, because planned replacement lenses are now available from many companies in an almost limitless range of parameters in both spherical and toric designs.

Non-steroidal anti-inflammatory drugs

Non-steroidal anti-inflammatory drugs (NSAIDs) were developed for the treatment of inflammatory disease, but unlike steroids, their use is not associated with the ocular adverse effects of raised intraocular pressure and cataract. Prostaglandins are pro-inflammatory chemical mediators and are implicated in the sensation of pain. NSAIDs inhibit the enzyme cyclo-oxygenase that produces prostaglandins from arachidonic acid; in low doses they produce analgesia, while in higher doses they relieve inflammation. Well-known over-the-counter examples of NSAIDs are aspirin (acetylsalicylic acid) and ibuprofen. Since prostaglandins have a protective function in the gastric mucosa, treatment with NSAIDs can result in upper gastrointestinal ulceration and gastritis. The use of NSAIDs is generally considered to be contraindicated in patients with a history of sensitivity, or adverse reactions, to aspirin.

The analgesic property of diclofenac, flurbiprofen and ketoprofen has made them useful in the area of anaesthesia as alternatives or adjuncts to opioids for the relief of postoperative pain, and for this purpose they can be administered orally or by injection. The anti-inflammatory action of these drugs is beneficial in the treatment of rheumatic disease. Topical NSAIDs are utilized primarily in the context of ophthalmic surgery and, in contrast to steroids, they do not inhibit healing or increase the risk of infection (Tables N.4 and N.5). If prostaglandins were released during surgery, they would cause miosis. While NSAIDs have no intrinsic mydriatic property, their mode of action in reducing the level of prostaglandins can ensure pupil dilation during cataract extraction.

NSAIDs can provide prophylaxis and reduction of post-operative inflammation and associated symptoms that may follow, e.g. cataract surgery, strabismus surgery or argon laser trabeculoplasty. The pain associated with corneal epithelial defects after photorefractive keratectomy, radial keratotomy or accidental trauma can also be alleviated by NSAIDs. In addition to their perioperative use, NSAIDs are sometimes employed in the treatment of conditions such as episcleritis and diclofenac is licensed for the treatment of seasonal allergic conjunctivitis.

Table N.3 • Ultraviolet radiation and the eye (courtesy of Blackwell Publishing Ltd, Oxford, 1985).

Spectral domain		Wavelength (nm)	Sources	Site of ocular damage
Biological	Physical			
UV-C	Far UV	200–280	Sunlight, lamps – arc, germicidal and mercury, excimer laser	Corneal epithelium resulting in photokeratitis, corneal opacity
UV-B	Far UV	280–315	Sunlight, sunlamps, welding arc, excimer laser	Corneal epithelium resulting in photokeratitis, corneal opacity
		295–315		Lens epithelium and nucleus, resulting in cataract
UV-A	Near UV	315–380	Sunlight, UV-A sunlamp, sunbeds, excimer laser	Lens epithelium and nucleus, resulting in cataract

Visible radiation and the eye.

Visible wavelength (nm)	Sources	Site of ocular damage
400–780	Sunlight; incandescent, fluorescent and arc lamps Lasers – argon, krypton	Retinal pigment epithelium, haemoglobin, macular pigment photoreceptors, resulting in visual loss, colour vision problems, accelerated ageing

Infra-red radiation and the eye.

Spectral domain		Wavelength (nm)	Sources	Site of ocular damage
Biological	Physical			
IR-A	Near IR	780–1400	Sunlight, furnaces, arc lamp, electric fires, neodymium-YAG laser	Pigment epithelium of retina, iris, lens, resulting in visual loss and cataract
IR-B	Far IR	1400–3000	Sunlight, furnaces, erbium laser	Corneal and lens epithelium, resulting in corneal opacity, aqueous flare and cataract
IR-C	Far IR	3000–10 000	Furnaces, carbon dioxide laser	Corneal epithelium, resulting in corneal opacity

Table N.4 • Topical NSAIDs: preserved multidose preparations.

Non-proprietary name	Proprietary name	Formulation	Preservative
Diclofenac sodium	Voltarol® Ophtha Multidose	Drops 0.1%	Benzalkonium chloride 0.005%*
Ketorolac trometamol	Acular®	Drops 0.5%	Benzalkonium chloride 0.01%*

* with disodium edetate

Notified bodies
- See *Medical Devices Directive*.

Nystagmus

Nystagmus is a regular, repetitive, involuntary movement of the eye whose direction, amplitude and frequency is variable. It is rare, with various estimates placing the prevalence at between 1 in 1,000 and 3 in 10,000. There are several factors that complicate the evaluation of nystagmus. It is a particularly difficult condition to evaluate, for the following reasons:

- Nystagmus is not a condition, but a sign. Many different ocular anomalies can cause nystagmus, or it can be idiopathic, with no apparent lesion as a cause.

Table N.5 • Topical NSAIDs: unpreserved single dose preparation.

Non-proprietary name	Proprietary name	Formulation
Diclofenac sodium	Voltarol® Ophtha	Drops 0.1%
Flurbiprofen sodium	Ocufen®	Drops 0.03%

- Attempts to classify the type of nystagmoid eye movement by simply watching the patient's eye movements often do not agree with the results of objective eye movement analysis.
- The pattern of nystagmoid eye movements cannot be used with certainty to predict the aetiology of the nystagmus. Some general rules exist, e.g. congenital nystagmus (CN) is usually horizontal. However, there are exceptions (e.g. when CN is not purely horizontal), and there are many cases of horizontal nystagmus which are not congenital.
- The same patient may exhibit different types of nystagmoid eye movements on different occasions. Congenital nystagmus is often worse when the patient is under stress or tries hard to see.
- Visual loss in nystagmus is only loosely correlated with the type of nystagmoid eye movements. There may be an underlying pathology causing poor vision resulting in nystagmus. Pathology may be causing, independently, the nystagmus and the poor vision. Pathology (hypothesized in congenital

Table N.6 • Characteristics of congenital, latent and acquired nystagmus.

Congenital nystagmus	Latent nystagmus	Acquired nystagmus
Presents in first 6 months of life	Usually presents in first 6 months of life, and almost always in first 12 months	Onset at any age and usually associated with other symptoms (e.g. nausea, vertigo, movement or balance disorders)
Family history often present	May be family history of underlying cause (e.g. congenital esotropia)	History may include head trauma or neurological disease such as cerebellar degeneration or multiple sclerosis
Oscillopsia absent or rare under normal viewing conditions	Oscillopsia absent or rare under normal viewing conditions	Oscillopsia common; may also have diplopia
Usually horizontal; although small vertical and torsional movements may be present. Pure vertical or torsional presentations are rare	Always horizontal; and, on monocular occlusion, saccadic, beating towards the uncovered eye	Oscillations may be horizontal, vertical, or torsional depending on the site of the lesion
The eye movements are bilateral and conjugate to the naked eye	Oscillations are always conjugate	Oscillations may be disconjugate and in different planes
Jerk or pendular nystagmus, eye movement recordings show accelerating slow phase	Jerk nystagmus, eye movement recordings show decelerating slow phase	Jerk, pendular, or saw-toothed waveform
May be present with other ocular conditions: albinism, achromatopsia, aniridia, optic atrophy	Usually or always secondary to an early-onset interruption of binocular vision, particularly congenital esotropia; may be associated with dissociated vertical deviation	Results from pathological lesion or trauma affecting motor areas of brain or motor pathways
A head turn may be present, usually to utilize a null zone, although nystagmus is present in all directions of gaze	May be a head turn in the direction of the fixing eye	There may be a gaze direction in which nystagmus is absent, and a corresponding head turn
Intensity may lessen on convergence but it is usually worse when fatigued or under stress	More intense when the fixing eye abducts, less on adduction	
Pursuit and optokinetic reflexes may be 'inverted'		Peripheral vestibular disease (e.g. Meniéres disease) usually generates linear slow phases and worsens if fixation is removed

idiopathic nystagmus) may be causing the nystagmus which causes poor vision. It seems that amblyopia also develops secondary to early onset nystagmus.

There are two fundamentally different approaches to classifying nystagmus, based on the aetiology (congenital, latent, acquired and other eye movement phenomena types) or on eye movement characteristics (pendular or jerky). Children with new nystagmus, or nystagmus which has not been previously investigated, should be referred to a paediatric ophthalmologist. Since specialist investigative techniques are required for the evaluation of CN, such cases are best referred to a tertiary centre with the appropriate facilities (e.g. pattern and flash visual evoked potential testing, electro-retinography, objective eye movement analysis). Perhaps, the most important clinical judgement for the optometrist is whether the nystagmus is congenital, latent, or acquired. The characteristic features of these conditions are summarized in Table N.6, to aid differential diagnosis.

Objective refraction

This term refers to the measurement of refractive error of a patient by a means requiring no patient response. An objective refraction is carried out in general practice by retinoscopy or by autorefraction. The ease of technique and accuracy makes objective refraction useful in most assessments as it provides a baseline measurement of refractive error from which to begin subjective refraction. This speeds up assessment and also improves accuracy in the many cases where a patient is uncertain in response. There are several instances where objective refraction is the main, or indeed sole, method of assessment. This may be where the patient has a learning or cognitive impairment, a behavioural difficulty, is very young or has serious communication difficulties. In screening, particularly for ametropia in the young, the accuracy and speed of the objective assessment make it the most important technique. See *Retinoscopy; Autorefraction*.

Obliquely crossed cylinders

Cylindrical lenses in combination, where the axes are not parallel or mutually perpendicular, are referred to as being 'obliquely crossed'. Any pair of cylindrical lenses (with associated sphere, if present) can be resolved into a single sphero-cylindrical combination. This calculation is somewhat more complex than resolving obliquely crossed prisms.

The effective power at a given angle θ to the axis of a cylinder with power 'F' is F/sin^2. Thus, along the axis, the power of a cylinder is at a minimum, and is at maximum perpendicular to the axis. In Figure O.1, two cylindrical lenses are shown, F_1 and F_2. Their axes are separated by an angle a. A resultant power component C has an angle of B from the axis of F_1. The effect of the two cylinders F_1 and F_2 at F can be calculated from:

$$F_A = F_1 \sin^2 B + F_2 \sin^2 (a - B)$$

Perpendicular to the axis of C the power is:

$$F_B = F_1 \sin^2(90-B) + F_2 \sin^2 (90-a - B)$$

This can also be written as:

$$F_B = F_1 \cos^2 + F_2 \cos^2 (a - B)$$

If these two values are the maximum and minimum, then the cylinder power of the resultant sphero-cylinder is:

$$C = F_B - F_A$$
$$C = F_1 \cos^2 B + F_2 \cos^2 (a - B) - [F_1 \sin^2 B + F_2 \sin^2 (a - B)]$$

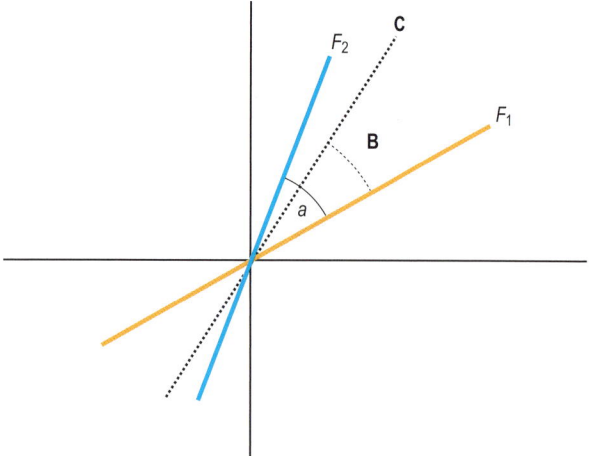

Figure O.1 • Resolution of obliquely crossed cylinders

If this expression is made equal to zero and differentiated, this gives the value of the relative axis of the cylinder as:

$$\tan 2B = \frac{F_1 \sin 2a}{F_1 + F_2 \cos 2a}$$

Assuming that we are finding the plus cylinder transposition, then the resultant sphere power can be found from:

$$S = F_1 \sin^2 B + F_2 \sin^2(a - B)$$

The resultant cylinder is:

$$C = F_1 + F_2 - 2S$$

Examples of the calculation method are shown in Table O.1. This calculation technique is of use to predict the effects of placing corrective cylindrical lenses at an incorrect axis before an eye.

Oblique rigid bitoric contact lenses

- See *Cylindrical power equivalent rigid toric lenses.*

Ocular adnexa

The ocular adnexa are those structures that support and protect the eye, and include the eyelids, conjunctiva and lacrimal system. They play an important role in the formation of the pre-ocular tear film, and collectively defend the eye against antigenic challenge.

Ocular defence mechanisms

The eye has a number of inherent protective mechanisms to resist infection. Potential pathogens are present in the tear film of 5% of a population at any time, yet the prevalence of ocular surface infection falls far short of this value. The tear film and the blinking process play an important role in the resistance of infection. Basal tear production is of the order of 1–2μl per minute and the overall tear volume is about 7μl, which confirms the rapid turnover of tears at the ocular surface with the consequent removal of micro-organisms.

Bacteria in the tear film must also breach the defence provided by proteins in the tear film, such as lysozyme, lactoferrin and transferrin, for an infection to be established. Furthermore, immunoglobulins such as secretory IgA, IgG, IgE and IgM can act to resist infection.

Ocular surface mucus provides a physical barrier to infection because it binds strongly to bacteria, thereby enhancing their removal from the ocular surface (Figure O.2). A bacterium that is able to defeat all the above systems is still hampered in its quest to invade and infect the cornea because of the presence of fibronectin at the epithelial surface, which is known to reduce the bacterial adhesion to epithelial cells in mucosal systems.

Contact lens wear adversely affects a number of these defence mechanisms. Perhaps the most significant effect is the prevention of clearance of debris and micro-organisms from the ocular surface by the blinking mechanism. The

Table O.1 • Calculation technique for predicting the effects of placing corrective cylindrical lenses at an incorrect axis before the eye.

OBLIQUELY CROSSED CYLINDERS		Example 1	Example 2	Example 3
Sphere 1	S_1	1.00	0.00	0.00
Cylinder 1	F_1	1.00	2.00	3.00
Axis 1	A_1	0.00	60.00	0.00
Sphere 2	S_2	0.00	−3.00	0.00
Cylinder 2	F_2	−1.00	3.00	−3.00
Axis 2	A_2	120.00	120.00	30.00
Angle between cylinders	$a = A_2 - A_1$	120.00	60.00	30.00
	$\tan 2B = (F_2 \sin 2a)/(F_1 + F_2 \cos 2a)$	0.5774	5.1962	−1.7321
Angle B	$B = (\tan^{-1}(2B))/2$	15.00	39.55	−30.00
Induced sphere	$S = F_1 \sin^2 B + F_2 \sin^2(a - B)$	−0.87	+1.18	−1.50
Resultant sphere	Sphere $= S_1 + S_2 + S$	+0.13	−1.82	−1.50
Resultant cylinder	Cylinder $= F_1 + F_2 - 2S$	+1.73	+2.65	+3.00
Resultant axis*	Axis $= A_1 + B$	15	100	150

Note that the angle A_2 must be larger than the angle A_1 in standard notation.
*If resultant axis is negative, add 180 to give final answer

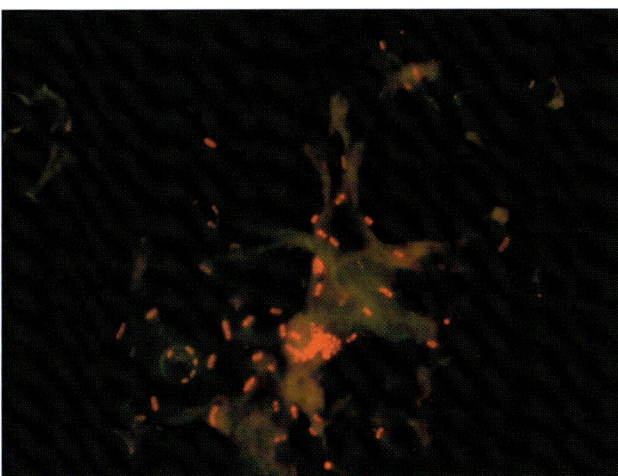

Figure O.2 • Pseudomonas bacteria (orange) bound to mucus (green), which is cleared from the eye during blinking. This forms an effective ocular defence mechanism against infection.

level of fibronectin is possibly reduced during contact lens wear, thereby increasing the likelihood of bacterial attachment.

A key reason for the increase in ocular infections amongst contact lens wearers is from the bioburden of micro-organisms introduced to the ocular surface when lenses are inserted. The risk of infection with Acanthamoeba is significantly increased when no contact lens disinfection is adopted by the lens wearer, or when weak disinfection systems (e.g. chlorine) are employed. The appropriate use of a suitable disinfection system can reduce the incidence of microbial infection of the eye.

Ocular dominance

Measurement of the ocular dominance or sighting preference is useful in establishing which eye to correct for distance vision during monovision contact lens fitting, or whilst making adjustments during simultaneous contact lens fitting. Ocular dominance can be determined using preferential looking tests, or alternatively by the +2.00D test. The former is carried out by sitting opposite the patient and asking the patient to look, through a hole in a piece of card, at an open eye of the practitioner. Whichever eye the patient lines up with the open eye of the practitioner is the dominant one. The latter test involves placing the best binocular distance refraction in the trial frame and, while the patient looks at the lowest line that can be read, a +2.00D lens is placed alternatively in front of each eye. The patient indicates when the vision is clearest. If the +2.00D lens is in front of the left eye when the image is reported as clearest then the right eye is considered as distance dominant, and vice versa. Unsuccessful wearers sometimes become successful after switching near and distance corrections contrary to the dominance as measured by traditional methods, but rarely do so contrary to the +2.00D test.

Ocular hazards

There are two main groups of ocular hazards: mechanical and non-mechanical (Figure O.3). The mechanical hazards may cause damage to the eye and orbit, ranging in severity from superficial foreign bodies to contusion or perforating injuries. Non-mechanical hazards can cause a wide range of injuries, including corneal scarring, cataracts and retinal burns.

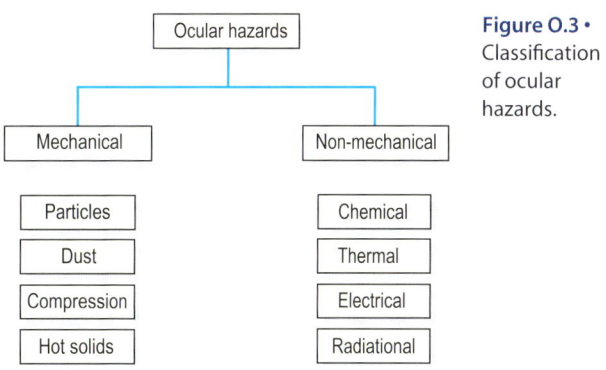

Figure O.3 • Classification of ocular hazards.

Ocular lens light absorption

Selective absorption of short wavelengths in the ocular lens increases systematically with age and has a significant effect on blue-green hue discrimination ability and threshold short wavelength sensitivity after about 55 years of age. The influence of ocular lens density makes the identification of acquired Type 3 (Tritan) colour deficiency more difficult in older patients, especially those with diabetic eye disease and glaucoma. The ocular lens suffers from chromatic aberration. Long wavelengths have a longer focal length than short wavelengths. In emmetropia long wavelengths are focused behind the retina and short wavelengths are focused in front of the retina. This difference is exploited in bi-chromatic methods of refraction which are effective for colour deficient people even when red and green are confused.

Ocular lubricants

- See *Artificial tears and ocular lubricants*.

Ocular motility

Testing for ocular movements is essential in any binocular vision assessment. There should be smooth movements throughout the motor field of action of the extra-ocular muscles within the binocular field (and also in the monocular field where the eyebrows or nose may be restricting the view).

The test for ocular motility is designed to elicit over- or under-action of the extra-ocular muscles and to identify any incomitancy. A non-focused pen torch at 33cm is used for fixation. The patient is asked to look directly at it. The pupil reflexes should be observed for symmetry and where they appear to be monocularly, since the pupil centre and position of the line of sight through the optical components of the eye may not coincide, resulting in non-central pupil reflexes. Once the position of the reflexes is known, they can be observed for any departure from normal as the test proceeds.

The light is moved along each of the diagnostic (primary) directions of gaze. The patient can be asked to report any diplopia; however, careful observation needs to be maintained since long-standing strabismus often leads to inhibition of the image belonging to the non-fixing eye.

The pen torch should be moved in an arc in front of the patient as in a perimeter until the point is reached where the patient's eyes stop moving. Repeating the test with a near fixation card (in the shape of a tongue depressor) as the target, will allow the patient to observe any tilting more easily. This helps to identify any torsional element of the deviation. It should be noted that the vertical meridian is not a diagnostic direction of gaze. However it is still useful to test in this direction, since it will help to identify some A patterns (greater divergence on downgaze) and V patterns (greater divergence on upgaze).

The horizontal meridians will only involve the lateral and medial recti and it is often convenient to start with these. The observer should look out for narrowing of the palpebral fissure and also lid lag, which can be signs of Duane's syndrome or hyperthyroidism. The diagonal meridians should then be tested.

The practitioner should also look for an over-action or under-action of the muscles. If unsure it is worthwhile performing a cover test in the nine cardinal points of gaze. In incomitant deviations, patients may report diplopia. The image seen furthest away belongs to the eye with the under-acting muscle that pulls in that direction.

Oedema, contact lens-induced

Oedema refers to an increase in the fluid content of tissue, and in the contact lens field 'oedema' is usually taken to mean excess fluid in the corneal stroma. Since the cornea is only able to swell in the anterior-posterior direction (as a result of the collagen fibre structural network in the stroma), the physical dimensions of the cornea can only increase in that dimension – that is, in thickness. The human cornea experiences about 2–4% oedema during sleep. With current generation hydrogel and rigid lenses, daytime corneal oedema typically varies between 1% and 6%, and the level of overnight oedema measured upon awakening generally falls in the range 5–13%. Silicone hydrogel lenses induce about 4% overnight oedema, which is about the same or only slightly more than occurs when sleeping without lenses.

Clinicians can estimate the magnitude of corneal oedema via careful observation with the slit-lamp biomicroscope, as a number of structural changes can be identified that correlate with various levels of oedema. Using direct focal illumination, striae appear as fine, wispy, white, vertically oriented lines in the posterior stroma when the level of oedema reaches about 5% (Grade 2). Striae are thought to represent fluid separation of the predominantly vertically arranged collagen fibrils in the posterior stroma. Folds can be observed – using specular reflection technique – in the endothelial mosaic as a combination of depressed grooves or raised ridges, or as a general area of apparent buckling, when the level of oedema reaches about 8% (Grade 3). It is thought that folds indicate a physical buckling of the posterior stromal layers in response to high levels of oedema. The stroma takes on a hazy, milky or granular appearance when the level of oedema reaches about 15% (Grade 4); such high levels of oedema are often associated with other signs and symptoms of ocular distress (Figure O.4).

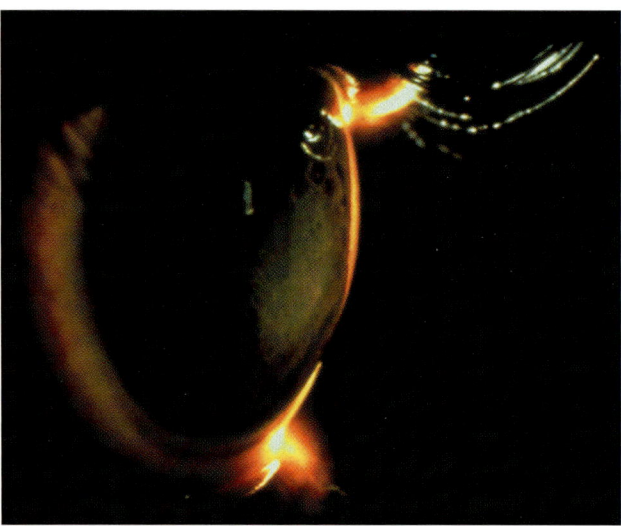

Figure O.4 • Severe central corneal oedema, resulting in 'clouding'.

Contact lenses restrict corneal oxygen availability, creating a hypoxic environment at the anterior corneal surface. To conserve energy, the corneal epithelium begins to respire anaerobically. Lactate, a by-product of anaerobic metabolism, increases in concentration and moves posteriorly into the corneal stroma. This creates an osmotic load that is balanced by an increased movement of water into the stroma. The sudden influx of water cannot be matched by the removal of water from the stroma by the endothelial pump, resulting in corneal oedema.

The key strategy for reducing the oedema response is to increase corneal oxygen availability during lens wear. Rigid lens oedema can be alleviated by increasing lens oxygen transmissibility, or by fitting a lens of flatter base curve, greater edge lift or smaller diameter so as to increase lens-mediated tear exchange. Soft lens oedema can be alleviated by fitting lenses of higher oxygen transmissibility, flattening the base curve or reducing lens diameter. General strategies for reducing oedema include changing from extended to daily wear, changing from soft to rigid lenses, fitting silicone hydrogel lenses, or reducing wearing time.

In general, the prognosis for recovery of the cornea from lens-induced oedema is excellent. The oedema induced when a patient wears a contact lens for the first time will resolve within 4 hours of the lens being removed. Chronic lens-induced oedema can take up to 7 days to resolve.

One-day contact lenses

- See *Daily disposable contact lenses*.

One-step hydrogen peroxide disinfecting solution for contact lenses

- See *Hydrogen peroxide disinfecting solution for contact lenses*.

Opaque contact lens backing

The matrix of a lens can be tinted with a translucent dye, and an iris pattern and black pupil applied to the back

Table O.2 • Features of direct ophthalmoscopy compared to indirect ophthalmoscopy.

Advantages	Disadvantages
High magnification view (15×)	Magnification varies with patient's refractive error: higher in myopes
Relatively good imaging through a small pupil	Very small field of view (10° in an emmetrope): difficult to scan fundus
Readily portable: good for domiciliary use	Monocular view
Relatively inexpensive	Difficult to use on small children
View of fundus is correct way up and non-reversed	Image degrades significantly with media opacities
	Poor at showing colour and elevational changes
	Close proximity to patient essential

surface of the lens using opaque paints. In this way, the entire back surface of the lens is rendered opaque; light reflects off the opaque layer and the coloured appearance is created from the translucent tint in the lens body. See *Tinted contact lenses*.

Ophthalmoscopy, direct

In routine optometric practice, the mainstay of ocular examination is the direct ophthalmoscope. This technique has various advantages and disadvantages, as detailed in Table O.2.

Direct ophthalmoscopy is particularly useful for examination through a small pupil for specific fine features, for example neovascularisation of the disc and microaneurysms. It is least useful when a stereoscopic view is required, such as in macular oedema or in the assessment of depth of cupping in potentially glaucomatous discs. It is also of little value when an overall view of the posterior pole is required, as is the case in diabetic retinopathy.

Ophthalmoscopy, head-borne binocular indirect

This technique involves examination of the ocular fundus through a dilated pupil using a head-borne illumination and binocular observation system in conjunction with a hand-held condensing lens. A scleral depressor is required if scleral indentation is attempted. The condensing lens captures the emergent light from the patient's eye and presents this for binocular viewing. The larger the lens and the bigger the pupil, the wider the field of view obtainable. The lower the condensing lens power, the greater the magnification and the smaller the field. Higher-power lenses are held closer to the patient. The view is a bright wide field (about 10° wider than that of direct ophthalmoscopy). There is reasonable stereopsis and negligible alteration in magnification with the refractive error of the patient or examiner. An addition of +2.00D or +2.50D is incorporated in the viewing system, so that presbyopic examiners can view the aerial image comfortably. The image is upside down and laterally reversed. The most peripheral part of the image seen is in the opposite direction to the patient's gaze, so that on looking up the superior periphery is seen at the bottom of the image.

Having optimally adjusted the headset and viewing system, the observational technique requires several weeks of practice and experience before the practitioner becomes confident. The procedure is as follows:

- Instruct patients that their eyes are going to be examined using a bright light, but that it will not be harmful. Both eyes should remain open throughout the examination.
- Lie patients down in a darkened room so that they are at waist height and their head is in front of the examiner.
- Start by examining the superior periphery. This will entail the patient looking up and the examiner standing 180° in the opposite direction (i.e. towards the patient's feet).
- Once the red reflex is seen, insert the lens with the steeper curvature of the bi-aspheric lens facing the examiner. The side facing the patient has a silver or white band at the edge.
- Hold the lens parallel to the patient's iris plane and a short distance from the cornea with the fingers steadied on the patient's forehead or cheek.
- If necessary, hold the lids apart with the fingers of the other hand.
- The anterior segment of the eye should be seen through the lens with a red reflex in the pupil.
- Move the lens away from the eye until the fundus image fills the lens, but not so far that an inverted minified image of the anterior segment is seen.
- Adjust the illumination, if necessary, to the minimum that permits clear visualization of the fundus details.
- Progressively cover all peripheral quadrants by asking the patient to adjust the direction of gaze and moving to a position opposite to the gaze direction. The lens needs to be re-aligned each time. Tilting the lens can improve the image dramatically by moving the lens' surface reflections out of the examiner's way.
- Examine the posterior pole, limiting exposure time to reduce dazzle.
- Release the lids before each re-fixation to allow the patient to blink and separate as necessary to improve your view.

Ophthalmoscopy, scanning laser

The principle of scanning laser ophthalmoscopy (SLO) is that the laser is focused to form a highly collimated beam that is passed through a series of mirrors, including a rotating polygon mirror, to pivot in the plane of the pupil and form a raster at the patient's retina. Light is then reflected back through the system and passed through signal amplification (and other devices to reduce reflections) to form an image via a computer and specifically designed software or to a video device. The main advantage of this system is that it can be used to carry out retinal investigations in ways that enable the observer to gain more information about the retina than can be obtained from conventional imaging techniques. The Panoramic 200 is designed to enable an area of up to 200 degrees of the fundus to be produced as one image and without the use of collaging or pupil dilation.

The SLO tends to be superior to standard imaging methods when cataract is present and can be used for both fluorescein and indocyanine green angiography. A further function that can be performed by a scanning laser system is that of retinal tomography or three-dimensional imaging to allow quantitative data to be obtained. For these measurements, a confocal system is needed whereby the laser beam is focused onto a flat reference plane on the retina. Such instruments (e.g. the Heidelberg Retinal Tomograph (HRT)) are able to compare topographic profiles so obtained with statistics gained from studies of a wide variety of patients. This data can indicate if the profile of any aspect of the fundus, such as the optic disc, falls outside that assessed as normal. Scanning laser tomography is particularly sensitive in detecting changes in profile over time.

Another type of retinal assessment is the use of retinal laser polarimetry, as performed with the GDx Nerve Fiber Analyzer. The laser beam double-passes through the retinal nerve fibre layer (RNFL) which is birefringent because of the presence of the retinal ganglion cells. The birefringent property of the RNFL causes the beam to be split into two parts, which are plane polarized at right angles to each other. One of these beams continues to obey the laws of refraction (the ordinary beam), while the other (the extraordinary beam) does not. This results in a phase-shift between the two beams. A polarization detector is used to measure the change in polarization and Fourier analysis is used to calculate the phase shift or retardation that has occurred. This retardation is proportional to the thickness of the RNFL. Reduction in the density of the RNFL (e.g. as can occur on primary open-angle glaucoma) over time is detected this way, often well before any corresponding visual field defect is measurable.

Ophthalmoscopy, slit-lamp binocular indirect

Hand-held indirect lenses are used when a thorough binocular scan of the central region of the ocular fundus is required. Assuming that there is a slit lamp biomicroscope (SLB) to hand, all that is required is a suitable binocular indirect ophthalmoscopy (BIO) lens. As a general principle, the higher the lens dioptric power, the lower the magnification and closer the lens must be held to the eye, but the higher the field of view. Lenses are available with detachable yellow filters (which reduce the blue-light hazard in prolonged examination), lid adapters (which help separate the lids and set the correct working distance), graticules to record the size of features, and mounts which steady the lens at the SLB. A stereoscopic low-magnification wide-field view of the fundus is obtained. The image of the fundus is laterally reversed and upside down, so care must be taken when considering and documenting any features of interest.

The technique for performing an examination using SLB indirect ophthalmoscopy is as follows.

- Instill a mydriatic as necessary. For the general routine examination of a young patient, a mydriatic is not essential, especially for the higher-powered lenses with shorter working distances. However, for older patients and for all instances in which a thorough binocular examination of the central fundus or foveal area is required, a mydriatic should be used.
- Position the patient comfortably at the SLB. Ensure the lens is clean and that the magnification is set to low.
- Select a beam height approximately equal to the patient's pupil diameter and a width of about 3mm.
- Pull the SLB back towards the practitioner and laterally align the slit beam so that the blurred slit-beam illuminates the centre of the patient's pupil.
- Interpose the BIO lens centrally and at about 2cm from the eye. It is generally not important which way round the BIO lens is held.
- The SLB should then be moved forwards towards the patient and focused on the aerial image of the patient's inverted pupil. Then continue moving forwards to focus through the pupil onto the retina. This image is between the BIO lens and the aerial image of the pupil/iris.
- The BIO lens should then be moved forward towards the patient to enlarge the pupil image and, by doing so, increase the field of view.
- The practitioner should then scan over the fundus using the same approach adopted when scanning the cornea.
- The patient should be instructed to look in the different directions of gaze (eight positions) and the lens repositioned each time to optimize the view, tilting where necessary to avoid reflections.
- The magnification can be increased where necessary. The amount of magnification will be limited by the particular slit lamp used.
- Finally, the patient is asked to look towards the practitioner's ear (right ear for right eye, left ear for left eye), which enables visualization of the optic disc.
- If the vitreous is to be examined, the microscope must be pulled back and the focus shifted onto the feature being examined (e.g. floater or hyaloid membrane). Visualization of the vitreous is difficult and the practitioner is recommended to begin with patients who have widely dilated pupils and who have suffered posterior vitreous detachment.
- If necessary, the field of view can be increased by moving the lens either vertically or horizontally in the frontal plane. The lens is moved in the same direction to the region that requires investigation. For example, if more of the superior fundus needs to be imaged, then the patient is instructed to look up as far as possible and the lens is moved upwards.

The technique has various advantages and disadvantages, as detailed in Table O.3.

As is highlighted, slit-lamp BIO is particularly useful for stereoscopic examination of the disc and macula,

Table 0.3 Features of hand-held slit-lamp indirect ophthalmoscopy compared to direct ophthalmoscopy.

Advantages	Disadvantages
Wide field of view, relatively easy to scan fundus	View of fundus is upside down and laterally reversed
Image degrades significantly less than direct image with media opacities	Magnification limited by quality of slit-lamp optics
	Very difficult to use with a small pupil
Good at showing colour and elevational changes	Difficult to use on small children
Relatively inexpensive if slit lamp available	Unsuitable for domiciliary use
Magnification does not vary with patient's refractive error	Takes some practice to become comfortable with technique
	Less pleasant for patient
Comfortable distance from patient maintained	Reflections are a problem
	Scanning of fundus required to build up general picture

especially to assess the depth of cupping in glaucoma and to detect subtle macular oedema in diabetics. With further experience, the vitreous can be inspected and the hyaloid membrane visualized. It is certainly not an easy technique to master and requires practice.

Optic nerve head

The optic nerve head (ONH) represents an area of considerable specialization where axons from retinal ganglion cells leave the eye. The thickness of the nerve fibre layer increases from the periphery of the retina towards the disc, where it is elevated above the plane of the retina (giving rise to the alternative term for the disc 'optic papilla'). Fibres from the nasal, superior and inferior retina follow a direct course to the ONH. Fibres from the nasal side of the fovea (papillomacular bundle) also take a direct route. By contrast, axons from ganglion cells temporal to the fovea take arcuate paths to enter the ONH at its upper and lower margins. Axon bundles in the nerve head show a considerable degree of spatial order. Ganglion cells from the central retina generally have axons near the centre of the optic nerve; peripheral ganglion cells have axons near the periphery of the nerve.

At the ONH approximately 1 million ganglion cell axons leave the retina through the scleral canal. The outermost half of the sclera is reflected backwards to become continuous with the dura mater, whilst the innermost half is modified to form the lamina cribrosa (cribiform plate). The lamina cribrosa offers a conduit for retinal blood vessels and provides mechanical support for ganglion cell axons as they pass through the scleral canal. The lamina also serves as a convenient reference point for localization purposes, such that the ONH can be resolved into 3 distinct regions (Figure O.5):

- Pre-laminar zone
- Lamina zone
- Post-laminar zone.

At the interface with the vitreous, the ONH is covered by a canopy of astrocytes (the so called 'internal limiting membrane of Elschnig'). This membrane is thickened centrally and thins towards the periphery of the disc, where it is continuous with the inner limiting membrane

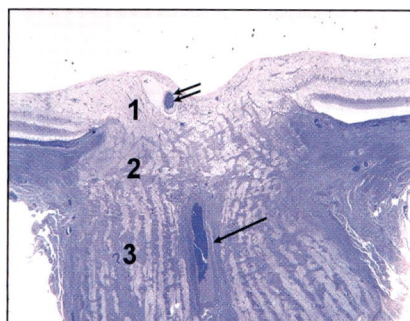

Figure O.5 • Microscopic view of the optic nerve head sectioned longitudinally. The pre-laminar (1), laminar (2) and post-laminar regions (3) are indicated. The central retinal artery is visible (arrow) and also branches of the central retinal vessels at the surface of the disc (double arrow).

of the retina. Within the prelaminar region, glial columns that extend forward from the lamina cribrosa maintain fasciculation of axons. Further glial tissue is interposed between ONH axons and the choroid (border layer of Jacoby). This extends forward to form the intermediary tissue of Kuhnt, which separates ONH axons from the outer layers of the retina.

The lamina cribrosa consists of a meshwork formed by interlinked connective tissue plates (cribiform plates). Central retinal vessels and bundles of axons pass through a series of round or oval apertures within the meshwork. The 300 to 400 pores that transmit axon bundles show a considerable variation in size, with the largest pores typically found in the superior and inferior quadrants.

Axons within the post-laminar optic nerve are myelinated, which principally accounts for the doubling of the optic nerve diameter from 1.5mm at the pre-laminar and laminar level to 3.0mm in the post-laminar region. Oligodendrocytes, that are responsible for myelination of the nerve axons, are numerous. Fasciculation of the myelinated nerve axons is maintained by connective tissue septa that are continuous with the lamina cribrosa. Within the post-laminar region, meningeal sheaths invest the optic nerve – a thin pial layer, a middle arachnoid layer and a thick collagenous dural layer.

The regional variation of the ONH vasculature is complex. The main source of arterial blood to the ONH is the posterior ciliary arteries, which derive from the ophthalmic artery. The number and site of entry of these arteries is variable, although typically 2 to 3 posterior ciliary arteries lie to the medial and lateral side of the optic nerve. Prior to entering the sclera, they divide into multiple smaller branches: 10 to 12 short posterior ciliary arteries (SPCAs) pierce the sclera close to the optic nerve, and 1 to 2 long posterior ciliary arteries penetrate further away. SPCAs contribute to an intrascleral arterial circle, the circle of Zinn and Haller, from which centripetal branches enter the laminar ONH. The circle is typically supplied by either medial or lateral SPCAs and is frequently incomplete, indicating that the circle functions as an end arterial system.

The arterial supply to the ONH is segmental:

- Small branches from retinal arterioles and cilio-retinal arteries supply the superficial nerve fibre layer.
- Arterial branches from the peripapillary choroid and SPCAs supply the pre-laminar region.
- Centripetal branches from the SPCA or the circle of Zinn supply the lamina cribrosa.
- Centripetal branches from the pia mater supply the post laminar region.

Venous drainage occurs via the central retinal vein and there may also be some drainage into the peripapillary choroid.

Optic papilla

- See *Optic nerve head*.

Optical coherence tomography

Optical coherence tomography (OCT) is a relatively new non-contact optical imaging technique that is capable of high-resolution micrometer-scale cross-sectional imaging of biological tissue. The commercially available OCT used for ophthalmic applications uses 843-nm wavelength near-infrared radiation, which provides a longitudinal resolution of 10–20µm. The technique uses Michelson interferometry to compare a partially coherent reference beam with one reflected from tissue. The two beams are combined and interference between the two light signals occurs only when their path lengths match to within the coherence length of light. The magnitude and distance within the tissue of the reflected or back-scattered light at a single point are determined using a mirror system. A tomographic image is generated by simultaneously displaying 100 adjacent scans, whose acquisition time takes approximately 1 second.

The technique of OCT is thus analogous to ultrasound B-mode imaging, except that it uses light rather than sound and performs imaging by measuring the back-scattered intensity of light from structures within the tissue. Strong reflections occur at boundaries between materials of differing refractive indices. The OCT two-dimensional scans are subsequently processed by a computer, which corrects for any axial eye movement artefacts that have occurred during the acquisition time. The scans are displayed using a false colour representation scale in which warm colours (red to white) represent areas

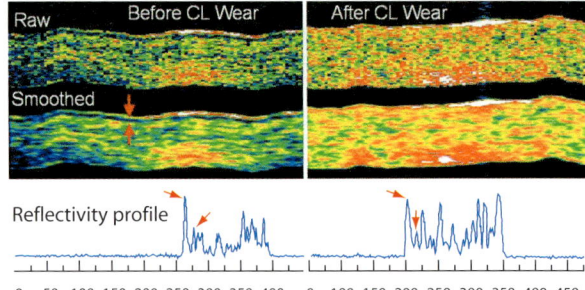

Figure O.6 • Optical coherence tomography (OCT) image, before and after closed-eye wear of a thick polyHEMA contact lens. The upper two-dimensional false-colour image indicates the plot obtained from the OCT, the smoothed image being that obtained once background noise is eliminated from the raw image. The lower plot indicates the reflectivity values obtained through the cornea. The data obtained indicate that the cornea has swollen substantially and that the water absorbed has resulted in an increase in the thickness and reflectivity of the corneal tissue. By determining the distance between two peaks from the reflectivity profile, corneal and epithelial thickness can be obtained. (Adapted from L. W. Jones (2002) Clinical instruments.)

of high optical reflectivity and cool colours (blue to black) represent areas of minimal optical reflectivity. The image obtained represents a cross-sectional view of the structure under investigation, similar in appearance to a histological section (Figure O.6).

This technique can be used to examine the retina and cornea. It has proven useful in determining epithelial and total corneal thickness changes following refractive surgery procedures, in cases of corneal oedema, and in evaluating contact lens positioning on the ocular surface. Because OCT enables the non-excisional, in situ, real-time imaging of tissue microstructure, it is a powerful and promising technique for ocular imaging purposes.

Optical Consumers Complaints Service

The Optical Consumers Complaints Service (OCCS) helps members of the public with complaints over the optical services received from an optical practice. It is funded by optometrists and dispensing opticians through a special levy on annual subscriptions paid to the General Optical Council. Complaints must relate to services provided by a registered optometrist or registered dispensing optician. Patients are always advised to try to resolve a complaint within the practice and the OCCS will intervene only if this process has been exhausted or the patient feels unable to return to the practice.

Optical illusion

- See *Visual illusion*.

Optical transmittance of contact lenses

Transparency is an essential requisite of a hydrogel for contact lens use, but not all hydrogels are optically transparent. Translucence and opacity in hydrogels is associated with microphase separation of water, which produces regions of differing refractive index within the

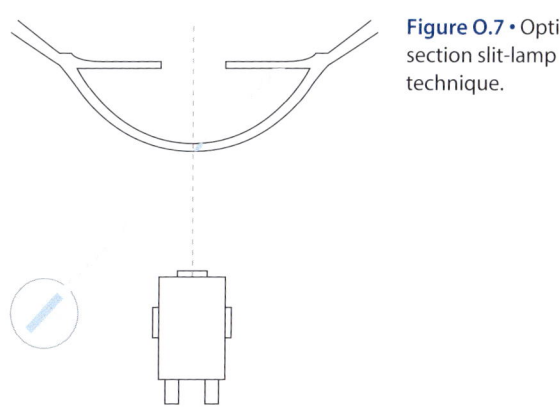

Figure O.7 • Optic section slit-lamp technique.

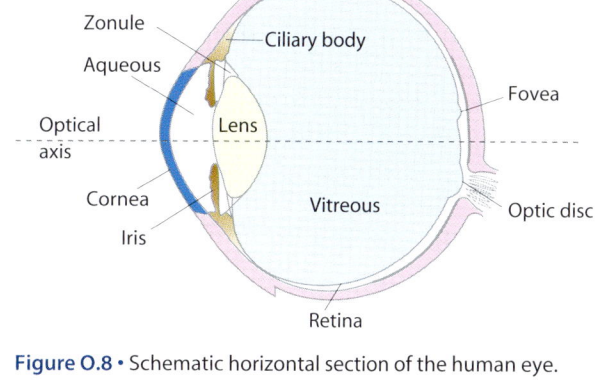

Figure O.8 • Schematic horizontal section of the human eye.

gel. Hydrogels that show this type of behaviour (typically synthesized by making co-polymers with large blocks or segments of hydrophobic and hydrophilic monomers rather then randomly dispersing them) do have advantages in terms of enhanced strength and permeability performance. Phase-separated hydrogels in which the domain sizes are small enough to retain optical transparency are of interest in applications in which strength and/or permeability are particularly important (e.g. extended-wear contact lenses and synthetic cornea). The lack of optical clarity in simple co-polymers of hydrophilic monomers such as HEMA and TRIS has been a major technical obstacle in the development of silicone hydrogel lenses.

Optic section, slit-lamp technique of

Once an area or object of interest is located when using the slit-lamp biomicroscope, the beam width can be narrowed to approximately 0.2mm to 'cross-section' the corneal tissue (Figure O.7). This provides the ability to assess accurately the depth of an object within the corneal layers. Typical uses include assessment of the depth of a foreign body, location of a corneal scar, and determining whether tissue within an area of staining is excavated, flat or raised.

Optics of the eye

The general structure and optical layout of the eye is shown in Figure O.8. About three-quarters of the optical power comes from the anterior cornea, with the crystalline lens providing supplementary power which, in the pre-presbyope, can be varied to focus objects sharply at different distances. The actual optical design is, however, subtle, in that all the optical surfaces are aspheric, while the lens (and probably also the cornea) displays a complex gradient of refractive index. There is little doubt that such refinements play an important role in controlling aberration.

Refractive indices of the media vary little between eyes, apart from the refractive index distribution across the lens, which changes with age as the lens grows throughout life. Each dimensional parameter is approximately normally distributed amongst different individuals. The values of the different parameters in the individual eye are, however, correlated so that the resultant distribution of refractive error is strongly peaked near emmetropia, rather than being normal. This correlation is thought to be due to a combination of genetic and environmental factors, visual experience helping to actively 'emmetropize' the eyes. The apparently greater incidence of myopia in recent times may be attributed to the greater prevalence of near tasks biasing this active process towards myopia rather than emmetropia.

Optometry

The word 'Optometry' is derived from the Greek: 'optikos' meaning 'of sight', and 'metron', meaning 'measure'. Optometry is an independent healthcare profession that is dedicated to measuring all aspect of eyesight and visual performance, prescribing corrective ophthalmic appliances, offering advice about ocular health and hygiene and the enhancement of visual performance, detecting eye disease, and in some cases, treating uncomplicated forms of eye disease.

Orbicularis oculi

The orbicularis oculi is the sphincter muscle of the eyelids, and can be divided anatomically into two main divisions – palpebral and orbital. Fibres of the palpebral division arise from the medial palpebral ligament and arc across the eyelids in a series of half-ellipses, meeting at the lateral canthus to form a lateral raphe. The lateral palpebral ligament also acts as an anchor point. The palpebral division can be further subdivided into marginal, pre-tarsal and pre-septal parts (Figure O.9). The marginal part (pars ciliaris), which is also known as Riolans muscle, is responsible for maintaining the apposition of the lid to the cornea during lid closure. A third part of the muscle (pars lacrimalis) is closely associated with the lacrimal outflow pathway. The pars lacrimalis (also known as Horner's muscle) encloses the canaliculus and provides attachments to the lacrimal sac and its associated fascia.

The orbital part of the orbicularis oculi lies outside the palpebral division and extends for some distance beyond the orbital margins. Muscle fibres arise predominantly from bone at the medial orbital rim, and appear to sweep around the lids without interruption as a series of complete ellipses. The muscle fibres of the orbital and palpebral divisions of the orbicularis are relatively short (0.4–2.1mm) and overlapping. The regional divisions of the orbicularis also show a functional distinction. The action of the palpebral part of the muscle is to produce the reflex or voluntary closure of the lids during

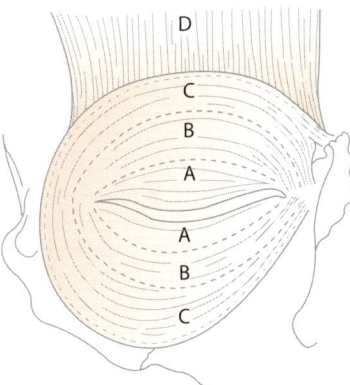

Figure O.9 • Schematic representation of the divisions of the orbicularis oculi and the frontalis. A = pre-tarsal; B = pre-septal; C = orbital; D = frontalis. Adapted from A. J. Bron, R. C. Tripathi, B. Tripathi (1997) Wolff's Anatomy of the Eye and Orbit, 8th edn. Chapman & Hall, London.

blinking. Contraction of the orbital division produces the forcible closure of the lids that occurs in sneezing or in response to a painful stimulus.

Orientation of toric contact lenses, soft

- See *Toric contact lens rotation, soft.*

Orthokeratology

This refers to a technique of fitting rigid contact lenses in such a way as to alter corneal morphology and thereby reduce the level of myopia. It is a technique that has been evolving since the 1960s, and the term 'modern orthokeratology' has been coined to distinguish previous approaches from current methods. More specifically, 'modern orthokeratology' refers to the practice of orthokeratology using reverse geometry lenses. Orthokeratology lenses can be made of highly oxygen-permeable materials, permitting the wearing of orthokeratology lenses on an overnight basis (i.e. overnight orthokeratology).

The advent and acceptance of keratorefractive surgery for the correction of refractive errors has ensured that interest in other non-surgical approaches, such as orthokeratology, has remained relevant. The resurgence of orthokeratology as a viable alternative to refractive surgery, or indeed traditional contact lens or spectacle corrections, is a consequence of three developments:

1. The availability of new lens designs, particularly reverse geometry lenses, and the ability to design and manufacture lenses to produce a specific tear layer thickness profile
2. The availability of videokeratoscopes to assist with contact lens design and evaluate corneal shape changes
3. The availability of new highly oxygen-permeable materials, allowing overnight lens wear.

The average magnitude of the refractive change using orthokeratology lenses is about 1.75D, and is subject to significant individual variability (Figure O.10). The issue

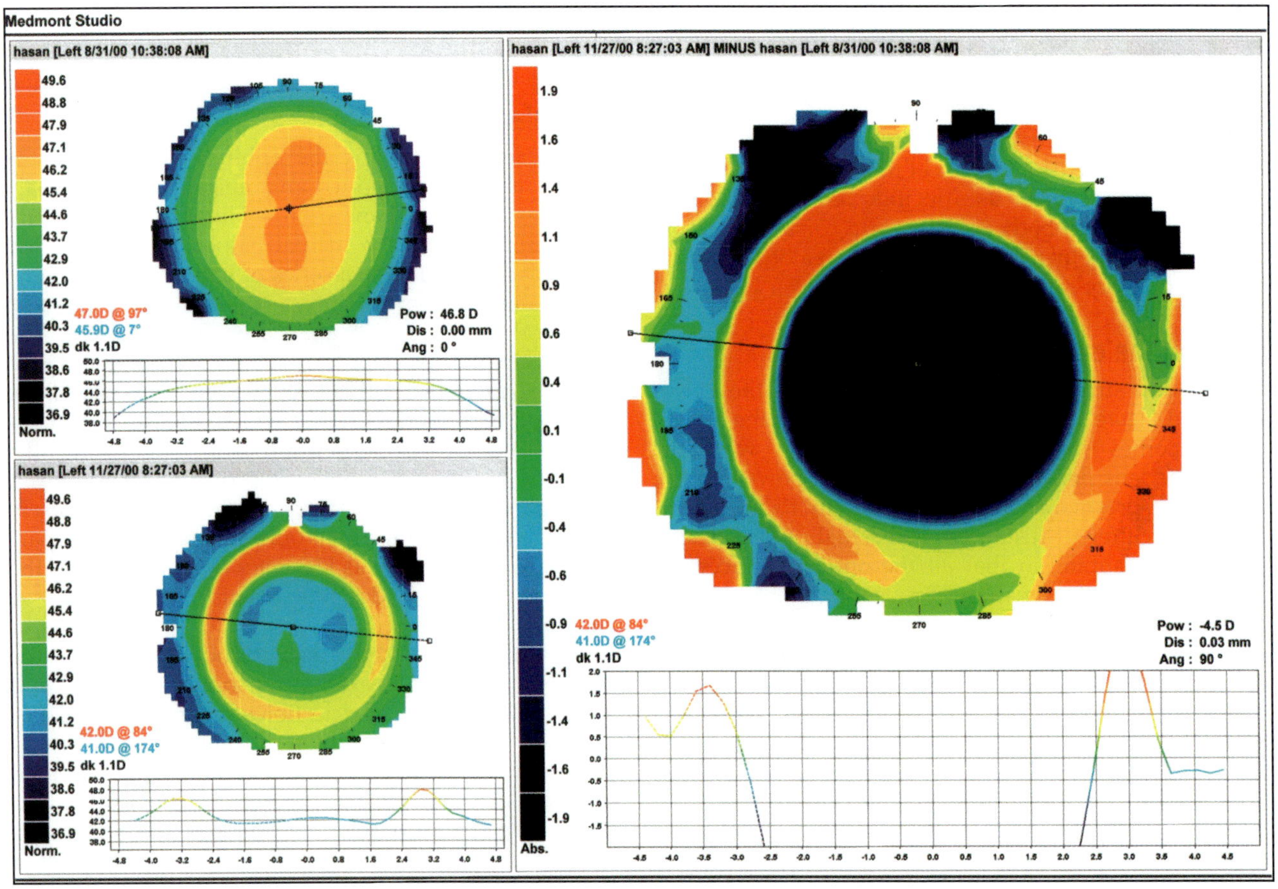

Figure O.10 • Corneal topography before (upper left) and after (lower left) wear of reverse geometry lenses in this example of a dramatic change of about 4.00D (difference plot, right) in corneal power.

of predictability of those changes is still an important and unresolved one. The corneal changes are not permanent, with significant regression occurring over a few hours. Ongoing use of contact lenses (sometimes referred to as 'retainer lenses'), whether for overnight or daily wear, is still needed to sustain the refractive changes.

The corneal curvature changes in orthokeratology appear to result from a combination of short-term corneal moulding and a longer-term redistribution of anterior corneal tissue. It has also been suggested that the tear reservoir generated by the steeper secondary curves leads to pressure changes, which are responsible for the corneal tissue redistribution.

Outcome measures, low vision

The prescribing of low vision aids (and the work of a low vision clinic in general) is aimed at removing activity limitations and participation restrictions suffered by the patient, in order that they can maintain their customary functional capacity. It is not aimed at reducing the visual impairment suffered: visual acuity and visual field, for example, will be unchanged by these interventions. In assessing the impact of the intervention, therefore, it is necessary to look for outcome measures which reflect global functioning, wellbeing and quality of life. The aim of these patient-centred measures is to give a more accurate assessment of the impact (either benefit or harm) experienced as a result of treatment. They may concentrate on the assessment of functional limitations, social interaction and relationships, or psychological adjustment, or attempt to combine all together. Such instruments are usually in the form of questionnaires in which the patient is asked to make a judgement about their own state. For individuals with a visual impairment, they are usually delivered face-to-face, or by telephone, rather than in printed format. Responses may be dichotomous (yes/no or true/false) or polytomous (choosing a rating from an ordered series of descriptors, such as different levels of difficulty or frequency, on a scale of 1 to 5).

The instrument may be divided into a number of different domains or dimensions, designed to capture information on several different aspects of life. Answers are then summed for domains and/or the whole instrument to provide a single global value to represent health status. Arriving at such a 'score' requires weighting the individual answers in some way (or assuming that they all carry equal significance), and it is unlikely that this will be equally appropriate for all responders; it also assumes that, for example, a 5-point difference in a high score means the same as a 5-point difference in a low score, and this is unlikely to be the case. A statistical item response model is required to convert scores into an interval scale form where each point on the scale has equal weighting, so as to facilitate mathematical manipulation and statistical analysis.

Generic instruments can be valuable in comparing the impact of different health problems, but many vision specific measures have been devised since Bernth-Petersen introduced the Visual Function Index in 1981 to measure the visual limitations before cataract surgery. One of the most widely used at the current time is the NEI-VFQ. Such questionnaires should be considered an important part of the audit of a low vision service to assess whether the patient has actually benefited from attendance (that is, has their score improved). Other types of questionnaire have also been used in this context: these might measure patient satisfaction with the service offered (often including questions such as the helpfulness of the personnel and clinic accessibility), or patient understanding of their eye condition, or the use of any low vision aids (e.g. how many times a day the aid was used, for which tasks, and any difficulties experienced). See *Low vision assessment*.

Overnight orthokeratology
- See *Orthokeratology*.

Overnight contact lens wear
- See *Extended contact lens wear*.

Over-refraction, contact lens

This is the standard technique for determining the power of the contact lens to be ordered for a patient. The over-refraction is conducted with the best fitting trial lens in place. The procedure is best performed using a trial frame and trial lens set. The technique of conducting the over-refraction is essentially the same as that conducted on a non-lens-wearing patient. A full sphero-cylindrical over-refraction is conducted first, and if the patient is to be fitted with a spherical lens, the best sphere refraction is determined. The result of the over-refraction is simply added to the power of the trial lens to determine the power of the lens to be ordered, after making any corrections for effectivity (see Appendix D). In toric soft lens fitting, the over-refraction can be used as an indication of the direction of cylinder axis mislocation.

Measuring the over-refraction during a rigid lens trial fitting not only helps to determine the final lens power but also gives an indication of whether the optimum fit has been obtained. An unexpected over-refraction suggests that either the lens is wrongly labelled or the fit is not perfect. The steeper the lens fit, the more minus power will be required in order to compensate for a relatively plus powered tear lens. Variable vision may indicate a decentred or flat fitting and relatively mobile lens fit.

Own-labelling, contact lens
- See *Contact lens supply routes*.

Oxygen permeability (Dk) of contact lenses

The term 'oxygen permeability' describes the ease with which oxygen may pass through a particular material under standard conditions. It is thus a property of a material, and not of a finished contact lens. Oxygen permeability of a material is a function of the diffusivity (D) and solubility (k) of oxygen in that material, and is represented by the term Dk. The diffusivity (D) refers to the speed at which oxygen molecules can pass through the material, and the solubility (k) refers to the number of oxygen molecules that can be absorbed into a given volume of material (Figure O.11).

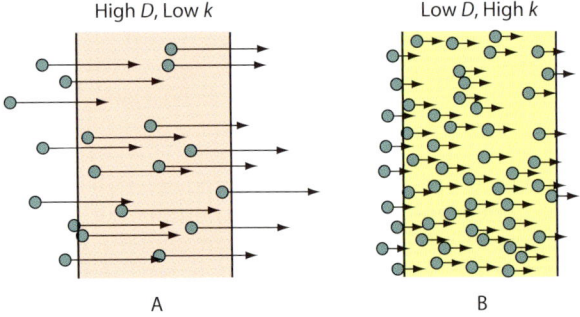

Figure O.11 • Schematic representation of the passage of oxygen through two infinitely thin sections of contact lens materials. Each circle represents an oxygen molecule. The length of the arrow indicates the distance moved per unit time. Compared with lens A, more oxygen molecules are observed in lens B (high oxygen solubility, k), but each molecule in lens B is moving at a slower speed (low diffusivity, D). It can be seen that both materials have the same permeability, since the same number of molecules pass through each section of material per unit time.

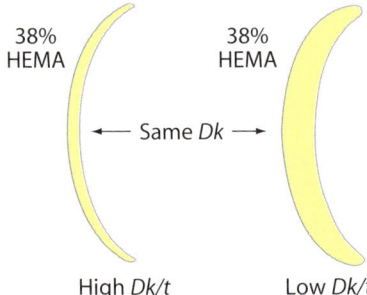

Figure O.12 • Illustration of the concept of oxygen permeability (Dk) and oxygen transmissibility (Dk/t). The Dk is an intrinsic property of the lens material. In this example, both lenses are made of the same material (38% HEMA); thus, they have the same Dk. However, the thicker lens will offer greater resistance to oxygen flow, and therefore has a lower Dk/t than the thinner lens.

In order to determine the oxygen permeability of a material at a given temperature, it is necessary to measure the rate (volume per unit time) at which oxygen passes through a sample of material of given dimensions (area and thickness) for a given gas pressure. The units of Dk take these variables into account, and are quite complex. It is common therefore to quote the value in 'Fatt units' (after Irving Fatt, who pioneered contact lens oxygen permeability measurement) or, more formally, 'Barrer', whereby:

$$Dk \text{ in Barrer (or 'Fatt units')} = 10^{-11} (cm^2 \cdot mlO_2)/(s \cdot ml \cdot mmHg)$$

The international standard unit for pressure is the 'pascal' (Pa). Because the term mmHg is now becoming obsolete internationally, it is being advocated that the closest accepted metric unit of pressure – 100Pa, or 'hectopascal' (hPa) – should replace the term mmHg. Indeed, this approach is specified in the international standard ISO 8321-2(2000). When hPa is used, Dk is quoted as:

$$Dk = 10^{-11} (cm^2 \cdot mlO_2)/(s \cdot ml \cdot hPa)$$

The difficulty here is that converting from the traditional Barrer or Fatt units to ISO units involves multiplying Dk by the constant 0.75. For example, a lens quoted with a traditional Dk of 40 units will have revised ISO Dk of 30 units.

For soft contact lenses, there is a well-defined relationship between water content (W, %) and Dk; this is given by the Morgan-Efron equation, where:

$$Dk = 1.67 \times 10^{-11} e^{0.0397W} \text{ (at 35°C)}$$

Silicone rubber has oxygen permeability several times greater than that of water and over 100 times greater than that of either PMMA or dehydrated polyHEMA. Its incorporation into a hydrogel therefore produces a marked gain in oxygen permeability. In such materials, as the proportion of silicone-based polymer is increased and water content consequently decreases, the Dk value rises to values well in excess of 100 Barrer.

Oxygen transmissibility (Dk/t) of contact lenses

The term 'oxygen transmissibility' describes the ease with which oxygen may pass through a particular material of given thickness. The oxygen transmissibility of a lens is a function of the oxygen permeability (Dk) of the material from which the lens is made, divided by the thickness of the lens (t) (Figure O.12). Thus, 'oxygen transmissibility' is represented by the term Dk/t, and describes the passage of oxygen through a finished contact lens.

The units of Dk/t are as follows:

$$Dk/t \text{ in Barrer/cm} = 10^{-9} (cm \cdot mlO_2)/(s \cdot ml \cdot mmHg)$$

When hPa is used, Dk/t is quoted as:

$$Dk/t \text{ in Barrer/cm} = 10^{-9} (cm \cdot mlO_2)/(s \cdot hPa)$$

To convert from the traditional Barrer or Fatt units to ISO units, Dk/t must be multiplied by the constant 0.75.

Contact lens oxygen transmissibility can be expressed as either the central or the average value. The central lens Dk/t is derived by dividing Dk by the centre thickness of the lens. The average lens Dk/t is derived by dividing Dk by the average thickness of the lens over a defined lens radius. The average Dk/t is always less than the central Dk/t for minus powered lenses (which become progressively thicker from the centre to the edge of the lens), and the converse is true for plus powered lenses.

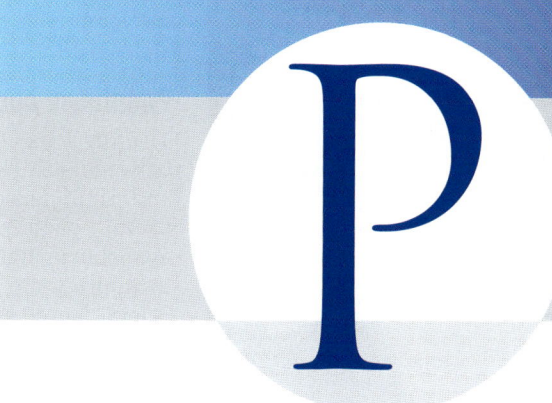

Pachometry, optical

Optical pachometry is based on the measurement of the apparent thickness of an optical section of the cornea, and its popularity is largely based on the commercial availability of a pachometer attachment for the Haag-Streit slit lamp. First, a split image device is inserted into one eyepiece of the slit-lamp biomicroscope. The method depends upon the relative rotation of two glass plates, which are placed on top of each other. Rotation of the upper plate moves the upper half of the image of the cornea with respect to the fixed lower half. When the corneal endothelium of the upper field is aligned with the epithelium of the lower field, the angle of rotation of the upper plate is read off an externally positioned scale. This measurement is proportional to the apparent thickness of the cornea, with true corneal thickness being determined by means of a conversion table.

Whilst perfectly acceptable for clinical purposes, the arrangement described above is too inaccurate for research purposes. A number of modifications to the technique have resulted in an accuracy of approximately 5µm being reported. Two such modifications include the use of two or four small light sources to ensure that the incident beam is normal to the corneal surface and an arrangement whereby the rotation of the glass plate is coupled to a potentiometer such that the angle of rotation is directly converted into an electrical signal, allowing immediate input into a computer program. This enables more rapid data collection, efficient file management, and more accurate, repeatable data collection (Figure P.1).

The Orbscan™ (Orbtek Inc., Salt Lake City) corneal topographer and pachometer is an advanced optical technique that operates by analysing the anterior and posterior boundaries of a corneal optical section as the incident slit scans over the cornea. The dedicated software quickly generates a two-dimensional pattern of corneal surface topography and thickness distribution. The Orbscan can also be used to measure thickness variations within a contact lens.

Pachometry, ultrasonic

The ultrasonic pachometer is based on traditional A-scan ultrasonography, where the recording is in one dimension only, as compared with B-scan instruments, which provide a two-dimensional view of the eye. Ultrasound is transmitted to the eye from a transducer. Sound is reflected back to the transducer from tissue interfaces, which possess different acoustic impedances, enabling the distance from the ultrasound probe at the anterior epithelial interface to determine the distance between itself and the endothelium-aqueous interface. The transducer determines the time difference between the pulse signals obtained at the two interfaces, and computes the corneal thickness based on this time delay and the velocity of sound in corneal tissue, which is approximately $1580 ms^{-1}$ at body temperature. A direct measurement

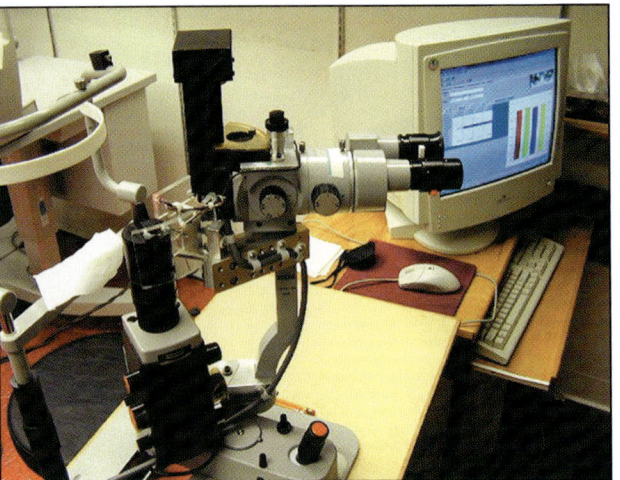

Figure P.1 • A computerized optical pachometer. The pachometer is connected to a potentiometer that is directly linked to a computer software program.

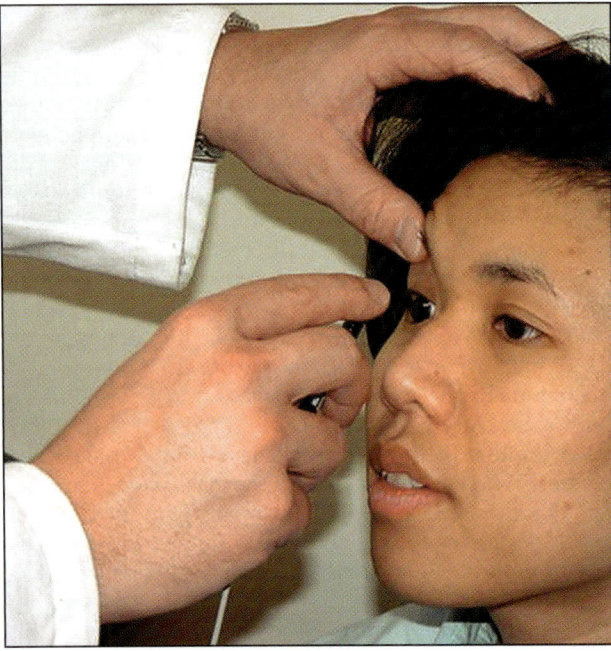

Figure P.2 • An ultrasonic pachometer evaluation. The eye is anaesthetized and the probe touched to the cornea. Readings are digitally recorded once the angle of inclination of the probe is correct.

of corneal thickness is then displayed on a digital readout.

Prior to undertaking ultrasonic pachometry, the cornea is anaesthetized and the patient slightly reclined (Figure P.2). Potential sources of error in measuring corneal thickness include holding the probe at an oblique angle to the cornea and measuring away from the central corneal apex, both of which would result in elevated readings of central corneal thickness (because corneal thickness increases from the centre to the periphery). The majority of modern instruments include a mechanism whereby a reading is not displayed if the probe is positioned such that there is excessive deviation from the perpendicular. The operator can use the pupil as a centring target, and using these adaptations the measurements obtained are valid for clinical use.

Paediatric contact lenses

The key lens choice in paediatric contact lens fitting is between soft hydrogel lenses, silicone elastomer lenses and rigid lenses. Silicone hydrogel lenses may have useful paediatric applications when they become available in high plus and high minus power ranges, and in appropriate paediatric parameters (for small eyes). Scleral lenses are rarely required, but may be used, for example, for prosthetic purposes.

Soft lenses are the most frequently used lens types in paediatric contact lens fitting. High water content soft lenses – or preferably silicone hydrogel lenses if available in the required parameters – are usually selected, as they can be worn for continuous or daily wear. Daily wear should be considered where possible to reduce the risk of infection, as oxygen transmission can be reduced through all forms of high powered lenses, such as those used to correct aphakia. However, as babies and young children sleep during the daytime, the lenses can remain in the eye during these periods. Lenses are usually fitted according to age, or based on keratometry readings and corneal diameter.

Advantages of soft lenses:

- they can be custom made in a range of radii, overall size, power and water content
- they are initially comfortable for the child
- parents/carers tend to be less apprehensive about inserting a soft lens into the eye of a baby or young child.

Disadvantages of soft lenses:

- they do not correct significant corneal astigmatism
- insertion can be difficult, especially for minus lenses, where there is considerable lid squeezing, or if there is a very small palpebral aperture
- they are prone to dehydration, which can be problematic in babies, who tend to have relatively dry eyes due to low blink rate
- there is frequent lens loss due to eye rubbing and dehydration.

Silicone rubber lenses are often used in the correction of refractive errors in babies and young children, and are particularly useful where there is frequent lens loss or a dry ocular surface (Figure P.3). The lens fit can be checked using fluorescein and UV light after a period of 30 minutes or so of settling.

Advantages of silicone rubber lenses:

- they have a very high oxygen permeability
- they are not susceptible to dehydration on the eye
- they are less susceptible to damage
- they are not easily rubbed out due to the negative pressure (eye suction) effect
- they are easier to insert than soft lenses due to their increased rigidity.

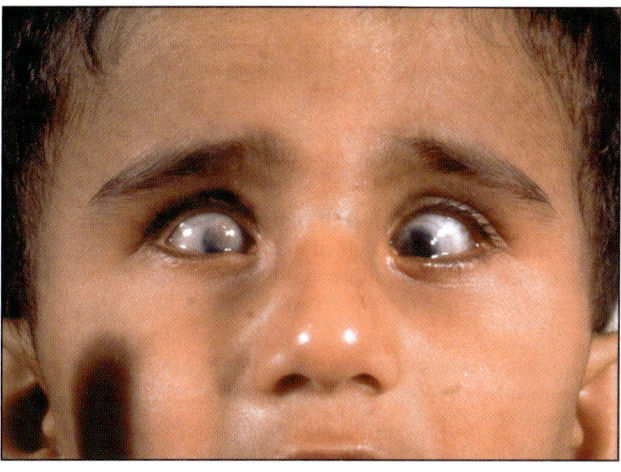

Figure P.3 • A silicone rubber lens fitted to the left aphakic eye of an infant with microcornea.

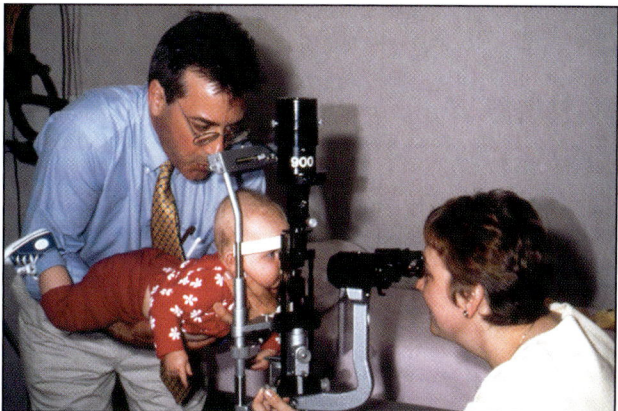

Figure P.4 • The 'flying baby' technique of child support for examining an infant at the slit-lamp biomicroscope.

Disadvantages of silicone rubber lenses:
- the range of parameters and availability is limited
- they need to be fitted precisely, and require more chair time due to longer settling periods
- negative pressure effects can cause adhesion to the cornea if the lens is too tight
- the surface coating can degenerate, resulting in an uncomfortable hydrophobic surface, so lenses have a relatively short lifespan
- they are more expensive than soft or rigid lenses.

The development of automated hand-held keratometry and improvements in rigid lens design has led to the increased use of rigid lenses for paediatric fitting. Rigid lenses have been successfully used for the management of aphakia in infants, and can be fitted without the need for general anaesthesia.

Advantages of rigid lenses:
- they are available in a large range of materials and parameters
- they correct corneal astigmatism
- durability
- their rigidity can help to ease insertion and removal.

Disadvantages of rigid lenses:
- they are not suitable for continuous wear
- parents/carers can be more apprehensive about inserting rigid lenses
- there is the risk of abrasion if insertion is difficult
- initial discomfort may be a problem in older children
- they are easy to dislodge.

See *Paediatric contact lens examination; Paediatric contact lens fitting.*

Paediatric contact lens examination

All the examination techniques that would normally be conducted on adult contact lens wearers also need to be conducted on the very young, but with an almost exclusive reliance on objective techniques of refraction.

The logistics of examination often need to be adjusted to obtain the necessary clinical data. The key aspects of the paediatric contact lens examination are:

1. Anterior segment examination. As with the adult patient, examination of the anterior segment in an infant is an important aspect of contact lens fitting and aftercare. A very simple method of determining the presence, location and severity of corneal staining or ulceration is to use an ultraviolet lamp with fluorescein. In babies, a major slit lamp can be used with the baby being held horizontally, belly down, and head facing towards the instrument (the 'flying baby' technique, Figure P.4). In the case of infants and young children, a hand-held slit lamp may be preferable for examining the anterior segment in more detail. Older children, from about 3 years upwards, are usually happy to position themselves at a slit-lamp biomicroscope by kneeling on a chair and grasping the headrest support bars.

2. Keratometry. A hand-held automated keratometer can be used to determine the corneal radius of curvature in young infants and in children who are too young to sit at a conventional keratometer.

3. Refraction. Determination of the refractive error or a contact lens over-refraction can usually only be performed objectively using retinoscopy and hand-held lenses; a paediatric trial frame may be more convenient in an older child. The use of a cycloplegic drug is recommended in those children with normal accommodative function. It is useful sometimes to dilate the pupil in aphakes or pseudophakes where there is a small or displaced pupil, or where significant media opacity is apparent (e.g. posterior capsular thickening).

4. Biometry. Prior to cataract surgery, the axial length of the eye can be measured with ultrasound and the corneal radius of curvature determined by keratometry. These measurements can be used to determine the power of the contact lens required post-operatively by using an IOL calculation formula, which can determine the ocular power at the corneal plane post-surgery. This is particularly useful as it allows a lens of more or less correct specifications to be ordered, which alleviates the need for many lenses to be used at the initial fitting and allows fewer lenses to be kept in stock.

See *Paediatric contact lenses; Paediatric contact lens fitting*.

Paediatric contact lens fitting

Contact lenses play an important role in the correction of complex refractive errors in the paediatric population, and in the management of deprivational amblyopia. Contact lenses also play an important role in prosthetic fitting.

Children over the age of about 12 years are generally capable of being examined, counselled and fitted like adults, albeit with parental guidance. However, there generally needs to be a specific indication for fitting children younger than this. The indications for fitting the very young are as follows:

1. Aphakia. Surgical removal of the crystalline lens results in aphakia. The most common reason for performing this procedure is congenital cataract, the incidence of which is about 2.1 per 10 000 live births and 7.7 per 10 000 children at 4 years of age. Of these cases, around 40% and 50%, respectively, have unilateral cataracts. Aphakia can also result from lens subluxation, as seen in Marfan's syndrome, or ectopia lentis. Trauma to the eye may result in the immediate loss of the crystalline lens or subsequent development of traumatic cataract, which may require surgical intervention. Refractive management of bilateral aphakia can be achieved with spectacles. However, the drawbacks of aphakic spectacles include the weight of the lenses and difficulty in achieving good frame fit in babies and young infants. In addition, the maximum power of lenses is restricted, even in lenticulated form, to around +26.00D. Since infants in the early stages of visual development require a focal length of around 30–50cm to see a face, the power of the selected contact is usually 2.00–3.00D greater than the ocular refraction. This over-correction should be reduced at 18 months to 2 years of age, when the toddler becomes more aware of distant objects. A reading correction or bifocal spectacles can be prescribed from around 3–4 years of age, when the child starts pre-school education.

2. Pseudophakia. The use of intra-ocular lenses (IOLs) in the management of congenital cataract is increasing, with IOL implantation being carried out in infants as young as 2 weeks of age. The aim of IOL implantation at this early age is to alleviate the need for contact lenses or aphakic glasses when the eye is fully grown. Typically, the young eye will be left 6.00–10.00D under-corrected with the implant so as to compensate for the expected ongoing 'myopic shift' during childhood. The resultant refractive error can then be corrected with a contact lens in the early months, with a 2.00D over-correction, gradually reducing lens power until the eye reaches an emmetropic state.

3. Myopia. Myopia is not uncommon in infants and young children, and correction with spectacles is the accepted practice. However, in high myopia, spectacles have the disadvantage of reducing the retinal image size, inducing peripheral distortion and reducing the effective visual field (especially with lenticulated lenses). Contact lens correction is warranted where spectacle correction is problematic or normal visual development is threatened. High myopia (>10.00D) may be present from birth, and may be related to a number of ocular and systemic conditions. Also, high myopia may be associated with craniofacial anomalies, which can make the wearing of spectacles difficult. The myopic eye is larger overall, and tends to have a flatter-than-average corneal radius and a larger corneal diameter than the emmetropic eye. Adult-sized lenses can often be used in young infants and children. Myopia can also result from buphthalmos, where the corneal diameter is much larger than normal (>12.5mm), and so requires a lens that is flatter and larger than an adult equivalent. Contact lenses in unilateral high myopia have been shown to be more satisfactory than spectacle lenses in the management of amblyopia, in regard to cosmesis, comfort and treatment.

4. Ocular motility disorders. Contact lenses can be useful in the management of ocular motility disorders. Applications include aniseikonia induced by anisometropia exceeding 6.00D, accommodative esotropia in older children, nystagmus, and occlusion.

5. Irregular astigmatism. This is derived from primary corneal ectasia, and is extremely rare in childhood. Most causes of corneal irregularity are secondary in nature – for example, following corneal infection or laceration. Neutralization of irregular astigmatism is important during the visual development period to prevent deprivational amblyopia. The optimum form of contact lens correction here is a rigid lens, although sometimes, if the irregularity is less severe, a toric soft lens may suffice.

6. Tinted prosthetic and therapeutic lenses. Tinted therapeutic lenses may be used in children to enhance visual performance by reducing the effect of photophobia. Tinted prosthetic lenses may be used for improving the cosmesis of the child by camouflaging a disfigured eye. The most common reasons for fitting prosthetic lenses in childhood are:

- albinism
- aniridia
- achromatopsia
- iris defects (e.g. coloboma)
- nanophthalmus or microphthalmus
- corneal anomalies (e.g. sclerocornea or Peter's anomaly).

A modified technique for insertion and removal is required in the young eye in view of the small palpebral aperture size of an infant **(Figure P.5)**. Some general points to consider when handling contact lenses in babies and young children are as follows:

1. Lenses are easier to insert and remove with the child lying down on a firm, flat surface, e.g. an examination couch.

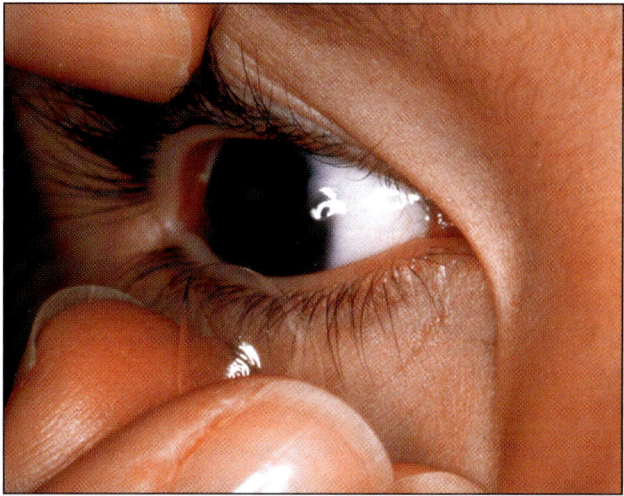

Figure P.5 • The small palpebral aperture of a child poses problems for lens insertion.

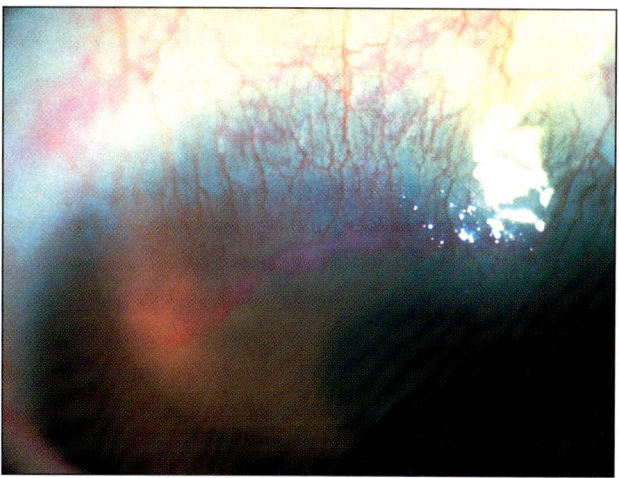

Figure P.6 • Contact lens induced fibrovascular pannus with a degenerative leading edge revealed by rose bengal staining.

2. Babies can be 'swaddled' in a blanket to make handling easier.
3. It is far easier to learn how to handle lenses on a young infant than on a more active baby or toddler. It is therefore important to encourage parents/carers to undertake lens handling from the outset of lens fitting.
4. Parents/carers should be advised to keep to regular times for handling, so that this becomes ritualized and accepted as part of daily routine.
5. If handling is difficult in young infants, lenses can be inserted or removed during sleep.
6. Handling often becomes more difficult from 18 months onward. Bilateral aphakes can start to use spectacles at this point, and anisometropes can use a spectacle correction when occluded.
7. Co-operation may be extremely limited in children aged between 2 and 5 years having lenses fitted for the first time. Spectacles may have to suffice at this age if the benefits of contact lenses are outweighed by the distress caused to the child by handling.

See *Paediatric contact lenses; Paediatric contact lens examination.*

Pain associated with contact lens wear

See *Discomfort, contact lens induced; Discomfort, investigation of.*

Pannus, contact lens associated

This is a particular type of corneal neovascularization characterized by a thick plexus of vessels typically observed at the superior limbus. Two forms of pannus may be observed in contact lens wearers; active (inflammatory) and fibrovascular (degenerative) (Figure P.6). An active pannus is initially avascular, and is composed of sub-epithelial inflammatory cells. In the later stages it may be associated with secondary scarring of the stroma.

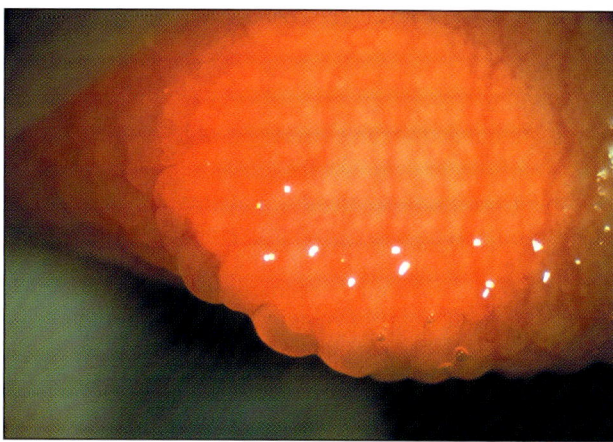

Figure P.7 • Papillary conjunctivitis induced by rigid lens wear.

Pantoscopic angle

The pantoscopic angle or tilt refers to the angle between the spectacle plane and the frontal plane of the face, whereby the top of the frame is further away from the face than the bottom of the frame. Ophthalmic lenses are generally designed to be set in front of the face with a pantoscopic angle of about 12 to 15°.

Papillary conjunctivitis, contact lens induced

This condition refers to the appearance of localized swellings, or 'papillae', on the tarsal conjunctiva. Papillae are primarily observed in the upper eyelid, and can only be viewed by everting the lid (Figure P.7). Rarely, papillae can be observed on the lower tarsus by pulling the lower lid firmly down. In soft lens wearers, papillae are more numerous; they are located more towards the upper tarsal plate (that is, closer to the fold of the everted lid), and the apex of the papillae take on a more rounded form (Figure P.7). In rigid lens wearers, papillae are flatter and are located more towards the lash margin, with few papillae being present on the upper tarsal plate. Papillae often appear as round light reflexes, giving an irregular specular reflection.

In the early stages (< Grade 1) of contact lens induced papillary conjunctivitis (CLPC), the tarsal conjunctiva may be indistinguishable from the normal tarsal conjunctiva apart from increased redness. In advanced cases (>Grade 2), papillae can exceed 1mm in diameter and often take on a bright red/orange hue. The distribution of papillae can be more readily appreciated with the aid of fluorescein. The hexagonal/pentagonal shape is lost in favour of a more rounded appearance, with a flattened or even slightly depressed apex or tip. A tuft of convoluted capillary vessels is often observed at the apex of papillae; this vascular tuft will typically stain with fluorescein. Other signs in severe CLPC (> Grade 3) include conjunctival oedema, excessive mucus and mild ptosis. The cornea may display punctate staining and superior infiltrates. Injection of the superior limbus may also be apparent.

There is general concordance between the severity of signs and symptoms. In the early stages of CLPC, patients may complain of:

- discomfort towards the end of the wearing period
- slight itching
- excess mucus upon awakening
- intermittent blurring
- a slight but non-variable vision loss while wearing lenses.

As the condition progresses, patients report itching, discomfort and excessive lens movement.

Key factors implicated in the aetiology of CLPC include lens-induced mechanical irritation, and immediate and delayed hypersensitivity. There is often a link with meibomian gland dysfunction, and atopic patients may be more susceptible to developing the condition. Treatment options include:

- altering the lens material
- replacing lenses more frequently
- altering or eliminating the care system
- improving ocular hygiene
- treating any associated meibomian gland dysfunction
- prescribing soft steroids (e.g. loteprednol etabonate)
- prescribing mast cell stabilizers (e.g. 4% cromolyn sodium)
- dispensing ocular lubricants for symptomatic relief
- reducing wearing time
- suspending or ceasing lens wear.

The prognosis for recovery from CLPC after removal of lenses and cessation of wear is good, with symptoms disappearing within 5 days to 2 weeks of lens removal, and redness and excess mucus resolving over a similar time course. Resolution of papillae takes place over a much longer time course – typically many weeks, sometimes as long as 6 months. The more severe the condition, the longer the recovery period. In the longer term, however, the prognosis is less good. The condition can recur, especially in atopic patients who appear to have a propensity for developing CLPC.

Parallelepiped, slit-lamp technique of

Using the same slit lamp set-up as for direct focal illumination, a 0.5–2.0mm wide illuminating beam is

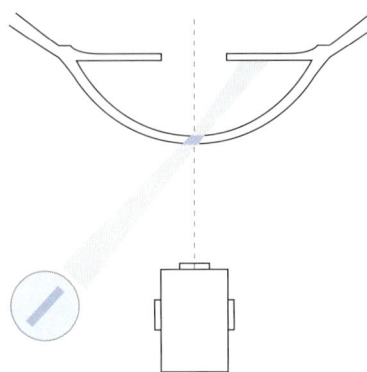

Figure P.8 • Parallelepiped slit-lamp technique. Adapted from L.W. Jones, D.A. Jones (2001) Slit lamp biomicroscopy. In: N. Efron (ed.) The Cornea: its Examination in Contact Lens Practice, pp. 1–49. Butterworth-Heinemann, Oxford.

scanned over the ocular surface. This permits assessment of the location, width and height of any object within the cornea or adjacent structures (Figure P.8). The parallelepiped is the most commonly used direct illumination technique, and is employed, for example, to assess corneal scarring, infiltrates, and corneal staining.

Partial sight
- See *Low vision*.

Party lenses
- See *Theatric tinted contact lenses*.

Patient discharge, contact lenses

A useful strategy to instil confidence in patients who have never worn lenses previously is to have the patient insert his or her lenses at the conclusion of the training session, and to discharge the patient from the practice wearing the lenses. The patient will then be forced to 'confront' the challenge of lens handling (at least lens removal in the first instance) rather than, as might occur, putting the lenses aside until enough courage can be mustered to wear lenses at a later date.

An appointment for the next aftercare visit should be made before the patient leaves the practice with the new contact lenses. The patient must appreciate that ongoing success with contact lenses is dependent upon several factors, such as adaptation to the lenses, compliance with the instructions given, and attending for regular aftercare visits. It should be impressed upon the patient that whilst good vision and comfort are indicators of success, they do not automatically prove there are no adverse ocular effects. All wearers must be made aware of the importance of regular biomicroscopic examination. The standard strategy for encouraging compliance with the requirement to return for regular aftercare visits is to restrict the supply of lenses issued to the patient to correspond with the desired time period between aftercare appointments.

Prior to being discharged, patients should be advised how to identify an emergency situation when wearing lenses. At the same time, new wearers need to be aware of normal adaptation symptoms, such as mild foreign body sensation and intermittent blurring of vision. If concerned that there is a problem, contact lens wearers can be advised to check that their eyes 'look good, feel good and see good'. This easy-to-remember adage refers to the following:

- 'look good' – there is no more ocular redness than normal
- 'feel good' – there is no discomfort prior to and after lens insertion
- 'see good' – there is no disturbance to vision (each eye checked monocularly).

Patients should be advised that:
- any significant redness when accompanied by pain needs urgent practitioner attention, especially if the redness and pain do not ease following lens removal
- visual losses should not automatically be put down to contact lens wear, as there may be some form of ocular pathology present that is unrelated to lens wear.

Patient education with contact lenses

The quality of instruction and advice given to a patient contributes to the success or failure of the new wearer. Proper and careful tuition of a patient at a dispensing visit will facilitate confident lens handling by the patient, and will help nurture a sound appreciation of how lenses should perform and how to manage various situations that can arise in contact lens wear. Certainly, poor patient education can result in premature discontinuation from lens wear and increase the likelihood of unscheduled visits to the practice.

The dispensing visit seeks to:
- teach the patient the correct methods of lens insertion and removal
- explain the methods that optimize lens comfort, such as understanding when a lens is inside-out, or how to remove post-lens debris
- inform the patient about the likely adaptation issues that may be encountered
- outline the correct use of the prescribed care regimen.

The use of diagnostic lens banks facilitates undertaking both the fitting and dispensing appointment on the same day. Some patients are so motivated following their first experience of contact lens wear that the dispensing can take place immediately after the initial trial fitting. On the other hand, rescheduling the dispensing visit for another day has the benefits of giving patients a break after the fitting visit, and allows them to read through some preliminary literature about their contact lenses.

A trained member of support staff (as opposed to the practitioner) commonly adopts the teaching role, and this person is sometimes referred to as the 'contact lens hygienist'. Having a trained member of the support staff undertaking this task can have several advantages. Some patients feel pressured to have to 'perform' in front of the practitioner, whereas they may feel more relaxed with a member of support staff. The delegation of this role requires careful selection of personnel who can be relied upon to provide accurate information to the patient and refer back to the practitioner when necessary.

Patients who have elected to wear contact lenses are often apprehensive about the process of lens insertion and removal. For this reason, the teaching room should be of a comfortable temperature and well ventilated, as many patients become quite anxious in their frustration

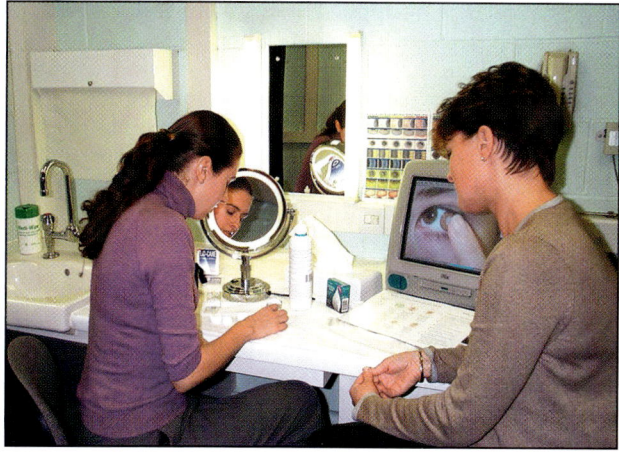

Figure P.9 • Suitable arrangement for contact lens patient education.

if they do not insert the lens on the first attempt. The area should be reasonably private – perhaps screened off from the rest of the practice – and it is essential that the instructor and the patient are free from incidental interruptions. Patients require careful attention when they first handle lenses, and the instructor must not be taken away or distracted from this supervisory task.

Good lighting is important, along with suitable seating for both the patient and the instructor, as flexibility to be able to sit on each side of the patient is needed (Figure P.9). The patient's chair should be set at a desk such that the knees of the patient can fit comfortably under the desk. This is helpful if the patient accidentally drops the lens during handling.

An illuminated, double-sided mirror (with one side that magnifies) that is height-adjustable and can be tilted is ideal. The teaching area must be prepared in advance of the lesson, so that all necessary items are to hand, including:

- contact lenses, cross-checked with the record card and spectacle prescription
- a lens case, which may be supplied with the solutions
- a trial pack of solutions, sufficient for the needs of the patient until the first scheduled aftercare visit
- additional saline, for rinsing during the lesson
- comfort drops (wetting solution), especially for rigid lens fitting
- a full box of tissues, with a spare box available
- hand washing facilities (soap in a pump dispenser and lint-free paper towels)
- a mirror, as described above, cleaned and free from fingerprints
- an appropriately-sized plastic bag, for the patient to carry away lenses, solutions and accompanying literature.

The full care regimen should be demonstrated from start to finish, explaining why each step is necessary as well as what could happen if the routine is not strictly adhered to. The patient should be handed written information about the care products being dispensed; this may be information that is supplied by the manufacturer and/or material prepared by the practitioner.

Contact lens handling can be a very frustrating experience for novice lens wearers. Accordingly, patience is the most critical personality trait of the member of staff chosen to instruct contact lens patients. The instruction session should not be rushed, and the patient should feel comfortable asking questions. See *Hygiene, practitioner and patient; Informed consent; Patient discharge; Wearing schedules.*

Patient instruction with contact lenses
- See *Patient education with contact lenses.*

Patient scheduling in optometry practice
Effective practice resource management without compromising clinical care is often dependent on the use of appropriate appointment scheduling methods. In particular, contact lens practice requires that a variety of appointment types are scheduled, such as general eye examinations, preliminary examination and initial fitting, evaluation after diagnostic lens wear (return), collection/education, routine aftercare, and unscheduled visits (urgent, emergency etc.). Three main approaches to patient scheduling can be employed to accommodate the various appointment types:

1. Individual appointments. Here, patients are booked in at regular intervals with equal times set aside for each consultation. For example, patients are booked in every 20–30 minutes starting and ending at a given time. This approach is simple, which is why it is used so often. However, it does not allow for patients who require longer consultations or patients who require less time. It is thus possible to end up with 'unproductive' portions of time when less time with a patient is needed, and long waiting queues should a patient require a longer consultation.
2. Block booking. This is not often used in optometry, but is found in hospitals and general medical practice. This method involves scheduling multiple patients in the same time slot – e.g. three patients may be booked at 9.00am and then none until 10.00am, when three more patients are booked, and so on. Individuals who have experienced this approach are often disgruntled to find that they have the same appointment slot as others.
3. A mixed system. Some practices find a mixture of traditional and block booking to be a workable combination, for example using the block system for scheduling shorter 15-minute visits for contact lens follow-up visits, and 20–30 minute individual scheduling for prescribing and fitting contact lenses.

The challenge is to schedule patients so that the 'downtime' and the time taken to 'settle in' in the consulting room does not curb the consultation time of the practitioner.

PD rule
- See *Interpupillary distance.*

Pemphigoid
- See *Cicatricial conjunctivitis, therapeutic contact lenses for.*

Pen-torch shadow technique
A very simple, though gross technique, involves shining a pen torch temporal to the patient's eye and interpreting the light and shadow across the iris front surface. This may be done as follows:

- The patient should be asked to stare straightforward in mesopic conditions.
- A pen torch is held at 100° temporal to the eye and brought around to 90°, at which point light is seen reflecting from the temporal side of the iris.
- The amount of iris that remains in shadow may then be interpreted as an indication of the depth of chamber. With a very narrow angle, the forward-bulging iris leaves much of the nasal iris in shadow, whereas a deep chamber with a wide angle allows reflection of light from most of the iris.

See *Appendix B.*

Penetrating keratoplasty, contact lens fitting following
- See *Post-keratoplasty, contact lens fitting.*

'Per case' contact lens supply
- See *Fitting rigid contact lenses.*

Peri-ballast
- See *Stabilization of soft toric contact lenses.*

Perimetry, blue-yellow
Blue-yellow perimetry, also known as Short Wavelength Automated Perimetry (SWAP), has been shown to be more sensitive to glaucomatous damage than conventional (white-on-white) perimetry. Blue-yellow defects (a) precede those for white-on-white perimetry, (b) predict which ocular hypertensive patients will develop white-on-white defects, and (c) are, on average, larger than those for white-on-white perimetry. The superiority of blue-yellow perimetry is believed to be due to either increased susceptibility of blue cones to glaucomatous damage or reduced redundancy in the blue mechanism. Reduced redundancy simply means that the relatively small number of blue cones makes the system very sensitive to even small losses.

A problem encountered when trying to test the blue mechanism is the relatively low sensitivity of blue cones. At 440nm, the blue sensitive cones are only marginally more sensitive than the red and green cones. Selective damage to the blue cones would have relatively little effect upon sensitivity as the red and green cones would simply up-regulate once the blue cone sensitivity dropped below that of the other receptors. To overcome this problem, the red and green cones are de-sensitized by adapting the eye to a yellow light. This increases the exposure of the blue sensitive mechanism to approximately 1.5 log units.

Blue-yellow perimetry is an option in both the 600 and 700 series of Humphrey Visual Field Analyzers. The background luminance is set much brighter than for white-on-white perimetry (100cd^2 rather than 10cd^2) and the standard stimulus is larger (Goldmann V rather than III).

Despite being more sensitive than white-on-white perimetry and readily available for routine clinical practice, blue-yellow perimetry has not been widely adopted. There are a number of possible reasons for this.

- The effect of lens opacities. Blue-yellow perimetry is particularly sensitive to lens opacities. The yellowing of the crystalline lens, a common occurrence in the elderly, selectively absorbs blue light and lowers the sensitivity to blue stimuli. There are a number of ways of compensating for lens absorption but these all involve additional measures that can be time consuming.
- Patients dislike the technique, even more than standard white-on-white perimetry.
- There is an increase in the variability of the responses.
- The main value of the technique, increased sensitivity, is only pertinent to a small percentage of patients attending for a visual field examination. Most patients seen in a glaucoma clinic already have visual field loss with white-on-white perimetry. There have been no studies demonstrating that blue-yellow perimetry is more sensitive at detecting progressive loss.

Perimetry, frequency doubling

Frequency doubling perimetry (FDP) is a clinical test that uses an alternating sinusoidal grating of low spatial frequency as a perimetric stimulus. The test is based upon an illusion in which an alternating sinusoidal grating of low spatial frequency (<4 cycles per degree) appears, at certain temporal frequencies (>15Hz), to have twice as many lines (doubled spatial frequency). The frequency doubling illusion is believed to be mediated by the magnocellular (M-cell) pathway and in particular by the large fibre diameter 'My' ganglion cells which constitute 1.5 to 2.5% of all retinal ganglion cells. Is has been suggested that these cells are particularly sensitive to glaucomatous damage either because of their small numbers or the nature of their large diameter fibres.

While the FDP uses the appropriate spatial and temporal frequencies for the frequency doubling illusion, the task presented to the patient is one of contrast sensitivity, i.e. the patient is being asked when he can detect the appearance of a target in the peripheral field, not when he sees the frequency doubling illusion.

The current FDP can use suprathreshold and threshold strategies (based on a modified binary search technique) and can test up to 17 test locations, 4 in each quadrant and one at the centre. The non-central stimuli are square and large (10×10°). Testing times vary, being approximately 5 min per eye for the threshold test and approximately 1 min per eye for the suprathreshold test. The FDP has many attractive characteristics for glaucoma screening. It is a small, self contained, portable instrument that is not sensitive to background illumination levels and does not require a corrective lens for refractive errors (results are reported to be independent of refractive error up to ±7.00D). The limited number of stimuli makes it less useful for monitoring visual field loss.

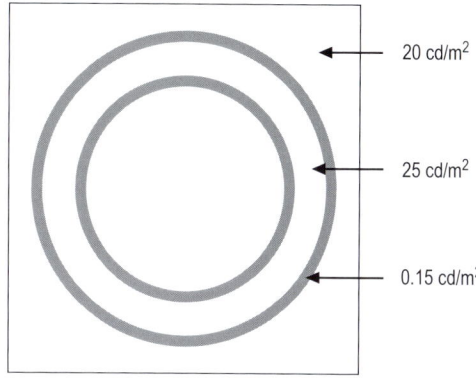

Figure P.10 • Ring stimulus used in high pass resolution perimetry.

Perimetry, high pass resolution

High-pass resolution perimetry is based upon the resolution of ring shaped targets of varying size rather than spots of varying intensity (Figure P.10). The overall intensity profile of the ring is such that when it cannot be resolved it cannot be detected. In the standard high-pass perimeter a repetitive bracketing strategy (one-reversal) is used to establish the minimum resolvable ring size at a series of 50 retinal locations within the central 30°.

High pass resolution perimetry has good sensitivity and specificity when compared to conventional (white-on-white) full-threshold perimetry. Its threshold variability is independent of sensitivity and it can detect progressive loss earlier than conventional perimetry.

High pass resolution perimetry is considerably faster than conventional perimetry, taking on average only 5.5 min to test 50 test locations (conventional full-threshold perimetry takes more than twice as long). On the negative side, the technique is sensitive to blur, either refractive or due to media changes, is unable to measure defect depth within small circumscribed lesions, and is unable to detect scotoma whose size is less than the local minimal test target. With the current monitor technology there is also a relatively small dynamic range of stimuli which limits the ability of the test to monitor loss in patients who have advanced defects but some important residual sensitivity.

Perimetry, oculokinetic

Oculokinetic perimetry is, contrary to what the name might imply, a form of static perimetry. It derives its name from the fact that the patient's eye moves to different fixation points while the test stimulus remains stationary. The test has been developed as a community based screening test for glaucoma. In practice the patient views a white tangent screen on which a series of numbers are printed along with a central black test stimulus. The patient's task is to look at each of the numbers in sequence and to note whether or not they can still see the central stimulus. They then mark any location where the stimulus could not be seen. An internet version of this test is currently available. Several different versions of this test have been developed, the most promising is a hand held version with just 23 test locations.

Peripheral fit, soft contact lens

- See *Fitting soft contact lenses.*

Personnel, optometric practice

Optometric practices rely on individuals to deliver their professional services and products to patients and customers. Thus, at a minimum level of practice activity, it will be necessary to employ someone to provide reception and general administrative support with respect to the day-to-day activities of the practice. At the other end of the spectrum, a large, busy practice may employ additional optometrists, dispensing staff, contact lens hygienists, technicians, optical receptionists/advisors, secretaries and cleaners. It is important to remember that as part-time employment increases, many more individuals will need to be employed to cover the practice requirements in terms of hours per day etc. The issues of managing the practice staff take more prominence as the size and the activity of the practice increase.

Once a vacancy has been identified and additional hours of staff time justified, it is essential to establish the duties of the new member of staff. Having decided on the qualifications, training needs and skills required to do the job, it is useful to prepare a job description and then to decide on the type of person who would ideally be recruited to fill this vacancy – i.e. a 'person specification' (Table P.1). A 'person specification' should take account of:

- physical make-up
- attainments
- general intelligence
- special aptitudes
- interests
- disposition and circumstances
- impact on others
- qualifications or acquired knowledge
- innate abilities
- motivation and adjustment or emotional balance.

Staff selection involves choosing the right person by interviewing short-listed candidates with a view to selecting the applicant who has the skills, abilities, aptitude and personal qualities to do the job. The job description and the person specification will decide the major selection criteria normally considered during the interview process.

A contract of employment needs to be issued to the staff member; this is simply the legal agreement between the employer and the employee, clarifying their mutual obligations. The law in the UK provides the employee with a number of employment rights and imposes some statutory obligations on the employer. Contracts do not have to be in writing. Employment law in the UK has gone a little further, and even with a verbal contract there is a requirement for employers to give any employee taken on for 1 month or more a written statement setting out the main employment particulars. This statement must be issued within 2 months of the starting date of employment. Covered by common and contract law, contracts of employment in the UK are governed by the Employment Rights Act 1996.

Table P.1 • Example of the job specification for a person whose primary role would be to provide contact lens patient education.

Essential qualities	Desirable qualities
1. Impact on other people	
(appearance, speech and manner)	
clean and tidy presentation	smart presentation
good writing and speech	gets on well with young adults
2. Qualifications and experience	
(education, training and work experience)	
GCSE English and mathematics	experience in medical reception, nursing assistance or pharmacy
able to work with a computer	experience of data input and output
3. Innate abilities	
(aptitude for learning)	
quick to grasp ideas and views	able to prioritize and decide on action
4. Motivation	
(consistency, determination and success in achieving goals)	
interested in health care and general cosmesis	interested in a potential career in optics
5. Adjustment	
(emotional stability, ability to handle stress and ability to get on with people) friendly and able to work as part of a team	comfortable with the pressures of day-to-day practice and the demands of patients and practitioners

A practice handbook that sets out basic information about the policies and facilities of the practice can act as a clear guide for all staff to providing optometric and contact lens services. It should be an easily accessible set of ground rules that promote a good working environment in the practice. Should a case of misconduct (breach of rules that merit disciplinary action) arise, the rules in the handbook regarding expected conduct will be invaluable.

Philosophy of fitting

- See *Fitting philosophy of contact lenses.*

Phoropter

As an alternative to placing trial lenses manually in a trial frame worn by a patient, a semi-automated instrument known as a phoropter or 'refractor head' may be used. A phoropter is a mechanical housing placed immediately in front of the patient, who looks at a distant or near target through sight holes set to the appropriate interpupillary distance. The phoropter contains a large number of spherical and cylindrical lenses, prisms, filters and occluders mounted in mechanical tracks that can be positioned in front of the sight holes by turning a series of dials. Toric lenses can be rotated to any orientation. A Jackson cross cylinder can be swung into position in front of each eye to determine the degree of astigmatism. The main advantage of a phoropter compared with a trial lens set is that it allows a subjective refraction to be undertaken much more rapidly. The main disadvantage is that the face of the patient is largely covered, thus depriving the clinician of the ability to observe facial reactions and expressions during the course of a subjective refraction.

Photochromic tints

Photochromic tints are available in glass and plastic ophthalmic lenses. Glass photochromic tinted lenses are capable of changing their tint density with the incident light, and also with temperature. Silver halide crystals doped with copper are mixed in with the glass at the time of manufacture, and in the borosilicate mixture used by Corning, the photochromic process can be represented as:

$$Ag^+ + Cu^+ + UV \Rightarrow Ag + Cu^{++}$$

The silver halide crystals are activated by ultraviolet (UV) radiation and blue light of the visible spectrum within the range 300 to 400nm, with maximum activation caused by light of wavelength 355nm. The influence of this radiation causes a colloid of metallic silver to appear. Once the UV light is removed, the reaction reverses, promoted by heat. In practical terms therefore, a photochromic lens darkens in sunlight and fades when not exposed to sunlight. A typical glass photochromic response curve is illustrated in Figure P.11. Note that the fading (recovery) rate is much slower than the darkening, and that the fading and darkening of photochromic lenses are affected by heat. The lenses go darker in colder conditions, and are less effective in hot climates. The time course is also thickness dependent, with thicker lenses taking longer to return to the faded state. Transmittance values should therefore be quoted for a specified temperature (preferably 25°C) and thickness (usually 2mm) to allow comparison between materials.

Photochromic lenses can be classified according to their transmittance in the faded (maximum transmittance) and darkened (minimum transmittance) states (BS 7394 part 2, 1994). For example, a photochromic varying between 90% and 25% transmittance would be described as a light/dark photochromic.

Photochromics with a narrow variation in transmission between the faded and darkened states are promoted for use 'in the city' where light conditions change quickly between outdoors and indoors. These lenses maintain a pale tint in their faded state. Photochromics with a wider variation in transmission between faded and darkened states are suitable for a narrower range of prescriptions as the variation in the tint density across the lens is more

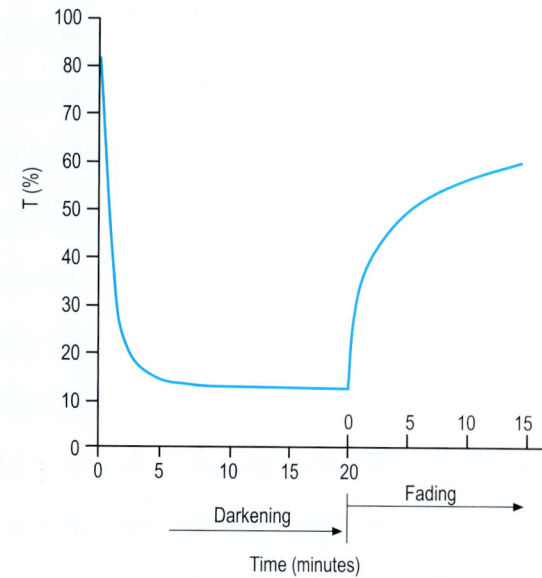

Figure P.11 • Transmission performance of a glass photochromic lens. The graph shows a lens that initially transmits 100% of the incident light through it. On exposure to light the glass darkens, reaching a minimum transmittance of around 10% of the incident light after 5 minutes. When the lens is removed from the light after 20 minutes, it gradually fades towards its initial state. Note that even after 15 minutes fading, the lens still only has a transmittance of 60%, as compared to its maximum original transmittance of 100%.

apparent. These lenses also take longer to change between states than photochromics with a narrower variation in transmission, particularly with thicker lenses.

Plastic photochromic tints can either be solid, or moulded into the front surface of the lens only, as in the Transitions material. Chemically, plastic photochromics are different to glass, being based on organic dyes. Although many early attempts were made to produce satisfactory lenses, it was not until the introduction of indolino spiroxazines in the early 1990s that lenses became available with a good fatigue life. The speed of reaction is similar to glass materials, although plastic materials appear to require more UV radiation for activation. Plastic photochromics also show temperature dependency, going darker in cold temperatures.

Photometric units

- See *Illuminance; Luminance; Luminous flux; Luminous intensity*.

Photorefractive keratectomy (PRK)

Photorefractive keratectomy (PRK) was the first of a number of laser-based surgical techniques to be developed to correct refractive error. In PRK, an excimer laser is used to sculpt the cornea. During this procedure, the central epithelium and approximately 25% of the stromal are ablated away. The technique can be used to correct myopia, hypermetropia and astigmatism. Higher refractive error corrections require a greater amount of tissue to be ablated. See *Laser refractive surgery, contact lenses following; Laser epithelial keratomileusis; Laser in-situ keratomileusis*.

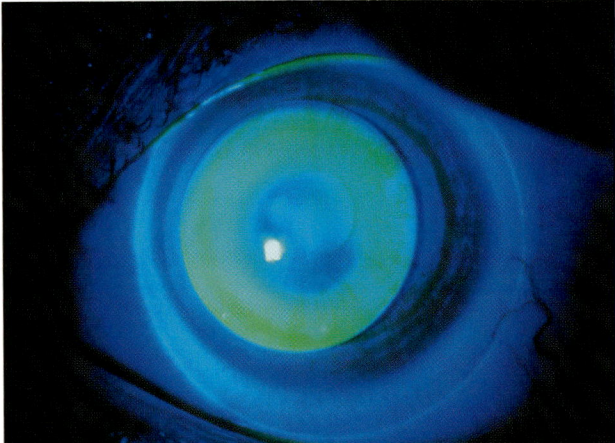

Figure P.12 • Piggyback fitting of a rigid lens sitting on top of a soft lens in a patient with keratoconus.

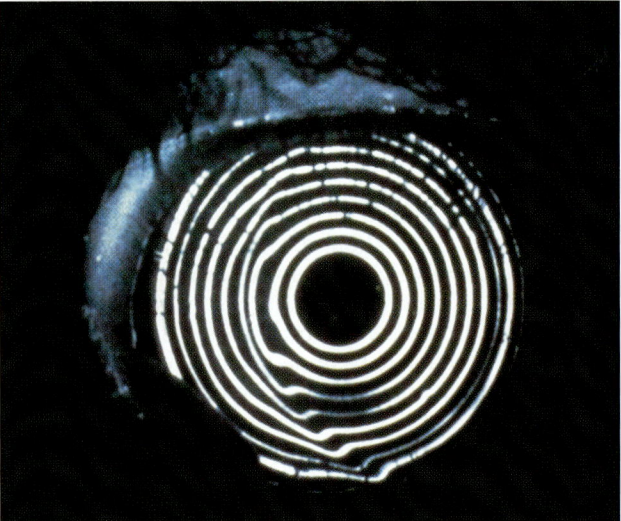

Figure P.13 • Placido disc image revealing a vertical arc of corneal distortion to the left of the corneal centre.

Pickford-Nicolson anomaloscope
- See *Anomaloscope*.

Piggyback contact lens fitting
This is when a soft lens is fitted to the eye and a rigid lens is fitted over the top of the soft lens (Figure P.12). An annular recess, slightly larger than the diameter of the overlying rigid lens, can be incorporated into the front surface of the soft lens to help the rigid lens locate centrally. Indications for piggyback lens fitting include the requirement for full corneal coverage of a distorted cornea, and as an aid to counteracting intolerance to rigid lens wear where a rigid lens is required due to corneal distortion.

Pingueculum
- See *Pterigium and pingueculum*.

Pinhole test
A pinhole in the centre of a black opaque disc can be placed in front of the eye, with or without any form of ophthalmic correction, of a patient with unexplained reduced visual acuity. Significant improvement of vision in the presence of the pinhole demonstrates that optical defocus was the probable cause of reduced vision. This is because a pinhole will reduce the size of the blur circle caused by optical defocus. Failure to improve vision in the presence of the pinhole demonstrates that optical defocus was probably not the cause of reduced vision, and that other possible causes, such as the presence of pathology, should be investigated.

Placido disc
This is the most basic reflective device for assessing corneal topography. It is simply a series of concentric black and white rings on a flat circular disc with a central sight hole. The disc is positioned in front of the cornea, and the reflections are observed (Figure P.13). Using this method, only gross irregularities in the corneal surface and very high astigmatism can be detected. Improved versions of the Placido disc include the internally-illuminated Klein keratoscope, the Loveridge grid, and the Tearscope-plus with corneal topography grid attachment.

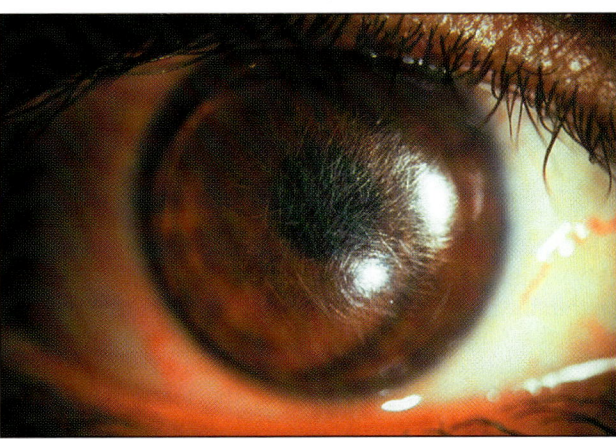

Figure P.14 • Heavy scratching on a rigid lens that had been used for 4 years.

Planned rigid contact lens replacement
Rigid lenses, irrespective of oxygen permeability (Dk) or material type, show a gradual deterioration in wettability and visual performance and an increase in surface scratching and deposition over time (Figure P.14). Some clinicians believe that re-polishing techniques can be applied to prolong the life of rigid lenses; however, caution should always be exercised with this procedure, as over-polishing can lead to reduced surface wettability and ultimately result in reduced comfort and visual performance. An alternative strategy is to replace rigid lenses more frequently; however, this is problematic because rigid lenses are manufactured using the lathe cutting method, which makes their unit cost significantly greater than that of soft lenses.

If it is accepted that higher Dk materials should be fitted for clinical reasons, that such lenses have a reduced life-expectancy and that all lenses show a deterioration in performance with age, then the planned replacement of high Dk rigid lenses would appear to be a logical modality to adopt.

Planned replacement of rigid lenses worn on a daily-wear basis results in significantly less corneal staining, limbal hyperaemia and tarsal conjunctival changes compared with identical lenses worn on a non-replacement basis. There is also less surface drying, surface scratching, mucus coating and surface deposition.

In extended-wear patients, planned rigid lens replacement results in less corneal and conjunctival staining and less corneal binding; however, this modality does not prevent the occurrence of tarsal conjunctival changes.

It is recommended that rigid lenses be replaced every 6 months, based on the argument that lenses should be replaced before any adverse ocular or lens surface changes would be expected to occur, and that this is an easy-to-remember calendar-based frequency – which would facilitate patient compliance.

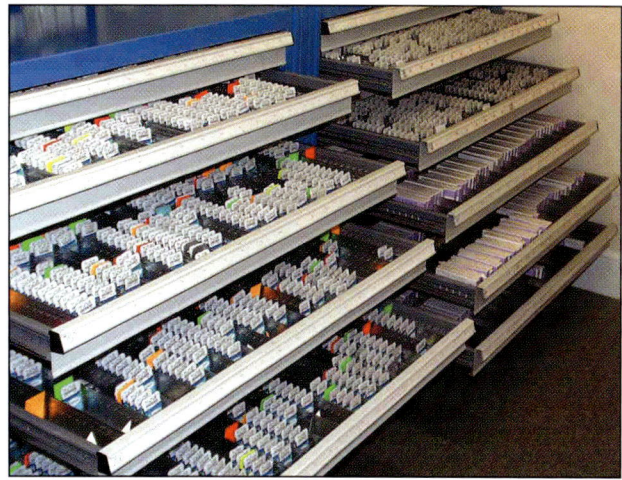

Figure P.15 • Single-use diagnostic lenses allow for convenient and accurate fitting assessment.

Planned soft contact lens replacement

The term 'planned replacement' refers to lens replacement intervals from 1 day to 12 months, and therefore includes all 'disposable lenses', which are defined as lenses replaced at least monthly.

Products replaced at least monthly have invariably been designed, packaged and promoted for replacement at specific intervals. However, the same is less true for lenses replaced 3-monthly, and is almost never true for lenses offered for biannual and annual replacement; such lenses are usually conventional lenses packaged in vials, and many of these lenses were developed prior to widespread use of planned replacement. This does not detract from the benefit of prescribing conventional soft lenses in this way, especially in view of the strong evidence supporting more frequent replacement intervals.

The rationale for the planned replacement of soft contact lenses is simple: cleaner lenses should produce fewer adverse ocular effects and afford better vision and comfort. All soft contact lenses suffer gradual spoliation from the environment and tear film components over time. Daily cleaning and periodic protein removal can slow this rate of deposition but not prevent its occurrence. By ensuring that soft lenses are replaced at a suitable pre-determined interval, one of the most enduring medical management axioms – that of prevention being better than cure – is brought to bear. In practice, patients who replace lenses regularly report fewer symptoms and exhibit less physiological changes, in most instances, compared with patients who do not replace lenses regularly.

The principal benefits of planned replacement soft lenses are as follows:

1. Use of higher water content materials. Higher water content lenses (i.e. >50% water) generally offer superior oxygen performance. However, such lenses are generally less durable than lower water content lenses. Planned soft lens replacement provides a rationale for the use of physiologically superior high water content materials; the increased fragility of such lenses is clinically inconsequential as long as the lenses will survive intact for the intended replacement period.

2. Simple lens care. Disposability obviates the need for prolonging the life of lenses with elaborate lens care systems. In cases where lens surface spoliation is a problem with monthly replacement, shortening the replacement interval to 2 weeks or even 1 day is likely to be a superior option.

3. Ready availability of replacement lenses. Lenses replaced weekly, fortnightly or monthly are normally supplied in three- or six-packs. Daily disposable lenses are usually provided in packs of 30 or 90 lenses. It follows that the loss or damage of a lens should not, in most cases, be an inconvenience to a patient wearing disposable lenses.

4. Enhanced compliance with aftercare schedules. Planned replacement protocols require patients to return at regular intervals for fresh lenses. Aftercare visits can be scheduled to coincide with lens collection.

5. Single use trial lenses. In the case of disposable lenses, new diagnostic or trial lenses are used with each patient and disposed of thereafter (Figure P.15). This eliminates the risk of cross-infection from a previous wearer of the lens. It also has the advantage of eliminating the time-consuming chore of trial lens cleaning, disinfection and storage.

6. Trial lens fitting with accurate prescription. With the ready availability of a comprehensive stock of trial lenses, it is nearly always possible to undertake a lens-wearing trial on a prospective disposable lens patient with the required lens parameters, especially with respect to lens power.

7. Lens parameters are easy to change. By the very nature of planned replacement, it is straightforward to modify the prescription of a patient, particularly with respect to changes in refractive error.

8. Superior comfort. Numerous factors can lead to lenses becoming less comfortable over time; these include the existence of microscopic lens defects, physical trauma and/or immunological reaction due to lens deposition, and progressive hypoxic effects due to lens ageing. Regular lens replacement avoids these problems.

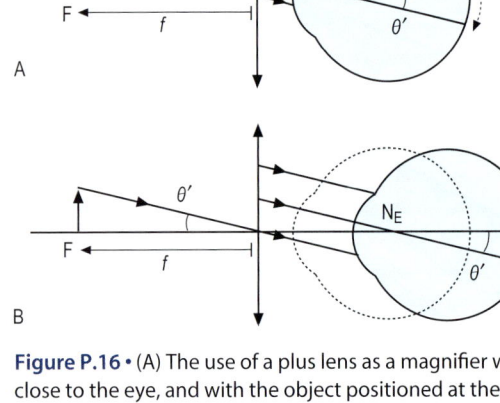

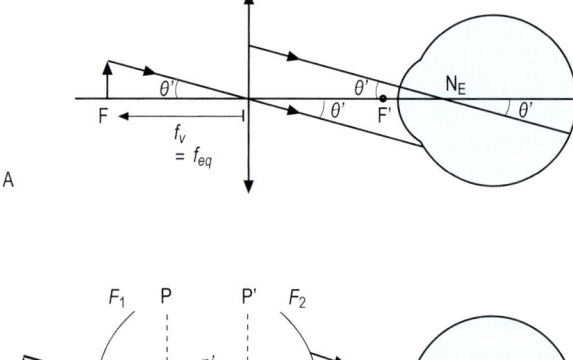

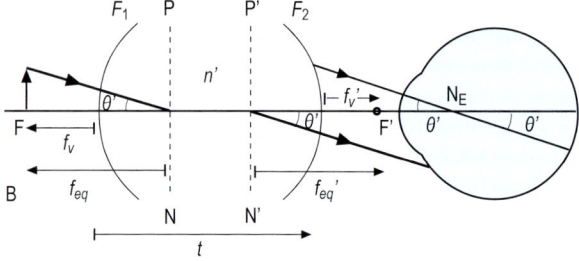

Figure P.16 • (A) The use of a plus lens as a magnifier when held close to the eye, and with the object positioned at the anterior focal point (f) of the lens such that parallel light enters the eye. (B) The same plus lens used with an increased eye-to-magnifier distance, showing the angle subtended at the nodal point; and that the retinal image size remains unchanged.

9. Superior vision. Deposit accumulation on lenses is associated with vision loss; this is avoided if lenses are regularly replaced.

10. Superior ocular response. Lens deposits can facilitate immunological, toxic and traumatic damage to the eye. Therefore, deposit-related problems such as corneal staining, corneal infiltrates and conjunctival injection will occur less if lenses are replaced more regularly.

See *Daily disposable contact lenses*.

Plastic, ophthalmic
- See *Spectacle lens materials*.

Plus lens magnifiers

A plus lens used as a magnifying aid allows the patient to obtain an increased retinal image size by holding an object close to the eye without requiring the accommodative effort that would usually be expected from viewing at this distance. This is achieved by placing the object at the anterior focal point of the positive convex lens, so that parallel light leaves the lens, the virtual image is at infinity, and the patient's accommodation can be relaxed (Figure P.16 a). It can be seen that the ray of light from the top of the object will pass through the optical centre of the positive lens, making an angle θ′ with the optical axis. Since all the rays of light leaving the lens are parallel to each other, they all make this same angle with the optical axis, including the ray which passes through the nodal point of the eye. Although the magnifier-to-object distance must be held constant and equal to the (short) focal length of the plus-lens, the magnifier-to-eye distance can be increased without affecting θ′ and so the magnification remains the same (Figure P.16 b). In this way it is possible to use a plus lens magnifier close to the eye, or remote from it; it can be spectacle mounted, hand held or on a stand, depending on the visual task requirements of the patient.

As it is the close viewing distance permitted by the plus lens which creates the magnified retinal image, then:

Figure P.17 • The angular subtence (θ′) at the nodal point of the eye (N$_E$) of an object placed at the anterior focal point (F) of a thin (A) and thick (B) plus lens. The thick lens is in air so the principal points (P, P′) coincide with the nodal points (N, N′). The front (f_v) and back (f_v') vertex focal lengths are measured from the respective lens surfaces, and the equivalent focal lengths (f_{eq}, f_{eq}') are measured from the principal points. Comparison of (A) and (B) shows that it is the angle subtended at the nodal point of the thick lens system which determines magnification.

magnification (M) = old object distance/new object distance

where the 'new object distance' will be the focal length of the plus lens. The 'old object distance' – the distance at which objects were habitually held – will be individual for each patient, but in order to allow the convenient labelling of magnifiers, some standard value must be adopted. Traditionally this is taken to be 25cm, and if this viewing distance was to be used by the patient he or she would require 4.00DS of accommodation, a +4.00DS reading addition, or some combination of the two. Thus the formula is restated as:

M = focal length of +4.00DS/focal length of magnifier lens

Or, since power is the reciprocal of focal length:

M = power of magnifier lens/+4.00 = F/4

As illustrated in Figure P.16, the retinal image size is determined by the angle subtended at the nodal point of the eye by the parallel beam of rays leaving the magnifier lens. This angle is that made by the ray entering the lens from the top of the object, which passes undeviated through the lens, and which makes an angle θ′ at the optical centre of the thin lens (Figure P.17 a) or at the nodal point (principal point) of the thick lens (Figure P.17 b). Thus, for a thick lens, the angle θ′ is inversely proportional to the equivalent focal length, and thus depends on the equivalent power. The magnification formula is therefore more accurately stated as:

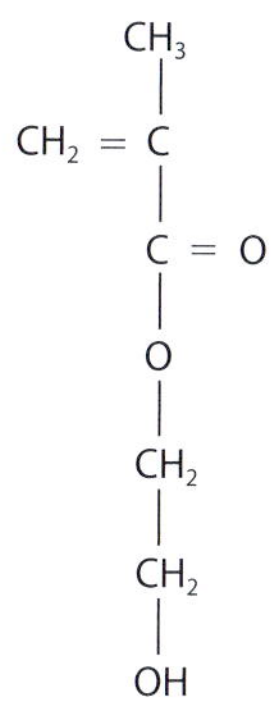

Figure P.18 • Chemical structure of 2-hydroxyethyl methacrylate monomer (HEMA).

M = equivalent power of magnifier/4 = $F_{eq}/4$

See *Hand held plus lens magnifier; Stand mounted plus lens magnifier; Spectacle mounted plus lens magnifier.*

PMMA
- See *Poly(methyl methacrylate).*

Polishing contact lenses
- See *Modification of contact lenses.*

Poly (2-hydroxyethyl methacrylate)
This hydrophilic material can be fabricated by the incorporation of hydroxyl groups into poly(methyl methacrylate) (PMMA), because hydroxyl groups have an affinity for water. That is, poly (2-hydroxyethyl methacrylate), or polyHEMA, is obtained by polymerizing the 2-hydroxyethyl methacrylate (HEMA) monomer (Figure P.18). In the absence of water polyHEMA is a hard glassy material, which upon hydration is transformed into the familiar contact lens material.

PolyHEMA
- See *Poly(2-hydroxyethyl methacrylate).*

Polymegethism, contact lens associated
- See *Endothelial polymegethism, contact lens associated.*

Polymers for contact lenses
The unique properties that polymers possess arise from the ability of certain atoms to link together to form stable bonds. Foremost among the atoms that can do this is carbon (C), which can link together with four other atoms of its own kind or alternatively with atoms of, for example, hydrogen (H), oxygen (O), nitrogen (N), sulphur (S) or chlorine (Cl). Silicon (Si) resembles carbon in this way, especially in its ability to link to carbon, hydrogen and oxygen. It is this property of carbon that forms the basis of what is called organic chemistry, or the chemistry of carbon compounds.

Most of the polymers that are encountered fall within the realm of organic chemistry as defined in this way. These polymers may be purely natural (such as cellulose), modified natural (such as cellulose acetate) or completely synthetic (such as PMMA). There is a much smaller family of polymers based on silicon rather than carbon. Their properties differ somewhat from those of the carbon-based polymers and they are best known in the form of siloxane polymers, in which silicon and oxygen alternate in the backbone. These materials are important in relation to contact lenses because both rigid lenses and silicone hydrogel lenses incorporate such units, which have the principal benefit of conferring enhanced oxygen permeability.

The single characteristic that unites silicon-based and carbon-based polymers is the fact that, as the name (poly-mer) suggests, they are composed of many units linked together in long chains. Thus if we can imagine a molecule of oxygen and a molecule of water enlarged to the size of a tennis ball (the molecular size of water is very similar to that of oxygen), a molecule of polyethylene or poly(methyl methacrylate) on the same scale would be of similar cross-sectional diameter but something like 60m in length. It is the vast length of polymers (sometimes called macromolecules) in relation to their cross-sectional diameter that gives them their unique properties, such as toughness and elasticity. The links between individual atoms are inclined to each other at an angle (the bond angle), which means that chains are not rod-like but 'kinked'.

The individual building blocks from which polymers are formed are termed 'monomers'. To indicate that a polymer contains more than one type of repeating monomer unit, for example when two different monomers are polymerized together, the description 'co-polymer' is used. 'Co-polymer' is a general term, and can be used to describe polymers obtained from mixtures of more than two monomers. Because most contact lens polymers are formed from monomers that are characterized by the presence of a carbon-to-carbon double bond that opens to form a linked chain, the process can be generalized. It is the way in which the structural and functional groups interact with each other and with their surrounding environment that governs the interaction of polymer chains and the resultant properties of the polymer itself.

Perhaps the best way of visualizing the way in which polymer chains arrange themselves is by taking several pieces of string to represent individual molecules. The most usual arrangement will be a random one in which the pieces of string are loosely entangled rather than being extended. It is the interaction and entanglement of the individual molecules in this way that gives polymers their characteristic physical properties. By changing the chemical nature of the polymer chain and their arrangement together, it is possible to change the physical properties and thus obtain either hard glassy behaviour or, at the other extreme, flexible, elastomeric behaviour. The best example of a hard glassy material is poly(methyl methacrylate), which is formed from methyl methacrylate monomer units. A widely known elastomeric material in the biomedical field is silicone rubber, which is based on the flexible silicon-oxygen backbone.

There is an important way in which a hard glassy polymer can be converted into a flexible material, and that is by the incorporation of a 'plasticizer'. This is a mobile component, often an organic liquid with a high boiling point, that will act as an 'internal lubricant'. Its presence separates the polymer chains and allows them to move more freely. A good example is poly(vinyl chloride), or PVC, which in its unmodified state is a rigid glassy material and will be familiar as the clear corrugated roofing material used on car ports, conservatories and similar domestic extensions. When a plasticizer is incorporated the material is converted into the flexible material used, for example, as 'vinyl' seat coverings in cars and general domestic applications. In these cases, pigments and various processing aids will also have been added in order to enable the polymer to be produced in a variety of colours and textures. An almost identical principle is involved in the formation of hydrogel polymers.

Poly(methyl methacrylate) (PMMA) contact lenses

The development of PMMA lenses (also referred to as corneal lenses or hard lenses) began as the result of an error in the laboratory of optical technician Kevin Tuohy. During the lathing of a PMMA scleral lens, the haptic and corneal portions separated. Tuohy became curious as to whether the corneal portion could be worn, so he polished the edge, placed it in his own eye and found that the lens could be tolerated. Further trials were conducted, leading to the development of the corneal lens or, in today's terminology, a rigid lens. Tuohy filed a patent for his invention in February 1948.

Lenses are made from PMMA by polymerization of methyl methacrylate with a free radical initiation system to form rods or buttons, from which lenses are fabricated by lathing and polishing. PMMA has a number of desirable properties, including optical clarity, ease of fabrication, acceptable surface wettability and excellent durability; however, it is impermeable to oxygen and is thus only used today for the fabrication of trial contact lens fitting sets.

Poor vision with contact lenses, investigation of

The causes of vision loss during contact lens wear are not always obvious, and a definitive diagnosis may be difficult due to the transient or inconsistent nature of the problem. In addition to measuring vision with and without contact lenses, additional descriptive information relating to symptoms of poor vision should be obtained from the patient (see Table P.2).

Other techniques for assessing vision may help to characterize the problem. These include:

- contrast sensitivity function – this may be suppressed during adaptation, but otherwise should be no different from that obtained with the best corrected spectacle prescription
- high- and low-contrast acuity charts – reduced acuity with a high-contrast chart suggests a refractive problem, and reduced acuity with a low-contrast chart indicates a 'non-refractive' problem (such as poor lens fit, ocular pathology or excess lens deposition)
- glare sensitivity test – a bright light is positioned next to a low-contrast eye chart facing the patient; reduced vision under this condition indicates 'glare sensitivity',

Table P.2 • Descriptive information relating to symptoms of poor vision.

Characteristic	Description
severity	mild or severe
consistency	constant or fluctuating
onset	immediate or delayed
proximity	distance or near
persistence	whether the problem persists throughout the period of lens wear and/or following lens removal
type	whether the problem is best described as blur, haze, glare, or some other descriptor

which can be due to conditions that scatter light, such as epithelial oedema, epithelial microcysts and anterior chamber flare.

After the symptoms of poor vision with contact lenses have been fully characterized, the following general strategies can be employed to help resolve the problem:

- restoration of vision immediately after lens removal (with a corrective trial lens before the eye) suggests a lens-related problem
- sustained vision loss after lens removal (with a corrective trial lens before the eye) suggests an ocular problem (which may or may not be related to lens wear)
- unilateral vision loss may be due to the lens or uniocular pathology
- bilateral vision loss may be due to a refractive cause or general ocular pathology (e.g. a toxic or allergic solution reaction), or to systemic disease (e.g. diabetes)
- worse vision immediately after a blink may signal excessive lens movement and either a flat fit (corrected by fitting the lens more steep) or inappropriate lens rotation in the case of a soft toric lens (corrected by employing better lens stabilization techniques); this indicator correlates with the appearance of keratometer mires before and after the blink
- improved vision immediately after a blink may signal a tight fit (corrected by fitting the lens more loosely).

The following causes of vision loss with contact lenses relate to spherical refractive error, and can be identified by the suggested strategies:

- patients may be unaware that the lens has become displaced from the cornea on to the sclera, or even lost from the eye, leaving vision uncorrected – inspect the eye
- shifts in refractive error can reduce vision – check the refraction
- lens power may have been ordered (and therefore supplied) incorrectly – check the record card against the power specified on the lens box

- lens power may have been ordered correctly but supplied incorrectly – check the record card against the power specified on the lens box
- lens power may be incorrect (manufacturing/packaging error) – measure the power of the lens and check this against the power specified on the lens box
- the tear layer beneath a rigid lens can have significant optical power – reconcile ocular refraction, over-refraction, keratometry readings, lens parameters and observed fluorescein pattern
- flexure of thick soft lenses can induce power shifts – fit lenses that are thinner and/or made of a material of lower modulus.

An uncorrected astigmatic component of a refraction with contact lenses can be due to:
- an astigmatic shift in refraction
- residual uncorrected astigmatism
- mislocation of toric lens cylinder axis
- the lens power may have been ordered (and therefore supplied) incorrectly – check the record card against the power specified on the lens box
- the lens power may have been ordered correctly but supplied incorrectly – check the record card against the power specified on the lens box
- the lens power may be incorrect (manufacturing/packaging error) – measure the power of the lens and check this against the power specified on the lens box
- corneal warpage.

Contact lens correction of presbyopia entails a variety of visual compromises, such as:
- monovision correction – degrades stereopsis at near
- alternating vision bifocal lenses – incomplete or improper lens translation will compromise vision
- simultaneous vision bifocal lenses – the visual system may have difficulty in processing clear and blurred images on the same region of retina; non-optimal pupil size will degrade vision.

Most non-optical causes of vision loss relate to problems of poor lens fitting, as follows:
- flat fitting lenses will decentre away from the pupil
- excessive post-lens movement can degrade vision
- steep fitting lenses may buckle in the centre and degrade vision
- hyper-thin soft lenses can dehydrate the epithelium, leading to vision loss
- lenses of low oxygen transmissibility can induce gross oedema, leading to vision loss
- poor lens surface quality (due to manufacturing problems, lens deposits or excessive surface drying) can degrade vision.

A variety of pathological and non-pathological ocular problems relating to lens wear can cause vision loss; these include:
- corneal infection
- corneal epithelial oedema
- corneal stromal oedema
- corneal stromal infiltrates
- corneal epithelial desiccation
- corneal neovascularization
- tear film dysfunction
- corneal warpage
- binocular vision problems.

Posterior limiting lamina of the cornea

The posterior limiting lamina of the cornea (Descemet's membrane) is the basement membrane of the corneal endothelium. It lies between the endothelium and the overlying stroma. At birth it is 3–4μm thick, and it increases to a thickness of 10–12μm in the adult. In the periphery of aged corneas the posterior limiting lamina displays periodic sections of thickening, which are known as Hassall-Henle warts. The anterior one-third of the posterior limiting lamina represents that part produced in foetal life and, under the electron microscope, is characterized by a periodic banded pattern. The posterior two-thirds, which are formed postnatally, have a more homogenous granular appearance. The posterior limiting lamina has a unique biochemical composition by contrast with other basement membranes. The major basement membrane collagen is type IV, whereas in the posterior limiting lamina type VIII collagen predominates.

Post-keratoplasty, contact lens fitting for

Corneal transplantation, also referred to as 'corneal graft' or 'penetrating keratoplasty' (PKP), is a surgical procedure by which diseased corneal tissue is removed and replaced by donor material. Corneal grafts are performed for the following reasons:
- optical – to restore visual function (e.g. in keratoconus)
- therapeutic – to treat disease (e.g. to treat an infection by debulking)
- tectonic – to restore, or preclude loss of, globe integrity
- cosmetic – to improve appearance (e.g. eliminate an unsightly scar in a non-seeing eye).

The main optical challenge following corneal transplantation is irregular surface astigmatism, which relates to the way in which the graft sits in the host cornea. It can be described as follows: 'nipple', or steep; 'proud', whereby the graft is totally or partially elevated above the host corneal surface; 'sunken', whereby the graft is depressed below the host surface; tilted; or 'eccentric'.

The indications for contact lens use following corneal grafts are post-operative irregular or high astigmatism, and anisometropia (e.g. as will occur in aphakia). Between 20% and 60% of post-PKP patients will benefit optically from wearing contact lenses. Contact lenses can be fitted when the graft is considered to have healed sufficiently to tolerate lens wear, which may begin as early as 3–6 months post-surgery, and often with one or more sutures remaining in situ.

Rigid lenses remain the overwhelming device of choice for the majority of PKP patients because they efficiently

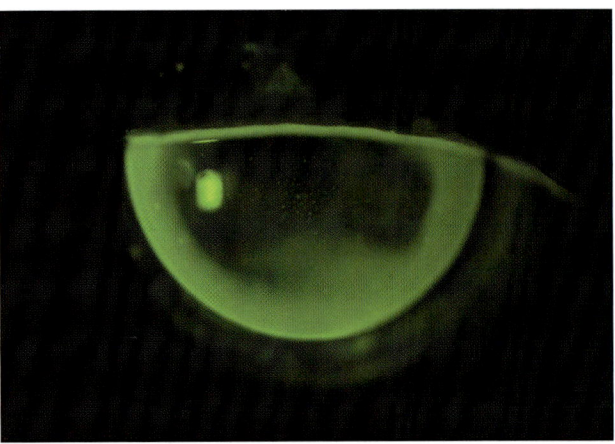

Figure P.19 • Fluorescein revealing points of corneal contact in respect of a 'plateau' rigid lens fit on a proud graft.

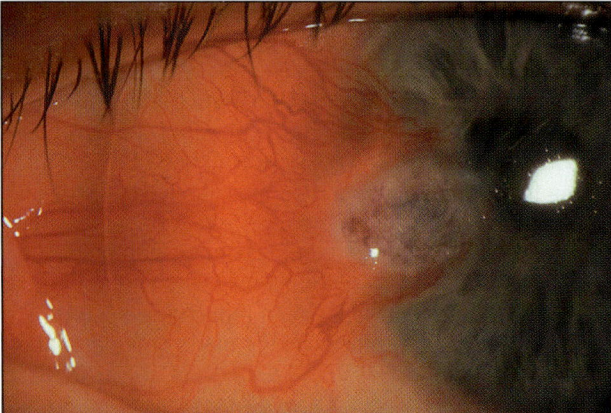

Figure P.20 • A 20.5mm diameter, high water content (77%) soft bandage lens covering a traumatic corneal wound sealed with histo-acryl tissue glue.

and effectively form an optical mask that neutralizes most regular and irregular astigmatism. Large-diameter lenses (9.0–11.0mm) that over-ride the entire graft without causing hypoxic difficulties allow enhanced stability and centration and often give good results; however, achieving a good fit may still be difficult, especially on sunken or tilted PKPs, as rigid lenses tend to 'ride' over the highest corneal point (Figure P.19). The back optic zone radius of a rigid lens should be selected, with initial assistance of keratometry or videokeratography measurements, so as to achieve some form of irregular corneal surface alignment with neither excessive touch nor pooling of tears.

Consideration needs to be given to edge design in fitting rigid lenses to graft corneas. Some corneal surfaces can be fitted with standard edge parameters. Many abnormal corneal shapes require flatter than standard, steeper than standard or even 'reverse geometry' peripheral lens designs to achieve mechanically acceptable corneal surface alignment and appropriate lens positioning. Toric and bitoric rigid designs can be helpful in fitting PKP corneas exhibiting relatively regular astigmatism, and occasionally in tilted and eccentric grafts.

Hydrogel contact lenses, both standard and in custom parameters, may sometimes be helpful, especially for patients who exhibit the following:

- high refractive errors with lesser degrees of astigmatism
- rigid lens intolerance
- acceptance of a less than optimal visual result.

Hybrid lens designs can be beneficial in post-PKP fitting; these include the following:

- 'piggyback', where a rigid lens is fitted upon a hydrogel lens
- Sofperm™ (former Saturn II), a lens with a rigid centre and hydrophilic periphery ('skirt')
- over-sized (scleral-like) rigid lenses.

The above hybrid designs will allow optimal vision, similar to rigid lenses, but such lenses are expensive to fit and may induce hypoxia, which in turn can increase the prevalence and severity of many complications (e.g. neovascularization).

Post-refractive surgery, contact lenses for

Fifty years of evolution in refractive surgery procedures has left in its wake a large group of patients with suboptimal visual results. Today, these patients are faced with three corrective options – glasses, contact lenses or further refractive surgery. For some of these individuals, contact lenses may provide the only option for visual rehabilitation and restoration of binocular vision. Past attempts with refractive surgery have included such procedures as keratophakia, keratomileusis, epikeratophakia, thermokeratoplasty, automated lamellar keratoplasty and radial keratotomy (RK), and, more recently, photorefractive keratectomy (PRK) and laser assisted in situ keratomileusis (LASIK). Each of these procedures modifies the corneal surface in a unique way, necessitating a rethinking of traditional lens designs and fitting techniques for optimal contact lens performance. See *Laser refractive surgery, contact lenses following; Radial keratotomy, contact lenses following*.

Post-surgery, contact lenses for

- See *Post-trauma, therapeutic contact lenses for*.

Post-trauma, therapeutic contact lenses for

Persistent or recurrent epithelial defects following trauma or surgery may heal more rapidly following the application of a soft bandage lens. A small aqueous leak following surgery or trauma can often be sealed with such a lens; if the anterior chamber is shallow or absent, a slightly flat lens will be needed, and this will have to be changed for a steeper lens as the chamber reforms. Custom-made lenses of over 20mm in diameter and with greater than 70% water content have been successfully used as bandage lenses to arrest leakage from trabeculectomy filtration blebs or traumatic wounds (Figure P.20). Corneal transplant problems such as loosening sutures or slippage of the donor disc are usually best dealt with by further surgery – for example, by suture removal and/or re-suturing.

Power changes of contact lenses
- See *Soft contact lens on-eye power changes.*

Practice location
In an optometry practice, the patient participates, in person, in the buying process. It is therefore important to locate the practice as conveniently for the patient as possible. The decision regarding the location of the practice is crucial, not only in terms of the ease of access for potential patients and customers, but also because a wrong or a poor decision cannot easily be reversed – unlike decisions on pricing or product choice. The costs of a mistake include the financial losses involved in acquiring and running a practice (e.g. fixtures and fittings, launch costs etc.) and, just as importantly to many businesses, the indirect cost of not keeping a competitor out of a better location. The suitability of a particular practice location is based on the estimated potential for attracting patients and customers in a given catchment area, and on the location of competitors.

Sophisticated models using a variety of information, including census data, family expenditure surveys, geodemographic characteristics etc., have been developed to help quantify catchment areas and the desirability of differing sites. Checklists with key considerations itemized may also be used to help in the decision-making process, with or without the computer modelling. Other good sources of information about an area include local authorities (e.g. planning department, electoral office, rating office, and clerk's office), estate agents, and the local and national press. Having decided on the location, it is important to ensure that the physical site will be able to accommodate a contact lens practice, including a waiting area, consulting and data collection rooms, spectacle and contact lens dispensaries, staff room, storage/stock room and washrooms.

Practice logistics, contact lens
There is no doubt that planned replacement, particularly when practised with disposable lenses, can generate a considerable extra workload in a practice. A critical issue is the maintenance of adequate stock levels.

As an example, a practice with 500 patients using 2-weekly disposable lenses will handle over 4000 six-packs of lenses per annum (ignoring new fits), or over 80 lens packs per week on average. Five hundred patients will also require 500–1000 aftercare appointments, depending on the preference of the practitioner. This takes perhaps as much as 30% of annual available chair time. If patients collect their supplies quarterly, practice staff will deal with nearly 40 collections per week.

Assuming the above level of activity, a reasonable stock or inventory of lenses will need to be kept in the practice to ensure good service to patients; however, such stocks can be expensive and can consume a considerable amount of space (Figure P.21). There are several approaches to deciding what levels of stock to maintain. The simplest involves keeping a few boxes of each parameter or 'stock kept unit' (SKU). As next-day delivery is usually available to UK practices it is not necessary to stock large numbers of lenses, although

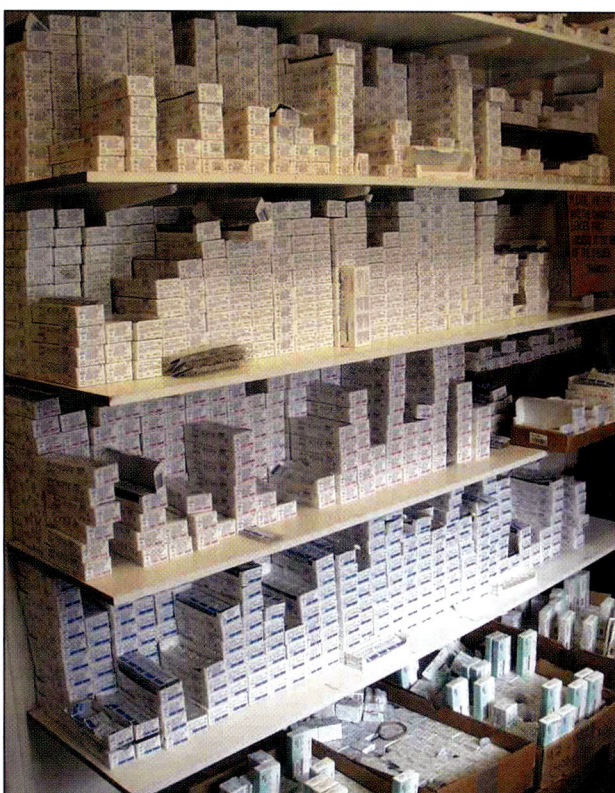

Figure P.21 • A considerable amount of storage space is required to carry extensive stocks of planned replacement lenses.

several spherical disposable lens brands now host parameter ranges of over 100 SKUs. Practices may wish to weight their stock towards the more commonly occurring prescriptions, such as the range from –1.00D to –5.00D. With very large patient bases it may be helpful to consult with suppliers, who can advise on an appropriate in-practice stock holding based on statistical stock models used to manage their own inventory.

Practices that are computerized may wish to model their stock on the actual prescriptions of their patient base. This approach can be tied in with the aftercare recall system. Due allowance needs to be made for unpredictable purchasing patterns, which can arise, for example, ahead of holiday periods. As well as holding sufficient stock for purchase, an adequate number of trial or diagnostic lenses are needed for ongoing fitting.

Practice management
Optometric practice embraces, amongst other products and services, the prescribing, fitting and dispensing of spectacles and contact lenses and associated products, and services.

Practice management may be defined as that activity concerned with planning, organizing and controlling the non-clinical activities of an optometric enterprise to ensure pre-defined outcomes and goals, through the effective use of the available physical, financial, and human resources. The supply of optometric goods and services ranges from very tangible goods (e.g. the supply of a contact lens case) to entirely intangible services such as a contact lens consultation (e.g. aftercare).

The key elements that determine the management issues in a primarily service-orientated enterprise such as an optometry practice can be categorized as per the following 'six Ps':
- practice location and the accommodation
- personnel at the practice
- products and services provided
- proper fees and charges
- promotional issues
- processes.

These issues have to be considered within the framework of the wider legal, political, economic and institutional environment within which optometry has to operate. Although optometry practice can be effected in a variety of settings, such as medical practices, hospitals, dispensing outlets etc., the principles of efficient management can be applied to all of these situations. See *Fees and charges, optometry; Financial management in optometry practice; Layout, optometry practice; Patient scheduling in optometry practice; Personnel, optometry practice; Practice location, optometry; Products and services, contact lens; Promotional issues in optometry practice; Staff training in optometry practice.*

Predicting magnification
- See *Prescribing magnification.*

Pre-formed scleral contact lens
- See *Fitting scleral lenses.*

Pregnancy and contact lenses
- See *Indications and contraindications for contact lens wear.*

Preliminary contact lens examination

This is the initial examination conducted on a prospective contact lens patient. It can be considered to be an extension of a general eye examination, with additional procedures and questioning introduced to allow the practitioner to evaluate suitability for lens wear, and to consider the most suitable options. If the preliminary examination is straightforward – which is often the case – a contact lens fitting can be conducted at the same time.

The procedures conducted at a preliminary consultation may include the following:
- general introductory discussion with patient
- history taking – general health, past ocular history and family ocular history
- vision testing
- general external ocular examination
- measurement of ocular dimensions
- refraction – objective (retinoscopy or automated refractometry) and subjective, at distance and near
- keratometry or videokeratoscopy
- slit-lamp biomicroscopy – with and without fluorescein
- binocular vision assessment
- supplementary tests as required – binocular indirect ophthalmoscopy, tonometry, visual fields, gonioscopy, cycloplegic refraction, colour vision analysis, low vision evaluation etc.
- contact lens fitting – if time allows.

Pre-ocular tear film
- See *Tear film.*

Preferred retinal locus

The fovea is the highest acuity region of the retina, and it is also the oculomotor reference point, whereby eye movements place the image of the object of regard onto the fovea, and keep it there. If the fovea is affected by disease, such that it no longer functions optimally, then another retinal area must be used instead. The area of retina chosen is called the preferred retinal locus (PRL), and it is possible for a patient to select one of several different PRLs, depending on the visual requirements of the task. If a patient has an absolute central scotoma with a well-defined margin, then central fixation no longer allows the target to be seen, and it is inevitable that the patient will adopt eccentric viewing and must place the retinal image on a PRL. In acquired pathologies it is more common for the central scotoma to be partial. The fovea may retain some function, although vision is patchy and distorted, or there may be a tiny preserved island of vision surrounded by a ring scotoma. Such a patient may not abandon central fixation spontaneously, and must be taught to eccentrically view, after careful assessment of which retinal region will offer the best chance of improved performance. The decline of visual acuity towards the periphery is well-known, so in general the area of preserved vision which is closest to the fovea should be used.

Locating a retinal area which has the best potential to be trained as a PRL is very difficult. It is necessary to control the patient's fixation, but a foveal or even parafoveal fixation target may disappear into the scotoma. The use of a large cross or radial spoke as a fixation target may make fixation more consistent. Secondly, visual field testing typically measures retinal sensitivity for the detection of single light targets. As the PRL will be required to perform more complex tasks, a more complex visual test will be needed (such as letter recognition), and the area selected must be large enough to perceive an extended object (several words if reading, for example). In the clinical situation, the location of the clearest area on an Amsler chart may represent the most practical method: if this is (for example) below the central area, then viewing upwards should be most successful. The Amsler chart sometimes gives false negative responses in individuals with a known scotoma, whereby the whole pattern is reported to be clear and complete.

Confirmation of the retinal area used for fixation can only be achieved using an instrument (a scanning laser ophthalmoscope or microperimeter) which allows the experimenter to project the visual target onto the area of retina to be tested, whilst simultaneously visualizing both the retina and the visual target. Even this is not perfect, since a severe fundus lesion can make it very difficult to identify the precise foveal location.

See *Eccentric viewing and steady eye strategy.*

Presbyopia

Refractive defect of the eye whereby there is insufficient accommodative capacity to focus on near objects. This is a condition that is progressive throughout life, and usually begins to become problematic during the fifth decade of life. Presbyopia is thought to be caused by a progressive sclerosing and hardening of the crystalline lens with age, rendering the lens unable to change shape to create more plus power. This condition is alleviated by introducing plus powered lenses before the eyes.

Presbyopic contact lens correction

One of the more challenging areas within contact lens practice is fitting presbyopic patients with contact lenses so as to allow them to fulfill the majority of their visual requirements. The number of newer designs available in recent years, as well as the availability of single-use disposable trial lenses, has resulted in an increased rate of prescribing of contact lenses for presbyopic patients by practitioners. With the presbyopic population growing in size at an ever increasing rate, practitioners can expect to see an increase in the number of presbyopic patients attending for this form of lens fittings, which should now be considered as an integral, routine part of contact lens practice.

The options for the correction of presbyopia for both existing and new contact lens wearers include:

- distance powered contact lenses and near reading spectacles
- monovision
- bifocal contact lenses – simultaneous vision or alternating vision.

Each option has different advantages and disadvantages, which vary with the lens type, the fitting approach used and the degree of presbyopia present. Distance powered contact lenses combined with near reading spectacles may be the simplest and least expensive option. However, this does not address the problem for the patient who does not wish to wear spectacles, and may even de-motivate an existing lens wearer. Nevertheless, the quality and stability of vision in this mode of correction is such that it may give the best optical correction when compared to bifocal or monovision contact lenses.

Patient motivation plays an important role in any form of contact lens fitting. However, it is often restricted to those patients who are aware of the contact lens options, which they are then keen to explore further. Perhaps more important is informed choice based on the advantages and disadvantages of the various options available, as the majority of patients are not aware that contact lenses are a possibility for the correction of presbyopia. This more 'proactive' approach may result in lower success rates but, inevitably, in a larger contact lens patient base.

Caution should prevail when considering patients with compromised binocular vision, amblyopia, distance acuity of less than 6/12, or exacting critical vision needs for either distance or near vision. High- and low-contrast visual acuity charts give more information about acuity. In particular, the difference in low-contrast acuity between spectacles and contact lenses may give some indication of possible success. It is important to have access to trial lenses to obtain an idea of potential success for any particular type of bifocal lens or fitting technique based on both patient subjective feedback and objective measurement.

Patients must be given realistic expectations about the likely level of vision, as is the case with any type of vision correction for presbyopia. It is necessary to ensure that they fully understand the basis of presbyopia, and their expectations should be set out in a positive but informative manner. This involves discussing the benefits of combined distance/near correction without the need for spectacles, as well as likely differences between the visual performance of monovision, simultaneous vision or alternating vision lenses. When compared to spectacles or single vision contact lenses, visual decrements may be noticed, such as reductions in visual acuity (especially in low luminance) and stereopsis, and reduced intermediate vision, depending on the type of lens fitted. It should also be explained that it is quite normal for fitting to require more than one appointment in order to try out alternative lens powers and fitting approaches. See *Alternating vision lenses for presbyopia; Bifocal and multifocal contact lenses; Monovision correction for presbyopia; Ocular dominance; Simultaneous vision lenses for presbyopia*.

Presbyopic spectacle lens correction

- See *Bifocal ophthalmic lenses; Progressive addition lenses; Trifocal lenses.*

Prescribing magnification

When a low-vision patient has been optimally refracted (see *Subjective refraction, visually impaired*), their acuity measured (see *Visual acuity measurement, low vision*) and a careful case history has identified the tasks they wish to perform, it should be clear whether refractive correction alone will be sufficient to improve vision to the required level, or whether magnification will be needed. If the patient wants to perform several different tasks, it is likely that each will require an individual strategy, and this prescribing procedure would be followed for each one:

1. Estimate the required acuity level for the identified task

Distance This will always be an estimate, but a reasonable starting point is 6/18 to watch TV, or read a blackboard, or 6/6 to read bus numbers.

Near Some reading tasks involve print sizes which are very familiar (telephone directories, novels) and easily determined. When the initial appointment is made, patients can be asked to bring samples of specific print with which they find difficulty, and the size can be measured. If a reasonable reading speed is required for 'high fluent' leisure reading, it is usually necessary to aim for an acuity reserve of 2:1. See *Reading requirements, low vision*: to read a book with text of N10 requires a target acuity of N5.

2. Predict the magnification

Predicting the magnification which will be required by a patient in order for them to achieve the target acuity means that a possible magnifier for the patient can be selected more quickly – it is tiring and time-consuming to try too many aids, and depressing for the patient if given a magnifier which is ineffective. Prediction can only act as a general guide, but if the achieved acuity is very different from that predicted, there may be additional problems which may require strategies other than magnification. In each case the optimum distance correction should be in place whilst predictions are made and tested, but it may not significantly affect performance, and may be discarded later.

Distance
Magnification required = required VA/present VA

For example, in Snellen notation to improve from 6/60 to 6/6,

Magnification required = (6)(60)/(6)(6) = 10x

or to improve from 2/36 to 6/18,

Magnification required = (6)(36)/(18)(2) = 6x

If visual acuity is measured in a logMAR notation, then each step between adjacent lines is 0.1 log unit steps = 1.25×, so:

Magnification = $(1.25)^n$

where n is the 'number of steps'. Thus, for example, if the current acuity is 0.5, and 0.1 is required, then:

Magnification required = $(1.25)^4$ = 2.4x

Near
It is important to use a word reading chart from which to determine present acuity. See *Reading tests, low vision*. The magnification formula:

$$M = F_{eq}/4$$

assumes that a standard '1×' magnification is achieved by using a viewing distance of 25cm, which is the focal length of the 'standard' +4.00D add. This means that acuity should be measured at that distance, with whatever reading addition is appropriate (on top of the full distance correction). The reading addition may be zero in a young adult, but the full +4.00D in an elderly person. The value of this addition does not affect the calculation:

Magnification required = present VA/required VA

In point notation, if the patient could read N24, for example, at a standard distance of 25cm (equivalent to magnification = 1), and the target acuity was N6, then:

Magnification required = 24/6 = 4x

3. Trial of magnification
Distance If the task is watching television, for example, then it may be practical to persuade the patient to sit closer to it. A magnification of 2 or 3× could easily be achieved without restriction in the field of view, and without wearing a heavy and uncomfortable spectacle-mounted aid. If it is not possible to get close to the task (for example, reading bus numbers or airport destination boards) then telescopic magnification must be used. See *Telescopes, distance*. An individual device may have the facility to change from the spectacle-mounting more appropriate in the long-duration task, to the hand-held version which is more suitable for quick 'spotting'. The clinician should view through the telescope to check that it is adjusted and focused for the distance to be viewed and then present it to the patient to try out. This allows the reaction of the patient to the limited field and unusual cosmesis to be noted, and the ease of manipulation and ability to hold it in the correct position can also be monitored.

Near This can be tried first using trial case lenses – by exchanging the +4.00D lens which had been used to give 1× magnification for a lens which would give (for the example quoted above) 4× magnification – to test that N6 acuity is actually achieved. For a plus lens magnifier,

$$M = F_{eq}/4,$$

so the lens would in this case be +16.00D. Of course, the reading material must be held at the focal length of the lens (6.25cm) and task illumination must be optimized. This not only allows a trial of the degree of magnification, but also allows an assessment of the reaction of the patient to the close working distance, giving an indication of the likelihood of success with a spectacle mounted plus lens magnifier. If it is not successful, higher magnification can be tried, but continued failure may suggest that a central scotoma is impairing performance and the patient needs to be taught eccentric viewing and steady eye strategy, or that contrast sensitivity is poor and contrast reserve is insufficient. See *Reading requirements, low vision*.

4. Select an appropriate low vision aid
The magnification required should then be 'fine-tuned' with suitable devices (see *Telescopes; Plus lens magnifiers*) and (where possible) the actual materials the patient wishes to see. This is more likely to be possible with near tasks, and samples of newspapers, maps, bank statements, timetables, handicrafts, screwdriver and plugs, music, pen and paper, books, labels from food packaging, needle and thread, price lists, bus tickets and crossword puzzles should all be available. The patient should feel free to make comments and choices without undue pressure from the clinician. The reactions of the patient to the magnifier are as important as the performance, since any reservations about the magnifier will reduce motivation. The deciding factor in the final decision must be the patient's own evaluation of the aids. See *Low vision aids, monocular versus binocular*.

5. Demonstrate and practise optimum use of aid
Testing performance with the aid may begin with the patient being assisted with positioning the magnifier and holding the task in the correct position, but at the earliest opportunity they should do this alone. When patients pick the magnifier up after taking a break, their ability to

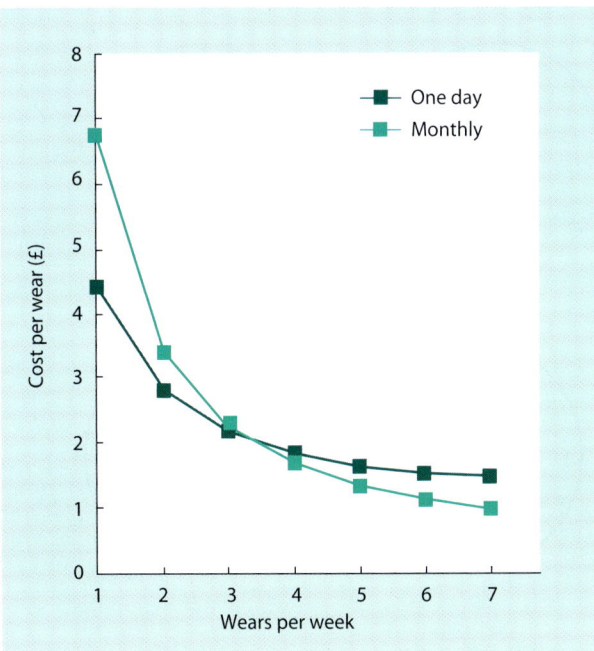

Figure P.22 • 'Cost per wear' of daily-disposable ('one day') versus monthly-disposable lenses based on the average number of days lenses are worn each week over a 12-month period. This model assumes an annual professional fee of £60 and solution costs.

remember how to position it correctly without guidance (which they will need to do at home) can be assessed. It may be necessary to demonstrate this repeatedly. Practical suggestions such as placing a newspaper on a clipboard to keep it flat, the use of a reading stand or typoscope, and improved illumination, may all be helpful. See *Low vision training*.

6. Loan aid for trial

If possible an aid should be loaned to the patient for trial to make sure it proves successful in the normal environment, before it is purchased. The patient must be seen again after a short period of time to assess progress, and to make any changes which are required. See *Follow up consultation, low vision*.

Pricing of contact lenses

A 'cost per wear' (CPW) model can be used to assist practitioners and patients when considering the cost implications of various lens replacement frequencies, tailored to the wearing habits of individual patients. The CPW is a simple calculation of the total cost of lenses (and solutions for non-daily lens replacement) and professional fees over a 12-month period divided by an estimate of the number of days lenses will be worn over 12 months (Figure P.22). This model demonstrates that monthly replacement lenses provide the cheapest option for the full-time wearer, although the difference in CPW between daily replacement and monthly replacement lenses is small. For part-time wearers, daily disposable lenses are usually cheaper than monthly replacement lenses.

Primary Care Trusts (UK)

Recent restructuring of the National Health Service (NHS) in England has seen the development of Primary Care Trusts (PCTs). Each Trust – currently there are some 300 – has responsibility for ensuring that the NHS services within its area are adequate to meet the needs of the local population. This means that, ultimately, the PCT is responsible for the provision of General Optical Services (GOS) and other local eye care initiatives. The funding for GOS is, however, still controlled centrally by the Department of Health.

Print tinting of contact lenses

Dye can be placed on the surface of a soft lens in a controlled manner using a printing process similar to that used for ink printing on paper. In this way, realistic iris patterns containing many colour elements can be applied, and the pupil region can be kept clear. See *Tinted contact lenses*.

Prism

A prism is defined as a lens causing deviation of light without changing its vergence. The deviation produced by a prism is given by:

$$d = (n' - 1)\, a \qquad \text{Equation 1}$$

where a is the apical angle of the prism, and n' the mean refractive index of the lens material. More usually, the deviation produced by a prism is expressed in terms of its prismatic power, P:

$$P = 100 \tan d \qquad \text{Equation 2}$$

where d represents the angle between the incident and emerging ray. The unit of prism power is the prism dioptre, given the symbol Δ. A prism with a power of 1^Δ will deviate light by one centimetre measured at a distance of one metre from the prism. In other words, the SI unit of prismatic power is cm/m.

It can be seen from Equation 2 that the relationship between deviation and prismatic power is not a straightforward one. The deviation of light in degrees by a prism of 1^Δ is $d = \tan^{-1}(1/100) = 0.57°$. Further, the apical angle of the prism is $a = 0.57 / (n-1) = 1°$ (to one significant figure) for crown glass. Also, the prismatic power of a prism that deviates light by one degree is $P = 100 \tan 1 = 1.74^\Delta$.

Prisms can be identified in several ways. Firstly, a prism consists of 2 flat planes inclined at an angle to form an apex and a base. The base end of a prism is therefore thicker by inspection than the apex end. Secondly, a plano prism deviates light but does not change its vergence. Thus there will be no transverse ('with' or 'against') movement of an image when a lens is moved against an object. Note that a prism always deviates the image of an object towards its apex.

A lens with focal power can be considered as a variable power prism. From Figure P.23 it will be apparent that the angle of deviation d varies with the distance from the optical centre of the lens c. The amount of induced prism P can be calculated from:

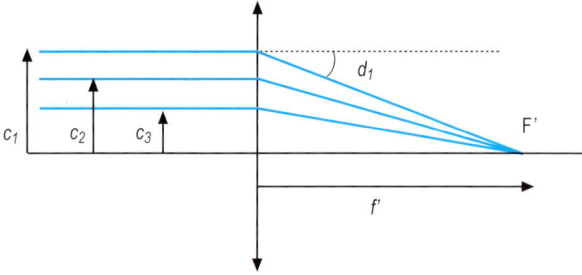

Figure P.23 • Deviation of light by a lens.

$P = cF$

This is known as *Prentice's rule* and gives the prismatic value in prism dioptres, assuming that the decentration c is in cm and the lens power F is in dioptres.

Prisms can be orientated in front of the eye using standard axis notation. The angle indicates the position of the base, and as prisms are not symmetrical about their mid-point, the full 360° protractor must be used. More commonly, prisms are only placed horizontally or vertically and oblique angle prisms are produced by resolving the prism into horizontal and vertical components. The prism is described as Base Up, Base Down, Base In or Base Out where 'In' refers to the nasal side of the eye.

If prisms are combined with their base-apex lines parallel, and with their bases in the same direction, then their effects are considered to be additive, just as with thin lenses. For example, if 3^Δ Base Up is combined with 2^Δ Base Up, then the resultant effect will be 5^Δ Base Up. On the other hand, if 3^Δ Base Up is combined with 2^Δ Base Down, then the resultant effect will be 1^Δ Base Up.

If the base-apex lines of the two prisms to be combined are not parallel, then the single effective prism can be produced by resolving the two prisms. For example, two prisms are placed in front of a right eye. One is 3^Δ Base Up (axis 90) and the other is 4^Δ Base In (axis 360). From Pythagoras' theorem, the power of the single prism that would replace these two is: $\sqrt{(3^2 + 4^2)} = 5^\Delta$. The base orientation is given by $\sin^{-1}(3/5) = 36.9°$. It is also possible to do the reverse calculation and find the two prisms aligned on major axes required to replace one oblique prism.

Prism ballast of contact lenses

- See *Stabilization of rigid toric contact lenses*; *Stabilization of soft toric contact lenses*.

Prism controlled bifocals

There are basically two types of prism controlled bifocals: prism segment bifocals and bi-prism bifocals.

Prism segment bifocals are downcurve solid bifocal lenses with the ability to incorporate prism into the segment, in 0.5^Δ steps between 0.5^Δ and 3.5^Δ. The prism is produced by tilting the reading portion relative to the distance portion of the lens, which has the added effect of making the segment more visible. In general, base up prisms are better cosmetically, and should be used where possible. However, if for example the amount of prism required is large (5^Δ base up right), the prism will have to

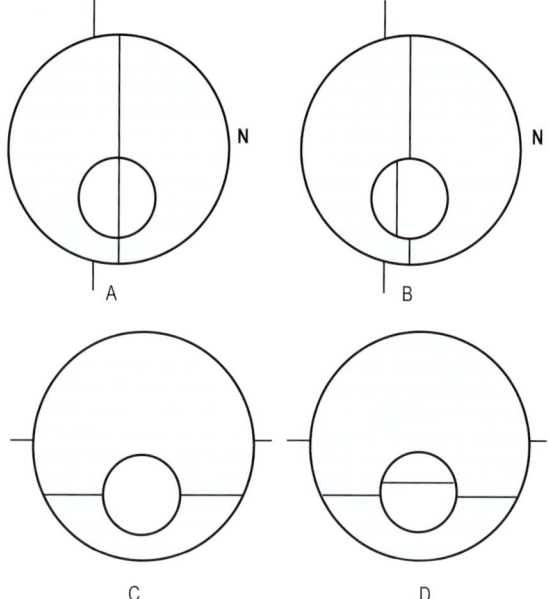

Figure P.24 • Effect of prism in downcurve solid bifocals. (A) No horizontal prism; (B) base in prism in segment; (C) no vertical prism; (D) base down prism in segment. In each case, the lens has been aligned so that the distance image is directed through the geometric centre of the segment.

be split between the two eyes, with 2.5^Δ base up being placed in front of the right eye, and 2.5^Δ base down being placed before the left. Prism segments have been available in a number of different diameters at various times, but at present they are only available as 30mm round glass segments.

Difficulty can arise when verifying the prism that has been incorporated into these lenses. One method used is to compare the incorporated prism with the prism induced by the distance prescription. The most practical way of measuring this is to neutralize any prismatic differences between the distance and near parts of the lens. In Figure P.24, lens A shows a vertical line seen through the geometric centre of a downcurve non-prism controlled segment, or alternatively a prism segment with no horizontal prism. Note that although there is displacement between the object line and the vertical image, indicating absolute prism, there is no deviation at the segment margin. In B a horizontal prism segment (base in) is shown, giving a horizontal displacement in the segment of a line in the distance towards the segment centre. The segment centre is chosen as the reference point as this is the optical centre of the addition in a non-prism controlled lens. The task is to use trial case prism to neutralize the displacement in B so that the final view is as in A. A similar situation for vertical prism is shown in C and D, with C being non-prism controlled, and D having base down prism in the segment. This method only works if the lens is spherical, or the principal meridians are vertical and horizontal in an astigmatic lens. Where there is an oblique cylinder, a distorted image will be seen, and thus the cylinder must first be neutralized before the prism is assessed. It is not necessary to neutralize the spherical component.

Bi-prism bifocals (also known as 'slab-off' bifocals) represent the best cosmetic solution to the problem of

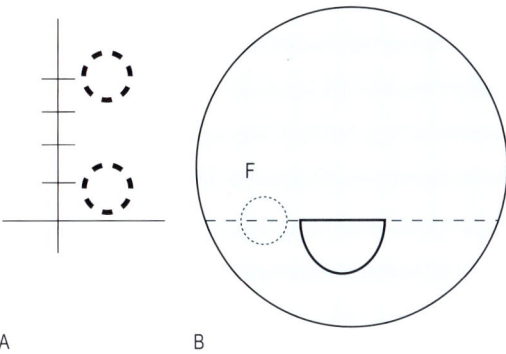

Figure P.25 • Verification of prism in a shaped segment.

anisometropically induced prism. They can be produced from glass semi-finished lenses, or in moulded plastic form. One method of producing an 'E' style lens or a fused 'D' segment bifocal is from a standard semi-finished uncut lens. Base up prism is first worked across the whole of the rear surface. Next, base down prism is worked on the distance curve of the front surface, on the top part of the lens only. This leaves a lens with zero prism at distance, and base up prism at near. The front surface is worked on a 'D' segment so that the line between the two parts of the front surface coincides with the top of the segment. It is usually recommended that the minimum prism worked is 2^Δ in order to obtain a clear dividing line between the two zones of the front surface.

The prism can simply be assessed in a bi-prism shaped segment as shown in Figure P.25, where the dividing line in the distance portion is placed mid-way across the focimeter aperture. This will give two vertically displaced focimeter images, the separation being the amount of prism worked on the segment, this being 3^Δ in Figure P.25.

Prismatic effects

When ordinary spectacles are worn and the visual axes do not pass through the optical centres, prismatic effects are introduced of the magnitude given by Prentice's rule P=cF, where P is the induced prism power, c the decentration in cm and F the lens power. If the corrections are the same for both eyes, these prismatic effects cause no problems for the spectacle wearer. In anisometropia, however, the prismatic effects will be different for each eye. For example, in reading, the visual axes of a young anisometrope would normally intercept the lenses of the distance correction at some distance below the optical centres. Assuming this distance to be 8mm and the corrections to be RE −3.00D, LE −6.00D, the prismatic effects would be RE 2.4D and LE 4.8D, both base-down. In this example, the difference in vertical prism power (2.4D) exceeds normal vertical fusional reserves, so that to avoid the problem the spectacle-corrected anisometrope would have to execute head turns during reading rather than simply depress the visual axes. This problem is absent with well-centred contact lenses.

Prismatic effects may arise as a result of a rigid lens either decentring or tilting, the latter often being due to pressure from the upper lid. To a reasonable approximation, the contact lens and the associated tear lens will both become decentred by the same amount with respect to the pupil centre; these effects can again be calculated using the Prentice rule. If, for example, F=±10.00D and there is 1mm of lens decentration, a 1^Δ prism can be induced, which will be of little importance if similar effects occur in both eyes – that is, if the correcting powers are similar and fitting has ensured that similar amounts of movement occur in the two eyes. See *Accommodation demand; Convergence demand*.

Private labelling of contact lenses
- See *Contact lens supply routes*.

PRK
- See *Laser refractive surgery, contact lenses following*.

Products and services, contact lens

Income generated in an optometric practice is derived from provision and sales of:

1. Eye examinations. The vast majority of patients attend for eye examinations, which is the key value driver in optometric practice. It is only after a complete eye examination has been conducted that contact lenses are prescribed and dispensed.
2. Spectacle dispensing. Regardless of how much contact lens activity a practice has, the supply of complete spectacles will almost always be a necessary part of contact lens practice.
3. Contact lenses. Apart from a stock of 'off-the-shelf' designs, the practice may need to have to hand specialist contact designs and products.
4. Accessories. A range of appropriate contact lens care systems and other accessories must be available, such as sunglasses, spectacle chains, contact lens and spectacle cases, etc.
5. Subscription schemes. Both contact lens and spectacle wearing patients benefit from 'service agreement' schemes, which enable them to obtain replacement products and specific professional services at preferential terms. Such schemes are now common, and maintain a degree of continuity to the practice.

The tangible products supplied by contact lens practices include all those products normally supplied in general optometric practice and, additionally, contact lenses, contact lens care systems and associated products. In view of concerns about contamination and cross-infection, the use of empirically fitted rigid lenses is now the preferred option, and the use of stock disposable soft lenses a practical alternative. It is thus necessary for contact lens practices to stock a variety of lens types for fitting and, possibly, initial supply. However it must be borne in mind that this stock, if paid for by the practice, is only creating value if sold. Similarly, the stocking of a variety of contact lens care systems and accessories is essential in providing a complete service. Like contact lenses, stock that is held in the practice only creates value if it is sold or supplied to patients and customers. Bar-coding of contact lenses and care systems will help manage the inventory of both contact lenses and solutions; however, the value of this process in the absence of a standardized bar-coding scheme is somewhat limited.

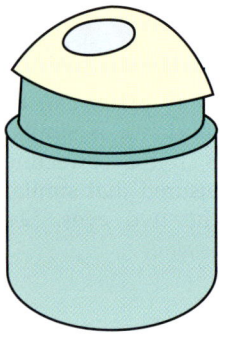 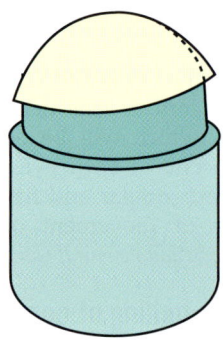

Figure P.26 • Estimation of soft lens BOZR using the template method. Left: the lens has a bubble beneath it, indicating that the lens BOZR is steeper than the curvature of the template. Right: the lens edge is lifting off the surface of the template, indicating that the lens BOZR is flatter than the curvature of the template.

Professional guidelines

Professional bodies have the right to make membership rules in the same way as any other society or club and members of the various organizations would be expected to abide by these. There is however a further area which is far less precise and this is guidance issued. In the past the College of Optometrists, the Association of British Dispensing Opticians, the Federation of Ophthalmic and Dispensing Opticians have all issued guidance on aspects of practice. The guidance as such is not statutory but may be used in cases of negligence or misconduct if it is shown to be a peer view. Of all the guidance issued, it is that of the College of Optometrists that has the biggest impact on the practice of Optometry and that of the Association of British Dispensing Opticians that has the biggest impact on dispensing.

Professional regulation

- See *General Optical Council*.

Profile matching, soft contact lens

The back optic zone radius (BOZR) of a soft lens can be estimated by placing the lens in a wet cell with its circular edge in contact with an optical flat. The lens is then illuminated from the side using a cold light projector, and a magnified profile of the lens back surface is projected onto a series of curves of varying radii. After correcting for magnification, the radius of the curve best fitting the profile is an indication of lens BOZR. Another similar technique (but one requiring contact with the lens) involves placing the lens on a series of perspex domes of known and varying curvature. This has been termed the 'template method' (Figure P.26). If the lens is steeper than the dome, an air bubble will appear between the lens and dome and/or central lens warpage will be observed. The lens is placed on progressively steeper domes until an air bubble no longer forms and the lens surface is smooth. If the lens is flatter than the dome, a section of the lens edge will be seen to lift off the periphery of the dome. This is a very crude although rapid method of radius assessment.

Progressive addition lenses

Progressive addition lenses (PALs) were a natural development from bifocal and trifocal lenses, having a continuous power change between the distance and near values of the prescription. The 'classic' progressive power lens can be summarized as follows:

- Stable (or nearly so) distance power in the top half of the lens.
- Stable reading area located in the bottom central area of the lens.
- Progressive power corridor joining the stable zones.
- Complete 'invisibility' of appearance giving single vision lens type appearance.

This type of approach is popular because it overcomes two inherent disadvantages found in bifocals and trifocals: poor cosmetic appearance due to the segment, and lack of continuous power change between distance and near. Hence this type of lens has the widest appeal as it can satisfy a number of requirements simultaneously. There are some disadvantages, the main ones being the aberration area on either side of the progressive corridor, and the fairly narrow near zone. However, the majority of wearers adapt to the lenses with little difficulty.

There are now many competing lens designs aimed at the 'general purpose' market. At one time it was common for manufacturers to have a specific design philosophy, for example minimum surface astigmatism, or optimum visual acuity across the lens. In recent years however, most lenses have become more of a compromise between the various concepts. A number of non-standard PAL designs have now appeared, to satisfy niche requirements of the PAL market. These can be summarized as follows:

- Short corridor lens – Most of the large manufacturers have now produced lenses with short progression lengths (typically around 12 to 14mm) for fitting into spectacle frames having a small vertical lens size. Shortening the progressive corridor does tend to increase the aberrational astigmatism on either side of the intermediate zone.
- Near vision lenses with enhanced depth of field – A near vision lens with a long progression extending upwards from the stable near portion, giving a small variation in power so that the range of clear vision is extended compared with a single vision lens of the same power.
- Bifocal with variable power segment – A bifocal lens where the 'D' shaped segment incorporates a progressive power change. The advantage of this construction is that by removing the requirement for invisibility of the power change, the optics of the progressive zone can be improved.
- Progressive power lens for high plus prescriptions – A blended aspheric lenticular which incorporates a progressive power change. The progression is shorter than in conventional progressive lenses.
- Progressive power lens for viewing VDU displays – Essentially a progressive lens with a long corridor, and small distance and near zones.

Projection magnifier, contact lens

The total diameter of soft and rigid lenses can be measured using a projection magnifier and a graduated scale (Figure P.27). Such devices typically have a

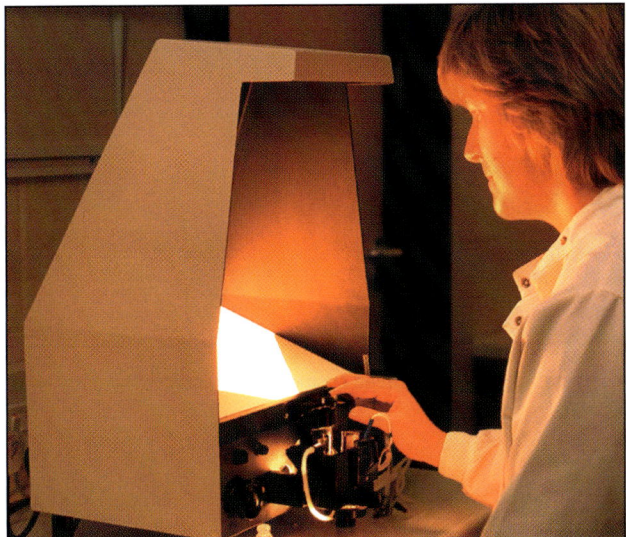

Figure P.27 • Projection magnifier in use.

magnification of between ×10 and ×20. The lens is placed in saline and illuminated with a cold light source, and the projected image is focused on to a fixed scale. The projected image can be checked for any optical defects and regularity of the circumference.

The same device can be used to check the optic zones, and the body of the lens and the lens periphery for physical defects. For toric, truncated lenses, the smoothness of edge transition can also be checked. The measuring device should be calibrated regularly.

Promotional issues in optometry practice

Communicating the availability of products and services that have been identified as 'needs and wants' by patients and customers, at a price that creates sustained value for the practice, is what promotions are about. A variety of options are open to the owner/manager of an optometry practice regarding communication with existing and potential patients and customers. The mix of these will often be determined by the stage at which the practice is in its life cycle. For example, a new practice with mostly new patients will rely more on external promotions, whilst an existing mature practice will rely more on internal communications and promotions.

Internal promotions embrace all aspects of communication to existing patients and include the spectrum from personal contact at the practice – which embraces the practice ambience and point-of-sale literature – through to special mailings. Personal communication is by far the most significant mode of internal contact with the patient, and can adopt the following guises:

- the recall letter – with careful database management, it is possible not only to send out recall letters for routine optometric review visits, but also to tailor promotions of specific products and services to patients by criteria other than clinical need
- special mailings – some practitioners will send patients thank-you cards for referrals, cards on the arrival of a new family member etc.
- practice newsletters, via both conventional mail and e-mail – these are increasingly used, and are indeed a good way of educating and maintaining contact with patients, and keeping them aware about the practice, its personnel, and its activities.

The use of a website as an internal communication tool merits some mention. Practice web sites and electronic mail will increasingly play a role in the following functions: facilitating patient education; e-mail recall letters; e-promotions and opportunities for patients to contact the practice to order sun wear, accessories and replacement products; to book an appointment; and even to submit medical history. Similarly, it makes sense to consider an appointment reminder communication via e-mail.

External promotions include all activities whereby potential patients might be exposed to the activities, personnel or products at the practice. These include national and regional newspapers, trade and professional magazines, radio and television broadcasts, telephone directories, exhibitions and health fairs, direct mail, public relations, speaking engagements and the Internet (world-wide web). This last method enables practices to broaden their catchment area, and to offer sun wear, accessories, frames and spectacles along with practice information and opportunities to book appointments on-line.

Prophylactic tints for contact lenses

The purpose of a prophylactic tint is to prevent the eye from injury or disease. The primary prophylactic application of tinted lenses is protection from excess ultraviolet (UV) light. Lenses with UV-protection tints may be beneficial to lens wearers who are frequently exposed to UV radiation, such as those who:

- have an active outdoor lifestyle, especially near snow, sand and sea
- work outdoors (such as professional tennis players)
- use photosensitizing drugs
- are often exposed to artificial UV sources during work or recreation
- are aphakic.

Some argue that everyone can benefit from UV tints to prevent chronic ocular damage, such as lens yellowing with age – although, paradoxically, an aged crystalline lens that has become yellow will intrinsically absorb UV light, obviating the need for UV protection later in life. Non-tinted lenses and lenses with standard cosmetic tints transmit light of wavelengths down to 230nm and thus do not provide UV protection. Lenses with special UV tints block light with wavelengths lower than about 350nm from entering the eye, thus affording the desired protective effect.

Patients must be warned of the limitations of UV-tinted contact lenses. For example, solar keratitis can occur in exposed regions of the cornea and conjunctiva in UV-tinted rigid lens wearers, and areas of the conjunctiva not covered by the lens are susceptible to solar damage in soft lens wearers. Accordingly, patients should be advised to wear UV-protecting sunglasses or goggles during prolonged periods of UV exposure, and to protect exposed regions of skin in extreme conditions. See *Tinted contact lenses*.

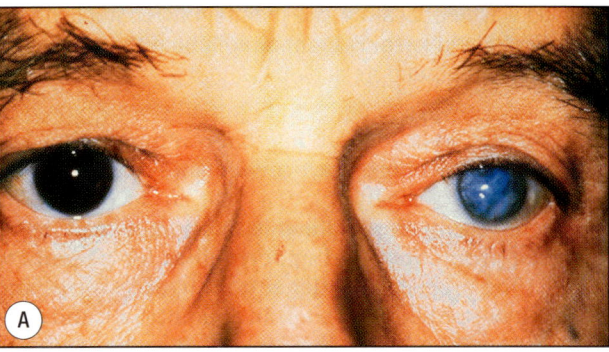 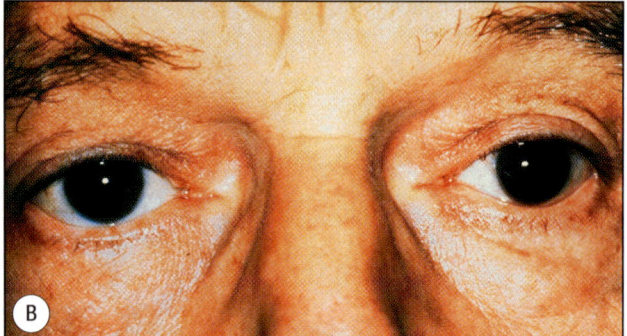

Figure P.28 • (A) Patient with severe opaque scarring of the cornea of the left eye. (B) Vastly improved cosmetic appearance with a prosthetic lens in the left eye that has a painted iris and black pupil.

Prosthetic tinted contact lenses

A prosthetic tinted lens can be defined as a lens that is designed to normalize an otherwise abnormal appearance. Typical cases for which such lenses are indicated include the aftermath of trauma, ocular disease and congenital abnormalities. Visible deformities of the anterior ocular structures – in particular the cornea, iris and crystalline lens – can be effectively masked using opaque tints (Figure P.28). Specific tinting configurations can be tailored for different circumstances – for example, a painted iris and clear pupil for a sighted eye with a disfigured iris; a painted iris and opaque pupil for a non-sighted eye; or a clear iris and opaque pupil for a non-sighted eye with a dense cataract. See *Tinted contact lenses*.

Protected titles

Protection of optometric titles is provided by the Opticians Act 1989 for specified titles applied to individuals and bodies corporate. The titles 'ophthalmic optician', 'optometrist', 'dispensing optician', 'registered optician' or 'enrolled optician' may only be used by those qualified for entry into the appropriate register. As a wider protection it is also a criminal offence to take or use any name, title, addition or description that falsely implies registration. Conviction for such an offence would result in the imposition of a fine.

Protein deposition on contact lenses

- See *Deposits, contact lens.*

Proteins in tears

- See *Tear proteins.*

Protein removal systems for contact lenses

Although surfactant cleaning may remove loose protein from the surface of soft and rigid lenses, it is less capable of removing denatured or bound tear proteins. The build-up of protein deposition has been linked to discomfort, visual compromise, and adverse reactions such as papillary conjunctivitis. Protein removal can be undertaken with enzymatic treatment, generally with products containing papain, pancreatin or subtilisin-A. When prescribed, they are used typically on a weekly basis. Traditionally, enzymatic cleaners were developed in tablet form and treatment was a distinctly separate part of the lens care process. More recently, Alcon has introduced the SupraClens product, which is a liquid formulation of purified pancreatin that is added to the overnight disinfectant on a daily basis. Other manufacturers also make protein removal tablets, which can be dissolved in either multipurpose or hydrogen peroxide solutions. Clinical benefits have been shown with regular enzymatic treatment, but the use of these products has declined with the use of more frequently replaced soft lenses, as the issue of protein spoliation is seen as less of a clinical problem.

Protein removal is arguably more important with rigid lenses than with soft lenses, in view of the fact that most soft lenses prescribed today are replaced more regularly than rigid lenses. With few exceptions, protein removal systems that were originally designed for use with soft lenses can also be used with rigid lenses. The frequency with which patients should be advised to use protein removal systems, and the way in which such systems should be applied to the lenses, will vary depending on the lens material and the strength of the active ingredient in the protein removal system. Advice on these issues should be obtained from the manufacturer.

Individual patient factors will also impact upon the way protein removal systems should be applied. Patients who display a propensity for depositing protein on lenses, and who wear their lenses more frequently and for longer periods of time, may need to treat their lenses more regularly. Typical frequencies of usage of protein removal systems vary from weekly to monthly.

Pseudoisochromatic plates

Pseudoisochromatic plates (sometimes described as 'PIC' tests) are the most widely used screening tests for abnormal colour vision. Pseudoisochromatic designs are essentially camouflage patterns consisting of printed patches of colour which aim to reproduce typical isochromatic colour confusions. The colour components of a figure appear 'falsely the same colour' as those in the background matrix of patches. If isochromatic colours are correctly reproduced the embedded figure cannot be seen in a specific type of colour deficiency. Screening designs are composed of small colour difference isochromatic colours and incorporate lightness differences (equivalent to differences in Munsell value and chroma) in order to eliminate perceived luminance contrast for both protans and deutans. Designs with larger colour differences aim to identify severe (significant) colour deficiency. However dichromats cannot be distinguished from anomalous trichromats using pigment tests because fully saturated colours are not available. Designs which utilize protan, deutan and tritan neutral colours on a grey background aim to classify the type of colour deficiency. Theoretically appropriate colour difference steps can be selected to correspond with the practical needs of a particular occupational task. Different designs are therefore used for screening (identifying abnormal colour vision), grading the severity of colour deficiency and classifying the type of colour deficiency (protan, deutan or tritan). Each design is viewed for about 4 seconds and the figure is identified verbally.

Only the Ishihara plates (Japan) and the American Optical Company plates (Hardy, Rand and Rittler) (USA) have gained worldwide acceptance. The Ishihara test has been shown to be the most efficient printed screening test available for identifying red-green colour deficiency. Ishihara plates identify red-green colour deficiency and aim to classify protan and deutan defects. Different types of design are used for screening which give both positive and negative confirmation of colour deficiency. The test has been reprinted many times but the format remains constant and all the editions are equally effective. The full, or standard, test has 38 plates. Twenty-five plates have numeral designs (Figure P.29) and 13 plates have pathways that the observer has to identify. Only the numeral plates of the standard Ishihara test are required for adult colour vision screening (Table P.3). Pathway designs are intended for the examination of non-verbal subjects but drawing over pathways prolongs the viewing time and reduces screening efficiency. The 'Ishihara test for Unlettered Persons' is preferred.

The serif design of the Ishihara numbers leads to misreadings due to 'filling in' of the loops of the design. Misreadings do not indicate colour deficiency especially when these occur on vanishing designs but have to be considered when determining the sensitivity and specificity of the 16 screening plates as a whole. Compared with the gold standard test (the Nagel anomaloscope)

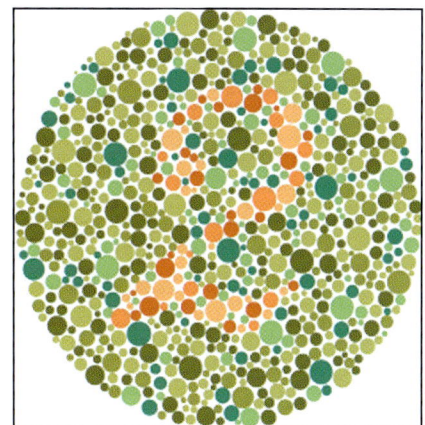

Figure P.29 •
Ishihara plate.

specificity is 100% if misreadings are distinguished from errors and sensitivity is 99% on the basis of 3 errors. Less than 6% of normals make as many as 5 misreadings. Although the Ishihara plates are not intended to grade the severity of colour deficiency, people with slight colour deficiency may make fewer than 8 errors. Two abridged versions of the Ishihara test containing 24 plates and 18 plates are available.

American Optical Company (Hardy, Rand and Rittler) pseudoisochromatic plates (AO HRR or HRR plates) contain vanishing symbol designs (circles, crosses and triangles) with 'neutral colours' with ranked colour difference steps. The test is intended to identifying red-green, tritan and 'tetartan' colour deficiency but has poor screening specificity and sensitivity. The 'tetartan' designs are superfluous. Classification of protan and deutan deficiency is good and is superior to that of the Ishihara plates when the test is failed. The plates are ordered with ranked colour difference steps which identify slight (minimal and mild categories) and severe (moderate and strong categories) red-green colour deficiency. Significant tritan colour deficiency is identified. Optimum use of the HRR plates is therefore to provide additional information when the Ishihara plates are failed by estimating the

Plates	Function	Design
1	Introduction	Seen correctly by all observers and therefore identifies malingerers
2–9 (Transformation)	Screening	A different number is seen by normals and by red-green colour deficient. (Sometimes severe colour deficient people see no number)
10–17 (Vanishing)	Screening	A number is seen by normals but cannot be seen by red-green colour deficient people
18–21 (Hidden digit) (These plates could be omitted)	Screening	Intended that the number can be seen by red-green colour deficient but cannot be seen by normals. These designs have poor sensitivity and specificity.
22–25 (Classification) Only used when screening plates identify colour deficiency.	Classifying protan and deutan deficiency	Protans only see the number on the right side and deutans see only the number on the left side of each plate. Colour deficient people with slight colour deficiency may see both numerals and protan/deutan classification is determined by comparing the relative contrast of the numbers: interpretation is as if the less clear number cannot be seen. Sometimes severe colour deficient people, especially protanopes, see neither number.

Table P.3 • Design and function of the 25 numeral plates of the standard 38 plate Ishihara test.

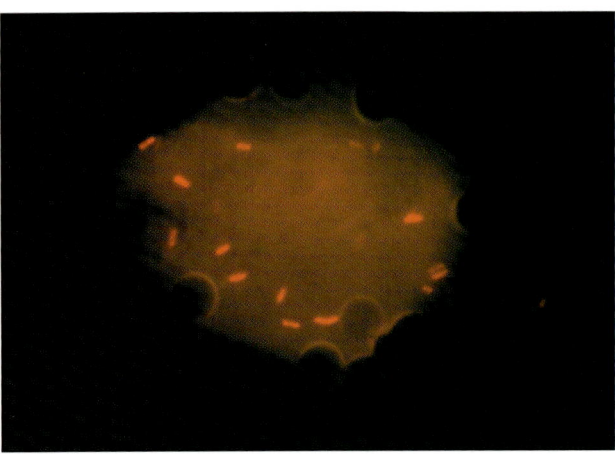

Figure P.30 • Pseudomonas bacteria adherent to a human corneal epithelial cell taken from a patient wearing extended wear hydrogel lenses.

severity of red-green colour deficiency and confirming the protan/deutan classification. Severe tritan defects are also identified. The AO HRR plates (first and second editions) are out of print and three new tests based on the original designs have been published. These are the HRR third and fourth editions Richmond HRR and Waggoner HRR plates. The Richmond HRR third edition is unsatisfactory and has been discarded in favour the fourth edition.

A number of other pseudoisochromatic plate tests have been produced in different countries but most of these have been discarded in favour of the Ishihara plates. Efficient tests are not easy to design and some published tests do not fulfil their intended function. The Standard Pseudoisochromatic Plates second edition (SPP2 plates) are intended for examining acquired colour deficiency. The geometric symbol designs in the Ishihara test for Unlettered Persons, the Colour Vision Testing Made Easy test, the AO HRR test and the Neitz Colour Vision Worksheet can all be used to examine young children. These require verbal identification which is always preferable to matching, tracing or sorting tasks. A selection of the numeral plates from the 38 plate Ishihara test can be used to examine children from about 4 years of age. Children over 7 years of age can usually complete the full Ishihara test. Young children should not be subjected to prolonged examination procedures. A useful guide is that the time taken for the examination should not exceed the chronological age of the child plus 2 minutes.

Pseudomonas aeruginosa keratitis during contact lens wear

Pseudomonas aeruginosa infection of the cornea can have a rapid and devastating time course, and be associated with anterior chamber flare, iritis and hypopyon. A mucopurulent discharge will be evident, although the discharge can sometimes be serous. If not properly treated, the corneal stroma can melt away, leading to corneal perforation in a matter of days.

Extended wear of hydrogel lenses increases Pseudomonas adherence to human corneal epithelial cells (Figure P.30). This bacterium does not adhere to the healthy cornea, because of the natural protective layers of the corneal surface; specifically, the mucus layer of the tear film and the epithelial cell surface glycocalyx (which also contains mucin molecules). The basolateral epithelial cell surfaces (the sides and the bottoms of cells) are much more susceptible to infection than the apical cell membrane (the top surface of cells). Notwithstanding these defence mechanisms, it is now known that some strains of Pseudomonas invade corneal epithelial cells during corneal infection. Once the bacterium is inside a cell it then has the potential to alter host cell function internally. Meanwhile, it is protected from factors of the host immune system and from most forms of antibiotic therapy – neither of which can enter epithelial cells.

Another important recent discovery is that there are two types of Pseudomonas that cause clinical disease, and that the pathogenesis of the two types is entirely different. One type, an invasive strain, invades corneal epithelial cells without killing the host cell, and probably causes disease largely via the host immune response. The other type, a cytotoxic strain, is cytotoxic for corneal and other epithelial cells; that is, these bacteria kill the host cell.

Pseudomonas infections may appear to worsen slightly during the first 24 hours after medication has commenced (see *Microbial keratitis*). The condition will gradually improve thereafter, with the micro-organism persisting for 14 days or longer.

Psoriasis
• See *Systemic disease, contact lens wear in*.

Psychological factors
• See *Indications and contraindications for contact lens wear*.

Psychophysical measurements of colour vision

Psychophysical measurements involve the measurement of a physical stimulus required to produce a 'criterion response'. These criteria are 'identity', where two stimuli are judged to be exactly the same, and 'threshold detection', in which a stimulus is perceived to be just noticeably different from another stimulus. All the test parameters, such as luminance and wavelength, are carefully measured and controlled. Cone function is measured with a field size no greater than 3° to avoid stimulating rod receptors. Psychophysical tests are used to define both normal colour vision and colour vision deficiency. Standard measurements include relative luminous efficiency, wavelength discrimination, detection thresholds and colour matching functions. Spectral anomaloscopes and computerized colour vision tests fulfill the criteria of psychophysical measurement. Computerized colour vision assessment requires accurate calibration of the luminance and chromaticity of the CRT display as well as control of ambient illumination affecting the appearance of the screen. Measurements are limited by the colour gamut of the display and fully saturated colours cannot be obtained. Therefore, although 'anomaloscope' type tests have been developed, dichromats cannot be distinguished from severe anomalous trichromats. Measurements of MacAdam Ellipses, isochromatic zones and luminance contrast deficits have been made on fully calibrated displays and have been applied to study of

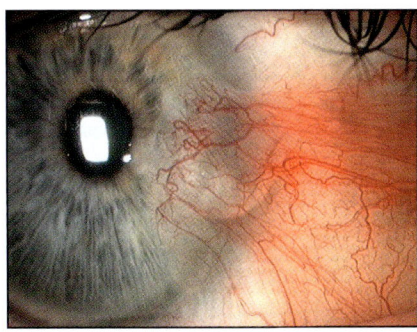 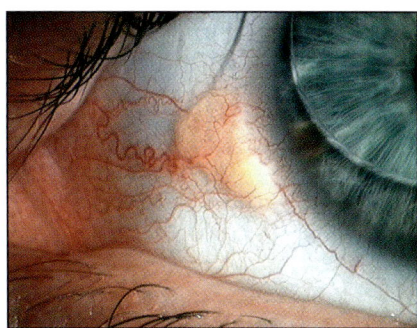

Figure P.31 • Pterigium (left) and pingueculum (right).

acquired colour deficiency. In addition computerized measurement of 'colour contrast sensitivity', or detection thresholds, using paired colours within protan, deutan and tritan isochromatic zones, has been used to study acquired colour deficiency in patients with glaucoma and diabetic eye disease. Pseudoisochromatic designs can be reproduced on calibrated cathode ray tube displays. For example, the design of the Cambridge Colour Test is based on ranked colour differences similar to the series of plates in the AO HRR plates.

Pterygium and pingueculum

Pterygium is a fibrovascular growth involving both the bulbar conjunctiva (the tail) and cornea (the head of the pterygium) (Figure P.31 left). Available epidemiological evidence suggests that they develop from excessive ultraviolet light exposure with damage to the conjunctival and limbal epithelium. Sidelight (albedo light), internally reflected through the cornea and focused at the limbus appears to be of particular importance in this process.

Pingueculum is a degeneration of the exposed interpalpebral conjunctiva (Figure P.31 right). It is also associated with chronic ultraviolet exposure and chronic irritation from wind and dust. The pathogenesis of pingueculum is a degeneration of the conjunctival stroma, with degeneration of the collagen fibres and some thinning of the overlying epithelium. Rather than the normal thin and transparent nature of the conjunctiva, there is focal thickening and opaque deposition.

Most patients with pterygium and pingueculum are asymptomatic, although they may at times become inflamed or irritated. Depending on the size and height of the lesion, ocular surface irritation with dryness and a foreign body sensation may occur. If pterygia are large or fibrotic enough, blurring of vision can occur from the induction of irregular astigmatism.

Pterygia commence with conjunctival scarring, thickening and distortion, followed by extension of this process onto the limbus with subsequent further extension onto the cornea. They are usually bilateral although may be quite asymmetric, are interpalpebral and usually medial. If present both medially and laterally and touching across the central cornea they are termed 'kissing pterygia'. When in an active growing phase the pterygium is fairly thickened, obscuring the underlying sclera and cornea. An avascular, slightly opaque area of epithelium termed a 'cap' also frequently precedes the head of an active pterygium. A corneal epithelial iron line termed a 'Stocker line' may occur just central to the leading edge of the lesion. Keratometry or corneal mapping may reveal central corneal distortion. Recurrent pterygia often appear slightly different to primary pterygia, being less well centred at the limbus and more distorted.

In contrast to pterygia, pinguecula appear as gelatinous deposits in the conjunctiva, adjacent to the limbus at the 3 and 9 o'clock positions, without corneal involvement. The lesion may be transparent, white or yellow, with calcification sometimes present. The surface of the deposit is usually raised and it may be round or triangular in shape (base toward limbus). While a pinguecula may be hyperaemic, it is not usually excessively vascularized, the vascularity being similar to or slightly higher than that of the adjacent uninvolved conjunctiva. If the apex of the lesion stains with fluorescein, then it is indicative that the pingueculum is creating an ocular tear film-surfacing problem. A corneal Dellen may occur if the pingueculum is sufficiently raised to disrupt the adjacent pre-corneal tear film. The condition is usually bilateral and reasonably symmetrical.

The incidence of pterygia may be as high as 20 to 30% depending on UV light exposure. Pinguecula are also very common (greater than 1/10) in older age groups, or in particular occupational or recreational groups of people with above average levels of UV exposure.

Patients with pterygia or pinguecula should be advised to wear wrap-around sunglasses or sunglasses with side-shields when outside in high UV conditions, both to limit further development of the lesions and to prevent them from becoming sore and inflamed. If there is any uncertainty in diagnosis/nature of the lesion, then the patient should be reviewed as appropriate. Ocular surface lubrication may be useful in alleviating some of the symptoms of ocular surface irritation. Older formulations of tear supplements preserved with Benzalkonium Chloride (BAK) should be avoided, unless for occasional use only. Mild hyperaemia or inflammation can be decongested with short-term palliative measures such as cold compresses or mild vasoconstrictors. Acute inflammation of a pterygium can be treated with topical corticosteroids such as fluorometholone or topical non-steroidal anti-inflammatory drugs (NSAIDs) such as ketorolac.

Excision of pinguecula is rarely required, usually for cosmetic reasons or if it is interfering with soft contact lens wear. A biopsy for more vascular or pigmented lesions may be indicated. The usual indications for offering surgical excision of pterygia are:

- Induced corneal astigmatism leading to decreased vision

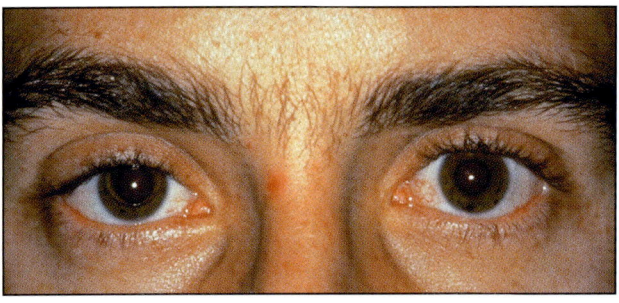

Figure P.32 • Unilateral ptosis of the right eye in a patient who had been wearing a rigid lens in that eye, and a soft lens in the contralateral eye, for 4 weeks.

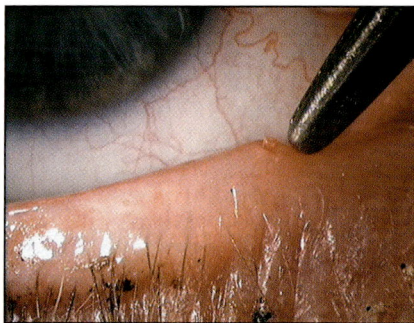

Figure P.33 • Collagen punctal plug being inserted into the lower eyelid.

- Chronic ocular surface irritation unrelieved by the moderate use of tear supplements
- Extensive pterygium threatening the central cornea
- Positional diplopia attributable to the tethering action of the pterygium (rare)
- Cosmetic concern.

Recurrence of the pterygia following surgical removal is common, especially in darkly pigmented races. Simple excision of the pterygium leaving the exposed sclera uncovered (bare scleral resection) leads to a high rate of recurrence of up to 70%. Adjunctive treatments such as beta-radiation and Mitomycin C are effective; however, both occasionally lead to significant postoperative complications including scleral necrosis and delayed epithelial healing. Surgical techniques employed to reduce recurrences include sliding conjunctival grafts, amniotic membrane transplants and lamellar keratoplasty. An autoconjunctival graft is now the most popular surgical procedure; using this method, recurrence rates are approximately 5% for primary and 10% for recurrent pterygia.

Ptosis associated with contact lenses

The classical appearance of ptosis is of a narrowing of the palpebral fissure and a relatively large gap between the upper lid margin and the skin fold at the top of the eyelid (Figure P.32). Rigid lenses can cause narrowing of the palpebral fissue by about 0.4mm, whereas soft lenses do not affect palpebral aperture size. Clinically significant ptosis occurs when the distance between the centre of the pupil and the lower margin of the upper lid is less than 2.8mm. Using this criterion, contact lens induced ptosis (CLIP) occurs in about 10% of rigid lens wearers. The ptosis takes 4–6 weeks to develop fully, and is generally noticed by patients in advanced cases. There are no associated signs or symptoms.

A number of mechanisms have been advanced as possible causes of CLIP. Those involving some form of dysfunction of the aponeurosis (see *Levator palpebrae superioris*) include forced repeated lid squeezing and lateral eyelid stretching during lens removal, rigid lens displacement of the tarsus, and blink-induced eye rubbing. Non-aponeurogenic causes of CLIP include lens-induced lid oedema, blepharospasm and papillary conjunctivitis.

To differentiate between these possible causes, patients demonstrating CLIP should be required to cease lens wear for at least 1 month (to detect any trends towards recovery) and perhaps as long as 3 months (to demonstrate complete resolution). If the CLIP partially or completely resolves after ceasing lens wear for 1 month, then the cause is lid oedema and/or involuntary blepharospasm, and the patient may need to be refitted with soft lenses (which do not induce ptosis). The eyelids should also be everted to determine if papillary conjunctivitis is involved, and if so, appropriate action should be taken to alleviate the condition. If the ptosis persists after resolution of the papillary conjunctivitis, or after ceasing lens wear for 1 month, then the cause is most likely damage to the aponeurosis, whereby surgical correction is the preferred option. Management strategies available to patients with severe CLIP who do not wish to undergo lid surgery include being fitted with a 'ptosis crutch'.

The prognosis for recovery from aponeurogenic CLIP is poor; the condition can only be reversed by surgical correction or other management options as described above. The prognosis for recovery from non-aponeurogenic CLIP is good. If the cause of ptosis is papillary conjunctivitis, the time course of resolution of the ptosis will parallel the time course of recovery of the papillary conjunctivitis. If a contact lens wearer presents with ptosis, the numerous other possible causes of this condition must be considered so that the appropriate course of management can be adopted.

Punctal plugs

The use of punctal plugs can be an effective step in treating moderate to severe dry eye that is unresponsive to artificial tear drops and ointments. The tears drain into the nose via the tear ducts and blocking this outflow is a reasonable strategy to keep the tears in the eye for longer. The term 'puncta' refers to the opening of the tear ducts on the eyelid margin. Plugs that can be inserted inside the tear ducts to block them are called 'punctal plugs'. Punctal plugs increase the comfort level and lower the frequency of artificial tear use in most dry eye patients. The decreased artificial tear use may be economically beneficial, considering the high cost of preservative-free artificial tears. Punctal plugs can be inserted either in the lower eyelid or in the upper eyelid or in both eyelids. Temporary punctal occlusion with collagen implants may be considered to ascertain if the punctal blockage will help reduce dry eye symptoms and also to rule out excessive tearing due to such blockage (Figure P.33). Most silicone punctal plugs are umbrella shaped and the top part of the punctal plug rests on the eyelid surface. A different type of punctal plug (Herrick plug) is completely embedded within the tear ducts. About 40% of punctal plugs are lost within 6 months of insertion. Most of the punctal plugs lost are due to spontaneous extrusion, and this happens usually within the initial 3 months post insertion. In addition, about 10% of patients may complain of local discomfort at the plug site or excessive tearing (especially if both upper and lower puncta are blocked); in such cases, the punctal plug may have to be removed. This is a simple procedure and is painless. Patients who have lost the initial plug are twice as likely to lose the replacement plug. Upper punctal plugs have a higher risk of loss compared with plugs inserted in lower puncta.

Pupil

The pupil is the aperture within the iris through which light passes from the outside world to the retina. It is located slightly nasal to the centre of the iris, and can vary in diameter from 2mm to 8mm. The pupils are typically slimmer in old age. The size of the pupil varies with ambient light levels (being smaller in brighter light) and constricts when gaze is directed to near objects.

Pupil, Adie's

This describes an anomaly whereby there is essentially no direct or consensual pupillary reaction to light, and a slow or delayed reaction to a near target. A reaction to light does occur only after prolonged exposure to light or dark. The condition is typically unilateral, and the affected pupil is usually larger. Adie's pupil is due to a disease or injury to the cilliary ganglion or short ciliary nerves. It can also be caused by diabetes, syphilis, or temporal arteritis in elderly patients.

Pupil, Argyll Robertson

This describes an anomaly whereby there is essentially no direct or consensual pupillary reaction to light, but a normal reaction to accommodation and convergence. The condition is bilateral and the pupil sizes are equal. The Argyll Robertson pupil is caused by neurosyphilis.

Pupil diameter

While the retinal image is always blurred by both aberration and diffraction, in ametropia and presbyopia it is often defocus blur that is the major source of visual degradation. Defocus will occur whenever the object point lies outside the range of object distances embraced by the far and near points of the individual. Even within this range small errors of focus will normally occur, due to the steady-state errors that are characteristic of the accommodation system. Such blur depends on the dioptric error of focus and the pupil diameter. For any object point and assuming that the eye pupil is circular, spherical defocus produces a 'blur circle' on the retina. It is easy to show that the diameter, dmm, of this blur circle is:

$$d = \Delta F \cdot D/K'$$

where ΔF is the dioptric error of focus with respect to the object point, D is the pupil diameter in mm, and K' is the dioptric length of the eye. If astigmatism is present, the blur patch is an ellipse, with major and minor axes corresponding to the focus errors in the two principal meridians.

The blur circle diameter can be expressed in angular terms as:

$$\alpha = \Delta F \cdot D \cdot 10^{-3} \text{ rads} = 3.44 \cdot \Delta F \cdot D \text{ min arc}$$

Thus, for a 3mm diameter pupil, the blur circle diameter increases by roughly 10min arc per dioptre of defocus. The impact of blur on visual acuity depends somewhat on the acuity target chosen and the criteria and observation conditions used. The minimum angle of resolution (MAR) would be expected to be somewhat smaller than the blur circle diameter. For errors of focus above about a dioptre, letter targets, a 50% recognition rate, and normal chart luminances of about $150 cd/m^2$ (giving pupil diameters of about 4mm),

$$MAR = 0.65 \cdot \Delta F \cdot D \text{ min arc}$$

With errors of focus smaller than about 1 dioptre, diffraction, aberration and the neural capabilities of the visual system are more important than defocus blur, and the MAR exceeds that predicted by the above equation.

The natural pupil diameter is chiefly dependent on the ambient light level. Pupil diameters at any light level tend to decrease with age (senile miosis) and with accommodation, as well as varying with a variety of emotional and other factors.

Reducing the pupil size results in smaller amounts of blur in the retinal image for any given level of defocus. Thus an uncorrected low myope may experience minimal levels of distance blur under good photopic levels of illumination, but may notice considerable blur when driving at night, when the pupil is large (Figure P.34).

Pupil, Hutchinson's

This describes an anomaly whereby a pupil is widely dilated and unreactive to all stimuli. It is caused by lesions to the central nervous system, and may be seen following head trauma.

Pupil reflex assessment

The response of the iris to light levels and with accommodation is a result of a neural reflex pathway that involves the iris, retina, visual pathway, midbrain and parasympathetic and sympathetic innervation of the eye. As such, clinical assessment of the pupil response to light elicits important information about the health of all these structures. If a pen torch is presented to one eye, the pupil will constrict (the direct reflex) as will that of the other eye (the consensual reflex). Both will constrict when a patient changes gaze from a distant target to a near one (the near reflex). Ambient lighting should be reduced to exaggerate the resting pupil diameter but be of sufficient levels to allow easy viewing of the pupil, particularly in patients with very dark irides. Disruption of the afferent pathway, such as may be caused by damage to the retina, optic nerve, chiasma, tract or superior brachium, will result in the loss or reduction of the direct and consensual reflexes. As the damage is often to only some of the pupillary fibres, there may well

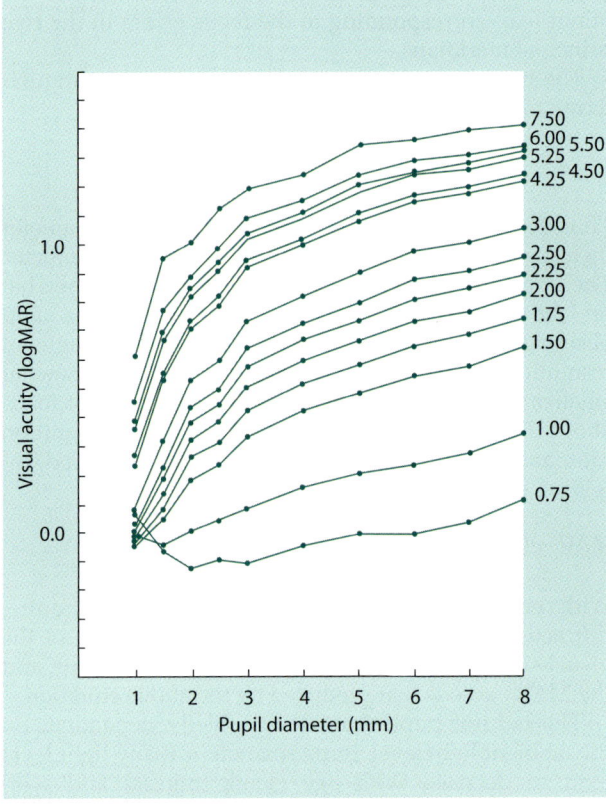

Figure P.34 • Effect of pupil diameter on visual acuity (logMAR) for uncorrected myopes at a constant retinal illuminance of 2150 trolands.

be a reduction in the pupil response that is only detectable when compared with the normal response; this is described as a relative afferent papillary defect (RAPD). This may also be found in patients with a very dense unilateral cataract as light scatter from the opacity may give an enhanced pupil response which appears as an RAPD in the contralateral eye. Some practitioners grade the RAPD by holding varying density filters before the normal eye until the contralateral direct reflex overrides the normal consensual reflex. With conditions where vision loss cannot obviously be traced to ocular signs, for example retrobulbar neuritis, it is essential to investigate anomalous pupil responses.

Pupillometer

An instrument that measures the diameter of the pupil is a pupillometer. This can take the form of a simple comparator gauge which is comprised of a series of black hemispheres of different sizes; the gauge is held close to the eye and the nearest match indicates the pupil size. Pupillometry can also be effected using digital image or video capture in conjunction with pre-calibrated electronic measuring tools. Some models of videokeratoscopes, aberrometers and autorefractors will give a readout of pupil size at the instant of measurement.

Pupil, Marcus Gunn

This describes an anomaly whereby stimulating the affected pupil will cause both pupils to constrict to a smaller extent than when the unaffected pupil is stimulated. The condition is easily observed when alternating the stimulating light from one eye to the other, whereby stimulation of the unaffected eye will cause constriction of both pupils whereas stimulation of the affected eye will cause dilation of both pupils. This condition indicates a lesion in the afferent pupillary pathway – typically the optic nerve. The Marcus Gunn pupil is observed in multiple sclerosis, optic neuritis and retrobulbar neuritis.

Puncta
- See *Lacrimal drainage system.*

Push-up test, soft contact lens
- See *Fitting soft contact lenses.*

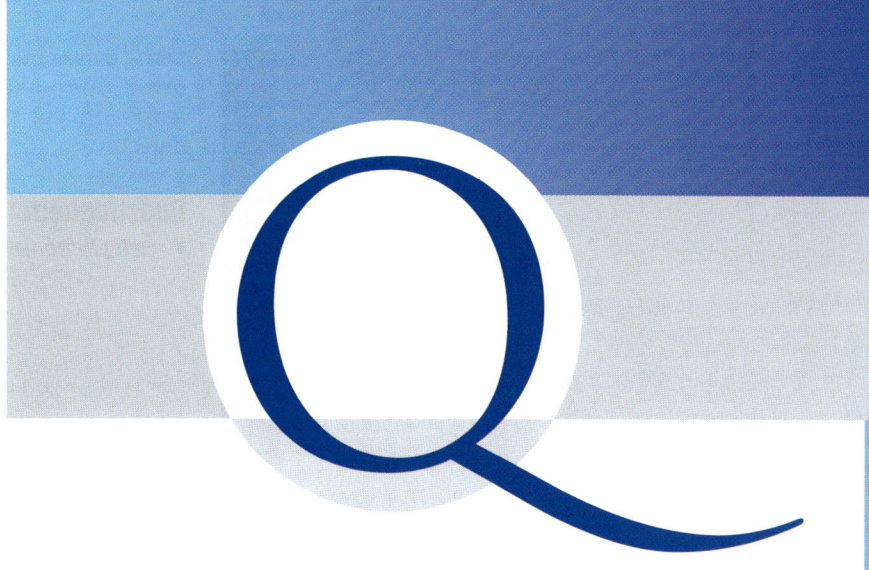

Quality, soft contact lens

Defects can sometimes be detected in soft contact lenses when observed at ×10–×20 magnification. These defects can be divided into two broad categories – edge defects and non-edge (body) defects (Figure Q.1) and four sub-categories, as follows:

1. Edge defects
- nick – small piece of lens material missing from lens edge
- tear – partial or full separation of lens material continuous with lens edge
- roughness – uneven edge profile
- excess material – lens mass or surplus material extending beyond lens circumference.

2. Non-edge (body) defects
- split – partial or full separation of lens material that is not continuous with lens edge
- blemish – hazy, low-transparency region of lens; may be on lens surface or within lens (Figure Q.2)
- eccentric optic zone – optic zone not concentric with lens perimeter
- multiple pieces – lens separated into sections.

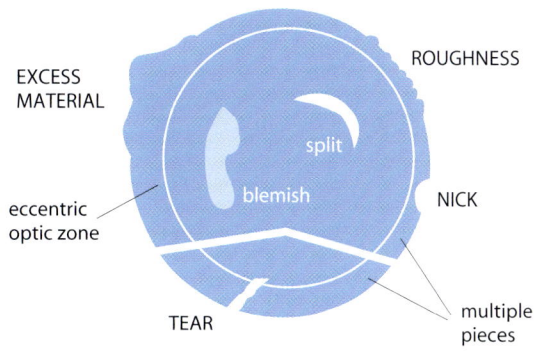

Figure Q.1 • Types of defects that can be observed on soft contact lenses. Edge defects are indicated in upper case and body defects in lower case.

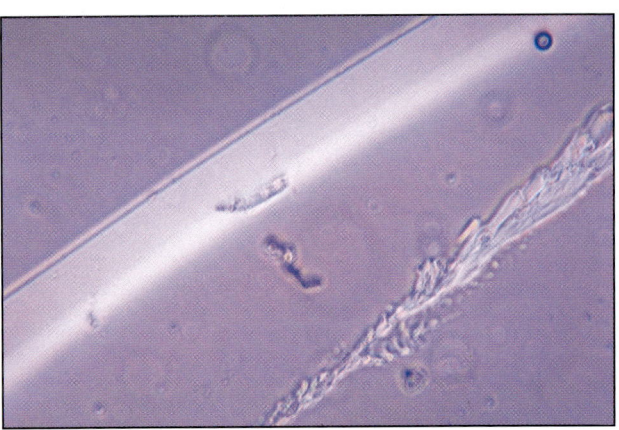

Figure Q.2 • Blemish on the surface of an early generation disposable soft lens, in the form of an irregular strip of excess lens mass lying parallel with the lens edge. Lenses containing such blemishes should be discarded.

Some lenses may contain more than one defect. Patients using disposable lenses should be urged to examine lenses on the tip of their finger to check for obvious defects.

Questionnaires, low vision

- See *Outcome measures, low vision.*

R

Radial edge lift, contact lens
- See *Edge lift of contact lenses*.

Radial keratotomy (RK)
Radial keratotomy (RK) is a surgical technique for the correction of myopia. It is largely being phased out in favour or more sophisticated and predictable laser surgical procedures. Nevertheless, RK is still indicated in certain circumstances, and patients may therefore occasionally present for supplementary contact lens correction having had the procedure performed some time previously. The surgical technique involves making a series of radial incisions from the mid-peripheral cornea to the limbus, leaving a central clear optic zone. The procedure is performed under local anaesthesia.

When the radial incisions are placed into the mid-peripheral cornea, the wounds gape open under the force of the intraocular pressure and stresses from within the corneal tissues. The gaping incisions are first filled with an epithelial plug, which is eventually replaced by a permanent wedge of fibroplastic scar tissue. This results in an overall increase in corneal surface area although the corneal diameter remains unchanged. There is a common misconception that the mid-peripheral cornea steepens following radial keratotomy. However, as the anterior cornea displaces to accommodate the gaping incisions, virtually the entire cornea, from limbus to limbus, flattens. The flattening effect is simply greater in the central cornea than in the periphery, resulting in the false impression of mid-peripheral steepening.

The degree of wound gape and the resultant amount of corneal flattening (and thus the amount of myopia corrected) are dictated by a number of surgical and biological factors including the following:

- the number, depth and length of the incisions
- intraocular pressure forces
- stresses and biochemical properties within the corneal tissue
- patient age at the time of surgery
- individual wound healing responses.

Radial keratotomy, contact lenses following
Following RK, the cornea may exhibit significant corneal flattening with only minimal mid-peripheral flattening (approximately 0.1–0.2mm flatter than its pre-operative curvature). Therefore, in the fitting of a rigid lens (Figure R.1), a back optic zone radius (BOZR) should be selected to align with the 'more normal' mid-peripheral cornea, approximately 4.0mm from the centre, along the horizontal meridian. The radius of the post-operative mid-peripheral cornea can be determined through corneal mapping or peripheral keratometry. Alternatively, the fit of a diagnostic lens with a BOZR that is

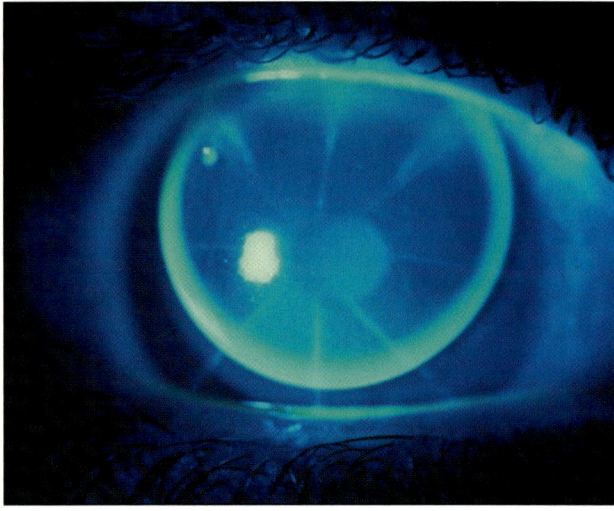

Figure R.1 • Rigid lens fitted to a patient post-RK.

0.1–0.2mm flatter than the preoperative flat 'K' reading can be evaluated. The appropriate BOZR should result in a fluorescein pattern that displays apical clearance over the flatter central cornea and a zone of mid-peripheral bearing at the 3 and 9 o'clock locations. The lens should display unobstructed movement along the vertical meridian.

Lens decentration is a common problem following RK. It is often the result of uneven wound healing, which creates geographic surface elevations on which the lens pivots. Lens decentration is best resolved by increasing the overall lens diameter to 10.0mm or larger. Final lens power is best determined by performing a spherocylinder refraction over a well-centered diagnostic lens. The cornea is malleable and prone to warpage for a period of up to 3 months following RK. Rigid lens fitting should not be carried out during this period unless it is medically necessary for short-term use to aid wound healing.

Several months should be allowed to elapse after RK surgery before fitting soft lenses, to allow the cornea to stabilize; loose-fitting, high water content lenses are the best option. A flat lens fit will tend to align more closely with the corneal contour and will avoid corneal compression following RK.

Incisional neovascularization is a common complication associated with the use of soft contact lenses following RK. This is especially true in the case of incisions that extend to or beyond the limbus. More modern surgical techniques in which the incisions terminate short of the limbus may be less prone to this complication. Today, incisional neovascularization can be minimized through the post-surgical fitting of high oxygen permeability silicone hydrogel lenses used on a daily wear basis.

Radiation injuries

- See *Ionizing radiation; Non-ionizing radiation.*

Radiuscope

The radiuscope (microspherometer) is the standard instrument for checking the back optic zone radius (BOZR) (Figure R.2). In Figure R.3, rays from an

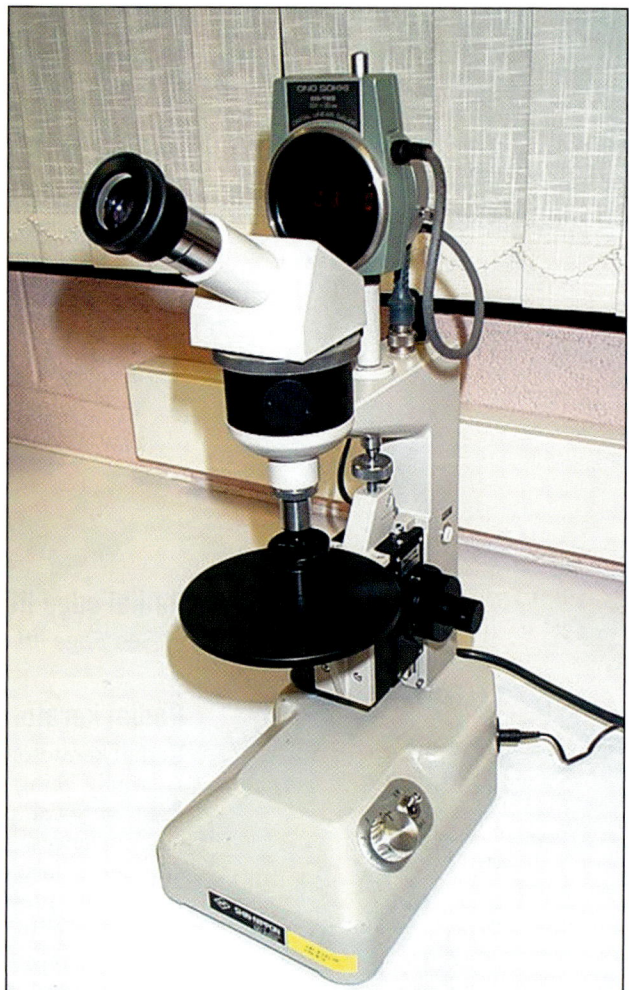

Figure R.2 • Radiuscope.

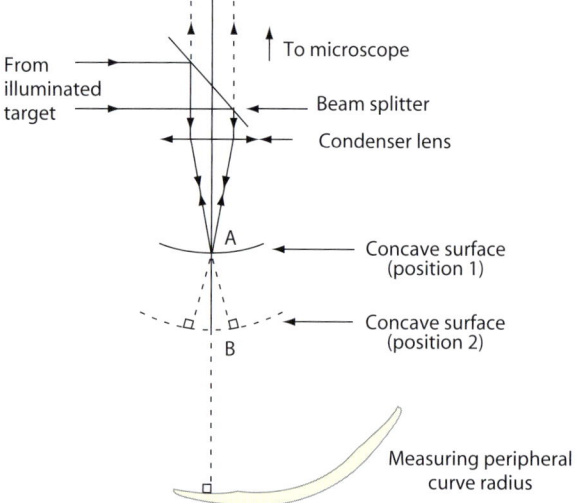

Figure R.3 • Basic optical arrangement of the radiuscope (Drysdale method) for measuring a concave (back) lens surface.

illuminated target are focused on a point A, and a travelling microscope is focused on this same point. The rays are directed towards the back surface of a rigid lens. For a spherical surface, a sharp clear image of the target

Table R.1 • The stimulus requirements to achieve different reading speeds (wpm).

Visual requirement	Optimum reading of normally-sighted individual (>300 wpm)	High fluent (leisure) reading (≈160 wpm)	Spot (survival) reading (≈40 wpm)
Acuity reserve	6:1	2 or 3:1	1:1
Contrast reserve	30:1	10:1	3:1
Scotoma diameter(°)	0	4	30
Field of view (characters)	12–15	12–15	1

will be observed in two conditions – when the travelling microscope is focused on the back surface of the lens, and when the lens is moved away from the microscope and the incident rays are perpendicular to the surface.

For the former condition, the reflected light again passes through point A and the distance AB is the BOZR of the lens. To reduce the effects of unwanted reflections, the lens front surface reflectivity is greatly reduced by immersing the lens in water. This optical arrangement, known as the Drysdale method, is employed in most contact lens radiuscopes. Using cross-shaped targets, the radiuscope can measure both spherical and toric surfaces. This technique is valuable not just for checking new lenses, but also for monitoring changes in lens shape due to flexure.

For aspheric surfaces, the measured BOZR is the radius over the chord diameter. By extending the size of the target, it is possible to focus different parts of the reflected image, thus allowing a rapid check for asphericity. This is not the best quantitative method for numerically evaluating an aspheric surface; nevertheless, it is useful as a quick check for regularity. Peripheral curves can be assessed in multicurve lenses by tilting the lens.

The device used to hold the lens could inadvertently distort the lens and affect the regularity of lens surface and quality. This can cause the reflection to appear fuzzy, which will in turn affect radius measurement. The radiuscope can also be used for checking the front surface of the lens.

Reading addition, determination of
- See *Near addition, determination of*.

Reading requirements, low vision

To be able to read is the primary requirement of most low-vision patients, and difficulty with reading is one of their most common complaints. To help determine whether, and by what means, a patient can best be helped, it is necessary to relate this to the reading tasks they wish to perform. To read for leisure (paperback novels, for example) requires 'high fluent' reading of approximately 160 words per minute (wpm). Very slow reading can impair understanding of the message conveyed, but it is the frustration of their slow progress that is more likely to disillusion the keen reader, and they may prefer to resort to books or newspapers on audiotape or CD. The so-called 'survival' or 'spot' reading strategy (used, for example, for reading price tags or personal correspondence, for which there is no audio alternative) can be usefully performed at a speed of only 40 wpm, since the tasks are usually of short duration. Experimental work has shown that reading is slow when the stimulus is close to threshold (small size or low contrast), but increases as the print size and contrast become progressively suprathreshold. As might be expected, the size of any central scotoma, and the field of view (the number of characters visible at any one time) also influence the reading rate. The optimum stimulus requirements are summarized in Table R.1.

The field of view requirement quoted in Table R.1 is not that required for the reading task itself, but is determined by the need for the patient to perform 'page navigation'; that is, to track along a line without missing any words, and then to move from the end of one line to the beginning of the next. The field of view may be limited by the patient's own eye condition, or by the magnifier (optical or electronic) which they are using.

The required size of the print is expressed in terms of an 'acuity reserve', which is the ratio of the size of the stimulus to the patient's acuity threshold. The patient can perform spot reading with an acuity reserve of 1:1 – i.e., at threshold, but to read faster requires print of 2 to 3 × the size (or 2 to 3 × greater magnification). This required acuity reserve can be determined clinically for each individual patient. The size of print required to read at optimal speed is called the critical print size, and it can be found using the MNREAD test (see *Reading tests, low vision*). Similarly, contrast reserve is the ratio of stimulus contrast to the contrast threshold. Although the contrast threshold should be determined for a target of the same size, it is more usual clinically to determine the peak contrast sensitivity from a test such as the Pelli Robson chart, and derive contrast threshold from that.

The required print contrast in order for an individual with given contrast sensitivity to read are shown in Table R.2. It is obviously impossible to achieve contrast beyond 100%. Comparison with Table R.3 shows the likely contrasts available in common reading materials. It can be seen that, for example, an individual with log contrast sensitivity 1.05 may struggle with newsprint, whereas laser printed letters may be possible. Another patient with log contrast sensitivity 0.60 may require books on audiotape, although they might still perform 'survival' reading of their personal correspondence using an optical magnifier. Good illumination will always optimize available contrast, and should always be used whenever possible. A halogen lamp, and/or an internally illuminated magnifier should always be considered for patients with poor contrast sensitivity.

Table R.2 • Contrast sensitivity (threshold), the contrast required for leisure reading (contrast reserve 10:1) and spot reading (contrast reserve 3:1) and the likely effect on reading performance of these thresholds.

Log contrast sensitivity	Contrast threshold (%)	Theoretical print contrast required (%) Leisure Reading	Spot Reading	Consequence of threshold in this range
0.00 to 0.45	100 / 35.5	>100 / >100	>100 / >100	Unlikely to access any print visually
0.60 to 1.05	25.1 / 8.9	>100 / 89	75.3 / 26.7	Survival reading achievable, but fluent reading unlikely
1.20 to 1.65	6.3 / 2.2	63 / 22	18.9 / 6.6	Fluent reading possible, but optimize contrast using good lighting
1.80 to 2.25	1.6 / 0.6	16 / 6.0	4.8 / 1.8	Normal, no restriction on performance

Table R.3 • The contrast of the letters in text presented in various formats.

Subject matter	Typical print contrast (%)
Video display	100
Laser printer	90
Magazine	80
Paperback	75
Newsprint	70
Dot matrix printer	48
Blackboard	30

Reading tests, low vision

There are many different reading charts available, and they differ in both the format of the test, the notation used to specify print size, and the purpose for which the test was designed. The range of word lengths used often varies, and some use meaningful sentences and paragraphs whilst others employ unrelated words. It is important to have variations of word length when testing patients with a central scotoma, since they usually read short words accurately but cannot manage long words, or read only part of them. Patient performance in a test which uses meaningful paragraphs of print may be better than for unrelated words as the likely meaning of the sentence can be interpreted and missing words (or parts of words) which cannot be seen can be guessed.

Four tests that have been designed specifically for the assessment of low-vision patients are:

- The Bailey-Lovie Word-Reading Chart – this test has letters of sizes logMAR 1.6 to 0.0 (6/240 to 6/6 equivalent) at 25cm in steps of approximately 0.1 log units. This translates in point notation to sizes of N80 to N2 (or 10M to 0.25M) (see *Near acuity*). There are between two and six unrelated words per line depending on the letter size, and word lengths between 4 and 10 letters are used. The weakness of the chart design is the limited number of words at large sizes (only two in each case), which makes reading speed hard to calculate above N20.
- The MNREAD Acuity Chart – this consists of a series of 19 sentences printed at progressively smaller sizes (logMAR 1.3 to –0.5 for a viewing distance of 40cm). Each sentence is laid out in three relatively short lines, and the same number of characters per line are used at each print size. With the tester revealing the sentences one at a time, starting with the largest size, patients read the sentences as quickly and accurately as possible. A score sheet is provided where incorrect and missed words and sentences, and the time taken for each sentence, can be recorded. This allows a calculation of threshold reading acuity, which is the smallest print size read without significant errors. The critical print size (the smallest print size which can be read at the maximum speed) is determined by plotting the reading times on the graph provided. The ratio between threshold acuity and critical print size represents the acuity reserve necessary for that individual to read fluently (see *Reading requirements, low vision*).
- The Pepper Visual Skills for Reading Test (VSRT) – this test is designed to evaluate the performance of patients with central scotoma, in terms of both reading speed and the text presentation which caused them difficulty. The test is available in print sizes 1M to 4M (N8 to N32) with each page having print of a single size. Within the page there are 13 lines of print, beginning with single letters, then on successive lines progressing to 2 and 3 letter and finally larger unrelated words. The spacing between the words and the lines also progressively decreases. The test is not designed to measure the threshold acuity: this is determined beforehand and the test is then administered at the next larger size than the patient's threshold. The reading speed forms a baseline value of

performance before the patient is, for example, trained to use a magnifier more effectively. If the patient does not reach the end of the page and complete the test, the position at which difficulties occur can be used to develop reading materials to help in this rehabilitation. If the patient can only read words up to 3 letters long, for example, then training materials with words of this size would be used initially, progressing to longer lengths later.
- The Low Vision Reading Comprehension Assessment (LVRCA) is a test designed to measure the ability of individuals to understand and extract meaning from the reading material, which will be essential if they are to regain ability in 'high fluent/leisure reading' (see *Reading requirements, low vision*). The test is produced in Palatino font to represent that seen in books and newspapers, and is available in 4 different print sizes (9 to 24 point, 1 to 3M). The size chosen should be appropriate to the task required by the patient (e.g. newspaper text is 9 point; textbook print 12 point, etc.). The test is structured as follows: a word which could be determined from the context is deleted from a meaningful sentence, and the reader is required to supply the missing word using the clues from the remainder of the sentence. Correct completion requires combining the visual information with cognitive information stored in memory, and represents good comprehension. A series of increasingly complex sentences are presented, such that the level of understanding required to correctly complete the sentences increases through the test. This forms a basis for determining the type of reading material that could currently be understood by the patient, and for planning and monitoring the effects of a training programme to improve it.

Re-branding contact lenses
- See *Contact lens supply routes*.

Recurrent erosion syndrome, therapeutic contact lenses for
Minor trauma to the cornea may predispose to this condition. Very often, corneal epithelial basement membrane dystrophy (such as Cogan's microcystic dystrophy or map-dot-fingerprint dystrophy) is found to be present; this is a bilateral condition, so both eyes should always be carefully examined. The eye with the erosion often becomes acutely painful when the eyes are opened during the night or when waking. At these times tear production is minimal and friction is maximal, and so the lid margin pulls on the unstable patch of epithelium, sometimes causing epithelial disruption. A contact lens interposed between cornea and lid can reduce the friction (Figure R.4).

Record keeping
Accurate and complete record keeping is an essential part of optometric practice. Consider, as an example, record keeping relating to a contact lens patient. During the whole process of the initial assessment, history taking, ocular examination, fitting, and aftercare, information is being gathered upon which clinical decisions as to patient

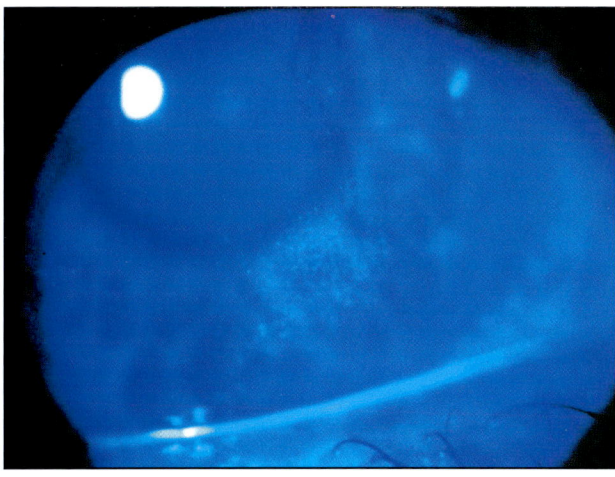

Figure R.4 • Recurrent corneal erosion in soft contact lens wearer with dry eye symptoms.

suitability and well-being with respect to contact lens wear will be made. As with all clinical processes, suitable records are essential. These records not only offer insight into the status of the patient, but also give credence to the clinical decisions being made. In the event of a dispute with the patient, clinical records can be invaluable in showing the maintenance of good clinical management and the provision of the standard of care expected.

In essence, record keeping should include all relevant patient information relating to the primary and significant secondary complaints, as well as all the tests conducted in response to that information. The records should clearly indicate the clinical decision being made and the basis of that decision (i.e. diagnosis). A written record of all the advice offered to the patient should be included. As a general rule, it should not be forgotten that potential and existing contact lens wearers are just as prone to general ophthalmic problems as the rest of the population, and non-contact lens causes of visual and ocular problems should not be overlooked.

Practitioners should conduct all the appropriate examination procedures necessary to test their working clinical hypothesis about the cause of the presenting problems. Where testing suggests that the hypothesis is flawed, the data should be re-examined and other possibilities assessed through further testing. At a minimum, the records should reflect this process and include all test results that rule a probable or possible diagnosis in or out of consideration. If this procedure is followed, there can be no doubt about whether the standard of care has been delivered.

Red dot test
- See *Confrontation test*.

Red eye, contact lens associated
Conjunctival redness is so obvious and easily observed that it is perhaps the only sign of contact lens wear that is also reported as a symptom by patients (Figure R.5). Indeed, excessive eye redness is cosmetically unsightly and is generally perceived as a potential disadvantage of wearing contact lenses. It is recognized in eye care that

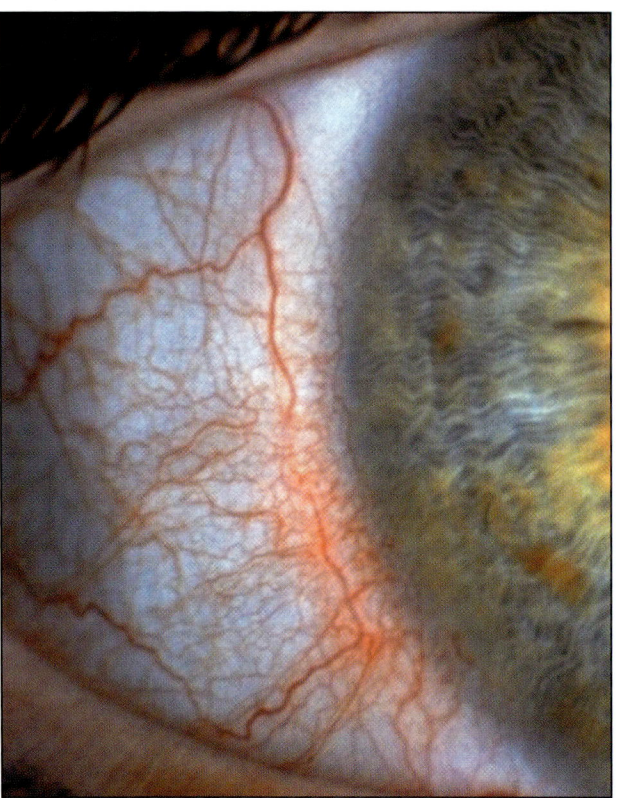

Figure R.5 • Bulbar conjunctival redness caused by a defective soft lens irritating the ocular surface.

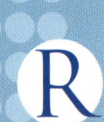

the clinical presentation of a 'red eye' can be one of the most difficult cases to solve, due to the numerous possible known causes. This problem may be even more complex in a contact lens wearer because there are also many other contact lens related causes of red eye.

Throughout the literature, the terms hyperemia, injection, vascularity and redness are used as synonyms. These terms are defined as follows:

- hyperemia – increased blood in a part, resulting in distension of the blood vessels
- injection – a state of hyperemia
- vascularity – the quality of vessels
- redness – of or approaching the colour seen at the least-refracted end of the spectrum, of shades varying from crimson to bright brown and orange.

Strictly speaking, 'hyperemia' or 'injection' is the cause and 'redness' is the effect. That is, an increased volume of blood in the conjunctival vessels (hyperemia or injection) causes an increased appearance of redness. The term 'vascularity' is somewhat ambiguous, and could represent both the cause and effect.

When a contact lens wearing patient presents with a red eye as a primary complaint, the initial diagnostic step is to determine whether or not the problem is related to lens wear. This can often be established by simply removing the lens; eye redness should dissipate rapidly if the problem is purely lens-related. However, the possibility that the lens was somehow exacerbating a complication unrelated to lens wear itself should not be discounted.

Another differential diagnosis that may be necessary when presented with an extremely red eye is to determine to what extent the redness is due to conjunctival injection or ciliary flush. Two simple tests can be applied. A sterile cotton bud can be held lightly against the bulbar conjunctiva in the region of redness and gently moved from side to side. The conjunctival vessels will move, but the ciliary vessels will remain in a fixed position. It can then be determined whether the redness relates primarily to the 'moving' vessels (indicating conjunctival involvement) or the 'static' vessels (indicating ciliary involvement).

An alternative test is to instill a decongestant into the eye. The effect of a decongestant is limited to the superficial conjunctival vessels; these drugs have no effect on the deeper ciliary vessels. Thus, if the instillation of a decongestant alleviates eye redness, the condition is primarily conjunctival. If the decongestant has no impact on eye redness, then the redness can be attributed to excessive ciliary flush.

A subconjunctival haemorrhage can be easily differentiated from conjunctival and/or ciliary hyperemia because of the stark appearance of an intensely 'blood-red' eye and the lack of hyperemia around the limbus. Small haemorrhages of individual conjunctival vessels can also increase conjunctival redness, but again these are self-evident and differential diagnosis from vascular engorgement is clear.

Assuming that a given case of eye redness is lens-related, it is necessary to determine whether the source of the problem is the cornea or conjunctiva. Conjunctival redness associated with a quiet limbus and absence of pain indicates a primary conjunctival problem. Conjunctival redness associated with an injected limbus and corneal pain indicates corneal involvement, or indeed a problem that is related exclusively to the cornea. Redness of both the limbus and bulbar conjunctiva may indicate the co-existence of corneal and conjunctival pathology. Careful examination of the anterior ocular structures with a slit-lamp biomicroscope, and inspection of the lens at high magnification, will generally reveal the cause of the problem. It may also be necessary to prescribe different care systems and differentially diagnose the effects of various solutions over time.

If the red eye is deemed to be unrelated to lens wear, then all other possible causes must be investigated. This may involve a full ocular examination, involving the use of direct and indirect ophthalmoscopy, tonometry etc.

Refraction

See *Autorefraction; Best vision sphere, determination of; Binocular balancing; Cross-cylinder technique; Duochrome test; Fan and block technique; Refraction end-point; Cycloplegic refraction; Objective refraction; Subjective refraction; Retinoscopy; Retinoscopy, dynamic; Retinoscopy, Mohindra technique; Subjective refraction with contact lenses.*

Refraction end-point

The refraction end-point is usually determined once the cylinder has been established during the course of a subjective refraction. During determination of the astigmatic component of the refraction using the cross-cylinder technique, the spherical component of the refraction may have been deliberately under-plussed so as to allow the patient to accommodate slightly to maintain the circle of least confusion on the retina. Thus, following that procedure, a small amount of plus power will be required to bring the circle of least confusion on the retina.

After the fan and block method, the sphere may need to be reduced to gain best acuity. The final sphere may be determined by introducing a fogging lens (typically a +1.00D lens) to ensure that the fog resulting is that expected for the lens (four lines for the +1.00D lens). As an additional check, the patient can be asked to confirm that the targets on the duochrome are equally clear. The final sphere chosen may be influenced by a number of factors. In cases of accommodative esophoric movement, the maximum plus may be introduced. It is generally considered preferable to adopt a slightly over-minussed refraction for younger actively accommodating patients, to guarantee sharp vision in the far distance at the insignificant physiological expense of having to exert a small amount of accommodation (remembering that the end point of refraction determined using a 6 m chart will result in the patient being over-plussed by 0.17D). There may also be a need to modify the final sphere in cases where a chart has been used at less than 6 metres (for example −0.25D will need to be added for a 3 metre chart).

Refractive error
- See *Ametropia*.

Refractive index
The refractive index of a lens material is an indication of how much it bends light in the yellow-green region of the spectrum (sometimes called the mean refractive index), and is defined as the velocity of light in a vacuum divided by the velocity of light in the material. In practice, the refractive index is measured in air, and for spectacle lenses the difference in refractive index is not significant. For lenses of high power it is obviously desirable for a material to bend light as much as possible, so that very steep curves, giving thick and heavy lenses, are avoided.

In the UK the mean refractive index (n_d) has traditionally been measured at a specified wavelength of 587.56nm, which corresponds to the helium 'd' line. Unfortunately, there is not yet universal agreement as to the wavelength for refractive index measurement; a wavelength of 546.07nm, corresponding to the mercury 'e' line (labelled as index n_e), is being used commonly in continental Europe. An international standard (BS EN ISO 7944:1998) recognizes both wavelengths, but it is expected that a revised version of this standard will eventually settle on one wavelength. For commercial reasons, this is likely to be that of the mercury *e* line. To put the matter in perspective, the values for three lens materials are shown in Table R.4.

The problem that can be caused by the use of two potentially ambiguous wavelength standards is that a lens manufacturer may calculate the surfacing curves for a lens base on one refractive index, while a user may measure the same lens on a focimeter calibrated for

Table R.4 • Refractive indices for three ophthalmic lens materials determined with the helium 'd' line (n_d) and the mercury 'e' line (n_e).

Material	Refractive Indices	
	n_d	n_e
Ophthalmic crown	1.523	1.525
CR39	1.498	1.500
Corning D0035	1.700	1.704

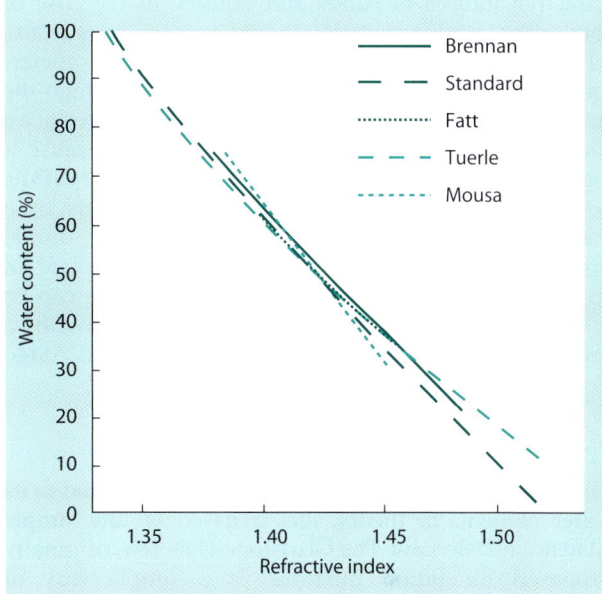

Figure R.6 • Relation between water content (%) and refractive index for hydrogels, as determined by various authors.

another. For example, if a plano-concave spectacle lens is manufactured with a back vertex power of −10.00DS, using a crown glass material n_d = 1.523, then this will have a radius of curvature for the concave surface of 52.3mm. If this same lens is checked on a focimeter calibrated for the mercury line (n_e), then the power will read −10.04DS. Thus, for high power lenses, it can be important to know the wavelength used for calculating the lens power.

Refractive index is measured using by material manufacturers using specialized equipment, e.g. the Abbe refractometer, in order to obtain a high precision of measurement for quality control. BS 3062:1985 (an obsolete standard mainly for glass materials) specified a tolerance in refractive index of ±0.001 for values up to 1.59, +0.001 to 0.0015 for the range 1.59 to 1.69, and ±0.0015 for values over 1.69.

Refractive index, contact lens
In soft lenses, refractive index decreases progressively with increasing water content (Figure R.6). The variation is almost linear with water content, and the results for hydrogels of the various types used in contact lenses lie within a fairly narrow, almost rectilinear band, decreasing from 1.46–1.48 at 20% water content to 1.37–1.38 at 75%

water content. It is for this reason that refractive index measurement can be used as a rapid method of determining the approximate water content of an unknown gel. In rigid contact lenses, fluorosilicone acrylates tend to have refractive indices lower than 1.458, and some silicone acrylates and fluorosilicone acrylates have refractive indices between 1.458 and 1.469. Refractive indices greater than 1.469 indicate silicone acrylate materials. See *Refractometer, rigid contact lens; Refractometer, soft contact lens.*

Refractometer, rigid contact lens

Refractometers are commonly used to measure the refractive indices of solids and liquids. In the case of solids, the sample material should have a flat surface, which is placed in contact with the refractometer-measuring prism. A contact fluid can be used when the surface is irregular. It may not be desirable to introduce a contact fluid beneath a finished contact lens because it may prove difficult to remove due to its steep curvature; however, by placing the convex surface of the lens onto the measuring prism and applying gentle digital pressure, the surface will flatten slightly and create an area of contact sufficient for measurement. This can be achieved using a hand-held refractometer, with a precision of ±0.001 (Model N3000 Refractometer; Atago Co. Ltd, Japan). See *Refractive index, contact lens.*

Refractometer, soft contact lens

The refractive index of a hydrogel is directly related to its water content. In theory, this is based on the simple Gladstone-Dale Law. The Gladstone-Dale law, originally proposed for liquid mixtures, is a simple way of predicting the final refractive index of a solution (N) based on the refractive indices of the solvent (N_1), the solid (N_2), and their relative proportions, as follows:

$$N = N_1 \cdot X_1 + N_2 \cdot X_2$$

where X_2 is the relative proportion of solid present in the mixture as a percentage (a), and X_1 is the relative proportion of solvent in the mixture (100 − a).

Measurement of soft lens refractive index to infer water content is an accepted simple, rapid, non-destructive technique with universal appeal. Of the several ways one can measure refractive index, a hand-held optical refractometer is probably the simplest and most economically viable (Atago Soft Lens Refractometer, Atago, Japan; Figure R.7). The resolution of refractometry to indirectly infer lens water content can be very high. A +0.001 unit increase in refractive index is equivalent to a 20.7% drop in water. Because this is a surface measuring technique, it is assumed that the refractive index at the surface is the same as the refractive index throughout the lens matrix. However, it is not possible to measure the water content of certain types of cast-moulded lenses which, as a result of the curing process, end up with a slight refractive index variation throughout the lens matrix. See *Refractive index, contact lens.*

Refractor head

- See *Phoropter.*

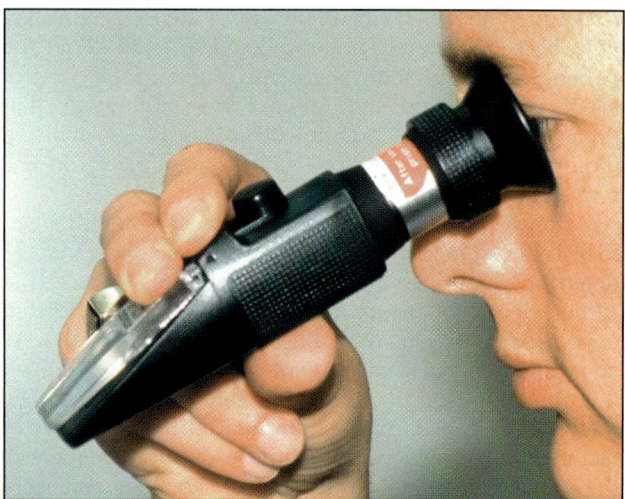

Figure R.7 • The Atago CL-1 Soft Contact Lens Refractometer, which is used to determine the water content of soft contact lenses.

Registered visual impairment

All developed countries have a system of social care where certain groups in society are identified as requiring financial benefits or access to appropriate services. The visually impaired and blind are one such group, and they are 'registered' in order to show their eligibility for special attention. Registration is undertaken in order to:

- assess what health and social work resources will be needed for the number of visually impaired people in a particular area
- act as the patient's passport to appropriate welfare benefits.

Registration requires a definition of 'legal' blindness, so as to stipulate a level of visual acuity and/or extent of visual field which the patient must not exceed if they are to be certified officially as 'blind'. Such standards are also required to prevent fraud. There are many different definitions of legal blindness used worldwide, with each country adopting its own unique system.

In the UK, there are two levels of visual acuity and/or visual field at which an individual may be registered with their Local Authority Social Services Department:

Partial Sight (or Sight Impairment) – this term is used to describe a persons who are 'substantially and permanently handicapped by defective vision caused by congenital defect, or illness or injury'. They will usually fall into one of the following categories:

- 3/60 to 6/60 with full fields
- up to 6/24 with moderate field contraction
- 6/18 or better with gross field defect (hemianopia or marked contraction such as that due to retinitis pigmentosa or glaucoma).

Blindness (or Severe Sight Impairment) – this is defined as 'so blind as to be unable to perform any work for which eyesight is essential' (National Assistance Act 1948 Section 64(1)), and the corresponding visual performance may be:

- below 3/60, if also poorer than 1/18
- 3/60, but less than 6/60, with very contracted field (excluding long-standing conditions without marked field loss)
- 6/60 or above, with a contracted field, especially in the lower part (excluding hemianopia if 6/18 or better).

Although registration has in the past been shown to be important in increasing individuals' awareness and use of available services, it is not essential to be registered in order to receive practical help and assessment by a rehabilitation officer (see *Multidisciplinary team, low vision*). Patients whom it is believed would benefit from assessment, yet whose acuity is not poor enough for registration, can be referred to social services by the consultant/hospital outpatients clinic, or be encouraged to self-refer using a letter obtained from their optometrist. Registration is necessary, however, to have access to some financial benefits, and most of these are only available to those registered as blind, rather than partially sighted.

Registers, professional

The primary task of the General Optical Council in 1958 was the establishment of registers of qualified opticians. These registers are still maintained and it is the job of the General Optical Council in relation to the registers to:
- Control applications for registration.
- Require notification of changes in the particulars shown in the lists.
- Prescribe an annual fee for registration.
- Register additional qualifications.
- Refuse to enter or maintain a name if a registration fee is not forthcoming.
- Record the death of registered opticians.
- Publish from time to time information from each register in such form (including electronic form) as considered appropriate.

There are five lists published in the Register, and they relate to:
- Optometrists
- Dispensing opticians
- Students undertaking training as optometrists
- Students undertaking training as dispensing opticians
- Corporate bodies carrying on business as an optometrist or a dispensing optician or both.

Regulations relating to contact lenses
- See *Food and Drug Administration; General Optical Council; Medical Devices Directive*.

Reis-Bückler's dystrophy
- See *Dystrophies of the corneal epithelium, therapeutic contact lenses for*.

Relative luminous efficiency

Relative luminous efficiency is defined as the sensitivity of the visual system to different wavelengths in an equal energy spectrum. The relative luminous efficiency curve

Table R.5 • Colour names associated with different wavelength bands.

Colour	Wavelength band
Violet	380nm–450nm
Blue	451nm–490nm
Green	491nm–560nm
Yellow	561nm–590nm
Orange	591nm–630nm
Red	631nm–780nm

(V-λ) is measured psychophysically using flicker photometry. The visible spectrum extends from about 380nm to 780nm. Colour names associated with different wavelength bands are given in Table R.5.

In normal colour vision, the wavelength of maximum relative luminous efficiency is 555nm in photopic viewing and 500nm in scotopic viewing. The latter corresponds with the sensitivity of the rod receptors. The change in relative luminous efficiency from photopic to scotopic viewing is known as 'the Purkinje shift'. Relative luminous efficiency is only slightly altered in deutan and tritan colour deficiency. In protan deficiency the wavelength of maximum relative luminous efficiency is at 535nm in photopic viewing. This results in marked differences in relative colour contrast and in so-called 'shortening of the red end of the spectrum'. The latter is a major occupational handicap.

Relative spectacle magnification

The relative spectacle magnification (RSM) is the ratio of the retinal image size in the corrected ametropic eye to that in a specified emmetropic schematic eye. Theoretically, the specification of RSM has the advantage of putting retinal image size on an absolute basis. However, in most clinical work it is the changes described by spectacle magnification that are of interest, and RSM is of limited practical use.

Relief of pain, therapeutic contact lenses for

Corneal epithelial pain can be severe and disabling. A simple corneal abrasion usually heals quickly and needs no help from the clinician, but a persistent or recurrent epithelial failure may benefit from the fitting of a soft 'bandage' lens, which acts as a barrier between the injured corneal surface and the lid.

Removal of contact lenses

See *Insertion and removal, rigid contact lens; Insertion and removal, scleral contact lens; Insertion and removal, soft contact lens*.

Replacement frequency, contact lens

The ideal lens replacement frequency would be one selected on the basis of the rate of lens spoilation of each patient, and would be such that comfort and vision does not deteriorate throughout the life of the lens. This rate will depend upon the lens material and the tear film quality of the patient. In general, a high water content

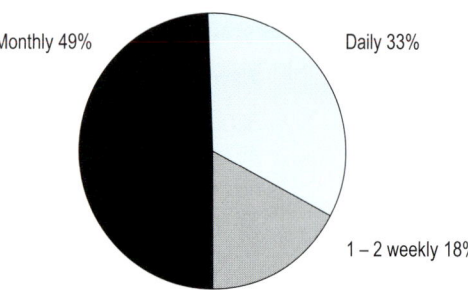

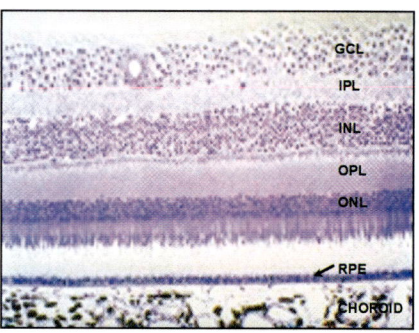

Figure R.9 • Transverse section through the retina. IPL= inner plexiform layer, INL= inner nuclear layer, OPL= outer plexifom layer, ONL= outer nuclear layer, RPE= retinal pigment epithelium.

Figure R.8 • Replacement frequency of soft lenses fitted to new patients in the United Kingdom in 2006.

ionic material (FDA Group IV) requires at least monthly replacement, and a high water content non-ionic material (FDA Group II) requires at least 3-monthly replacement. These are guidelines only, as individual patient variation can have a significant impact. Monthly or more frequent replacement ensures consistent performance over the period of use of the lens in terms of subjective comfort and visual performance for FDA Group I and Group IV lenses. Rigid lenses are best replaced every 6 to 12 months.

In practice, it is not straightforward to identify the ideal lens replacement frequency for a given patient. Instead, an appropriate replacement interval can be chosen from one of the seven 'standard' replacement intervals (generally based on convenient and easily remembered calendar intervals) formulated for various products by contact lens manufacturers – that is, 1 day, 1 week, 2 weeks, 1 month, 3 months, 6 months and 1 year. Such a decision is made after consideration of the lens type, desired pattern of wear and the contact lens history of the patient. Monthly and daily lens replacement are the most popular soft lens replacement frequencies in the United Kingdom (Figure R.8).

Reproducibility, soft contact lens

Practitioners who prescribe lenses that have been manufactured using mass-production technology, and patients who wear such lenses, need to be assured that a series of lenses of identical specifications are indeed all the same, or very nearly so; this characteristic can be described as 'reproducibility'. Studies that have examined this characteristic have all found lenses to be within acceptable tolerance ranges for providing wearers of these lenses with consistent vision and fit. Reproducibility is generally slightly worse for lenses of higher power, but is still clinically acceptable.

Residual astigmatism with rigid toric contact lenses

The term 'residual astigmatism' is often used loosely, and is frequently confused with induced astigmatism or corneal astigmatism. Residual astigmatism has been defined in various ways, but the simplest definition states that residual astigmatism is the component of the spectacle (ocular) astigmatism that is not due to the cornea. In the context of rigid lens fitting, a better definition would be that residual astigmatism is the astigmatic component of a lens required to correct fully an eye wearing a spherical powered rigid contact lens with a spherical back optic zone radius.

Sometimes the axis of the residual astigmatism does not correspond exactly with one of the principal meridians of curvature of the cornea. If the difference between the axes of the spectacle refraction and the principal meridians of the cornea is marginal (less than 20°), it can be assumed that the axes of the spectacle refraction over the lens do correspond with the principal meridians of corneal curvature. By doing this, the need for any complex oblique cylinder calculations is obviated and the resulting error in the power calculations is usually not significant. If there is a large difference between the cylinder axis of the ocular refraction and the axis of the corneal astigmatism, then an oblique bitoric lens (where the principal meridians of the toroidal front and back surfaces are not parallel) will be required. See *Compensated rigid bitoric lenses; Cylindrical power equivalent rigid toric lenses; Induced astigmatism with rigid toric lenses; Stabilization of rigid toric lenses; Toric lens design, rigid; Toric lens, rigid.*

Retainer contact lenses
- See *Orthokeratology*.

Retina

The retina is the innermost of the three coats of the eye. Its principal function is 'phototransduction', whereby light imaged onto the retina is converted into a series of electrical impulses (action potentials) that are transmitted to higher centres for processing and interpretation. All vertebrate retinas show the same basic structural organization: two synaptic layers (outer and inner plexiform layers) sandwiched between three nuclear layers (outer, inner and ganglion cell layers) (Figure R.9). Light entering the eye passes through these layers and is captured by photopigments that are contained within the outer segments of specialized neurones known as photoreceptors. Rod photoreceptors mediate vision in dim light and cones function in bright light and are also responsible for colour vision. In addition to photoreceptors, the retina contains five other types of neurone: horizontal, bipolar, amacrine, interplexiform and ganglion cells. The cell bodies of photoreceptors and horizontal cells are located in the outer nuclear layer, whereas those belonging to amacrine, bipolar and interplexiform cells are found in the inner nuclear layer.

Visual information passes from photoreceptors to second order neurones (bipolar cells), then on third order neurones (ganglion cells). Ganglion cell axons then relay the information to the brain along the optic nerve. Within the retina, the transfer of information from one neurone to the next occurs within the plexiform layers. However, it is important to emphasize that this transfer does not simply reflect a simple relay of information, since significant processing of visual information occurs at each stage. The outer plexifom layer contains the synaptic connections between photoreceptors and bipolar cells (with some lateral interactions from horizontal cells). Within the inner plexiform layer the situation is more complex, with amacrine, bipolar, interplexiform and ganglion cell interactions.

In addition to neural cells, the retina contains three classes of glia: Müller cells, astrocytes and microglia. The Müller cell is the principal retinal glial cell. These cells span most of the retina. As well as a general supporting and nourishing role, these cells are also responsible for modulating neural activity by regulating the concentration of neuroactive substances in the extracellular space.

The retinal pigment epithelium plays a critical role in retinal function. This is a single layer of hexagonal cells that lies between the neuroretina and the choroid. The retinal pigment epithelium acts as a selective permeability barrier between choroid retina; it absorbs stray light and is also involved in the phagocytosis of photoreceptor outer segments and recycling of visual pigment.

The oxygen and nutrient requirements of the retina are met by the choroid, which primarily serves the photoreceptors. An intra-retinal blood supply, which derives from the central retinal artery, supplies the neurons of the inner retina.

Retinal detachment

A retinal detachment (RD) refers to the condition where the neurosensory retina lifts off and separates from the underlying retinal pigment epithelium (RPE).

Possible causes of an RD include:

1. Rhegmatogenous: where a full-thickness retinal break (tear or hole) allows liquid vitreous fluid to enter between the sensory retina and the RPE, thereby causing the retina to lift off. Possible predisposing factors include lattice degeneration, posterior vitreous detachment, trauma, intraocular surgery, and myopia.
2. Tractional: where another retinal disease such as proliferative diabetic retinopathy, or retinopathy of prematurity, leads to direct fibrotic or fibrovascular traction on the retina without a break.
3. Exudative: due to the accumulation of exudative material, serous fluid, or blood beneath the retina, without a retinal break or tear having occurred.
4. Therapeutic: miotic therapy, such as pilocarpine, used in glaucoma therapy may precipitate RD.

Symptoms include a sudden or dramatic onset characterized by:

1. an increased number of floaters;
2. increased flashes of light (photopsia) which does not diminish;
3. loss of peripheral or side vision;
4. the appearance of a curtain or blind coming down over vision;
5. cloudy vision, or the observation of cobwebs or shadows.

The retina appears elevated and undulating or billowing with eye movements. While retinal blood vessels may be visible, the underlying choroidal detail is obscured. When the RD is recent, the retina may be relatively transparent, but with time the separated tissue becomes more opaque. If the detachment has been static for some months, the posterior border may be pigmented. A rhegmatogenous RD is indicated by the presence of a retinal break – often a tear – which is more obvious with scleral indentation. There may be pigment cells in the vitreous (Shafer's sign), as well as reduced intraocular pressure and a relative afferent pupillary defect (RAPD). Peripheral visual field testing (30 to 60°) may be required to detect field loss.

Peripheral retinal lesions which are not considered a predisposing condition for RD include:

- Bear tracks or peripheral grouped
- Paving stone or cobble-stone degeneration.

Signs that uncommonly lead to RD include:

- Lattice degeneration, but only if extensive
- Snail track degeneration
- Peripheral cystoid degeneration
- Asymptomatic operculated tears, pigmented breaks or atrophic holes
- Post-inflammatory chorioretinal scars
- White without pressure.

Signs with significant risk for RD, in conjunction with vitreo-retinal traction, include:

- Retinoschisis
- Symptomatic tears with persistent traction, horseshoe tears, giant tears
- Symptomatic operculated tears or atrophic holes, or asymptomatic lesions with other risk factors as listed
- Asymptomatic flap or tears
- Retinal dialysis, post-traumatic tears or commotio retinae.

Other risk factors include aphakia, pseudophakia, high myopia, personal or family history of retinal detachment, use of miotics. The incidence of RD is low (approximately 1 in 10,000) in the general population, although more common in specific risk groups as mentioned above.

Macular-threatening rhegmatogenous retinal detachment is an ocular emergency needing treatment within 24 hours. If the macular has already detached, then treatment is still urgent, and should be undertaken within 48 to 96 hours. B-scan ultrasound may be used to evaluate the vitreous cavity if the fundus is difficult to visualize. Ocular coherence tomography may be helpful in differential diagnosis. Fluorescein angiography can assist in evaluating exudative retinal detachment.

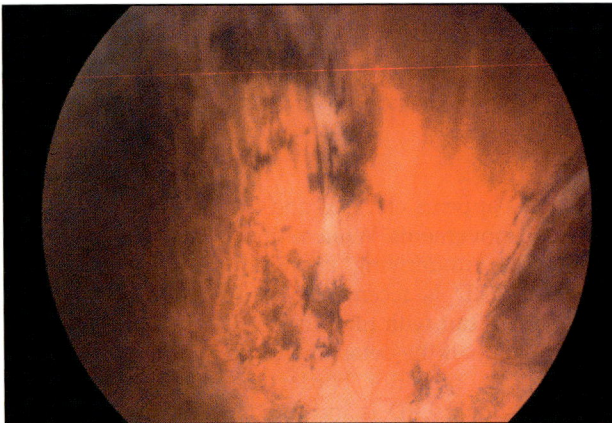

Figure R.10 • Old retinal detachment showing scar tissue. The visual acuity of the eye is light perception only.

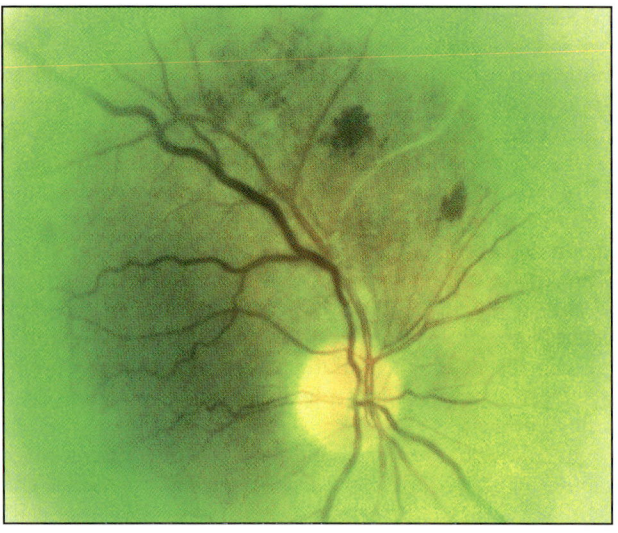

Figure R.11 • Asymptomatic branch retinal vein occlusion, shown in red-free illumination. The superior-temporal vein is a white ghost vessel and surrounded by several blot haemorrhages.

For symptomatic lesions, two or three rows of laser photocoagulation can be made around tears or holes located posteriorly. Such an approach is also appropriate to prevent progression of rhegmatogenous retinal detachment if the patient is asymptomatic and the detachment is not threatening the macula (mainly pre-detachment disease). Cryotherapy is more useful for anterior lesions, cloudy media and cases where there is significant sub-retinal fluid (mainly pre-detachment disease). Surgical options include scleral buckle, pneumatic retinopexy, pars plana vitrectomy and drainage of sub-retinal fluid. If there are underlying conditions, for example in exudative retinal detachment, then the underlying condition should be treated. If vitreoretinal traction is present, surgery to relieve the traction may be considered. (Figure R.10).

Retinal vascular occlusions

Retinal vascular occlusions are the second most common vascular disease affecting the retina, after diabetic retinopathy. They show a strong association with systemic diseases, such as atherosclerosis and carotid artery disease, hypertension, diabetes, hyperlipidaemia, temporal arteritis, and hypercoagulation or vasculitis disorders. Retinal artery occlusions may be directly the result of atherosclerosis, where atheromatous plaques break free into the blood stream, most often from the carotid artery, and cause a blockage downstream. Emboli may also be cholesterol (Hollenhorst plaques), calcifications, impurities injected into the blood from IV drug use, and many other factors. Venous occlusions can also be related to arterial disease, since there is a tendency for blockages to occur at arteriovenous crossings, where the stiff-walled atheromatous artery may compress the lumen of the adjacent thin-walled vein, creating blood turbulence and thrombotic build-up. Central retinal vein occlusions have an association with primary open-angle glaucoma, since raised intraocular pressure (IOP) is thought to compress the central retinal vein, making the narrowed lumen of the vessel more vulnerable to blockage.

Retinal vascular occlusions are usually unilateral and may, or may not, be noticed by the patient, particularly if the non-dominant eye is affected. Visual symptoms are more likely in branch vein and artery occlusions if a large area of retina is affected or is in close proximity to the macula. A sudden painless loss of vision may be reported with a central retinal vascular occlusion. There may be a history of previous brief loss of vision (amaurosis fugax), transient ischaemic attack (TIA), or stroke (cerebrovascular accident).

Retinal vascular occlusions can be classified as follows:

- Branch Retinal Vein Occlusion (BRVO) (Figure R.11). Initial signs are dilated and tortuous veins, flame haemorrhages, dot and blot haemorrhages, retinal oedema and cotton wool spots. Later signs may include hard exudates, macula oedema and neovascularization. BRVOs may be characterized in terms of the occlusion location, specifically, distance from the disk or proximity to the macula. The occlusion location dictates the size of the affected area of retina and the likelihood of macula oedema, which in turn affects the visual prognosis.
- Branch Retinal Artery Occlusion (BRAO). Arterial occlusions cause retinal infarction (whitening) rather than the haemorrhagic signs associated with venous occlusions. The arterioles and venules are narrowed and the retinal tissue whitens due to ischaemia. BRAOs may be characterized in the same way as BRVOs.
- Central Retinal Vein Occlusion (CRVO). Venous occlusion affecting the entire retina is attributed to a blockage in the central retinal vein at the level of the lamina cribrosa within the optic disc, or perhaps to atherosclerosis of the adjacent central retinal artery. A complete blockage is termed an ischaemic CRVO. If the vein bifurcates posterior to the lamina cribrosa, then a hemi-retinal vein occlusion may occur.
- Central Retinal Artery Occlusion (CRAO). A superficial whitening of the retina occurs due to the retinal nerve fibre ischaemia and infarction. There is a characteristic cherry-red spot at the macula, since the nerve fibre layer is thin and the choroidal circulation is more visible. A positive relative afferent pupil defect (RAPD,

Marcus Gunn pupil) is present, and vision loss is usually severe.
- Venous stasis retinopathy. A partial occlusion of the retinal veins leads to a slowing of the blood flow but not a complete blockage.
- Cilio-retinal artery occlusion. The small cilio-retinal artery supplies the posterior pole retina and derives from the posterior ciliary circulation.
- Ophthalmic artery occlusion. Both retinal and choroidal circulation is obstructed.

Whilst overall vascular occlusions are uncommon (1:1000), they are relatively common (1:100) in specific at-risk groups such as people over 50 years. Vascular occlusions are not only vision threatening, they are a harbinger of potentially life-threatening systemic conditions such as stroke. For CRAO seen within 24 hours, emergency treatment may be attempted, and is aimed at dislodging the emboli, decreasing IOP and improving the retinal perfusion. Strategies include ocular massage for 5 to 15 minutes, intravenous Acetazolamide 500 mg, a topical beta-blocker (e.g. timolol 0.5%, one drop), and if required an anterior chamber paracentesis, to reduce the intraocular pressure. Unfortunately, such treatment is often unsuccessful.

Patients need a full blood workup to treat any underlying systemic disorders such as hypertension or cardiovascular disease. Prior to considering laser treatment, two to three months is allowed to elapse after a BRVO for the haemorrhages to clear. The presence of macular oedema with good macular perfusion and reduced vision is an indication for grid laser treatment. If neovascularization of the iris, angle, retina or optic nerve develops following CRVO, then pan-retinal photo-coagulation may be indicated.

There is no proven ocular therapy for CRAO or BRAO. In CRVO, consideration should be given to discontinue oral contraceptives, and reducing IOP if elevated. Patients should be reviewed at 1 to 2 month intervals for the first 12 months to check for macular oedema or neovascularization.

Retinoblastoma

Retinoblastoma is a malignant tumour of the retina, that may be unilateral, bilateral or multifocal. It is a rare but potentially fatal condition, primarily affecting young children before the age of 2 years. For this reason, a presentation with early onset paediatric strabismus or amblyopia requires a fundus examination with mydriasis for a full assessment. Retinoblastoma arises from primitive retinal cells before their final differentiation, and consequently the onset is usually before 1 or 2 years of age. Retinal detachment, pseudohypopyon, iris neovascularization or vitreous haemorrhage may be present. These conditions may be seen as leukocoria, or a white pupillary reflex (Figure R.12). An opacity in the lens, vitreous cavity or at the retina causes the abnormal white pupil appearance. While leukocoria may occur for a variety of reasons, retinoblastoma is perhaps the most notable condition.

Since retinoblastoma predominantly affects infants, the condition is detected by a parent or carer seeing the white pupil; however, in some cases the underlying

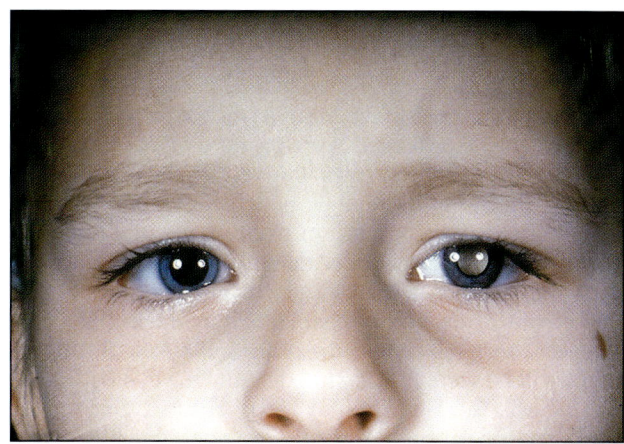

Figure R.12 • Leukocoria in the left eye caused by extensive retinoblastoma.

condition causes a secondary strabismus and the cause is found during dilated fundus examination. A family history may be present.

Initially a retinoblastoma presents as a flat or elevated white lesion. With growth, several forms occur:

1. endophytic tumour – a white nodular mass extending into the vitreous, with prominent feeder vessels;
2. exophytic tumour – a mass lesion underlying a retinal detachment;
3. diffuse infiltrating tumour – a rarer form more resembling a chronic uveitis.

Congenital cataract, if bilateral, can affect eye movements (nystagmus) or if asymmetric or unilateral can cause a strabismus. There is a range of forms and densities of cataract that may develop. Due to the range of conditions that may be present, a fundus examination with mydriasis is a necessary step in assessment of paediatric strabismus.

Leukocoria is a rare condition (approximately 1/10,000), primarily affecting young children before the age of 2 years. Retinoblastoma affects about 1 in 20,000 live births. In a large city there may be only a handful of cases per year, and in the United States it is estimated there are about 300 cases per year.

Urgent hospital evaluation and treatment is indicated if retinoblastoma is suspected. Special investigations include: B-scan ultrasound, computed tomography (CT) scan, and intravenous fluorescein angiogram. A CT scan can also detect calcification associated with retinoblastoma. There is a range of possible therapies, dependent upon the tumour size and location within the eye. Therapies include transpupillary thermotherapy with a diode laser, laser photocoagulation, cryotherapy, plaque radiotherapy, chemotherapy, and external radiotherapy. Enucleation may be required for large tumours. Cataract extraction and intraocular lens (IOL) implantation in children with congenital cataract is a controversial issue and is only indicated if the cataract is highly visually significant. However, with the advent of the foldable IOL and small incision surgery, an IOL can be implanted in children as young as 1 year of age.

Retinoblastoma has a genetic heredity in 40% of cases. In such cases there is a significant risk of siblings being affected. DNA analysis may assist in management.

Retinoscopy

Retinoscopy is a method of objective refraction. It involves the interpretation of the movement of a projected beam of light across the retina of a patient (or the shadows around the illuminated patch, more correctly called skiascopy) which indicates the refractive error of the patient. For a highly myopic patient, the point focus of the reflected light will fall in front of the practitioner's retinoscope and hence the beam will appear to move in the opposite direction to that in which the projected beam is moved (an 'against movement'). For hypermetropia where the point focus is behind the practitioner a 'with' movement will be seen. A lens placed before the eye will move the focus to the plane of the retinoscope (positive for the hypermetrope, negative for the myope) at which point no movement will be apparent ('neutralization' or 'reversal'). This may occur with different lenses for different meridians for astigmatic patients. Once reversal is reached in all meridians, the final result is obtained by adding the appropriate sphere to move the point focus from the plane of the retinoscope to infinity. A typical 'working distance' for retinoscopy (i.e. distance from the retinoscope to the patient's eye) is two thirds of a metre. This is far enough away to reduce error due to working distance variation while close enough to allow the lenses before the patient to be reached for alteration. This requires the addition of $-1.50D$ to the retinoscopy result to obtain the distance refractive error. If the working distance is less – e.g. if the practitioner is of small build or if the reflex is difficult to interpret, as with a cataract patient – then small variations during assessment will result in greater errors in dioptric terms. Moving from 10 to 12cm for example will represent a dioptric shift of almost 2 dioptres.

It is also important for the practitioner to make the assessment as close to the visual axis of the patient as possible. Not doing so will result in a false cylindrical result. The main source of error in retinoscopy, however, is due to failure to control the accommodation of the patient. Without resorting to cycloplegia, this potential error is usually overcome by ensuring the patient stares at a non-accommodative distance target, typically the green of the duochrome. The opposite eye to that under examination should also be fogged such that the point focus is in front of the retinoscope (so showing an against reflex). This ensures a degree of fogging such that any attempt to accommodate will result in blurring of the patient vision and hence will be avoided. If the practitioner occasionally moves to obscure the duochrome target, this serves to check that the patient is looking at the correct distance target (in this case the patient will report that their view is blocked) and that the practitioner is close to the visual axis.

The procedure as described, with the patient viewing a distance target while in a fixed position relative to the practitioner throughout, is often described as static retinoscopy. Variations on the procedure include dynamic retinoscopy, where the distance between patient and target or practitioner vary, and near fixation retinoscopy (also known as the Mohindra technique).

Retinoscopy assessment, soft contact lens
- See *Fitting soft contact lenses.*

Retinoscopy, dynamic

Whereas static retinoscopy relies on control of the patient's accommodation, dynamic retinoscopy is a technique where the accommodation is stimulated by moving either the retinoscope or the fixation target relative to the patient. Most typically the technique is used to measure accommodative lag. If a patient (and it is usually a child where this technique is useful) is fully corrected and asked to look at a target in the plane of the retinoscope, a neutral reflex is expected. However, this is rarely the case and most often a 'with' movement is seen, suggesting the patient is under-accommodating by a small amount. This amount is described as the 'lag' and is measured by moving the retinoscope away from the target until neutrality is reached, and the distance to do so measured. If the target is held at 25cm (+4.00D demand), but the neutral point seen at 33cm (+3.00D demand), then the measured lag would be 1.00D. Another method is to keep the retinoscope with the target and use spheres to gain the neutral reflex (in this example +1.00DS would be needed). This might be described as a form of near fixation retinoscopy. If the neutral point is further from the patient than the target, so requiring plus lenses to neutralize, this is said to be a positive lag. A negative lag would describe the situation where the neutral point is closer to the patient than the target, so requiring negative lenses.

Retinoscopy, Mohindra technique

The Mohindra technique is a variation of near fixation retinoscopy and is sometimes used as an alternative to cycloplegic retinoscopy; however, there is some debate as to how well the results of these two techniques correlate, particularly with higher refractive errors. The Mohindra technique involves the patient viewing the retinoscopy light, something many infant patients do automatically, and $-1.25D$ is added to the final result once neutralisation has been reached. This is performed on each eye with occlusion introduced for the opposite eye to that refracted.

Reverse-geometry contact lenses

Such lenses were originally developed for the fitting of eyes with keratoconus; they have a secondary curve radius that is steeper than the back optic zone radius (BOZR). When used for the purpose of orthokeratology, these lenses offer the prospect of improved centration (and hence less corneal distortion), and a capacity to induce significant corneal shape change.

Reverse geometry lenses have secondary curves that are steeper than the BOZR (Figure R.13). These lenses are manufactured in a range of optic zone diameters and with secondary curves that are of variable width and steepness compared to the BOZR. This design allows for the lenses to be fitted with a much flatter central cornea relationship than usual, while maintaining good lens centration. The fitting of these lenses is based on corneal sagittal height measurement so that an improved balance between central touch and tear layer thickness can be established.

Reverse telescopes
- See *Field expanders.*

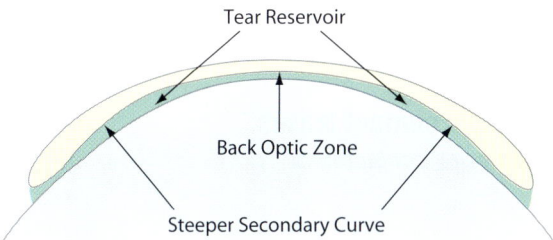

Figure R.13 • Reverse-geometry lens design, showing the steeper secondary curve and related tear reservoir.

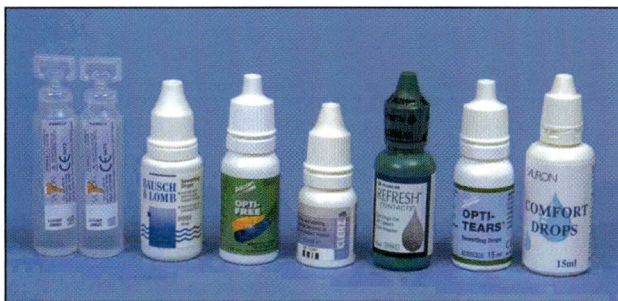

Figure R.14 • Soft lens re-wetting solutions.

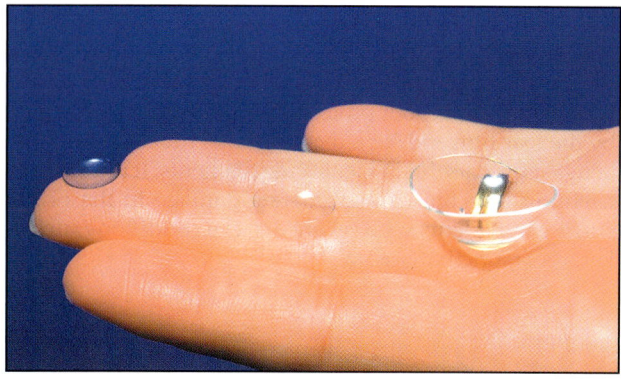

Figure R.15 • A rigid lens (left), shown in comparison to a soft lens (centre) and scleral lens (right).

Re-wetting solutions, soft contact lens

Contact lens wearers can complain of numerous symptoms, including dryness and general discomfort; such symptoms are the primary reasons for the discontinuation of contact lens wear. A common method of the clinical management of ocular discomfort is the prescription of soft lens re-wetting solutions, which are also known by the synonyms of 'lubricants' and 'comfort drops' (Figure R.14). Although these products are often well received by wearers, and comfort is improved for at least 6 hours after their instillation, their effect is not much different from that of saline. Furthermore, the mechanism of symptomatic relief is unclear, and does not seem to be due to an enhancement of the pre-lens tear film.

Some re-wetting solutions are in 'unit-dose' form, which can be advantageous in clinical situations where the introduction of solution preservatives to the ocular surface is contraindicated. The packaging required for this approach is relatively expensive. Most re-wetting solutions are supplied in multi-use bottles, and therefore contain preservatives to prevent contamination of the solution. These preservatives are similar to those found in other soft lens solutions.

A number of products contain viscosity-increasing agents, such as methylcellulose, which promote the adherence of the solution to the lens and enhance the contact time of the solution at the ocular surface. Other components that are commonly found in re-wetting solutions include sodium chloride and buffering agents.

RGP contact lens

- See *Rigid contact lens*.

Rheumatoid arthritis

- See *Systemic disease, contact lens wear in*.

Richmond (Hardy, Rand and Rittler) pseudoisochromatic plates

- See *Pseudoisochromatic plates*.

Rigid contact lens

A rigid contact lens is a contact lens made from a rigid or inflexible material that is incapable of being folded so that opposite edges can touch together. The diameter of such lenses is smaller than that of the cornea (12mm; see Figure R.15). All rigid lenses, apart from PMMA, are made from materials that are permeable to gases. Prior to the demise of PMMA as a contact lens material that is prescribed to patients, non-PMMA rigid lenses were referred to as 'rigid gas-permeable' or 'RGP' lenses – a term that is now redundant.

The readily discernible trend in the development of rigid contact lens materials described in the patent literature is one of increasing oxygen permeability balanced against the retention of acceptable dimensional stability and ocular compatibility (characterized by wettability and deposit resistance). The essential structural developments have centred on three areas. The first is the TRIS component, characterized by attempts to incorporate higher proportions of more highly branched siloxy derivatives, giving rise to silicone acrylates. The second is the use of fluorocarbon comonomers in the place of hydrocarbon-based components such as methyl methacrylate, giving rise to fluoro-silicone-acrylates. The third is the improvement of wettability by incorporation of hydrophilic co-monomers, or subsequent surface modification of the formed lens. Because rigid lens materials necessarily contain much higher levels of cross-linking agents than do soft lenses, it might be reasonable to add the development of cross-linking technology as a fourth area. Such materials have Dk values many times greater than that of PMMA.

Terms, symbols and abbreviations used to describe rigid (and soft) contact lenses are given in Appendix H.

Rigid gas-permeable contact lens

- See *Rigid contact lens*.

Rosacea keratopathy

- See *Degenerations of the corneal epithelium, therapeutic contact lenses for*.

Rose bengal stain

A purple-red dye that can be introduced into the eye as a drop or from an impregnated paper strip. Staining occurs wherever there is poor protection of the surface epithelium by the tear film and/or a dysfunctional mucus layer. Rose bengal is also useful in identifying filaments. It is especially useful in detecting and evaluating damage to the ocular surface in patients with severe dry eye conditions such as keratoconjunctivitis sicca.

Rotation of toric contact lenses, soft

- See *Toric lens rotation, soft.*

Rust spots on contact lenses

- See *Deposits, contact lens.*

Sag, contact lens

The radius of curvature of a circle can be calculated by measuring the height, or sag, of the curve over a fixed chord diameter. In Figure S.1,

$$R = (y^2 + s^2)/2s$$

where R is the radius, s is the sag height and y is half the chord diameter. By differentiating this formula, the minimum change or difference in s required to detect a change or difference in R of +0.05mm can be calculated as:

$$dR/ds = 0.5 - (y^2/2s^2)$$

For y = 5mm and s = 2mm, ds = –0.019mm. Hence, 'sag' methods should be capable of measuring apical height to within a tolerance of 0.019mm. Clearly, if y is reduced, then ds will also reduce in order to maintain the tolerance in R.

Instrument manufacturers have used this approach to develop several devices for determining lens back surface radius. Using an appropriate calibration curve, the BOZR can be estimated. The apical height can be measured using mechanical or ultrasonic probes, either in air or saline. In ultrasonic devices, the sound beam is reflected from the back surface; the BOZR of mass-produced disposable lenses can be measured to within ±0.1mm of the stated value using this technique.

Sag can be measured using a mechanical probe. The lens is immersed in temperature-controlled saline, and a magnified side view profile of the lens is projected on to a viewing screen. The mechanical probe is manually raised until the observer witnesses slight lens movement, indicating that the probe has come into contact with the posterior pole of the lens. This device tends to measure BOZR slightly less than stated when used on most lenses. In a variation of this approach, the lens is placed on a cylindrical column and a central probe is gently raised until it touches the back surface of the lens. On contact, an electrical circuit is completed. The height of the probe is electronically monitored and displayed; once the probe touches the lens back surface, the displayed figure is 'frozen'. This figure is the sag height of the lens, and by using a calibration chart the BOZR corresponding to the recorded sag height can be determined.

The sag method assumes that the lens back surface is spherical over the chord diameter of measurement. If the surface is aspheric, the estimated BOZR can be noted as the 'equivalent sphere'. If it is suspected that a particular lens design has an aspheric back surface, it is possible to estimate the asphericity of the surface by measuring the apical height over more than one chord diameter.

Saline solutions for soft contact lenses

Many contact lens wearers are prescribed a saline rinsing solution when they commence lens wear. These products are particularly helpful to the new

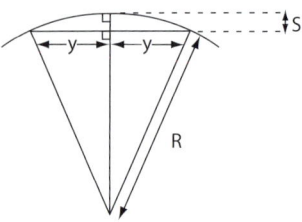

A Diagram of 'sag' theory

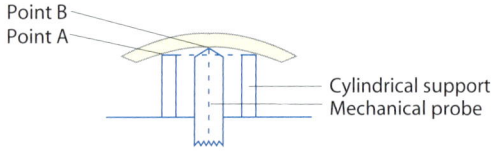

B Mechanical sag-based system (in air; wet cell systems are available)

Figure S.1 • Sag method for determining back optic zone radius (BOZR). (A) Sag theory. (B) Mechanical sag-based system.

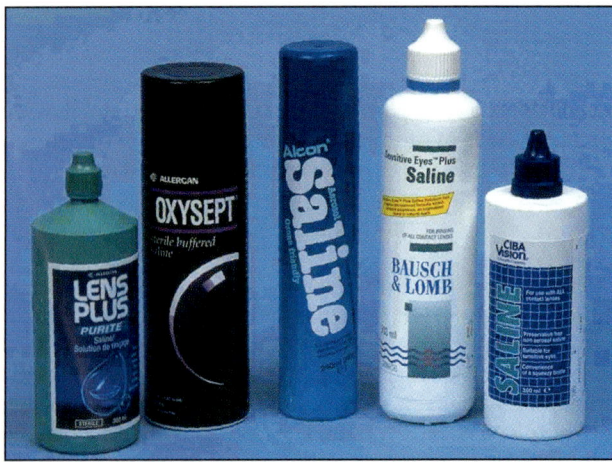

Figure S.2 • Examples of saline supplied in aerosol cans and 'squeezy' bottles.

wearer, who tends to handle lenses more frequently and requires more attempts at lens insertion, leading to increased contamination from the fingers. Some hydrogen peroxide users remove any residual hydrogen peroxide with a saline rinse to reduce any stinging on insertion. The rinsing process can also play a significant role in the removal of micro-organisms from the lens surface.

Homemade and unpreserved saline have been associated with serious ocular surface infections and are not recommended. There are three types of saline solutions available on the market: aerosol, unit-dose and 'squeezy' bottle formats (Figure S.2). The pressure within aerosol saline canisters prevents contamination, although it is recommended that the user eject a small amount of saline before use as contamination of the spray tip has been associated with corneal infections. These are usually buffered to retain a consistent pH, and tend to be relatively expensive and bulky. Unit-dose products are non-preserved and can be useful in some circumstances, such as travel to warm climates or in-practice use.

More recently, preserved saline solutions have gained popularity in their 'squeezy' bottle format. With these products, the active ingredient serves only to prevent contamination of the solution, rather than play any role in contact lens disinfection. Examples of these products include Purite saline (Allergan), which contains chlorine dioxide; Bausch & Lomb saline, which contains sorbic acid; and CIBA Vision saline, which contains 60ppm hydrogen peroxide.

Salzmann's nodular degeneration
• See *Degenerations of the corneal epithelium, therapeutic lenses for.*

Scheduling of patients
• See *Patient scheduling in contact lens practice.*

Sclera
The sclera forms the largest part of the fibrous outer coat of the globe. It is pierced by two large foramina: the anterior scleral foramen filled by the cornea and the posterior scleral foramen penetrated by the optic nerve. It is also crossed by a number of smaller channels for the various nerves and blood vessels that enter the eye. The sclera can be resolved into three distinct layers: episclera, scleral stroma and the lamina fusca. The episclera is a loose vascular connective tissue layer that lies beneath Tenons capsule, to which it is attached by fibrous bands. Its internal surface merges with the underlying scleral stroma. Like the cornea, the stroma is composed of densely packed collagen embedded in a matrix of proteoglycans. However, there are key differences: in the sclera, collagen fibrils show a large variation in diameter and spacing and lamellae branch and interlace extensively. This results in the increased light scatter that is responsible for the opaque dull white appearance of the sclera. The particular fibril arrangement imparts a high tensile strength to resist the pull of the extra-ocular muscles. The high tensile strength of the sclera also contains the intra-ocular pressure. The lamina fusca is a pigmented layer located at the inner aspect of the sclera at the interface with the choroid. It contains numerous melanocytes and a small amount of elastic tissue.

Scleral contact lens
Scleral lenses have retained a small but valuable place in modern contact lens practice four decades after the introduction of corneal and hydrogel lenses (see Figure R.15). Originally they were made from glass, until polymethyl methacrylate (PMMA) was introduced in the 1940s. From the mid-1980s, rigid gas-permeable materials transformed scleral lens practice, allowing simpler fitting processes and improved patient tolerance, and expanding the therapeutic application of these lenses so that they could be used for more subtle forms of ocular pathology. The essential advance is that gas-permeable scleral lenses can be 'sealed' in most cases; that is, there is no need to introduce small holes (known as 'fenestrations') into the lens to aid tear exchange and corneal oxygenation.

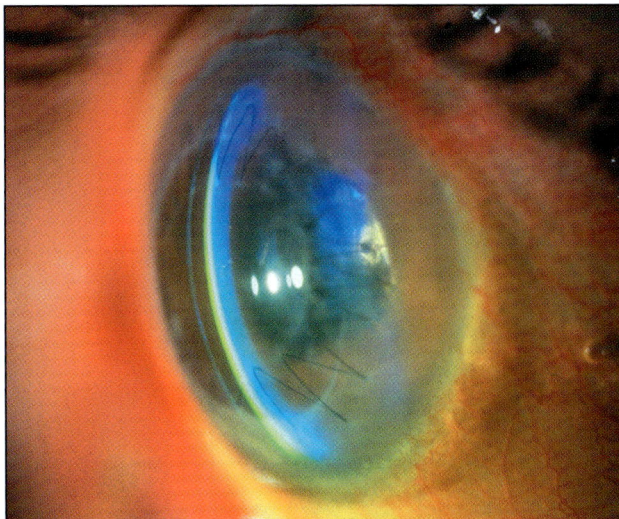

Figure S.3 • The extent of corneal clearance is revealed by the thickness of fluorescein-stained tears between the scleral lens and the cornea.

Advantages of scleral lenses include the following:
- they fit on the sclera and are held in place by the eyelids, and therefore can be used for almost any corneal topography
- high powers are possible
- they are robust and easily maintained
- handling may be easier for patients who have difficulties with soft or rigid lenses
- they are surprisingly comfortable because the lids are never in contact with the lens edge
- foreign bodies under scleral lenses are rare.

The primary disadvantages of scleral lenses are as follows:
- full coverage of the anterior eye reduces the oxygen available to the cornea
- scleral lens manufacture is labour intensive and therefore expensive
- there may be a subjective feeling of bulk in the eye
- scleral lenses can induce a slightly proptosed appearance during wear
- the lens size intimidates some patients.

The two primary indications for fitting scleral lenses relate to vision and therapeutic applications:

1. Vision. Keratoconus or other primary corneal ectasia is the largest single group for which scleral lenses are indicated. Other applications for which scleral lenses can provide significant improvements in vision include post-keratoplasty, high refractive errors and the correction of high astigmatism.
2. Therapeutic applications. The pre-corneal fluid reservoir (Figure S.3) maintains corneal hydration in serious dry eye conditions such as Stevens-Johnson syndrome and cicatricizing pemphigoid, and creates a favourable environment for corneal healing in some situations. Tear film evaporation is prevented when lid closure is poor or if the lids are absent, and there is excellent corneal protection from trichiasis or lid margin keratinization. Some ocular surface disorders – e.g. Salzmann's nodular dystrophy – cause gross corneal irregularities, which can be optically neutralized to improve vision. 'Ptosis props' can be fixed onto scleral lenses to assist in management of ocular myopathy or other causes of poor lid elevation. A painted iris can be encapsulated into a scleral lens to cover an unsightly blind eye, or to relieve intractable diplopia.

Scratch resistant coating for plastic lenses

Many plastic lenses are now supplied with a scratch resistant coating as standard. Although these coatings can be considered optional for thermosetting plastics such as CR39, they are essential for thermoplastic materials such as polycarbonate and acrylic. There is a problem with all hard coats, in that if they are too hard and inflexible they will crack under pressure or impact. In addition, it is difficult to get a coefficient of thermal expansion match between the coat and the lens substrate, which causes stress in the coating if the lens is placed in extreme temperatures. There are a number of different methods of application:

Dipping. Lenses are dipped into hard coat solution and the surplus material is allowed to drain off. An example of a liquid hard coat is a mixture of alcohol pyrrolidone, acrylate ester and butyanol. As in all coating procedures, the lens must be scrupulously clean before coating takes place. This process is used in the mass production of lenses, but is not suitable for coating straight top solid bifocals as streaks of hard coat will form at the visible edge of the segment.

Spin coating. For small-scale production, a liquid hard coat is dripped on to the front of a lens on a spinning holder. The spinning action spreads out the coating evenly across the lens.

Vacuum hard coat. A silica coat can be deposited onto the lens surface in a vacuum chamber. This method requires expensive equipment and the hard coat cannot be subsequently tinted. However, this type of hard coating is often used prior to the application of an anti-reflection coating.

Hard coating 'in mould'. This type of hard coat is introduced into the mould at the time of basic lens manufacture. The resultant lenses are difficult to tint, so the hard coat is usually only applied to the front surface of a lens.

Hard coatings are typically 10 to 20 times thicker than anti-reflection coatings. Coating thickness and refractive index are critical, as unwanted interference effects, including enhanced surface reflections, may occur if the wrong combination is used.

Sealed scleral contact lenses
- See *Fitting scleral lenses.*

Services, contact lens
- See *Products and services, contact lens.*

Sessile drop measurement of contact lens surface wettability

The wettability (or surface affinity for water) of a biological polymer can be measured using the sessile drop method (see Figure C.1). This is one of the simplest laboratory tests to perform, and is also commonly referred to as the 'water in air' method (when water is used as the probe liquid). It involves introducing a drop of water (or saline) onto the material or lens surface and measuring the angle at the solid/liquid/air interface. The introduction and measurement are both carried out in air, which means that the liquid will be in equilibrium with its vapour.

In theory, measurement of the contact angle by this method requires minimal specialist equipment, since the drop produced can be photographed or projected and the angle readily measured from the image produced. In practice, a fairly inexpensive piece of equipment named a goniometer is usually used. The goniometer consists of a telescope at the end of which is a platform where the sample is placed. The telescope has a crosshair in the eyepiece, which is rotated until it corresponds to an imaginary tangent to the profile of the droplet. The value of the contact angle is then simply read from a graticule to the nearest 1°.

This laboratory test is difficult to perform in a clinical environment, and it does not predict how well a material will perform on a specific eye.

Settling time, contact lens

Soft lenses alter their fitting characteristics during a period of equilibration due to differences in temperature, pH and osmolarity between the lens storage solution and eye. Lenses tend to show less movement after this period of settling. In some cases, lenses exhibit gross tightness immediately after insertion and are unlikely to show sufficient improvement on settling. Many fitting guides recommend a long settling period before assessing lens fit, particularly in the case of high water content lenses (e.g. 30 minutes); however, this is frequently impractical and unnecessary. High water content ionic lenses stabilize within a 10–15-minute period. In most cases, lens fit can be assessed 5 minutes after lens insertion. A fast blink rate appears to quicken lens settling.

The initial reaction of new patients to rigid lenses can give an indication of how easily they are going to adapt to rigid lens wear. Clearly, those showing little or no lacrimation, and who are able to move their eyes without apparent discomfort, are the most promising candidates for successful rigid lens wear. In these cases, the lens fit can be assessed immediately. However, in most cases it will be necessary to wait 5–10 minutes for excess lacrimation to subside. This period can be used to discuss aspects of the process, such as costs, hygiene, lens maintenance etc., and to answer any questions.

In a few cases when fitting either soft or rigid lenses, it may be some time before lacrimation subsides enough to allow examination. It is necessary, however, to consider other possible reasons for the discomfort. This might be due to a foreign body attached to the lens (the tears usually clear any loose foreign bodies), or the fit might be so poor as to be causing some mechanical trauma to the cornea or conjunctiva. Having ruled out other causes of discomfort, it might be necessary to allow a longer settling period, e.g. 10–30 minutes. It is preferable that the patient does not leave the practice during this period.

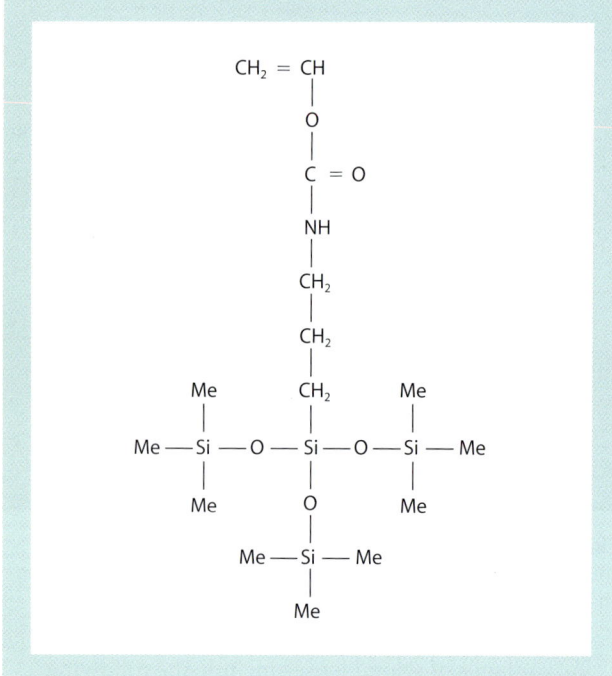

Figure S.4 • Vinyl carbamate derivative of TRIS molecule (TRISCV). Me = CH3.

Sight impairment
- See *Low vision.*

Silicone acrylates
- See *Rigid contact lens.*

Silicone elastomer
- See *Silicone rubber.*

Silicone hydrogel contact lenses

Owing to their silicone content, these soft lenses have oxygen permeability values that are far in excess of conventional hydrogel lenses. A major hurdle in developing these lenses was to work out how to combine the elements of hydrophobic silicone rubber with those of a typical hydrophilic hydrogel-forming monomer such as HEMA, to form a co-polymer that combines the properties of both. The logical answer was to combine HEMA with the monomer that has been so successfully used in the preparation of rigid lens materials, commonly referred to as TRIS; however, this presented the same fundamental difficulty as trying to combine oil and water to form an optically clear product. Phase separation occurs and the optical clarity of the product is impaired.

PureVision (balafilcon; Bausch & Lomb) is based on a substantially homogeneous co-polymer of a vinyl carbamate derivative of TRIS (Figure S.4), giving a water content of 35%, a Dk of 110 Barrer, and a water transport slightly (10%) in excess of that of polyHEMA. Focus Night & Day (lotrafilcon; CIBA Vision) is described as a lens that contains both ion transport and oxygen transport phases running from the anterior to the posterior surfaces. The biphasic structure of the material is produced by co-polymerizing a fluoroether macromer with TRIS monomer and N,N-dimethyl acrylamide (which acts both as a hydrophilic monomer and a polymerizable solvent) in the presence of a non-polymerizable diluent. The resultant material is a fluoroether-based silicone hydrogel with a water content of 24% and a Dk of 140 Barrer.

Both of the lenses described above are treated using gas plasma techniques, but whereas Bausch & Lomb has opted for plasma oxidation, CIBA Vision has chosen to apply a plasma coating. In the former case (PureVision), oxidation of TRIS produces hydrophilic glassy silicate islands on the surface, whereas the surface of Focus Night & Day is coated with a 25-nm thick, dense, high refractive index coating. These differences are at an atomic level, and are not evident on clinical inspection of the lenses.

Because of their extremely high oxygen performance, silicone hydrogel lenses can be used for extended wear without inducing excess oedema – a factor that has severely limited the application of hydrogel materials as extended-wear lenses.

Silicone rubber

Silicone rubber belongs to a group of materials, known as synthetic elastomers, that are not only flexible but show rubber-like behaviour – i.e. they are capable of being compressed or stretched, and when the deforming force is removed they instantaneously return to their original shape. They consist of polymer chains that possess high mobility and are cross-linked at intervals along the polymer backbones. Because of this chain mobility, oxygen is able to diffuse rapidly through the structure. These polymers have oxygen permeabilities more than 100 times greater than that of PMMA. Silicone rubber is the most significant member of the group, with an oxygen permeability around 1000 times greater than that of PMMA. This extremely high oxygen permeability arises from the backbone of alternate silicone and oxygen atoms, which confers not only great freedom of rotation but also a much higher solubility for oxygen than rubbery polymers with simple carbon backbones.

Silicone rubber lenses, surface treated to enhance wettability, were developed in the mid-1960s and found clinically to have little deleterious effect on corneal respiration. However, the problems of maintaining adequate surface properties (Figure S.5), which were initially encountered during routine clinical use, have never been fully overcome. Furthermore, silicone rubber lenses tended to develop tremendous suction forces and were very difficult to remove from the eye. As a result, silicone rubber lenses are used only rarely today. The uniquely high oxygen permeability of the silicon-oxygen backbone has, however, been harnessed in two distinct types of contact lens material: silicone hydrogel lenses and rigid lenses.

Simultaneous vision contact lenses for presbyopia

A variety of simultaneous lens designs are available in both rigid and soft materials. The recent availability of single-use disposable soft trial lenses and empirically ordered individually based aspheric rigid lenses has resulted in increased prescribing of this form of lens correction.

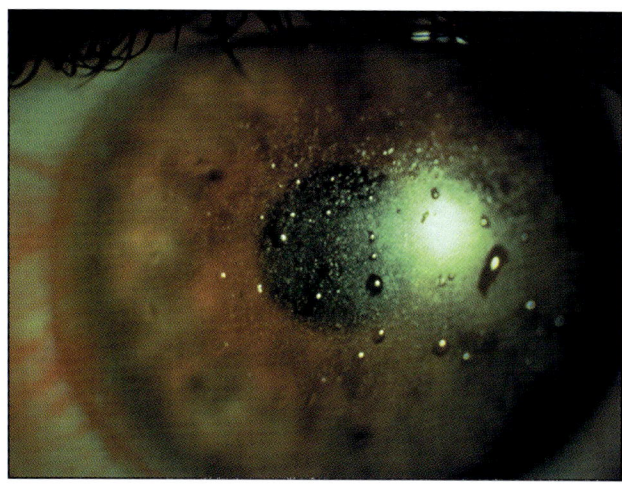

Figure S.5 • Poorly-wetting surface of a silicone elastomer lens.

In simultaneous vision designs, the distance and near correction zones are both positioned in front of the pupil in every direction of gaze so that light from either a distant or near object passes through both zones. As fixation is directed to either a distant or a near object, one zone produces a focused image while the other produces a blurred image that overlaps the same retinal elements as the focused one. The simultaneous images placed on the retina by any optical system rely on the visual system being able to select the clearer picture and to ignore the out-of-focus image, whether a distant or near object is being viewed.

The spread of light from the defocused image reduces the contrast of the focused image. As a result, the fitting of a simultaneous vision lens is likely to result in a reduction in image quality in comparison to that resulting from a single vision correction. The extent of contrast loss will depend upon the relative amounts of in-focus to out-of-focus light striking the retina. If equal contrast is to be achieved for both near and far viewing, the refractive system should allow approximate equality of the area of the two portions of the lens transmitting to the pupil. Lens performance may be affected by many factors, which include pupil size, lens design and centration of optics relative to the pupil.

The following simultaneous vision lens designs are available:

> **1.** Bi-concentric designs. Early soft and rigid simultaneous vision bifocal lenses were bi-concentric in design, consisting of two discrete zones of distance and near power. A centre-distance design has the central portion of the optical zone for distance vision, which is surrounded by an area containing the near power. The ratio split between light forming the distance image to that forming the near image can be controlled for a given pupil size by altering the diameter of the central segment. As the pupil is a dynamic structure, a fundamental concern with such a design is its dependency on the pupil size. The near pupil reaction means that, as a near object is brought into view, proportionally less of the pupil allows light in from the near zone of the centre

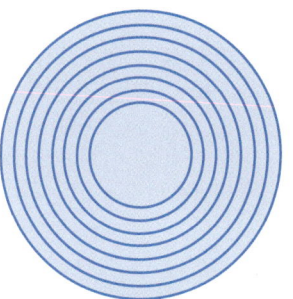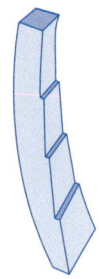

Figure S.6 • Diffractive design of simultaneous vision lenses for the correction of presbyopia. Left: concentric design of facets. Right: Each facet is 3μm deep.

distance design. In addition, as the eye ages the pupil naturally decreases in size, resulting in less light from the near portion of the lens and a reduction in near-vision quality. In low luminance levels the pupil naturally dilates, resulting in more light proportionally from the near zone and a reduction in the quality of distance vision. In centre-near designs the optical principle is the same as for the centre-distance lens but reversed, so that the central portion of the lens focuses the light from close objects and this is surrounded by a distance powered area. The design remains pupil-dependent; therefore, in bright conditions giving pupil constriction, distance vision becomes progressively less clear. Bi-concentric designs in both soft and rigid materials are still available, but are now used less frequently due to the availability of more advanced, easier to fit designs, and single-use disposable lenses.

2. Multi-zone concentric designs. A consequence of the above discussion is that benefits should be possible if the dependency of lens function on pupil size could be minimized, especially in relation to different lighting conditions. One approach is to increase the number of concentric zones and to power these zones alternatively for distance and near vision. The width and spacing of the zones is based on the variation of pupil size in different illuminations within the presbyopic population. Theoretically, this lens design favours distance vision in extreme high and low lighting conditions, and provides a more equal ratio of light division in ambient illumination conditions.

3. Diffractive bifocal contact lenses. These use refraction to correct distance vision, and a combination of refraction and diffraction to correct near vision. This is achieved by a diffractive 'zone plate' on the back surface of the lens, which is able to split the incident light passing through into two discrete focal points. Individual facets ('echelettes') are etched in a concentric ring pattern onto the posterior lens surface (Figure S.6). Each facet is only 2–3μm deep and therefore will not traumatize the epithelium. As with any simultaneous vision lens, incident light is divided between the distance and near foci so that the intensities of these images are reduced and the images are superimposed on each other, resulting in a reduction in retinal image quality. In addition, approximately 20% of incident light is lost to higher orders of diffraction, leaving 40% of light to make up each image. This may explain the greater reduction in low-contrast acuities with such lenses when compared to monovision correction. Diffractive lenses are largely independent of pupil size; however, like aspheric designs, they are dependent on lens centration.

4. Aspheric designs. With aspheric designs, the refractive power gradually changes from the geometric centre of the lens to the more peripheral area of the optic zone. Such lenses are best described as 'multifocal' due to the progression of powers, but can also be considered as a type of concentric design as the power distributions are concentric around the centre of the lens. By the nature of their design, lens function will vary with changes in pupil size. This will lead to variation in distance- and near-vision image contrast similar to that described previously for bi-concentric designs. Power distribution is produced by the use of a continuous aspheric surface of fixed or variable eccentricity. As with bi-concentric designs, aspheric lens designs can be subdivided according to whether the power distribution is most plus (least minus) centrally, resulting in a centre-near design, or most minus (least plus) centrally, resulting in a centre-distance design. Both options are available in soft and rigid materials.

Single-use contact lenses
- See *Daily disposable lenses*.

Skin tumours around the eyes
There are numerous types of skin tumour that can present around the eyes. Depending upon the histopathological changes within a tissue, a variety of terms are used:

- Metaplasia: when one adult cell type is replaced by another. e.g. conjunctival mucosa becoming keratinized in dry eye (squamous cell metaplasia)
- Dysplasia: the abnormal growth of a tissue, but where normal tissue architecture is retained.
- Neoplasia: an abnormal growth of a tissue with uncontrolled multiplication of cells and loss of normal tissue architecture. Also referred to as tumours or cancer.

A neoplasia signifies the irreversible loss of control of cell growth, frequently due to alteration of oncogenes. Oncogenes are a gene sequence that affect cell growth and signal transduction. Related genes in normal cells are called proto-oncogenes. There are also tumour suppressor genes, e.g. the absence of such a gene causes retinoblastoma.

There are three main forms of neoplasia:
- Benign – whereby lesions only grow by expansion, affecting the local tissue and having limited growth potential. Examples include seborrheic keratosis, actinic (solar) keratosis, naevi, keratoacanthoma, viral wart (papilloma), cutaneous horn, pyogenic granuloma, strawberry naevus and port wine stain.

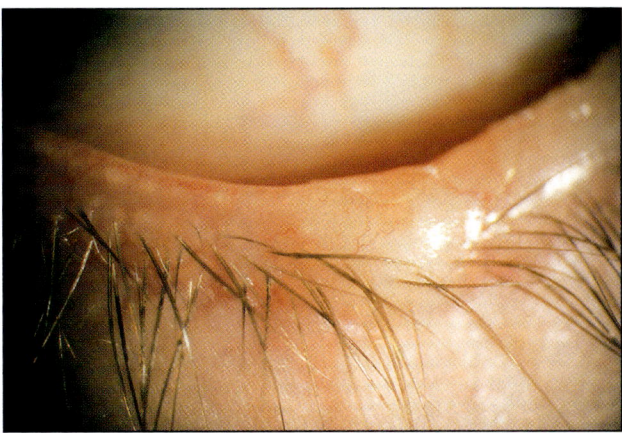

Figure S.7 • Early nodular basal cell carcinoma, showing the pearly smooth translucent surface and mild telangiectasia over the margin. The lesion is firm to palpate but asymptomatic.

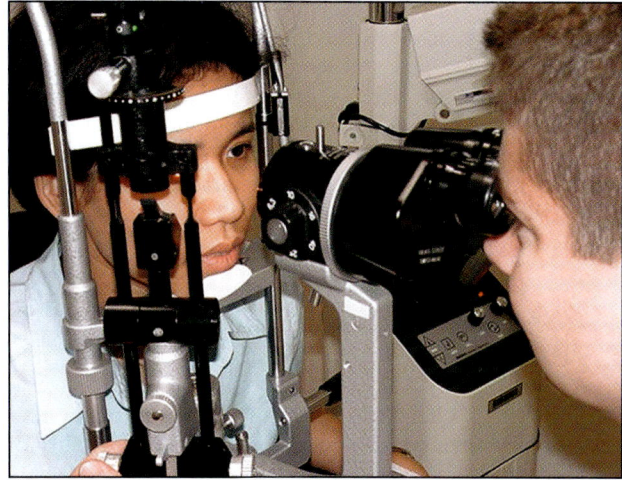

Figure S.8 • Slit-lamp biomicroscope.

- Malignant – indicating a lesion that grows and invades adjacent tissues. Examples of such lesions around the external eye include conjunctival intraepithelial neoplasia (CIN), basal cell carcinoma (BCC) (Figure S.7), squamous cell carcinoma (SCC), sebaceous gland carcinoma (SGC), melanoma, Kaposi sarcoma and Merkel cell carcinoma.
- Metastatic – in which the cells of a neoplasm infiltrate the blood vessels and lymphatics, to be spread throughout the body. e.g. melanoma, SCC and SGC.

The terminology refers to the tissue affected by the neoplasm: carcinoma refers to tumours from epithelia e.g. BCC; adeno- infers glandular; and sarcoma- refers to neoplasms derived from connective tissue.

The patient may have cosmetic concern for a mass or lesion. They may have noticed a change in its size, or noted pain and tenderness. Skin tumours tend to be unilateral and asymmetrical. Common findings with malignant tumours of the eyelid include skin ulceration, inflammation and distortion of the eyelid anatomy. Other findings suggestive of malignancy include abnormal colour or texture, persistent bleeding and madarosis (loss of eyelashes). Induration of the lesion signifies a feeling of hardness on palpation, as well as the impression that the lesion extends deeper than it appears to. Further signs which may be used in assessment include: rapidity of growth, pigmentation, telangiectasia and skin surface texture including whether scaly, waxy/oily, or verrucous (wart-like).

Naevi are usually even in colour, with a regular shape and border. Naevi should be distinguished from a malignant melanoma. The 'ABCDE' mnemonic is useful for assessing for the possibility of malignant melanoma:

A = Asymmetrical shape and elevation
B = Border is irregular or scalloped
C = Colour is mottled and variable. Melanoma may be vascularized.
D = Diameter is usually large (greater than 5mm)
E = Evolutionary change (in size or pigmentation).

Benign neoplasms are very common (approximately 1/10) in all age groups. Malignant neoplasms are less common. Malignant lesions can be locally invasive and cause significant tissue destruction and loss of function. Metastatic lesions are potentially life threatening.

The specific management depends upon the nature of the neoplasm. Benign lesions may simply be documented and monitored. A photograph can provide more information than a drawing. The advent of digital photography has made it easier to document a lesion and can facilitate discussion with the patient. A biopsy is indicated if there is doubt about the nature of the diagnosis, or the distinction between benign and malignant. Excision is usually indicated for malignant lesions and may be indicated for larger benign lesions. Additional systemic treatments are likely to be required for lesions with a risk of metastasis. A review at 6 to 12 month intervals is indicated for patients with a history of multiple skin lesions or as required if there is any concern by the patient. After surgery, review may be weekly to monthly to ensure full healing.

Slab-off bifocals

- See *Prism controlled bifocals*.

Slit-lamp biomicroscope

The slit-lamp biomicroscope plays an essential role in the preliminary assessment and aftercare of the prospective and existing contact lens wearer. The instrument consists of a separate illumination system (the slit lamp) and viewing system (the biomicroscope), which have a common focal point and centre of rotation (Figure S.8). A height control moves both systems simultaneously, and focusing and lateral movements are achieved via a joystick. This common control feature facilitates rapid and accurate positioning of the slit beam on the area of interest, and ensures that the microscope and illumination system are simultaneously in focus.

Virtually all slit-lamp manufacturers have adopted the Koeller illumination system, which is optically almost identical to that of a 35-mm slide projector. A bright illumination system (producing approximately 600 000lux) is a fundamental requirement for a slit lamp if subtle conditions are to be seen clearly. While halogen or xenon lamps are more expensive than tungsten lamps, they are the preferred illumination source as they provide a brighter light, last longer, have better colour rendering, and generate less heat. Illumination brightness is controlled by a rheostat or multiposition switch that allows brightness to be adjusted to obtain the correct balance between patient comfort and optimal visibility of the area of interest. The slit within the illumination system must have sharply demarcated edges, and desirable features include the ability to:

- adjust slit width and height
- graduate the slit width
- rotate the lamp housing
- offset the slit beam.

A number of filters can be incorporated into the illumination system, which serve to enhance the visibility of certain conditions. These include:

- a green ('red-free') filter, which enhances contrast when looking for corneal and iris vascularization
- a neutral density (ND) filter, which reduces beam brightness and increases comfort for the patient
- a polarizing filter, which reduces unwanted specular reflections
- a diffusing filter, which diffuses the illumination source over a wide area
- a cobalt blue filter, which provides a suitable means of exciting sodium
- a Kodak Wratten 12 (yellow) filter, which is placed in front of the viewing system to enhance the contrast of any fluorescent staining observed with the cobalt blue light.

A key prerequisite for a slit-lamp biomicroscope is a viewing system that provides a clear image of the eye and has sufficient magnification for the practitioner to view all structures of interest. Ideally magnifications of up to ×40 should be possible, and this may be achieved through interchangeable eyepieces and/or variable magnification of the slit-lamp objective. Zoom magnification systems have the advantage of allowing the practitioner to focus on a particular structure without losing sight of it during changes in magnification. See *Slit-lamp biomicroscopy*.

Slit-lamp biomicroscopy

Slit-lamp biomicroscopy refers to the technique of using the slit-lamp biomicroscope. In the preliminary examination, biomicroscopy is used to assess the health of the anterior eye, and more specifically to screen for conditions or features that may be relevant to contact lens wear. Any observed signs should be reconciled with symptoms and assessment of the corneal curvature. Characteristics of the normal anterior eye, and the severity of any abnormalities that are detected, can be recorded with the assistance of grading scales. In fitting and aftercare examinations, slit-lamp biomicroscopy is also used to assess the fit of contact lenses and the effect of lenses on the anterior ocular structures. A normal technique is to use a variety of illumination methods – such as direct focal illumination, indirect illumination, optic section, parallelepiped, retro-illumination, sclerotic

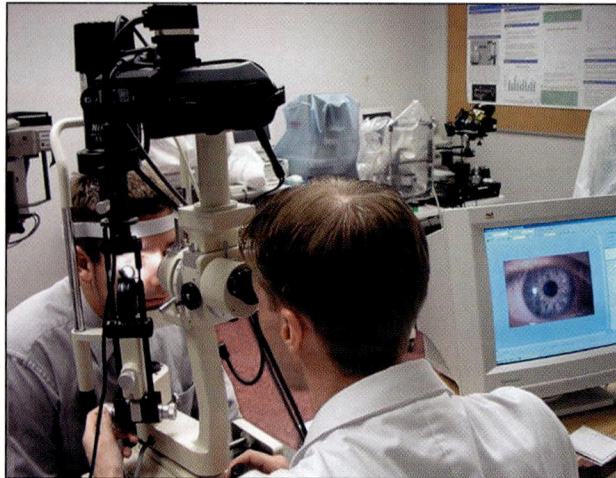

Figure S.9 • Equipment for slit-lamp digital image capture.

scatter, and specular reflection – and cobalt blue light for fluorescein staining.

Slit-lamp digital image capture

The basic principle of digital imaging is that a light-sensitive silicon computer chip is used instead of film in a camera. The silicon chip is known as a 'charge-coupled device' (CCD), and forms the light-sensitive element in video and digital cameras. The image can be instantly displayed on a computer screen, viewed by the practitioner and patient, then stored or printed (Figure S.9). The image digitization can take place at the camera or computer.

A digital image may be characterized in three main ways:

> 1. Image resolution. This refers to the image dimensions (width x height) in units of the number of dots (pixels). Common resolutions are 640 × 480 or 800 × 600, although a smaller image to fit into a digital record card – such as 320 × 240 – may also be acceptable.
> 2. Colour depth. This is the number of colours that may be specified for each pixel. For true colour, this should be in the thousands or millions.
> 3. File format. This describes the way an image is saved on disk and affects its compatibility with different programs for viewing, e-mailing etc. The Internet standard image file format is JPEG, and carries the benefit of small file size, high definition and broad compatibility with Internet e-mail and browser software.

There are numerous advantages to using digital photography instead of conventional 35-mm film photography. These include the following:

- reduced cost – once a digital imaging system is set up, an image can be captured instantly and at no additional cost
- instant imaging – digital imaging avoids the delay required for film processing in conventional photography, and thus any error in image focus or exposure can be immediately corrected

- patient education – there is a benefit in patients immediately seeing their own condition (for example, limbal neovascularization)
- live preview – with a video-based system the image may be previewed on screen and if necessary optimized before it is saved onto a hard disk
- no media costs – with digital imaging there is no ongoing cost for film or processing; although Polaroid photography gives a virtually instant result, it is relatively costly per print and the quality is limited
- ease of upgrade – many conventional slit lamps can be modified for digital imaging, by the addition of a beam splitter and camera; a normal slit lamp may be used with a flash rather than needing a specialized photographic slit lamp.

Digital image capture has a distinct advantage in that the captured images are in an electronic format; this opens up the following possibilities:

1. Image transfer. Increasingly, clinicians are communicating by electronic mail. A digital image is already on the computer, and this makes attachment to an e-mail easy. Images can be transferred by computer and modem to anywhere – this is the basis of 'telemedicine'.
2. Presentations. Images can be transferred to computer presentation programs, which are used for training and delivering lectures.
3. Web pages. Digital images can be readily transferred onto Internet web pages, and a similar approach used for storage and retrieval via an internal practice intranet.
4. Video movies. Dynamic conditions such as contact lens fittings or certain dynamic forms of pathology evaluation can be captured as a short movie on the computer. For example, a movie enables recording of the intricacies of lid interactions and the effects of lens centration on fluorescein patterns. See *Slit-lamp photography*.

Slit-lamp photography

Traditionally, the imaging system of choice for contact lens practice was a photographic slit-lamp biomicroscope using 35-mm or Polaroid film. A photographic slit lamp differs from a conventional slit lamp in that a flash tube is built in to the illumination system. The flash is necessary to provide sufficient illumination for correct exposure of photographic film. The camera is mounted on the slit lamp with a beam splitter attached to the observation system. See *Slit-lamp digital image capture*.

Small field tritanopia

About 2% of foveal cones, in the central retina, are comprised of short wavelength (blue) sensitive photopigment. All individuals therefore exhibit 'small field tritanopia', and make tritanopic colour matches and colour confusions, for field sizes subtending less than 0.5°.

Soft contact lens

A small, circular transparent device that is placed directly onto the cornea to correct optical defects of vision. It is soft, it can be folded in half, and it is made from hydrogel materials. Syn: hydrogel lens.

Soft contact lens on-eye power changes

When a soft lens is worn, its inherent flexibility allows it to 'drape' so that the shape of the posterior surface approximates closely to that of the anterior cornea. Although this greatly simplifies fitting, any associated changes in the curvatures of the lens surfaces and lens thickness may result in the on-eye power of the lens differing slightly from that measured off-eye.

Although draping implies that the tear lens between the contact lens and the cornea ought to have zero power, this may not always be the case. A tear lens of about 10μl in volume may sometimes exist and contribute about –0.15D of power to the combined lens-eye system. Although low minus lenses may entrap only a small volume of tears (about 5.5μl), thicker, low plus lenses may entrap a greater volume (about 9.5μl), giving a correspondingly greater tear lens effect (up to –2.00D).

Changes in hydration – which are a function of the lens design and material, the wearer, the visual task and ambient environmental conditions – will affect the refractive index and geometry of any soft lens, and hence its power. Typically, hydration may fall by up to 8% after the first hour of lens wear. Thinner lenses reach equilibrium after about 5 minutes, whereas thicker, high-power positive lenses may continue to dehydrate for 30 minutes or more after insertion. Effects appear to be material-dependent; in particular, high water content lenses dehydrate more and reach equilibrium sooner than lower water content lenses of comparable thickness. Greater dehydration may occur during near work, due to reduced blinking, and when atmospheric humidity is low. Water loss can occur by several pathways, including evaporation into the atmosphere, drainage into the nasolacrimal system, and, possibly, absorption into the conjunctival capillaries.

As the corneal temperature is around 32–35°C, while the room temperature is normally about 20°C, there is a change in temperature when the lens is put on the eye; this affects all the lens parameters, including hydration and the refractive index. However, the associated power change would only be about 0.25D for a ±10.00D lens.

Theoretical and empirical models have been developed to allow overall on-eye power changes to be predicted. Among the more mathematically sophisticated models of flexure alone are those based on the concept that the flexed lens always retains constant volume or that the arc length of the back optic zone of the lens remains constant. Any power changes are small for negative lenses, but larger, clinically significant changes, which increase with the lens power, occur for positive lenses. For practical work the most sensible approach is to conduct a trial lens fitting, since, after suitable equilibration, the trial lens will display similar on-eye effects to those of the ordered lens of the same design and power.

Soilation

- See *Deposits, lens*.

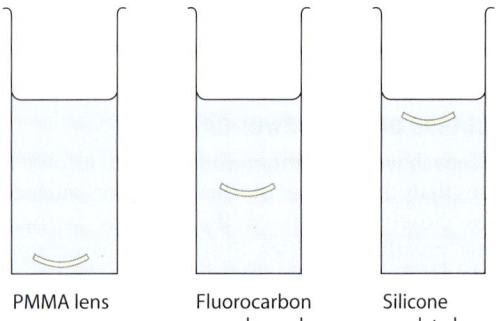

PMMA lens   Fluorocarbon co-polymer lens   Silicone acrylate lens

Figure S.10 • The three tubes each contain a solution with a specific gravity (SG) of 1.1. The lens in the centre tube has a SG of 1.1 and displays 'equiflotation'. The PMMA lens in the left tube has a SG of 1.2 and sinks to the bottom. The silicone acrylate lens in the right tube has a SG of less than 1.1 and floats to the top.

Specific gravity, rigid contact lens

The specific gravity (SG) of a material is a ratio defined as its density divided by the density of water (thus, the SG of water is unity).

The density of hydrogel polymers depends upon both the water content and the monomer composition. Typical contact lens co-polymers containing HEMA and the more hydrophilic monomers decrease progressively from a specific gravity around 1.16 at 38% water content to around 1.05 at 75% water content (all at 20°C).

If a rigid lens is placed in a saturated saline solution, it will float on condition that the SG of the lens is less than that of saturated saline (1.197). Adding distilled water to the saline reduces the G, and the lens will sink when the SG falls below the SG of the lens material. By adding saturated saline to the solution the SG will gradually increase and the lens will start to float again. At this point, no more saline is added. The SG of the lens material is the same as the SG of the surrounding saline. Using a hygrometer, the SG of the saline (and hence that of the lens material) can be measured, and the material identified from a table. This simple technique, which is referred to as 'densitometry', is dependent upon ambient conditions, and is limited by the available range of SG of the saturated immersion fluid.

An alternative approach is to use 20 tubes containing progressively changing concentrations of calcium chloride solution to give specific gravity readings between 1.00 and 1.20. The principle underlying these techniques is shown in Figure S.10.

Spectacle correction, plus lens magnifiers

In the case of a spectacle-mounted plus lens magnifier, the lens is obviously worn instead of the refractive correction and so this will need to be taken into account. For example, a −4.00DS myope requires 3× magnification, which is provided by a +12.00DS add, so the final lens is (−4.00) + (+12.00) = +8.00DS. For the uncorrected +4.00DS hypermetrope to achieve 3× magnification with a +12.00DS add would require a +16.00DS lens. Cylinders can be incorporated into such lenses when they are individually prescribed, but many come 'ready-glazed' with only spherical powers. This will not usually impair performance since cylinders up to 1.50DC are probably not subjectively appreciated. This should be confirmed by subjective acuity testing with the patient.

For hand-held plus lens magnifiers, it is assumed that the object is at the focal point of the magnifier lens, and thus parallel rays of light leave the lens and the image is at infinity. This allows the user to obtain a clearly focused retinal image whilst wearing the distance refractive correction, and with the accommodation relaxed. It is likely, however, that the patient will not intuitively use the magnifier in this way. It would be natural for the pre-presbyopic patient to converge and accommodate for the physically near location of the object, and presbyopic patients using a hand-held or stand-mounted magnifier for reading may well expect to wear their reading spectacles. In order to now create a focused retinal image, the rays of light must be divergent when leaving the magnifier lens, and the converging effect of the reading addition or the accommodation will bring the rays to parallel. This will require the lens-to-object distance to be decreased, so the object will be closer to the lens than its focal point. In either situation, the magnifying system is no longer the single plus-lens magnifier; it is now a combined system of two spaced elements, one being the positive magnifier and the other being the positive accommodation or reading addition. The magnification produced by this combined system depends on its equivalent power, and this is given by:

$$F_{eq} = F_M + F_A - zF_MF_A$$

where z = the separation of the two elements in the system – either the distance of the magnifier (F_M) from the cornea in the case where accommodation provides the second component (F_A) in the system, or the distance of the magnifier from the reading spectacles (F_A). This value of equivalent power can then be used to calculate the magnification:

$$M = F_{eq}/4$$

When z is small (and the magnifier is close to the spectacle plane), there is an increase in the combined power over that expected when using the magnifier with the object at the focal point. When the two components are separated by a distance equal to the focal length of the magnifier lens, the magnification is not affected by the power of the reading addition and is only dependent on the magnifier power. It is when the separation z becomes greater than the focal length of the magnifier that the combined power of the system begins to diminish in proportion to that separation. The effects can be extreme; for example, a +40.00DS magnifier combined with 6.00DS of accommodation gives an equivalent system power of +46.00DS if the two components are touching, but only +10.00DS if they are separated by a distance of 15cm. To avoid this potential power loss, it is recommended that hand magnifiers should be used with distance correction, unless the magnifier is held in contact with the spectacles, when the reading correction could be used. This is the basis of the 'trade magnification' formula, which assumes that the magnifier is used in conjunction with a +4.00DS addition. The magnification of the two-component system is then:

$M = F_{eq}/4$
where $F_{eq} = F_M + F_A - zF_MF_A$

F_M is the magnifier power, F_A is the reading addition (+4.00DS in this case) and z is the separation of the two components. If it is assumed that the magnifier is held in the spectacle plane, touching the addition lens (so z = 0), then:

$F_{eq} = F_M + (+4.00) - 0.F_M(+4.00) = F_M + 4$
and $M = (F_M + 4)/4$
Thus, $M = (F_M/4) + 1$

Although this approach is commonly used, it is not very realistic, since there is no reason to assume that the patient always has a +4.00DS reading addition (or equivalent accommodation), and it is not likely that the magnifier will be held in contact with the spectacles.

When considering stand-mounted plus lens magnifiers, the variable focus designs allow the patient to place the object in any desired position, and they should be considered in the same way as hand-held magnifiers. For the fixed focus type, however, the stand height is usually less than the focal length of the lens. The object is closer to the lens than the focal point, and divergent light leaves the lens. Thus the image is not at infinity, but at some finite distance from the eye. The patient must therefore accommodate, or, if presbyopic, wear a reading addition appropriate to the apparent distance of the image in order to neutralize the divergence and focus the image clearly on the retina. The accommodation or reading add required depends on the design of the magnifier (how much shorter the stand height is than the focal length) and the distance of the magnifier lens from the eye. If the add is too great, the image through the magnifier will be constantly blurred; if too low, the user will need to lift the stand off the page (hence moving the object closer to the focal point, and reducing the divergence of light leaving the magnifier). In addition there is no 'standard' reading addition or accommodative effort: manufacturers vary in the object position selected, and often vary within a particular range of magnifiers of different powers.

A very quick check can be performed by the clinician viewing some reading print with the magnifier placed in contact with it, and at the same eye-to-magnifier distance that the patient will use. If a trial lens equal to the patient's reading addition can be placed over the magnifier lens, and the print remain clear, then it shows that the presbyopic patient will need a reading correction. A genuine difficulty can arise with high-powered stand magnifiers, however, when the patient's reading correction is in the form of multifocal lenses. When the magnifier is held very close to the spectacles, as it must be in order to achieve a useful field of view with a small diameter lens, the patient's natural gaze is straight ahead, through the distance portion of the lens, and downward gaze through the reading portion can be difficult to achieve.

The magnification given by the manufacturers must be interpreted with caution because the equivalent power of the magnifier/spectacle combination will vary depending on how each individual patient uses the device.

Spectacle correction, telescopes

Distance telescopes which are hand-held or clip-on can be positioned over distance spectacles. The patient may find this awkward, especially if the vertex distance is large, and may appreciate the larger field of view when the telescope is held right up to the cornea. If the telescope is a focusing design then the separation of the lenses can be altered to compensate for moderate degrees of spherical ametropia. With high degrees of ametropia the magnification will be changed from the manufacturer's stated value if this re-focusing is carried out, since the telescope behaves as if some of the eyepiece power has been 'borrowed' to correct the ametropia. As the formula for the magnification is

$M = -F_E/F_O$,

then as F_E apparently changes, magnification alters as well (Table S.1) (see *Telescopes, distance*). If the telescope is used over the spectacles, the magnification is always exactly that stated by the manufacturer, regardless of the power of the refractive correction.

Any significant cylindrical correction would have to be worn as a spectacle behind the telescope, or be incorporated into a holder behind the eyepiece, although it has been found that powers less than 1.50DC usually do not affect acuity.

An intermediate or near telescope is designed to be worn over the distance correction, since compensation for the close working distance has already been made in the telescope itself. See *Telescopes, near/intermediate*.

Spectacle lens materials

A spectacle lens material must satisfy a number of conflicting requirements. Besides being transparent to visible wavelengths, and constant in properties (homogeneous), the material must not split light up into the constituent colours to any great extent, giving rise to chromatic aberration. Desirable properties of spectacle lenses include the following:

Table S.1 • The effect on magnification of focusing a telescope to compensate for spherical ametropia.		
Type of telescope	Galilean	Astronomical
Hypermetrope	Magnification increases if telescope refocused	Magnification decreases if telescope refocused
Myope	Magnification decreases if telescope refocused	Magnification increases if telescope refocused

Table S.2 • Spectacle lens materials.

GLASS

Name	n	V	Density (gm cm^{-3})
Crown	1.523	58	2.54
SW60	1.600	41	2.58
SF64	1.701	30	2.99
BaSF64	1.701	39	3.20
OF8035	1.800	35	3.56
Corning 1.9	1.885	31	3.99

PLASTICS

Name	n	V	Density (gm cm^{-3})
Acrylic (PMMA)	1.491	58	1.19*
CR39	1.498	58	1.32
Polycarbonate	1.586	30	1.20*
HL-II	1.560	40	1.27
Super 16	1.600	34	1.37
Teslalid	1.710	36	1.40

*Thermoplastic material

- High refractive index to give the thinnest possible finished lens.
- Low density so as not to give a finished lens that is too heavy.
- Hard surface so that it is robust enough to withstand the rough handling of daily use. Soft materials can have a hard coating applied to improve this property, but if a very hard coating is applied to a soft substrate there is always the risk of the coating cracking. Related to this is the ability of the material to be worked in the laboratory. Very hard material will take longer to surface or edge, and vice versa.
- Ease of tinting. Whereas at one time it was common to use glass dyed in the mass for tinted lenses, currently the vast majority of lenses are manufactured in untinted ('white') form, and subsequently tinted by surface coating.
- Resistance to chemical attack. Not only should a lens material be impervious to normal domestic solvents, it should also be resistant to atmospheric chemical attack, as well as to skin secretions. Some materials in the past have been prone to attack by common chemical agents, for example fruit juice and tobacco smoke.
- Must not cause adverse reactions in the wearer.

Spectacle lens materials can be readily divided into two categories – glass and plastics. (Note the description *plastics* to describe a material, the more common *plastic* being recommended for use as an adjective to describe the property of any material.)

There is a simple choice to be made with lens weight; for light lenses, use plastics materials. In general, plastics lenses are approximately half the weight of their glass counterparts. However, this simple approach conceals a more complex situation. The densities of both glass and plastics materials vary quite widely, as shown in the Table S.2.

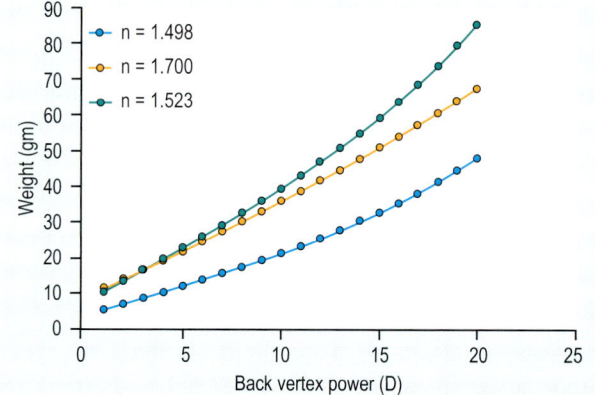

Figure S.11 • Calculated weights for lenses with the same characteristics as in Figure S.12 (from Charman, 1991).

It is not enough simply to compare lens weight and thickness imply on the basis of back vertex power. Other factors need to be taken into consideration, such as finished lens thickness and lens form. Figure S.11 shows a comparison of lens weights for three common lens materials. These values were calculated for circular uncut lenses, all made in plano-convex form with a fixed 1.0mm edge thickness. The three lens materials used are listed in Table S.3.

It will be apparent from Figure S.11 that although the high index glass is denser than crown, which is reflected in heavier lenses at low powers, at higher powers it actually gives lighter lenses. This is because the higher refractive index requires a smaller volume of lens material as a result of the flatter front surface curve on the lens. It should be pointed out, though, that except at

Table S.3 • Lens materials used to compare lens weight and thickness.

Material	n_d	V_d	Density (g.cm^{-3})
White ophthalmic crown glass	1.523	58	2.54
High index glass	1.700	30	2.99
CR39 plastic	1.498	59	1.32

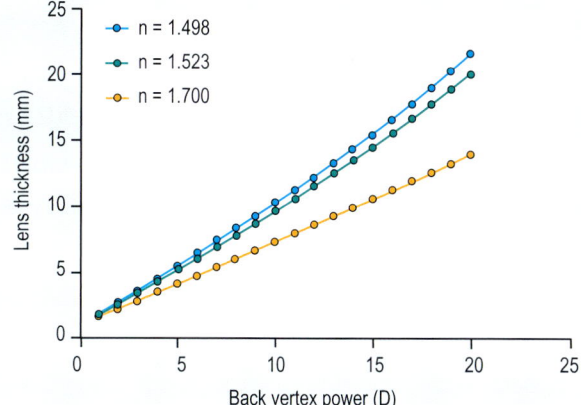

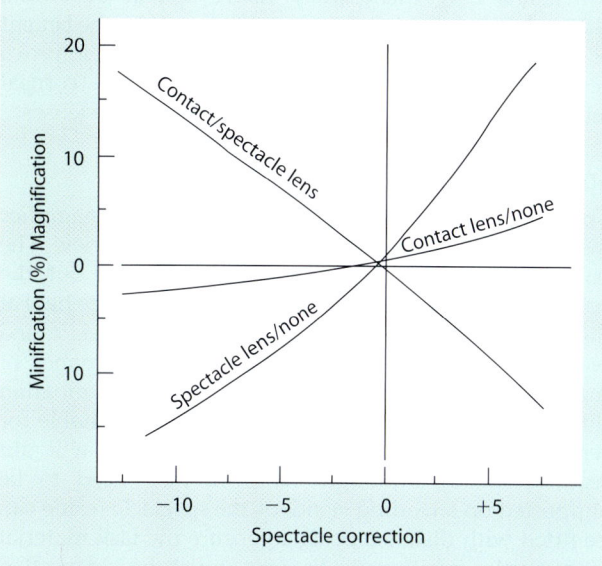

Figure S.13 • Typical values for spectacle magnification obtained with spectacle lens and contact lens corrections. The ratio of the two spectacle magnifications is shown. Effectivity has been allowed for, so that points on any vertical line refer to the same ametropia. Adapted from G. Westheimer (1962) The visual world of the new contact lens wearer. J. Am. Optom. Assoc. 39, 135–138.

Figure S.12 • Calculated thickness for a series of lenses made in materials CR39 ($n = 1.498$, density 1.32 gm cm^{-3}), crown glass ($n = 1.532$, density 2.54 gm cm^{-3}) and high index glass ($n = 1.700$, density 2.99 gm cm^{-3}). All lenses: 60 mm diameter, plano rear surface, 1.0 mm edge thickness (from Charman, 1991).

very high powers this weight saving is relatively small, and patients should not be promised significantly lighter lenses when using high refractive index glass.

The graphs for lens thickness (Figure S.12) are more straightforward. Lens thickness on the graphs is in order of refractive index for the conditions given here, where plus lenses are compared when finished to a common edge thickness of 1.0mm.

A comparison of minus power lenses is more difficult to make as these are not made to a standard centre thickness. CR39 lenses in negative powers are generally produced to a minimum thickness of 2.0mm, in order to retain mechanical stability. By comparison, glass lenses are surfaced down to 1.0mm or so at high minus powers. What is advisable as a centre thickness in minus lenses is a complex question, as thicker lenses will be less prone to accidental breakage, whereas thinner lenses will look better and weigh less. It will be noticed that some modern high refractive index plastic materials are more rigid than CR39 and can be made to a centre thickness in the order of 1.0mm in higher powers.

Spectacle magnification

Spectacle magnification, as its name implies, describes the ratio of the image size in the corrected ametropic eye to that in the uncorrected eye. It is particularly significant in cases of anisometropia (where after correction the differential magnification of the two retinal images may give rise to symptoms of aniseikonia) and with cylindrical errors (where the different magnifications in the two principal meridians caused by the correction may lead the patient to complain of distorted images).

The retinal images of any object in the eyes of an uncorrected ametrope have a size that is governed by the chief rays passing from the extremities of the object through the centres of the entrance and exit pupils of the eye. Each image point will, of course, be blurred. While placing a contact lens on the cornea does not affect the course of the chief ray, and hence does not alter the size of the retinal image, this is not the case with a spectacle lens. A positive correction increases the angle that the chief ray makes with respect to the axis, whereas a negative correction reduces it.

The spectacle magnification will be unity for contact lenses (vertex distance = 0), less than unity for negative, myopic spectacle corrections, and greater than one for positive corrections. Spectacle correction is often expressed as the percentage by which it differs from unity, so that a spectacle magnification of ×1.05 would be described as '5% magnification'.

In practice, corrections cannot strictly be treated as thin lenses and the entrance and exit pupils do not lie at the cornea. For practical purposes, the pupils may be taken as being situated about 3mm behind the cornea. Magnification is a function of both lens design and vertex distance (Figure S.13). Spectacle magnification is always close to unity for contact lenses, so that there are likely to be few magnification-related complaints from patients when moving directly from no correction to a contact lens correction, or from one contact lens correction to another. Casual contact lens wearers who normally wear spectacle corrections may theoretically notice spatial distortion, although for myopes this is counterbalanced by the benefit of relatively larger retinal images, which may improve acuity. Spectacle magnification effects after corneal refractive surgery are similar to those with contact lenses.

Spectacle mounted plus lens magnifiers

This type of magnifier has the shortest eye-to-magnifier distance, and consequently the largest field of view. The patient has both hands free to hold, or to carry out, the particular task. As the object being viewed must be held at the focal point of the magnifier lens, however, the limited working space is too restricted for the performance of most manipulative tasks, and makes task illumination difficult. Such magnifiers are therefore most suitable for reading (where the increased field of view will aid reading speed), although the print may need to be supported on a reading stand, or the spectacle frame can be fitted with distance posts, to ensure the task material is correctly positioned. Patients must be counselled carefully about why this restricted working distance is necessary. It may be appropriate for the patient to retain a pair of near spectacles or bifocals with a conventional addition (≤ +3.00DS) for near tasks such as preparing and eating food, checking money, etc.

Prescribing of spectacle-mounted plus lenses does not require any special equipment in the practice. The patient can be tested using standard trial-case lenses, and then the required lens form can be ordered from the prescription house. Various high-powered single vision (lenticular, aspheric, Hyperocular) and bifocal (solid, cemented, Franklin split) forms are available and can all be glazed into standard metal or plastic frames. This does not, however, allow the patient to see the cosmetic result of the finished spectacles or to try the device at home to judge its effectiveness, and the lenses will be expensive. It is better, if possible, to use a device ready-made in standard powers up to 20× magnification for patient evaluation, ordering prescription devices later if preferred. Such standard devices do not cater for the astigmatic patient, since cylindrical corrections are not incorporated, but it is possible to obtain clip-on aids to place over the patient's own spectacles. Typically, cylinder powers of less than 1.50DC do not influence the patient's acuity.

The patient using a spectacle-mounted plus lens will experience extremely blurred vision when looking up from the visual task, which may make them feel disorientated or nauseous. Bifocal, half-eye and clip-on/flip-up forms of these lenses are all available, and can help with this problem. See *Low vision aids, monocular versus binocular use*.

Spectacles

Spectacles, or glasses, are an optical appliance consisting of a pair of ophthalmic lenses mounted in a frame or rimless mount, resting on the nose and held in place by sides (sometimes called 'arms' or 'legs') extending from the outer edges of the frames or lens (if rimless) towards, and often curling around, the top of the ears. Spectacles are supported on the nose by a bridge containing nose pads or a plastic saddle. Spectacle frames are usually made from inert plastics or metal alloys.

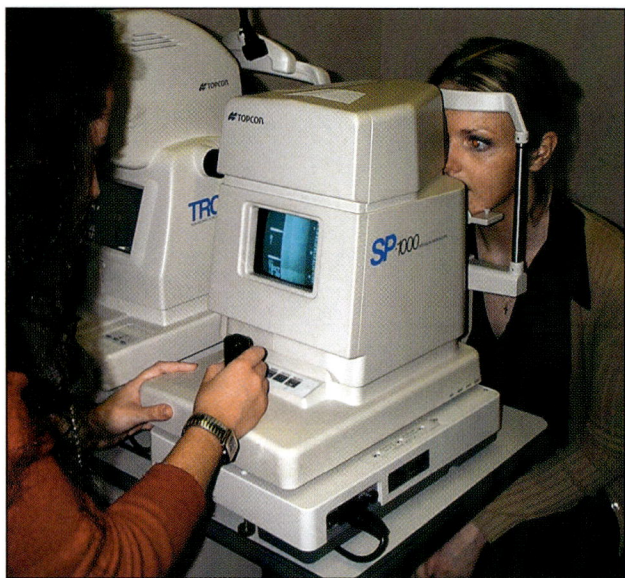

Figure S.14 • Specular microscope used for endothelial evaluation.

Spectacles with low vision aids
- See *Spectacle correction, plus lens magnifiers*; *Spectacle correction, telescopes*.

Spectrum Colour Vision Meter 712
- See *Anomaloscope*.

Specular microscope

The specular microscope allows viewing of objects illuminated from the same side as the light source, and the objective lens also acts as the condenser lens. Light passes from inside the microscope out through the objective lens to arrive at a focus near the focal plane of the lens. If this position coincides with a reflecting surface, the focused light is reflected back through the objective lens and is viewed through the eyepiece of the microscope. This technique enables high magnification images of the corneal epithelium and endothelium to be made, which would otherwise be difficult due to their transparency.

Early versions of the specular microscope used a contact dipping cone objective lens that was optically coupled to the cornea to provide higher magnification and resolution; however, most modern clinical specular microscopes can achieve equally high magnification without the need for ocular contact (Figure S.14). These instruments are primarily used to view and photograph the corneal endothelium and to monitor its morphology. By direct viewing with the specular microscope, an overall impression of the condition of the endothelium can be established immediately. In addition, some of these instruments allow corneal thickness to be determined by measuring the distance between the epithelium and endothelium.

Typically, the features looked for are the regularity of the endothelial mosaic, the size of the individual cells, the presence of intracellular vacuoles, and abnormal features such as corneal guttae and keratic precipitates.

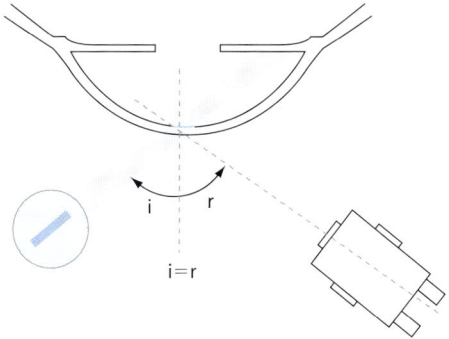

Figure S.15 • Specular reflection slit-lamp technique. Adapted from L. W. Jones, D.A. Jones (2001) Slit lamp biomicroscopy. In: N. Efron (ed.) The Cornea: its Examination in Contact Lens Practice, pp.1–49. Butterworth-Heinemann, Oxford.

From the images obtained, factors such as the number of cells per unit area, cell shape and cell area can be calculated, enabling the clinician to assess the endothelial appearance compared with that expected of normal age-matched individuals. This instrument can be used to investigate endothelial changes in a number of disease conditions, including posterior polymorphous dystrophy and Fuch's dystrophy, and in corneal surgery, refractive surgery and contact lens wear. In addition, deep stromal opacities such as glass foreign bodies, pigment deposits and corneal dystrophies can be imaged.

Specular reflection, slit-lamp technique of

This is a specific case of a parallelepiped set-up, where the angle of the incident slit beam is equal to the angle of the observation axis through one of the oculars (Figure S.15). At this angle (typically 40–50º) the illumination beam is reflected from the smooth surfaces of the anterior segment and provides a mirror-like reflection. Such specular images occur at every interface between structures of different refractive indices. The technique of specular reflection is typically used to view the endothelium, and may reveal changes such as endothelial blebs, guttae and polymegethism. However, even at ×40 magnification only a gross clinical judgement of the endothelium can be made as individual cells can be barely seen. The tear film lipid layer and the inferior tear meniscus can also be readily examined, as well as the anterior surface of the crystalline lens. If a contact lens is being worn, front surface wetting can be assessed and the post-lens tear film may be observed using specular reflection.

Spherical power equivalent rigid bitoric contact lens

- See *Compensated rigid bitoric lens*.

Spherical rigid contact lens designs

Spherical designs incorporating a spherical back optic zone with a number of flatter spherical peripheral zones are the most widely used and readily understood form of rigid lens. The peripheral zone is generally 1–2mm in width and is composed of one to four peripheral curves. Tricurve designs (i.e. a central curve plus two peripheral zones) are probably the most commonly used lens form.

Bicurve designs are occasionally used with small lenses (e.g. 8.5mm). Tetracurve and other multicurve designs are used with larger lenses, or where a smoother transition is required between the peripheral zones.

The front surfaces of most spherical designs are bicurve, incorporating an optic zone slightly larger than the back optic zone diameter (BOZD), and a front surface peripheral zone. The curvature of the front optic zone is governed by the required lens power, and that of the peripheral zone by the edge thickness, power and front optic zone diameter (FOZD) of the lens; these parameters are invariably calculated by the manufacturing laboratory. Monocurve front surface designs (single-cut) are occasionally used in small, low-power lenses, but most lenses are lenticulated (i.e. made with a thinner peripheral zone) in order to reduce mass and overall thickness. Multicurve front surface designs are occasionally used with higher-power lenses in order to reduce peripheral thickness.

Spin casting

This process can be used to manufacture soft lenses. A convex 'male-shaped' stainless steel tool, or 'insert', is produced on a high-precision engineering lathe and lapped to provide an accurate surface that matches the dry dimensions of the proposed anterior surface of the contact lens. The final surface shape of the steel master is verified using interferometry. Any given tool can be used to make millions of moulds. The steel tool is impressed against heated liquid polypropylene, which then cools and sets to form a solid plastic concave female mould. A series of about eight tools is used to produce eight moulds simultaneously.

The xerogel lens form is created by pouring liquid monomers into the concave moulds, which spin at a high rate about the central mould axis. This takes place in a controlled atmosphere of carbon dioxide at high temperature. The shape of the mould defines the form of the front surface of the lens. The shape of the back surface is governed by centrifugal force generated by the rate of spin of the mould, surface tension and friction forces between the mould and polymer, and the effects of gravity. A greater speed of rotation of the mould will result in more polymer mass being shifted towards the lens periphery, and more negative lens power.

As the mould spin rate stabilizes, a catalytic monomer is added and ultraviolet radiation is introduced to initiate polymerization. The lens is removed from the mould, and the mould is discarded. The edges of the lens are polished, and the lens is inspected, hydrated, re-inspected, packaged and autoclaved. In modern industrial settings (Figure S.16), spin casting can produce a much higher lens yield than lathe cutting, but still can not match the high volume of lenses that can be produced by cast moulding.

Spoilation, contact lens

- See *Deposits, lens*.

Sport, contact lenses for

Sport and recreation are often cited as key reasons for seeking contact lenses. With modern contact lens

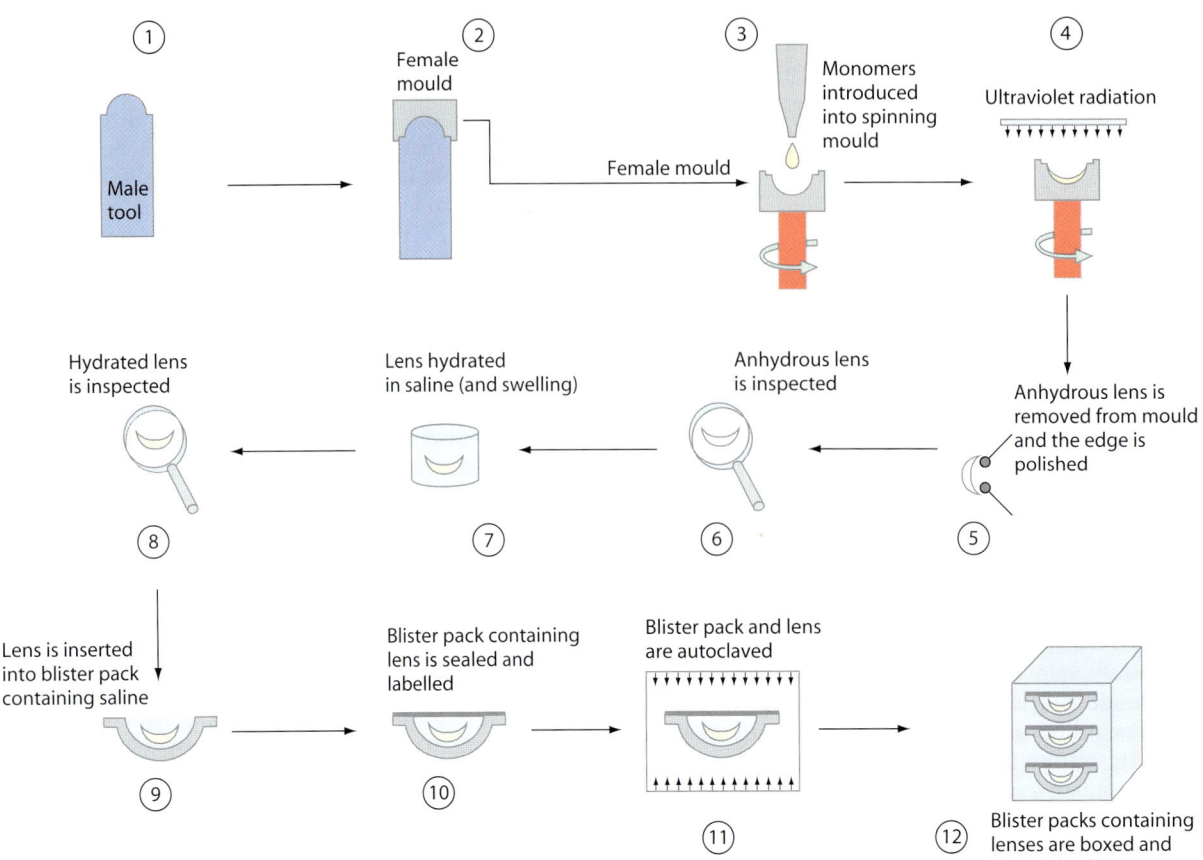

Figure S.16 • Schematic representation of a production line for spin cast manufacturing of soft contact lenses.

technology, there is no reason why an ametropic sportsperson cannot compete with a normally sighted opponent on an equal basis from the standpoint of visual function. The three primary vision correction options are soft contact lenses, rigid contact lenses, or spectacles. Scleral lenses are sometimes prescribed, but only if circumstances dictate the necessity. A comparison of the key features of the three primary options is presented in Table S.4. Refractive surgery, of course, represents a more radical alternative.

The choice of contact lens for use in a given sport must be made with reference to the length of time that it takes to play the sport, the environment in which it is played, and the general physical demands of the sport. The majority of sports are completed within 2 hours, which equates to a total period of lens wear of 4 hours, allowing for pre- and post-match activity during which lens insertion and removal would be impractical and/or undesirable. Even when these factors are understood, the lens of first choice may not be obvious. The most appropriate lens is sometimes only determined by trial and error.

Sports are played in almost every environment. Perhaps the only environment that is not sought for the playing of sport is extreme heat. The most suitable lenses for various environmental conditions are as follows:

- cold – large-diameter, medium water content soft lenses
- altitude – high oxygen performance silicone hydrogel lenses
- dirt and dust – large-diameter soft lenses; rigid lenses are prone to trap debris beneath the lens and are clearly contraindicated
- aquatic sports – large-diameter, medium water content lenses; goggles worn over contact lenses will, in the same way as worn by a non-lens wearer, ensure good vision, and help to preserve ocular health and reduce lens loss
- sub-aquatic sports – silicone hydrogel lenses, to facilitate the escape of nitrogen gas from beneath the lens; good blinking is important
- ultraviolet light – goggles with UV-absorbing tints, to be worn over UV-absorbing contact lenses, constitute an extra precaution for periods when the mask is removed; skiers should be reminded to also apply UV-protection creams to the remaining exposed skin on the face and neck. See *Prophylactic tints*.

The most suitable lenses for various physical situations are as follows:

- extreme body movements – large-diameter soft lenses; rigid lenses are contraindicated
- body contact – large-diameter soft lenses, with supplementary eye and face protection via the use of helmets and masks; rigid lenses are contraindicated
- air flow – large-diameter, medium water content lenses with enclosed goggles; rigid lenses are

Table S.4 • Comparison of soft lenses versus rigid lenses versus spectacle lenses for the sportsperson.

characteristic	soft lenses	rigid lenses	spectacle lenses
field of view	full	full	restricted
stability of vision (post-blink)	excellent	good	excellent
glare	none	in low light	none
glare protection tint possible	cosmetic only	no	yes
UV protection tint possible	yes	yes	yes
initial comfort	good	poor	good
long-term comfort	good	good	good
adaptation required	very little	yes	sometimes
suitability for intermittent use	yes	not usually	yes
disposability viable	yes	no	no
risk of loss	low	moderate	low
risk of dislodgement during wear	low	moderate	high
risk of damage during wear	low	low	high
risk of damage with handling	high	low	low
ease of care	multiple-step	fewer steps	simple
initial cost	moderate	high	high
ongoing costs	high	moderate	none
cost to correct astigmatism	high	low	low
bifocal correction possible	compromise	very difficult	yes
use in rain	good	good	poor
susceptibility to fog up	no	no	yes
susceptibility to dirt up	no	no	yes
risk of complication	low	negligible	none

contraindicated, and good blinking activity is required if goggles are not worn
- gravitational forces – large, tight-fitting soft lenses.

The following points are of particular relevance to the prescription and aftercare management of those involved in sport:
- for young sportspersons participating in outdoor sports, prescribe minimum plus power to facilitate sharp far-distance viewing
- silicone hydrogel lenses worn on an extended-wear basis are indicated for endurance events of such as rally car driving
- contact lenses are contraindicated (in favour of spectacles) for sports requiring critical static visual acuity, such as archery and shooting
- for routine contact lens care, the best time is immediately following the conclusion of the season
- athletes often come into contact with grip rosin, grease, tape dressings and ointments that are toxic to the eye and highly irritative, as well as dirt, soil or general contaminants; thus, hygiene and general compliance must be emphasized
- since contact lenses will not shield the eye from potential trauma, the usual protective eyewear or headgear used in a given sport should also be used by sportspersons wearing contact lenses
- for presbyopic sportspersons, monovision is generally contraindicated, and a spectacle over-correction is often the best option.

Squamous cells of the epithelium
- See *Corneal epithelium*.

Squint
- See *Esotropia; Exotropia; Hypertropia and hypotropia*.

Stabilization of rigid toric contact lenses

Three techniques are used to stabilize rigid toric lenses:

1. Toroidal back surface. With lenses incorporating a toroidal back surface, rotation is generally not a problem due to the stabilizing effect of the toric back surface on the toric cornea (provided there is sufficient corneal toricity).

2. Prism ballast. This is the most commonly used method of lens stabilization for rigid lenses that have toroidal front surfaces combined with spherical back optic zones. With prism ballasting, the lens is prescribed in the normal manner with the addition of between 1 and 3^Δ. When ordering the lens, practitioners assume that the weight or prism ballast orientates the lens in a certain fixed position on the cornea and order the cylinder axis with respect to this position. To avoid recording the prism base position as 'down along 90' or 'down along 100', its actual location is recorded as being at 270 or 280, respectively. Prism ballast may also be used in combination with a toroidal back surface where the corneal astigmatism of the patient is too small

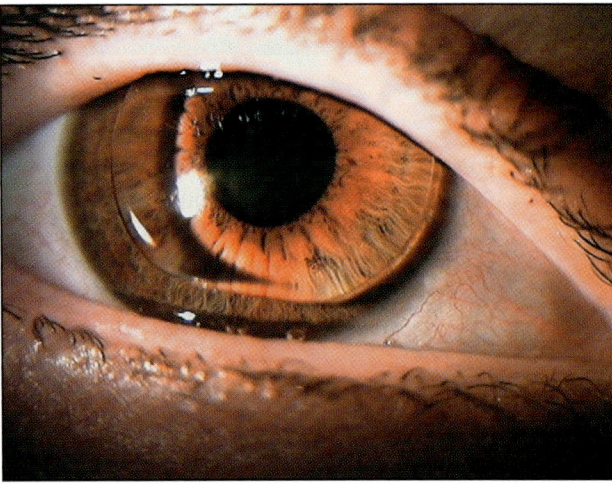

Figure S.17 • A prism-ballasted rigid toric lens with a single truncation designed to align with the lower lid.

(< 2.00D) to maintain the proper position of a bitoric lens but large enough (>1.00D) to cause a front toric lens to become unstable. Prism ballasting can often cause rigid lenses to sit inferiorly, causing patients to experience symptoms of discomfort and flare.

3. Truncation. A truncation is created by slicing off the bottom of the lens in such a way that when the truncation rests against the lower lid, the lens will adopt the correct orientation in the eye (Figure S.17). Truncations can also be added to front surface toric lenses if prism ballasting is insufficient to stabilize the lens. Truncations can be uncomfortable for the patient, and they are not always successful in preventing lens rotation. Consequently, a soft toric contact lens is generally preferred to a rigid toric contact lens when fitting patients who have significant residual astigmatism but negligible corneal astigmatism.

See *Compensated rigid bitoric lenses; Cylindrical power equivalent rigid toric lenses; Induced astigmatism with rigid toric lenses; Residual astigmatism with rigid toric lenses; Toric lens design, rigid; Toric lens, rigid.*

Stabilization of soft toric contact lenses

All forms of soft toric lenses need to be stabilized so that the toric optics of the lens can be maintained in the correct orientation so as to correct the ocular astigmatism. The aim is to minimize rotation from the ideal in-eye orientation. The orientation of a soft toric lens on the eye must be predictable and consistent, otherwise sub-optimal vision will result. The following stabilization techniques can be employed:

1. Toroidal back surface. It is thought by some that a soft toric lens with a toric back surface will generally locate better than a front surface toric lens, because it is believed that the back toric surface is more likely to align with, or 'lock on' to, the matching toroidal corneal surface. However, experience has shown that a toroidal back surface alone is insufficient to achieve lens stabilization.

2. Prism ballast. The theory of prism ballast is that base down prism is incorporated into the lens so that the lens will be heavier at the prism base (due to excess lens mass). Gravity then acts to cause the prism base to locate inferiorly. This effect, however, is minimal. Prism ballast lenses work not because of the extra weight of the prism base, but because the thin apical zone is squeezed between the upper lid and eyeball.

3. Peri-ballast. This method of lens stabilization features a lens with a minus carrier (peripheral zone), with the carrier being thicker inferiorly. In other words, the prismatic thickness profile changes are confined to the lens carrier, where the carrier is thinner superiorly (prism base down).

4. Truncation. Truncation refers to the technique of slicing off the bottom of the lens, so as to form a 'shelf' that will rest upon (and therefore align with) the lower lid. There are problems with the use of truncation in soft toric lens fitting. The truncated edge can make the soft lens uncomfortable to wear, and the measurement of the lid angle can be difficult and imprecise. Quite often the truncation does not work, with the lid angle appearing to have no effect on the positioning or location of the truncated lens. Instability can occur with oblique cylinders because of the uneven thickness produced by them. For these reasons, soft toric lens truncation is rarely used today.

5. Dynamic stabilization. The technique of dynamic stabilization is currently the most commonly used method of stabilization for soft toric lenses (Figure S.18). With this technique, the dominant lens orientation effect is achieved by pressure from the upper lid (primarily) and the lower lid. The pressure exerted on the thin zones of a lens between the upper lid and globe and between the inferior lid and globe causes the lens to orientate correctly, with the thick zone of the lens lying horizontally between the lids.

See *Toric lens fitting, soft; Toric lens rotation, soft; Toric lens, soft.*

Staff, optometry practice
- See *Personnel, optometry practice.*

Staff training in optometry practice

Staff training embraces the identification and development of employee potential for job satisfaction, improvement, practice value creation and ultimately improved patient care. It can often be the driver of improvements, and has the potential to bring about reduced costs, increased value and practice profitability. Ultimately, training is about getting people to do different things or to do things differently.

For training to be effective for the practice, however, it must be:

- valid – i.e. relevant to jobs in the practice, and to the overall style of the practice (e.g. a specialty contact lens practice)

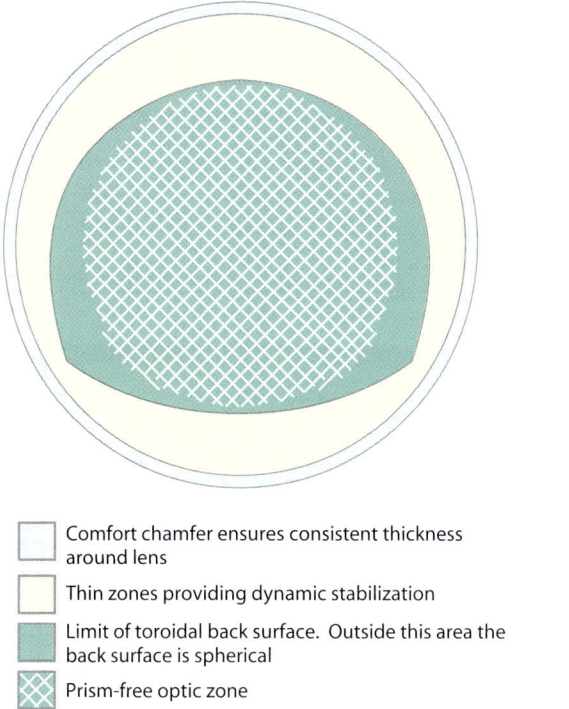

Figure S.18 • Design features of a soft toric lens that help to minimize lens rotation by dynamic stabilization. Note the prism-free optic zone in the toroidal region of the lens.

- capable of solving problems identified as needing resolution in practice
- focused on objectives, either at the individual or at the job/practice level
- measurable, with results that can be gauged directly or indirectly.
- Improvements that training and development bring should result in reduced costs and increased value and profits through (for example):
- improved efficiency – doing the job correctly, accurately and with care at the outset reduces replacements, unplanned rescheduling and revisits to the practice by patients, and this improves utilization of resources and practice output overall
- improved quality – this enhances the reputation of the practice, and reduces complaints, costs of returns, refunds and credits
- less wastage and re-working – this leads to less material being wasted, but the greater cost saving is in the staff costs, the time for which the equipment is occupied, and the ancillary costs in re-working the job by the laboratory (e.g. a complete pair of spectacles, alternative set of contact lenses etc.)
- improved consulting room and equipment utilization – consulting room occupancy and equipment use dictates the capacity of the practice to conduct eye exams and contact lens consultations; an unnecessarily occupied or indeed unoccupied consulting room is costly
- reduced time taken to do jobs – less time taken to produce same or better quality products will translate to reduced staff costs relative to sales revenues
- improved time management – this translates to improved patient scheduling and staff usage, which will lead to reduced staff costs relative to sales revenues
- reduced staff turnover – this means that costs of recruitment, selection, training and reduced efficiency are not unnecessarily incurred
- reduced accidents and equipment 'downtime' – this reduces costs to the practice in terms of sick pay, 'down time' of equipment, compensation claims, insurance premiums, unscheduled service costs and replacements
- reduced sickness and absenteeism – greater job satisfaction means better staff morale and efficient teamwork.

Training alone is not the driver of these benefits. Other factors that affect these issues include economic, political and employment situations locally and in the country. An important decision for the practice owner/manager is to decide what training can be done by the practice itself and what external support will be required.

Stand mounted plus lens magnifiers

In order to maintain image clarity and optimum magnification, a plus lens magnifier must be kept at a precise distance away from the object being viewed. This positioning is very critical, with slight alterations in object distance producing large changes in the vergence of light leaving the magnifier, usually creating a noticeably blurred image for the patient. A simple solution is to place the magnifier lens on a stand so that an accurate working distance is easily maintained; this is particularly useful when the patient has hand tremor or weakness. It is especially beneficial in high-powered lenses where depth of field is restricted. This is the principle of the stand magnifier, of which there are two main categories:

Variable focus – these are usually large diameter, low-powered lenses, held on an adjustable or flexible stand, sometimes with illumination incorporated, or suspended around the neck on a cord. The patient can freely select the position of the object plane but maximum magnification is achieved by placing the object as far behind the lens as possible before it starts to blur. The fact that the lens is supported leaves the patient's hands free, and avoids fatigue. These lenses are used most frequently by those wishing to write or do handicrafts.

Fixed focus – these magnifiers are usually designed so that the magnifier-to-object distance is less than the anterior focal length of the lens, and the object is closer to the lens than its focal point (Figure S.19). The height of the stand is fixed. Stand design and construction are critical to the success of the device. A firm and robust stand completely surrounding the lens is best for accurate location of the lens, but prevents access to the working plane for manipulative tasks. The bottom of the stand should not be visible to the patient as they look through the lens, or it will further restrict the limited field of view. As the stand is likely to obstruct ambient light falling on the task, these magnifiers are most commonly available with built-in illumination, which avoids the need to arrange separate task lighting. The stand – and the power supply in the case of an internally illuminated design – may

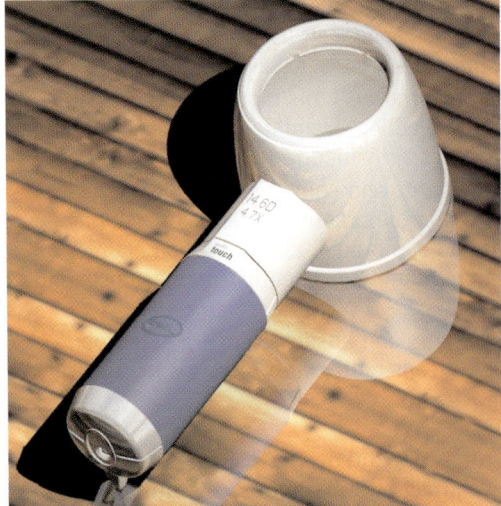

Figure S.19 • Fixed focus stand magnifier with built-in illumination (reproduced with permission of COIL Low Vision Products UK).

Table S.5 • x, y chromaticity coordinates for standard light sources.

Light source	x, y chromaticity coordinates	
	x	y
Source A (Tungsten)	0.448	0.407
Source B (direct sunlight)	0.348	0.352
Source C ('north sky')	0.310	0.316

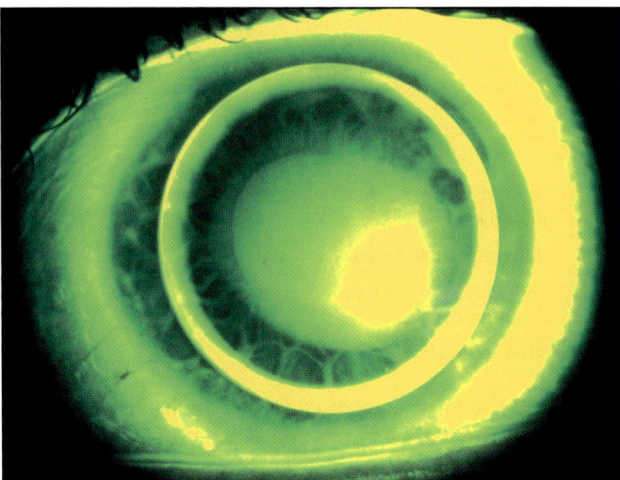

Figure S.20 • Steep-fitting rigid lens revealed by fluorescein.

make the magnifier heavy and unwieldy to carry around. See *Spectacle correction, plus lens magnifiers*.

Standard illuminants

Incandescent light sources contain substances which emit radiation when heated to high temperatures. The amount of energy released varies with temperature. Sources which emit a wide range of wavelengths appear white and are specified by the equivalent temperature of a perfect (black body) radiator.

The CIE has specified x, y chromaticity coordinates for different colour temperature whites (Table S.5). Source A represents tungsten emission (reddish-white) and has a colour temperature of 2856° Kelvin, Source B is equivalent to direct sunlight and Source C represents no direct sunlight equivalent to north sky illumination in the northern hemisphere (bluish-white) and has a colour temperature of 6700° Kelvin. Source D65 (6500° Kelvin) is similar to Source C but has additional ultraviolet content. See *CIE chromaticity diagram 1931*.

The choice of illuminant has implications with respect to colour vision testing because colour appearance varies according to the spectral content of the illuminant. Colour vision tests composed of pigment colours are designed to be illuminated with Standard Source C or Source D65 to preserve the intended colour design. Appropriate illumination can be achieved with natural daylight or an equivalent incandescent light source. The MacBeth Easel lamp is the illuminant of choice for colour vision tests but several other satisfactory illuminants are available including colour corrected fluorescent lamps with colour temperatures of at least 6500° Kelvin. Light sources with a colour rendering index close to 100 have good colour reproduction capabilities. The MacBeth Easel lamp is equivalent to Source C and provides 350 to 400 lux (approximately 100 candelas per square metre). Tungsten illumination is unsatisfactory for colour vision tests.

Steady eye strategy
- See *Eccentric viewing and steady eye strategy*.

Steep contact lens fit

A lens that has a curvature greater than that of the anterior eye (especially the cornea) is deemed to be fitting steep. The degree of steepness cannot be predicted simply by comparing the back optic zone radius of the lens with central corneal curvature, because the curvature of both the lens and the cornea can change dramatically towards the periphery. In general, a steep-fitting lens will appear to be tight. A steep rigid lens fit, when examined using fluorescein, will display a broad region of central clearance and substantial peripheral bearing (Figure S.20).

Stereopsis

Stereopsis is the perception of the relative depth of objects based on binocular disparity, and it can be assessed using qualitative (Lang two-pencil test) or quantitative (Titmus, Frisby, TNO and Lang stereo tests) methods.

Lang two-pencil test. This test investigates the presence of stereopsis by comparing the patient's response with both eyes open and with one eye covered. The patient holds a pencil vertically and is instructed to place it exactly on top of a pencil held by the examiner. The patient uses horizontal disparity clues to locate the correct position. The test is then repeated with one eye closed. If accuracy in locating the pencil is repeatedly better with both eyes open then stereopsis is present. If the response is similar with both eyes open and the squinting eye covered, the squinting eye is suppressed and binocular single vision is absent.

Titmus test (Wirt). The image seen by one eye is polarized at 90° to that seen by the other eye when viewed through

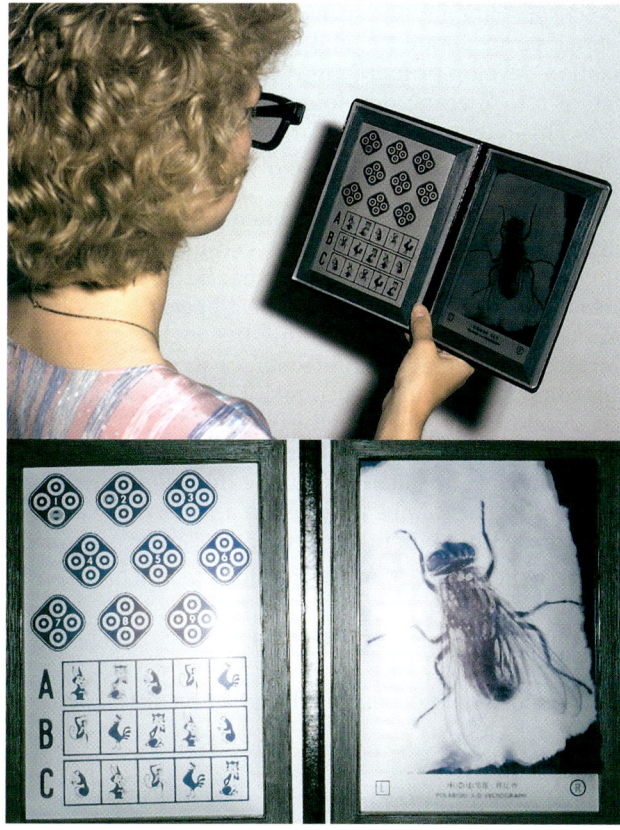

Figure S.21 • Titmus test.

Frisby stereotest. This is the only clinical test based on actual depth where random shapes are printed on three clear plastic plates of different thickness. The test does not require any form of dissociative glasses. Each plate has four squares of curved random shapes and one square contains a 'hidden' circle that is printed on the opposite surface to the squares. Disparities range from 600 to 15 seconds of arc. Care should be taken that neither the plates nor the patient's head significantly move during testing as this can provide monocular clues. The thickest plate is held in front of a plane white background and the patient is questioned as to the position of the hidden circle. The plate can be rotated or turned over to change the position of the circle to reduce false-positive responses due to learning. If the first plate is recognized successfully then the thinner plates are presented in the same fashion.

TNO test. This test is based on random dot stereograms and uses red and green glasses for dissociation. The disparities range from 1,980 to 15 seconds of arc. The test is performed at 40cm wearing the red and green glasses supplied and the plates are shown in sequence. This is probably the best test of stereopsis as there are no monocular clues or contours.

Lang stereotest. The targets consist of vertical sections that are seen alternately by each eye as they are viewed through the built-in cylindrical lens elements (Figure S.22). Displacement of the random dots creates the disparity which ranges from 1,200 to 550 seconds of arc on the Lang I card and from 600 to 200 seconds of arc on the Lang II card. The cards are held at the normal reading distance for the subject, who is asked to name or point to the pictures. Pre-verbal children are observed looking at the pictures or attempting to pick them up.

polarized glasses. The disparities range from 3,000 to 40 seconds of arc. The targets comprise a fly, animals and set of circles (Figure S.21). Monocular clues are present when viewing the first three sets of circles and animals. The test is performed at 40cm with the patient wearing polarized glasses. The patient is first asked to pick up the wings of the fly. The animals and circles are then presented until the stereoscope image can no longer be identified.

Stereo-acuity is reduced if suppression is present although it should be noted that 2 per cent of the binocular population are stereo-blind. The use of sensitive stereo tests will also confirm the presence of good vision since it is impossible to achieve good stereopsis without good acuity in both eyes.

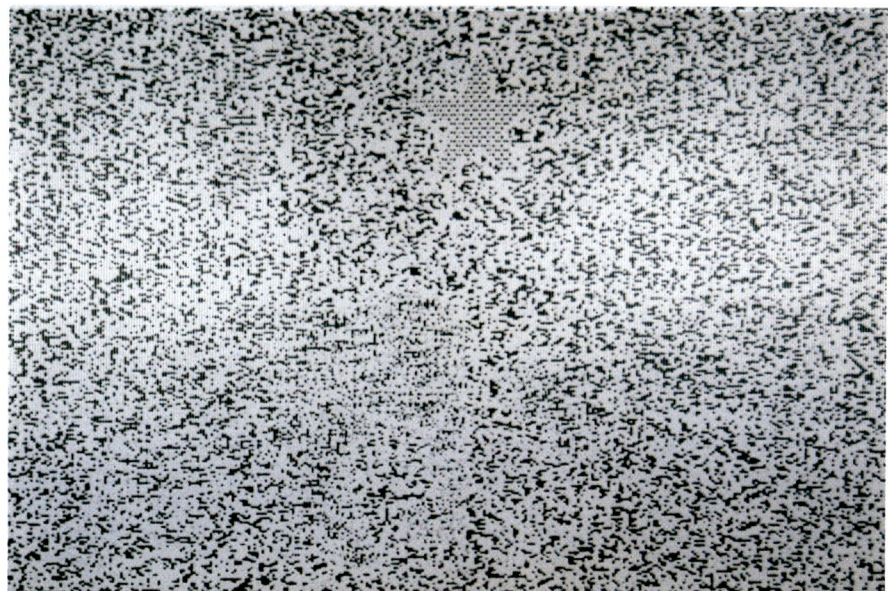

Figure S. 22 • Lang stereotest.

Stevens-Johnson syndrome
- See *Eyelid pathology, therapeutic lenses for*.

Stiles-Crawford effect
Cone spectral sensitivity is greatly reduced if light enters the eye obliquely at the pupil margin. Monochromatic light appears to change in both hue and saturation due to the wave guide properties of the cone receptors. This phenomenon is known as the Stiles-Crawford effect. Rods do not have directional sensitivity.

Stock kept unit, contact lens
- See *Practice logistics*.

Stock contact lenses
- See *Practice logistics*.

Storage case, contact lens
An important component of the complete lens care system is the case in which the lenses and disinfecting solutions are stored. Surveys have reported that up to 77% of lens cases are contaminated with bacteria and 8% with Acanthamoeba. Contamination appears to be unrelated to solution type, and it is now clear that the development of microbial biofilms in contact lens cases can reduce the effect of a disinfecting solution. Indeed, it has been speculated that long-term use of a solution might select a naturally resistant population of microbes that adapt to survive exposure to a disinfectant. Interestingly, some bacteria release catalase when their cell membranes are disrupted; this release could potentially act to neutralize local hydrogen peroxide and protect other bacteria within the biofilm.

The careful cleaning of lens cases has been advocated by some practitioners. This can include measures such as manually scrubbing the case (using a cotton-wool bud or new toothbrush) with cooled boiled water, or submersing the case in boiling water on a regular basis. However, with compliance acknowledged to be poor in a high proportion of lens wearers, this approach might be unrealistic. Certainly, rinsing the contact lens case with fresh disinfecting solution after lens insertion and leaving the case open to air dry is likely to be helpful. It is clear, however, that the regular replacement of contact lens cases for both soft and rigid lenses is an effective method of reducing this potential problem. Many manufacturers assist practitioners in this regard by supplying a new contact lens case with each bottle of disinfecting solution.

Strabismus surgery
The objective of strabismus surgery is primarily to restore comfortable binocular vision and/or to improve the patient's appearance. Whether or not both of these objectives are fulfilled depend largely on the age and binocular status of the patient at the time of surgery. If the level of co-ordination between the two eyes was poor during visual immaturity, then visual functions such as fusion and stereopsis will not have developed normally, and subsequently sensory adaptations to the ocular misalignment may occur.

Sensory adaptations such as suppression, anomalous retinal correspondence and amblyopia and eccentric fixation develop primarily in younger children. After the age of 6 to 7 years, development of these anomalies is rare. This suggests that ocular misalignment in visually immature patients is a strong incentive to perform corrective surgery.

Anomalous retinal correspondence will always be of clinical significance, primarily because any surgical alignment of the two eyes might not be accepted by the visual system and may cause post-operative diplopia. Another important factor is how the angle of deviation varies with the patient's direction of gaze. Whether the deviation is comitant or incomitant is largely dictated by the location of the lesion in the ocular motor system.

The goal of strabismic surgery is to correct ocular misalignment by altering muscle function or muscle mechanics. This can be achieved in a variety of ways but most procedures will fit into one of three main categories:
- Weakening procedures (decreasing the pull of the muscles)
- Strengthening procedures (enhancing the pull of the muscle)
- Transposition procedures (changing the direction of the muscle).

Stress test, contact lens
- See *Extended wear*.

Striae
- See *Oedema*.

Stroma
- See *Corneal stroma*.

Stromal edema
- See *Oedema*.

Stromal microdots
- See *Microdots*.

Stromal neovascularization
- See *Neovascularization*.

Stromal oedema
- See *Oedema*.

Stromal opacities
- See *Deep stromal opacities*.

Stromal thinning
Although low levels of stromal oedema during the day may appear to be harmless, there is a growing body of evidence indicating that chronic oedema may compromise the physiological integrity of the cornea. It is now clear that long-term extended wear of hydrogel lenses can induce a slight thinning of the stroma. Whereas the extent of stromal oedema varies with the prevailing level of

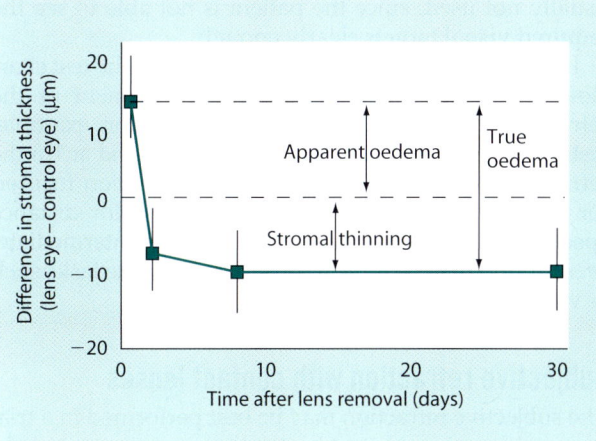

Figure S.23 • Change in corneal thickness of lens-wearing eyes (compared with 'normal' non-lens-wearing eyes; the dotted zero line) after ceasing wear of hydrogel lenses that had been worn on an extended wear basis for 5 years. When the lenses were removed (t=0), the lens-wearing eye was apparently about 14μm thicker than the normal eye. However, after 7 days, when all oedema had subsided, the cornea of the lens-wearing eye was about 25μm thinner than it had been originally, representing the true oedema. This suggests that long-term extended hydrogel lens wear induced 11μm of stromal thinning.

corneal oxygenation and dissipates upon removal of hypoxic stress, stromal thinning is a chronic and apparently irreversible tissue change observed in patients who have worn lenses for many years.

Extended wear of hydrogel lenses causes the stroma to thin at a rate of 2μm per year (Figure S.23). This phenomenon can be of clinical significance; for example, patients who have worn contact lenses for many years may be precluded from undergoing laser ablative refractive surgery if too much thinning has occurred.

The phenomenon of contact lens induced stromal thinning does not confound or invalidate interpretation of the clinical signs of stromal oedema. Striae, folds and haze represent a given level of oedema irrespective of whether or not the stroma has thinned.

It is presumed that stromal thinning is due to the effects of chronic oedema, and two mechanisms may be postulated to explain how this might occur. First, stromal keratocytes may lose their ability to synthesize new stromal tissue due to the direct effects of tissue hypoxia, and/or the indirect effects of chronic lens-induced tissue acidosis due to an accumulation of lactic acid and carbonic acid. Second, constantly elevated levels of lactic acid associated with chronic oedema may lead to some dissolution of the mucopolysaccharide ground substance of the stroma. Recent evidence obtained using confocal microscopy demonstrates a loss of stromal keratocytes following long-term hydrogel lens wear.

Subjective refraction

Subjective refraction might be defined as the measurement of a patient's refractive error by the use of corrective lenses to achieve the best possible image reported by the patient. This necessarily means that the accuracy of the measurement is dependent upon patient response, and therefore patient understanding of what is being presented to them and the degree to which they understand what is required of them in interpreting the presentation. Another potential source of error is inadequate control of the patient's accommodation during assessment which may lead to an over-minussed correction being prescribed. Typically lenses are presented either by placing them in a trial frame or within a phoropter in front of the patient. Care must be taken to note the back vertex distance of the main spherical lens and where the correction is greater than 5.00D, changes of a few millimetres between the examination distance and the final correcting appliance vertex distances may introduce significant error. The vertex distance may be underestimated when the lenses are not placed in the back cell of the trial frame and also when using a poorly positioned phoropter.

As far as possible, the refraction should be carried out in an environment as close to that in which the patient will be using any final corrective appliance – typically normal room illumination and binocularly. Too dark a consulting room, or indeed the use of an occluder, may lead to error due to aberrations from the dilated pupils. Binocular refraction has other advantages. The use of a positive fogging lens (typically to reduce visual acuity to around 6/12) in front of the non-assessed eye will act as a septum but still allow appreciation of a reduction in clarity upon accommodation. The patient is therefore forced to relax accommodation. This is essential for those with high accommodative reserve (children), pseudomyopes with a spasm of accommodation or latent hypermetropes who are used to constant accommodation. It also helps maximize visual potential in latent nystagmus and avoid the influence of cyclophoria if present. This latter point is essential in refraction prior to refractive surgery. As accommodation is controlled, binocular balancing is unnecessary which may speed up the refraction, again important where patient attention is a factor, such as with young children. Only where binocular refraction is impossible (as with markedly different acuities or very strong ocular dominance) or where the data from just one eye is needed (as with a monocular over-refraction of a contact lens) should monocular refraction be considered.

Whether using an occluder or fogging lens, subjective refraction follows a set sequence; measurement of the best vision sphere, the axis and power of the cylinder and finally a check of the sphere power again. This is carried out for each eye. After monocular refraction of each eye binocular balancing should be undertaken in patients who still have accommodation. See *Best vision sphere, determination of; Binocular balancing; Cross-cylinder technique; Duochrome test; Fan and block technique; Refraction end-point.*

Subjective refraction, low vision

Subjective confirmation of refractive correction is often unreliable or imprecise if acuity is poor, so it is important to assess the refractive error objectively if possible. The retinoscopic reflex can be made brighter by using radical retinoscopy at a very short working distance. A prescription may also be obtained from neutralizing previous spectacles, although the presence of a balance lens must be considered.

The patient should view a letter chart which contains circular letters which can be used for subjective confirmation of cylindrical corrections, and must view from a distance at which they can see a line of at least 5 letters. Full-aperture trial lenses placed in a trial frame are preferred since it is important that the patient can adopt different head and eye positions, and that these can be monitored. If the current spectacle prescription is >±10.00DS then it is more appropriate to conduct an over-refraction, placing any additional trial lenses in a Halberg Clip. This ensures that prescription changes are genuine and not simply the result of a difference in the vertex distance between the trial frame and the spectacle frame. With the final prescription present, the resultant combined power when added to the spectacles can be measured using a focimeter.

Spherical lens confirmation should begin with large steps of power. A starting point can be selected on the basis of the recorded vision, although this can be modified later. The denominator of the Snellen acuity at 6m should be divided by 60: thus 6/60 acuity would suggest 6°/60 = ±1.00DS steps; 2/60 when converted to 6m would be 6/180, giving 18°/60 = ±3.00DS steps. The test chart should be placed at a reduced distance so that the patient can read at least three to four lines of letters since this will give a better basis for comparison. All lens choices offered should be successive comparisons for a defined visual target within a short space of time (e.g. 'Is the second line of letters clearer with lens 1 or lens 2?'; 'Is the letter T more distinct with this lens or without it?') since alterations in the patient's gaze angle may produce spontaneous changes in acuity which do not relate to the lenses used. All results should be checked several times, and the size of the changes in lens power can be reduced if the patient is giving confident and repeatable responses. Nonetheless, it may only be possible to 'bracket' the final prescription, to determine, for example, that with a +4.00DS lens in place the patient reports that an extra −1.00DS improves vision, but with +3.00DS in place he or she prefers an extra +1.00DS, leading to a final prescription of +3.50DS. Any attempt to use smaller steps of power change to confirm this (±0.50DS, for example) may cause the patient to become unsure.

To check the cylindrical component, a ±1.00DC cross cylinder (which gives a 2.00DC difference between alternate positions) can be used to optimize the clarity of a circular letter of a size two lines above the lowest read. Alternatively, if the objectively determined cylinder is >1.00DC, simply increase the axis by 20° from its current position, and ask the patient to compare the shape and clarity of the target in the two positions; that is, at the original axis, or 20° from that. Repeat by rotating the cylinder between its original position and one with an axis decreased by 20°. If the patient is confident in their responses, the rotation can be reduced to 10°. When the axis has been fixed by bracketing, power increases and decreases at that axis can be tried. The patient should be given more opportunities to make each subjective judgement, allowing comparison of two alternatives repeatedly. Confirmatory refractive tests (such as the equality of appearance of targets on the red and green backgrounds in the duochrome test, or the expected degree of blurring produced by a +1.00DS lens) are usually not used, since the patient is not able to see the required visual targets clearly enough.

If the refraction has been carried out with the test chart closer than 6m, the final spherical component of the refractive error will be over-plussed – for example, testing at 2m gives a lens +0.50DS stronger, and at 1m the refraction will be +1.00DS over the prescription focused for infinity. This may need to be modified for distance spectacles, although the over-plussed 'intermediate' prescription may be more appropriate for some tasks such as watching television.

Subjective refraction with contact lenses

The subjective refraction may be best performed in a trial frame, since many contact lens patients are young and the trial frame may be less likely to induce accommodation than the phoropter. Even if 6/6 vision is achieved, it is useful to check the subjective refraction in each eye with the spectacles or contact lenses that the patient presents with, as they may reveal excess minus power that could account for symptoms unrelated to visual acuity (such as asthenopia or binocular vision problems).

It is necessary with non-presbyopic patients to adopt a technique with the refraction so as to relax accommodation. Measuring blur function is one such method, whereby the addition of 10.50D or 10.75D lenses is expected to blur the 6/6 line significantly. See *Over-refraction*.

Superficial cells of the epithelium
- See *Corneal epithelium.*

Superior limbic keratoconjunctivitis, contact lens induced

In its mild form, contact lens induced superior limbic keratoconjunctivitis (CLSLK) is easy to overlook. The condition is confined to the superior limbal area, and as such is hidden by the upper lid in primary gaze. The proper procedure for observing this condition is to lift the upper lid while the patient gazes down.

A myriad of signs are observed in the region of the superior limbus in patients with CLSLK (Figure S.24); these include:

- punctate epithelial fluorescein staining
- epithelial rose bengal staining
- intra-epithelial opacities
- sub-epithelial haze
- epithelial dulling
- microcysts
- infiltrates and irregularities
- stromal fibrovascular micro-pannus
- fine sub-epithelial linear opacities
- limbal oedema
- tissue hypertrophy
- vascular injection
- poor wetting, punctate staining, hyperemia, chemosis and irregular thickening of the superior bulbar conjunctiva
- papillary and follicular hypertrophy

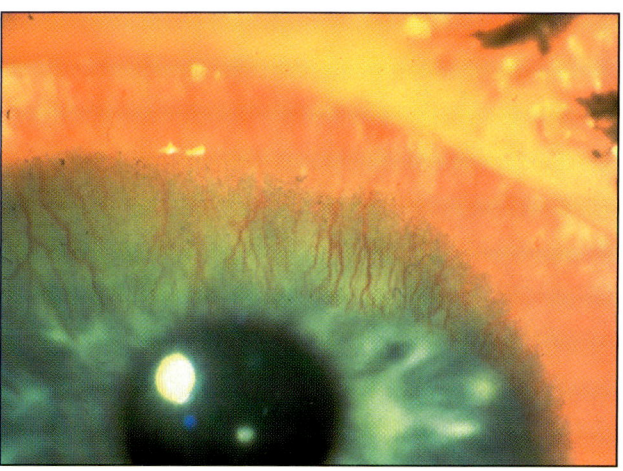

Figure S.24 • Superior limbic keratoconjunctivitis.

- hyperaemia and petechiae of the upper tarsal conjunctiva
- corneal filaments
- corneal warpage and astigmatism
- corneal pseudo-dendrites.

The tissue compromise progresses from the limbus to the centre of the cornea in a V-shaped pattern with the apex directed towards the pupil centre.

Symptoms of CLSLK include:

- increased lens awareness
- lens intolerance
- foreign body sensation
- burning
- itching
- photophobia
- redness
- increased lacrimation
- slight mucus secretion
- slight loss of vision.

This condition occurs mostly in soft lens wearers, it is almost always bilateral, and the specific signs often display symmetry between the eyes. There is considerable variability in the time course of onset of the condition; signs usually become manifest between 2 months and 2 years of commencing lens wear.

The primary aetiological factor in the development of CLSLK is thimerosal hypersensitivity. Provocative tests in thimerosal-sensitized patients result in general circumlimbal redness (not just confined to the superior limbus), meaning that contact lens wear must be impacting on the clinical presentation of CLSLK, which is confined to the superior limbus. Although other factors perhaps play a minor role by initiating, modulating or exacerbating the condition, it is unlikely that CLSLK will develop in the absence of ocular contact with thimerosal. Other factors implicated in the aetiology of CLSLK include:

- thimerosal toxicity
- mechanical effects
- lens deposits
- hypoxia beneath the upper lid.

Patients suffering from CLSLK may be advised to cease lens wear for 2–4 weeks if less than Grade 2, and up to 3 months in severe cases (greater than Grade 2). All previously worn lenses should be discarded. Refitting can be undertaken when the corneal haze has largely resolved and the corneal surface is smooth (less than Grade 1); however, a vascular pannus may be permanent. Lens wear can be resumed in the presence of a vascular pannus as long as the patient is monitored closely to check for the absence of further vascular encroachment. Thimerosal and any other potentially allergenic preservatives should be excluded from the care system. Single-use daily disposable lenses are the best option. Ocular lubricants in the form of drops or ointments may provide symptomatic relief during the recovery phase, further to affording a positive placebo effect in a naturally anxious patient. Clinical signs and visual acuity will generally resolve within about 4 months of cessation of lens wear, although this can vary from 3 weeks to 9 months.

Suppression

Suppression is considered to be an interocular (or binocular) inhibitory process, where information in one eye is inhibited to below threshold and, as a result, is not perceived by the suppressed eye. Binocular suppression may occur in both normal and anomalous vision. In normal vision, suppression occurs for two main reasons. The first is in order to eliminate confusion arising out of the presence of diplopic images. For fixation at a given distance, objects located on the horopter (the locus of points in space that have zero binocular disparity) will be perceived as single. Objects located nearer or further than the horopter will have images located on non-corresponding points and will be perceived as double. This normal feature of binocular vision is referred to as physiological diplopia and may be readily demonstrated using two pens:

Hold both pens together at some near fixation distance and binocularly fix on the tip of one of them. Now move the other pen away from the pen that your are fixing, moving it both nearer to you and away from you. As the moving pen crosses Panum's fusional limit you should perceive diplopia. Here the moving pen is imaged on non-corresponding retinal points.

Outside of Panum's area, physiological binocular suppression (sometimes also referred to as suspension) prevents the symptoms that would arise if the diplopic images were perceived in everyday viewing. Within Panum's area the normal processes of binocular sensory fusion operate. Binocular suppression may also occur in normal vision in cases where dissimilar objects are presented simultaneously, one to each eye, on corresponding retinal points and single vision cannot occur. In this case, the phenomenon of binocular retinal rivalry ensues comprising of an alternating suppression of the image of each eye.

Suppression may exist in patients with (a) decompensated heterophoria, (b) heterotropia as well as anisometropia, and (c) amblyopia. The presence of suppression should be suspected by practitioners until proven otherwise. In heterophoria, foveal suppression may occur as a consequence of perturbations in either sensory or motor processing. For example uncorrected anisometropia or aniseikonia or poor convergence may all lead to suppression. In these examples, the presence of suppression attempts to relieve some or all of the symptoms that would otherwise result from the sensory or motor disturbance. In heterotropia or strabismus with normal retinal correspondence, the object of regard is imaged on non-corresponding points, resulting in diplopia. This form of diplopia is referred to as pathological diplopia. An associated disturbance in strabismus is confusion, where the images from two separate and dissimilar targets are positioned on each fovea. The two targets have identical visual directions and are therefore perceived to overlap, one on top of the other. Suppression in this case acts to eliminate both the pathological diplopia and confusion. An alternative way to eliminate diplopia and confusion is to develop anomalous retinal correspondence.

Suppression shows particular characteristics that depend on whether or not it is associated with strabismus. Where suppression occurs as part of the sensory sequelae to strabismus, it rarely affects the whole region of the deviating eye; instead, only a portion of the retina is suppressed. Suppression occurring in strabismus exists in order to eliminate diplopia and confusion. Diplopia occurs when the fixation target is imaged onto non-corresponding points, i.e. the fovea in the fixing eye and a non-foveal point in the deviating eye. The non-foveal point in the deviating eye is referred to as the 'zero point' (zero measure, target point). In addition, in order to eliminate confusion where dissimilar targets are imaged onto each fovea, the fovea in the deviating eye is suppressed. Even in a patient with anomalous retinal correspondence (ARC), these two areas may be suppressed, and these suppression areas may be joined to resemble a 'D' shape. However, the precise size and shape of the suppression zone depends, amongst other things, on how it is measured. If a patient with a large angle strabismus does not demonstrate ARC and yet has no diplopia or confusion, then they must be suppressing the entire binocular field of their strabismic eye. Where suppression occurs in the absence of strabismus, such as in anisometropic amblyopia or decompensated heterophoria it is typically central, affecting the fovea and the region immediately surrounding it.

Suppression is also classified according to the size of the suppressed region and the intensity or depth of suppression. However, measures of the quality of suppression are dependent on the tests used to assess suppression. In general, suppression is regarded as central if the zone of suppression is 5° or less, and peripheral if it is greater than 5°. Measures of the intensity of the suppression zone are based on how close the test condition is to normal viewing. Suppression found under conditions that interfere minimally with normal viewing, such as the Bagolini lenses, is deemed to be shallow, whereas suppression that persists under less natural viewing conditions such as with stereoscopes is considered to be dense.

Surface damage, contact lens

All soft lenses are manufactured with a 'shelf-life', which primarily indicates how long the lens can be guaranteed to be sterile. In addition, there is the possibility of natural

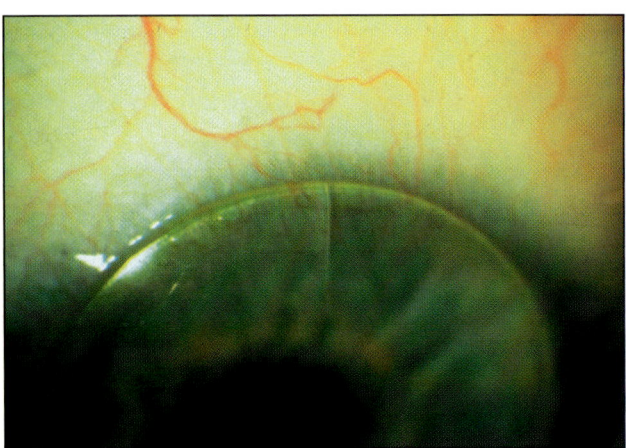

Figure S.25 • Split in a rigid lens.

polymer degradation over time, whereby clinically relevant changes may be noticed – typically on the lens surface – after about 5 years from the time of manufacture.

Physical trauma can also lead to a variety of lens defects. If a defect is obvious, such as a large piece of the lens breaking off, then the patient will typically notice this and discard the lens. If such a defect is not noticed, discomfort on insertion will normally alert the wearer to the problem. However, small defects may not be noticed, and this is potentially problematic because such defects can compromise ocular integrity at a subclinical level.

Rigid lenses can develop fine surface scratches over time (necessitating lens polishing), or fine splits (requiring lens replacement) (Figure S.25). Another ageing problem with rigid lenses is the development of crazing; that is, the appearance of interconnecting surface cracks that can extend deep into the lens. Crazing predisposes the lens to the development of secondary deposits, and the lens can become uncomfortable due to the crazing and/or the existence of deposits. Crazing can also be due to problems occurring during manufacture.

Surface properties, soft contact lens

It is apparent that soft lenses do not suffer deficiencies in terms of inherent wettability, provided that they are fully hydrated. However, two contributing factors influence their behaviour in the eye. The first is the fact that the anterior surface of the lens will progressively lose water, especially in adverse environmental conditions. The second is that the polymer chains are able to rotate rapidly in response to a changed interface. When in contact with aqueous fluids, the hydrophilic groups rotate to the surface. Conversely, when in contact with more hydrophobic interfaces, such as air or lipids, the hydrophilic groups 'bury' themselves within the gel and a more hydrophobic surface is exposed. Chain rotation is a dynamic process, whereas evaporative water loss is a progressive process. Molecular processes such as protein deposition and denaturation are well able to respond to the dynamic processes, which is why the eye presents such a challenging environment. The progressive dehydration has a more influential effect on the gross surface properties of the hydrogel, and is part of the complex process that produces end-of-day discomfort for many wearers.

Two surface properties that can be used to characterize hydrogels are surface energy (which manifests itself as wettability) and the coefficient of friction (which underlies the biotribological behaviour of the lens). Both of these properties are linked to the water-binding ability of the lens. Frictional studies show that both synthetic hydrogels and natural hydrogels (e.g. the cornea) are normally lubricated by a hydrodynamic (water) boundary layer. This dominates the dynamic coefficient of friction to the extent that when an intact lubricating layer separates the hydrogel and substrate, it is the properties of the solution rather than those of the material or substrate that govern the value of sliding friction. The simplest analogy is that of a car aquaplaning – the ease of sliding is independent of the rubber from which the tyres have been fabricated. When this water layer breaks down, there is an increase in the resistance to sliding. The surface energy of a hydrogel is a more progressive property. It rises rapidly up to a water content of around 30%, and much more slowly thereafter. As previously stated, however, at a hydrophobic interface the surface energy drops dramatically because of chain rotation.

The clinical consequence of these facts is relatively simple to state, but complex to relate to direct measurement. All conventional hydrogels have very adequate wettability and frictional behaviour when fully hydrated, no matter what the initial water content. Problems only arise because of progressive dehydration and the dynamic responsiveness of the lens material to air and lipids (caused primarily by tear break-up). These processes in turn influence the irreversible deposition of tear components and the onset of symptoms such as end-of-day dryness, which are linked to biotribological phenomena.

Surface wetting of contact lenses

A stable, uniform tear film over the surface of soft and rigid lenses is required to maintain good, stable vision. A surface with poor wetting characteristics will break up the prelens tear film, creating sources of light scatter, which will depreciate optical transmission and hence visual quality. High oxygen permeability (Dk) silicone-based lens materials have intrinsically poor wetting properties. The wettability of the surfaces of lenses made from these materials can be improved using a variety of manufacturing and chemical techniques, such as plasma treatment. Lens surface wetting properties are measured using a variety of techniques – e.g. the captive bubble, Wilhelmy plate and sessile drop methods. The wettability of a lens is typically expressed as the 'wetting angle' or 'contact angle', which is the angle between the test surface and the tangent of a fluid drop or air bubble in contact with the surface.

The friction from high-speed polishing may singe the lens surface and thus affect wettability. Chemical conditioning solutions may improve lens wettability in vitro, but not necessarily in vivo. Placing the lens on the eye and checking the stability of the pre-lens tear film using a tear break-up test is a useful in vivo clinical measurement of lens wetting. The Keeler Tearscope can assess lens wettability quantitatively and allow the clinician to categorize the structure of the pre-lens tear film (Figure S.26).

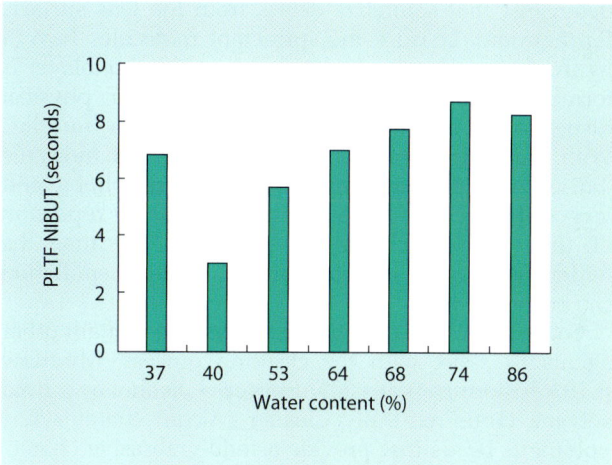

Figure S.26 • Pre-lens tear firm (PLFT) non-invasive break-up time (NIBUT) of hydrogel lenses of various water content, determined using a Tearscope.

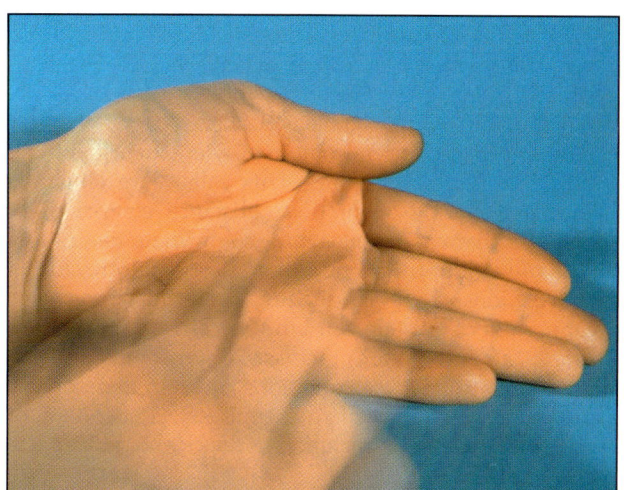

Figure S.27 • Surfactant cleaning a soft lens.

Surfactant cleaning of contact lenses

There are two key reasons why a contact lens should be cleaned with a surfactant solution. First, a wide variety of intrinsic debris (tear-film products such as proteins, lipids and mucus) and extrinsic debris (environmental pollutants and cosmetics) can adhere to the surface of a contact lens. This can lead to lens distortion, discomfort, an unsightly cosmetic appearance (as soiled lenses can show marked discoloration clearly visible to an onlooker), ocular surface and eyelid pathology, and vision loss. Secondly, a cleaning action supplements the disinfection process by reducing the levels of microorganisms on the contact lens. The processes of rinsing and rubbing lenses in the course of surfactant cleaning also lead to a reduction in the bioburden on the lens.

A common method of lens cleaning is to use a 'standalone' surfactant cleaner. The lens is placed in the palm of one hand, a few drops of surfactant cleaner are introduced into the concavity of the lens, and the forefinger of the other hand rubs the cleaner into the lens (Figure S.27). Agents that contain surfactant cleaners are detergents that solubilize debris from the lens surface. Furthermore, because the surfactant molecules have a hydrophilic end and a hydrophobic end, a monolayer is formed around lipid droplets created after physical dispersion of any lipid spoilation, creating a 'micelle'. With the hydrophobic end of the surfactant molecule 'buried' in the lipid droplet, and the hydrophobic end 'exposed', re-coalescence of the lipid due to repulsion of the electrical charges is prevented. Because the hydrophilic region is water soluble, the lipid spoilation can be emulsified.

Some surfactant cleaning products also contain other agents to assist with the cleaning process. Miraflow (CIBA Vision) contains 20% isopropyl alcohol as a lipid solvent. Opti-Free Daily Cleaner (Alcon) contains fine polymeric beads that provide a mildly abrasive characteristic, although this is not thought to affect the lens surface.

Most surfactant cleaners contain other agents such as preservatives to prevent microbial contamination after opening. In the case of Miraflow, the isopropyl alcohol acts as a preservative in addition to its lipid-removing characteristics. Other preservatives include sorbic acid and potassium sorbate. Due to the hypersensitivity reactions to thiomersal and chlorhexidine, these preservatives are rarely found in modern soft lens cleaners.

A number of cleaners contain ethylene diamine tetraacetic acid (EDTA), or one of its salts, as a chelating agent. A chelating agent is a substance comprised of molecules that can form several co-ordinate bonds to a single metal ion. In the case of contact lens care, EDTA removes ions such as calcium, resulting in a lens-cleaning effect (protein can bind to calcium on the lens surface, and therefore increase deposition) and an antimicrobial effect (calcium ions are required for cell wall metabolism by micro-organisms). Phosphate or borate buffers are also included in the cleaner to stabilize solution pH.

Generally, rigid lenses are cleaned with a separate solution to the disinfectant and wetting product. An exception to this is Solo-Care Hard (CIBA Vision), which is analogous to a soft lens multipurpose solution because it contains a surfactant cleaner. Rigid lens cleaning solutions can be more intensive than their soft lens equivalents because there is less opportunity for the solution to enter the lens material with the subsequent possibility of toxic reaction. For example, Total Care Daily Cleaner (Allergan) contains three cleaning agents and Boston Advance cleaner contains a silica suspension of microscopic beads that act like a gentle polish on the lens; this is beneficial with deposits such as denatured proteins, which can otherwise be difficult to remove. This cleaner also contains an alcohol base, which assists in removing lipid type spoilation.

Swell factor of soft contact lenses

Since both the linear swell and volume swell that occur on hydration of hydrogels are a direct consequence of the volume of water absorbed, any phenomenon that causes a change in water content will cause a change in lens dimensions. The precise combination of monomers used can have a marked effect on the stability of the material.

Extremes of behaviour are observed with respect to the temperature dependence of the water content of hydrogels. Group I materials, particularly polyHEMA, show little temperature dependence, and Group IV materials show a significant drop in water content between 20ºC and 30ºC. These thermally induced changes take place rapidly, and the lens will quickly reach its new equilibrium water content on insertion into the eye. All lenses dehydrate over time in the eye, but that process is separate from thermal re-equilibration and is no better or worse for any particular class of hydrogels. The initial drop in water content will, however, significantly reduce the oxygen permeability of the lens material.

The sensitivity of water content to tonicity is similarly affected by monomer structure. In general, hydrogels show some small decrease in water content when the equilibration solution is changed from pure water to isotonic saline. Such a change, as with others induced by changing the nature of the storage solution, is much greater than those brought about by tonicity variations in the eye.

Variations in water content with respect to pH are more marked and are monomer-dependent. The pH ranges required to bring about such changes are, however, greater than those found diurnally or on a patient-to-patient basis in the eye, which lie well within one pH unit. High water content anionic hydrogels (FDA Group IV materials) suffer dramatic parameter changes in solutions of different pH; however, this is largely inconsequential if such materials are used to make disposable lenses. In order to maintain the stability of lenses during storage and to minimize dimensional changes between the storage medium and the eye, lenses are packed in buffered saline solution, which ensures that both pH and tonicity are controlled.

Swimming in contact lenses

Contact lenses can be worn safely in sea water, fresh water and chemically treated water, although swimming should be avoided if it is known that the body of water where the swimming will occur is subject to high levels of pollution (many seaside authorities routinely advise of the ambient pollution levels). Overall, the risk of infection as a result of swimming in lenses is extremely small.

There is a greater risk of lens loss when swimming in lenses; this risk will be minimized if large-diameter soft lenses are worn. The use of swimming goggles will prevent lens loss and further reduce the already low risk of infection. It is advisable not to wear contact lenses in spa baths due to the increased risk of acanthamoeba infection.

Swimmers should be advised to follow these guidelines for avoiding lens loss and preserving eye health when not wearing goggles:
- close the eyes on impact with water
- do not open the eyes fully when underwater; instead, squint and maintain the head position in the direction of gaze
- upon surfacing, gently wipe water from the closed lids before opening the eyes
- irrigate the eyes with fresh saline upon leaving the water
- remove, clean and disinfect contact lenses as soon as practicable after swimming.

Systemic disease, contact lens wear in

Patients with any systemic disease known to affect the anterior eye potentially face problems during contact lens wear. Conditions such as diabetes, thyroid deficiency, hyperthyroidism, rheumatoid arthritis, atopic eczema, psoriasis and acne rosacea may affect a patient's suitability for contact lenses. In general, these conditions, when managed, do not contraindicate contact lens wear but may influence the lens type or the wear schedule selected. Patients with allergies can achieve success with contact lenses but may require more frequent aftercare examinations, since these patients are more susceptible to lens-induced discomfort and lid problems. There is no contraindication to fitting contact lenses to patients who are HIV-positive providing the anterior eye is healthy. Practitioners should wear protective gloves if they have open skin lesions. If the patient has progressed to AIDS, the increased risk of opportunistic infection should be considered and contact lens fitting approached with extreme caution.

Restrictions of mobility, as in rheumatoid arthritis or 'diabetic hand syndrome' (Figure S.28), may make the handling of contact lenses difficult. Patients should be encouraged to handle their own lenses whenever possible. When handling becomes impossible, a relative or neighbour may provide assistance and periods of extended or continuous wear may be appropriate.

The ocular complications of both prescription and over-the-counter medications – such as decongestants, antihistamines and oral contraceptives – should be taken into consideration in the context of contact lens wear. Possible side effects of medications include dry eye, photosensitivity, corneal and contact lens deposition, punctate keratopathy, subconjunctival haemorrhage, and discoloration of contact lenses.

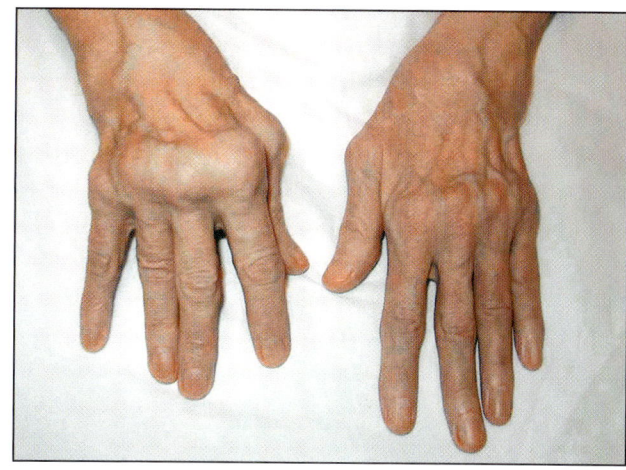

Figure S.28 • Deformation of the knuckles and finger joints in a patient with rheumatoid arthritis.

When considering whether to proceed with contact lens fitting in patients with systemic disease affecting the anterior eye, the practitioner needs to conduct a risk-benefit analysis. Where an increased risk of ocular complications has been ascertained, the patient should be informed of the risks and the benefits of contact lens wear. The importance of complying with recommendations for lens care and maintenance, wearing schedules and attending follow-up visits should also be emphasized. A thorough understanding of the ocular and systemic history, careful examination during fitting and follow-up to exclude the possibility of external eye disease, and the use of superior contact lens products will increase the likelihood of success for all prospective contact lens wearers. See *Diabetes, contact lenses for*.

T

Tarsal glands
- See *Meibomian glands*.

Tarsal muscles (of Müller)
The superior and inferior tarsal muscles are smooth muscles that arise from the lower border of the levator in the upper lid and the inferior rectus in the lower lid, and insert into the orbital margins of the tarsal plates. The role of the superior tarsal muscle is to assist the levator in maintaining the width of the palpebral aperture. A mild degree of ptosis results from damage to its sympathetic nerve supply (see *Horner's syndrome*).

TD
- See *Total diameter, contact lens*.

Teaching patients contact lens care
- See *Patient education*.

Tear break-up time
Rapid tear break-up can lead to symptoms of dryness and discomfort in both lens wearers and non-lens wearers. The tear film break-up time can be assessed by instilling fluorescein into the eye and timing how long it takes for breaks in the even fluorescent glow to appear (Figure T.1). One problem with this approach is that it is invasive in that the instillation of fluorescein in itself alters the quality and quantity of the tear film. See *Non-invasive tear break-up time*.

Tear electrolytes
Human tears contain approximately the same range of electrolytes found in plasma. During the process of secretion by the lacrimal gland there is a process of active electrolyte transport, which is coupled to the passive movement of water by an osmotic process. Acinar-derived fluid is essentially an isotonic ultrafiltrate of plasma. Its composition is altered as it passes along the ductal system, where further chloride and potassium ions are secreted. A variety of ion transport proteins have been identified in acinar cells, including sodium-potassium ATPase and potassium and chloride channels.

Tear film
The tear film is a complex fluid, which covers the exposed parts of the ocular surface framed by the eyelid margins. The physical characteristics of this fluid are summarized in Table T.1. Classically, the tear film has been regarded

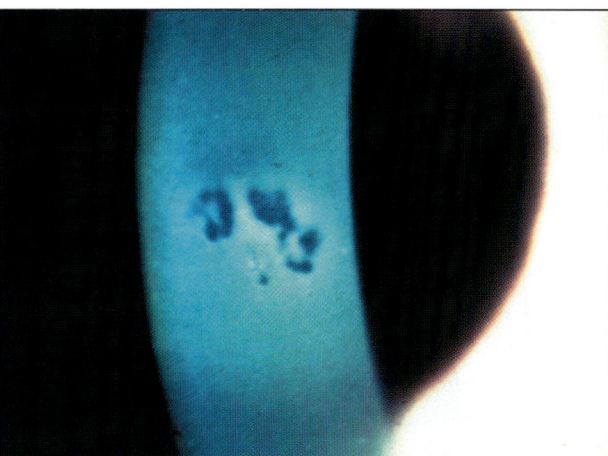

Figure T.1 • Dark spots in the illuminated slit beam indicate break-up of the pre-corneal tear film.

Table T.1 • Physical properties of the pre-ocular tear film.

Parameter	Value
osmolarity	302 (6 6.3) mOsmol/l
pH	7.45
volume	7.0 (6 0.2) μl
rate of production:	
unstimulated	1–2 μl/min
stimulated	.100 μl/min
refractive index	1.336

Table T.2 • Biochemical composition of the pre-ocular tear film.

Component	Concentration
Electrolytes[a]:	
Na^+	135 mEq/l
Cl^-	131 mEq/l
K^+	36 mEq/l
HCO_3^-	26 mEq/l
Ca^{2+}	0.46 mEq/l
Mg^{2+}	0.36 mEq/l
Major proteins[a]:	
lysozyme	2.07 g/l
secretory IgA	3.69 g/l
lactoferrin	1.65 g/l
lipocalin	1.55 g/l
albumin	0.04 g/l
IgG	0.004 g/l
Lipids[b]:	
wax esters	32.3% (dry weight)
sterol esters	27.3%
polar lipids	14.8%
hydrocarbons	7.5%
diesters	7.7%
triglycerides	3.7%
fatty acids	2.0%
free sterols	1.6%
Mucins[c]:	
MUC1	nd
MUC2	nd
MUC4	nd
MUC5AC	nd

Sources:
(a) Main and accessory lacrimal glands
(b) Meibomian glands
(c) Epithelial cells/goblet cells.
nd 5 not determined.

as a trilaminar structure, with a superficial lipid layer (secreted by the meibomian glands) that overlies an aqueous phase (derived from the main and accessory lacrimal glands) and an inner mucinous layer (produced mainly by conjunctival goblet cells). The tear film performs several important functions, which can be broadly classified as:

- optical
- metabolic support
- protective
- lubrication.

By smoothing out irregularities of the corneal epithelium the tear film creates an even surface of good optical quality which is reformed with each blink. The air–tear interface forms the principal refractive surface of the optical system of the eye and provides two-thirds (43D) of its total refractive power. Since the cornea is avascular, it is dependent on the tear film for its oxygen provision. When the eye is open the tear film is in a state of equilibrium with the oxygen in the atmosphere, and gaseous exchange takes place across the tear interface. The constant turnover of the tear film also provides a mechanism for the removal of metabolic waste products.

Tears play a major role in the defence of the eye against microbial colonization. The washing action of the tear fluid reduces the likelihood of microbial adhesion to the ocular surface. Moreover, the tears contain a host of protective antimicrobial proteins (Table T.2). The tear film acts as a lubricant, smoothing the passage of the lids over the corneal surface and preventing the transmission of damaging shearing forces. To facilitate this, tear fluid displays non-Newtonian behaviour with respect to shear. Newtonian fluids maintain a constant viscosity with increasing shear rates. By contrast, tear fluid has a relatively high viscosity between blinks to aid stability, and with increasing shear rates during the blink process the viscosity falls dramatically, thereby easing the movement of the lids over the ocular surface.

The classical trilaminar model of tear film structure has recently been challenged. Several pieces of evidence have suggested that the mucin contribution to the tear film is much greater than previously thought, and an alternative tear film model, which possesses a substantial mucinous phase, has been proposed. The nature of the mucinous phase has not been fully established, but is thought to consist of a mixture of soluble and gel-forming mucins. There is currently great uncertainty as to the overall thickness of the pre-corneal tear film. Published values, using several different techniques, lie in the range 3–40μm. Invasive methods (e.g. using fine glass filaments) usually give rise to thickness estimates between 4 and 8μm. Interferometric measurement gives values of around 40μm, but these data have been questioned on the basis of methodological and interpretational difficulties.

Tear layer
- See *Tear film*.

Tear lens beneath a contact lens

The power of the tear lens beneath a rigid lens, sometimes alternatively called the liquid, fluid or lacrimal lens, depends on the relative geometry of the optic zone of the back surface of the rigid lens and the anterior surface of the cornea. The tear lens may contribute negative, zero or positive power to the overall lens-eye system, depending upon whether the fitting of the rigid lens is flat, in alignment or steep.

From a clinical perspective it is important to determine the likely magnitude of the power of the tear lens and how it varies as the back optic zone radius (BOZR) of the lens is changed. As an approximate rule of thumb, for a rigid lens the tear lens power increases by about +0.25D for each 0.05mm that the BOZR of the lens is steeper than the corneal radius. Correspondingly, on any cornea the back vertex power (BVP) of the rigid contact lens needs to be changed by −0.25D for each 0.05mm that the BOZR is made steeper, to compensate for the extra positive power of the liquid lens. If the lens BOZR is made flatter by 0.05mm, the BVP needs to be changed by +0.25D.

Trial or diagnostic lenses are often used to find the BOZR that gives the required fit with a particular lens design – an over-refraction then being carried out to determine any additional power needed in combination with the trial lens used to give the patient clear vision. In this case the ordered lens power is simply the sum of the BVP of the trial lens and the over-refraction (assuming that the power of the latter is small enough for effectivity to be ignored). This is because the BOZR and corneal radii will be exactly the same as with the trial lens, so that the tear lens has equal power in both cases.

The situation may arise where a trial lens with a given BOZR is not available, in which case it may be necessary to order a lens with a BOZR that differs from that of the trial lens actually used. Since the BOZR in the two cases differs, so also will the power of the tear lens, and this in turn will influence the required BVP of the ordered lens.

Tear lipids

The source of lipids in the tear film is the meibomian glands embedded within the tarsal plates of each lid. The blinking process is an important mechanism in the expulsion of the secretion from the glands. Lipid is delivered directly as a clear oil onto the lid margins, and is spread over the tear film from the inner edge of the lid margins with each blink. The thickness of the lipid layer is variable (60–100nm) and, depending on thickness, gives rise to characteristic interference patterns when viewed in specular reflection. Meibomian secretion consists of a complex mixture of lipids, including wax esters, sterol esters, fatty acids and fatty alcohols (Table T.2). The primary functions of this secretion are to provide a hydrophobic barrier at the lid margin to prevent over-spill of tears, and to cover the surface of the tear film to retard evaporation.

Tear mucins

Mucins are a family of high molecular weight glycoproteins of which sugars contribute up to 85% of their dry weight. Structurally, they consist of a polypeptide backbone to which chains of sugar molecules attach via O-linkages to the amino acids serine and threonine. Mucins are a heterogeneous group of molecules, which can be subdivided into secretory and integrated-membrane varieties (see Table T.2). So far modern molecular biology techniques have identified nine mucin (MUC) genes, although only four of these (MUC1, MUC5AC, MUC4 and MUC2) are expressed on the human ocular surface. The epithelia of the cornea and conjunctiva express the transmembrane mucins MUC1 and (to a lesser extent) MUC4, which attach to apical microvilli, where they form a hydrophilic base to facilitate the spreading of the goblet cell-derived mucin MUC5AC. A secondary goblet cell mucin (MUC2) is present in only trace amounts. Mucins play a major role in stabilizing and spreading the tear film, and provide protection against desiccation and microbial invasion. The combined aggregation of mucins is known as mucus. Adjective mucous.

Tear production

The terms 'basic (basal)' and 'reflex' can be used to describe tear flow. The accessory lacrimal glands are the basic (minimal flow) secretors, and reflex secretion (i.e. in response to strong physical or emotional stimulation) is mediated by the main lacrimal gland. Alternatively, tear output can be thought of as a continuum whereby the rate of production is proportional to the degree of sensory or emotive stimulation. This concept would also mean that a functional distinction between main and accessory lacrimal glands, in terms of basal and reflex tear production, is unnecessary. Rather, it is more likely that tear flow is the combination of contributions from both glands, although the output from the accessory glands alone is sufficient to maintain a stable tear layer.

Tear proteins

Tear proteins are thought to originate from three main sources; the lacrimal gland, ocular surface epithelia and conjunctival blood vessels. The major lacrimal proteins include secretory IgA (sIgA), lysozyme, lactoferrin and lipocalin (formally known as tear-specific pre-albumin). IgA, which is the major immunoglobulin in tears, is secreted as a dimer by plasma cells in the interstices between lacrimal acini. It then binds to a receptor on the basolateral aspect of acinar cells, and is transcytosed across the cell and secreted into tear fluid. IgA is a constitutively secreted lacrimal protein whose rate of secretion is independent of flow rate. During sleep, the levels of IgA increase as sIgA production continues and

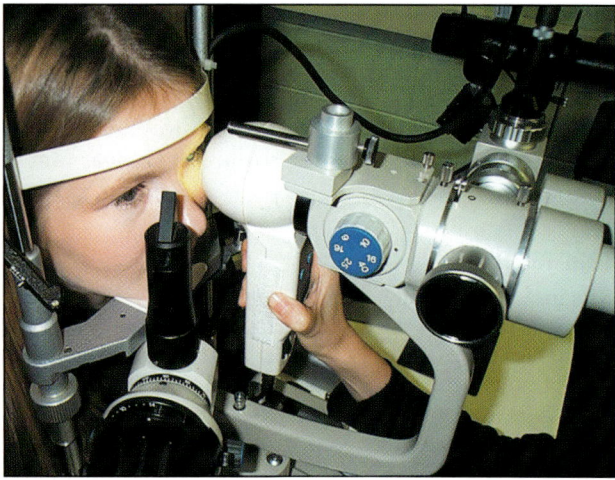

Figure T.2 • Tearscope Plus used in conjunction with a slit-lamp biomicroscope.

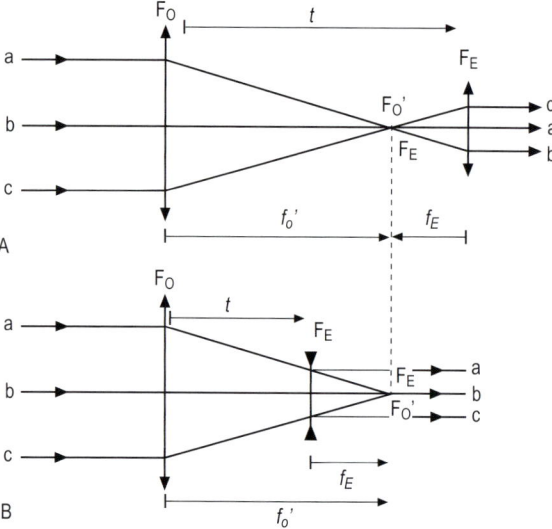

Figure T.3 • A schematic representation of the optical system of (A) an astronomical and (B) a Galilean telescope. In the astronomical telescope the top-most ray (A) entering the telescope becomes the lowest ray of the exiting bundle, so the image is inverted. In the Galilean telescope, the order of the rays is the same on entering and exiting so the image is erect.

as acinar secretion declines. IgA plays an important role in the defence of the ocular surface against microbial infection by preventing bacterial and viral adhesion, and inactivating bacterial toxins. Other immunoglobulins (e.g. IgG and IgM) are present in tears at much lower levels (see Table T.2).

Lysozyme, lactoferrin and lipocalin, by contrast, originate from acinar cells, and their rate of secretion roughly matches flow rate. Lysozyme is a well-known bacteriolytic protein, which has the ability to lyse the cell wall of several gram positive bacteria. Lactoferrin serves an important bacteriostatic function by binding iron and making it unavailable for bacterial metabolism. It also acts as a free radical scavenger, thereby reducing free-radical mediated cell damage. Lipocalins are a family of lipid-binding proteins with an affinity for a broad array of lipids including fatty acids, phospholipids and cholesterol. It has been suggested that tear lipocalins act as scavengers for a wide range of meibomian lipids, which could spill onto the corneal surface and perturb its wettability. Furthermore, lipocalin may promote lipid solubility at the aqueous-lipid interface to facilitate the formation of a thin layer of lipid on the surface of the tear film.

Tears

- See *Tear film*.

Tearscope-plus

An instrument known as a Tearscope-plus (Keeler, UK) can be used to observe certain characteristics of the tear film non-invasively. This instrument takes the form of a small white dome with a central sight hole, surrounded by a cold cathode light source. It can be held directly in front of the eye, or used in conjunction with a slit-lamp biomicroscope to gain more magnification (Figure T.2). The thickness distribution, quality and freedom of movement of the tears can be assessed by observing the reflected light from the featureless white dome, and the integrity of the aqueous and lipid phases can be inferred from colour fringe interference patterns.

Telescopes, distance

Telescopes are a very effective way of producing magnification (an enlarged retinal image) for visually impaired patients, for distance (street signs, bus numbers, blackboard), intermediate (television, music, playing cards) or near (writing, handicrafts) tasks. A disadvantage of telescopes is the very restricted field of view allowed by such devices. Also, telescopes can rarely be used whilst the patient is moving. It is common for a hand-held telescope to be used intermittently for spotting tasks outdoors, and for spectacle mounting to be reserved for sedentary use. See *Telescopes for mobility*.

The optical systems of the two types of telescope used in low vision work are illustrated simply in Figure T.3, which depicts (a) the astronomical and (b) the Galilean telescope. In the astronomical telescope, a ray from the bottom of the object forms the top of the image, and thus the image is inverted. This is obviously unsuitable for low-vision work, so an erecting system is always included to re-invert the image. In the astronomical telescope, the convex objective lens F_O forms an image of the distant object (i.e. focuses the incident parallel light) at F_O', the second focal point of this lens. The distance between the image and the objective lens is obviously the second focal length, f_O'. Light then diverges from this focus, and is refracted by the convergent eyepiece lens, F_E. If this lens is positioned so that its first focal point, F_E, coincides exactly with F_O' and the image, then parallel light will emerge from the system. For the Galilean telescope, the eyepiece lens F_E is negative and is positioned so that its first focal point is coincident with F_O': rays of light converging towards F_O' are intercepted before focusing, and emerge parallel from the system. The ray of light which left the top of the object emerges at the top of the image; the image is erect and no additional components are required to make practical use of the system.

Magnification = $-F_E/F_O$

where F_E and F_O are the powers of the eyepiece and objective lenses respectively. The negative value for magnification in the astronomical telescope indicates an inverted image.

The overall length of each telescope (t) is determined by the separation between the eyepiece and objective lenses, which is the sum of the respective focal lengths:

$t = f_O' + f_E'$

The astronomical telescope will then be longer than the Galilean system of equivalent magnification, since, for the Galilean telescope, f_E' is negative. The reflecting system, which the astronomical telescope requires to produce an erect image, may use prisms or mirrors. Although this adds to the weight and complexity of the system, and there is loss of light with each reflection, it has the advantage that the optical path length between the objective and eyepiece lenses can be 'folded' thus reducing the overall length of the astronomical telescope. In purely practical terms, the powers of both components should be high, so the corresponding focal lengths will be short and the overall length of the telescope minimized. The use of more powerful lenses will inevitably cause aberrations to affect the final image quality. Thus in high-magnification astronomical systems (up to 14× is available) the eyepiece and objective lenses each consist of up to four components to minimize aberrations. This large number of air/glass interfaces inevitably causes a loss of image brightness, even with anti-reflection coated lenses. By contrast, Galilean systems are not available beyond 4× distance magnification due to the poor image quality associated with the higher powers. This means that the objective and eyepiece lenses are generally of lower power than in the astronomical designs, and in the interest of producing compact and lightweight aids each component may be reduced to a single aspheric lens.

The optical systems described above are afocal, but it is possible to adjust the telescope to correct for the refractive error of the user (see *Spectacle correction, telescopes*) and for viewing at near or intermediate distances (see *Telescopes, near/intermediate*).

Telescopes for mobility

Although telescopes can be used to produce a magnified image of objects at any distance, they cannot usually be worn for prolonged periods and/or whilst mobile. Whilst weight and cosmetic appearance are obvious concerns, it is the limited field of view (approximately 10 to 15° at best) which is the most serious obstacle. There are two key solutions to this problem: bioptic and contact/intraocular lens options.

The bioptic telescope can be spectacle-mounted above the line of sight, such that the user views through a carrier lens (usually the distance refractive correction) for 90% of the time. When a magnified view is required, lowering the chin allows the user to view straight ahead through the telescope for a short period of time, before reverting to normal viewing once again. This bioptic telescope presents two different retinal images (magnified and non-magnified) to the user in rapid succession. If the system is fitted monocularly, the magnified image in one eye and unmagnified in the other eye can be available simultaneously. These telescopes can be manual-focus, or autofocus. The latter case will require a motorized system (and its power supply) which can alter the length of the telescope and, in the case of a binocular device, alter the angle between the two telescopes to take account of convergence. This adds considerably to the cost, weight and conspicuous appearance of the device.

The limited field of view in the conventional telescope occurs because the objective lens (the limiting aperture) is so far from the entrance pupil of the eye. There are therefore various contact lens and intraocular lens options where this distance is reduced, and field of view consequently increased:

- Contact lens telescope was a term used originally to describe a theoretical system in which a telescope was incorporated into a scleral contact lens. It is more commonly used, however, to refer to a system which uses a negative contact lens (≈ −25.00DS) as the eyepiece and a positive spectacle lens (≈ +15.00DS) as the objective of a Galilean telescope, with the length of the telescope being equal to the separation of the lenses (the vertex distance of the spectacles). The field of view of the telescope is determined by the diameter, power and position of the spectacle lens, and is equivalent to that of the highly hypermetropic spectacle wearer. Due to the prismatic effect of the lens edge, there is a ring scotoma following the shape of the lens periphery; this can be avoided by the use of a blended aspheric lens. Even when the contact lens power, spectacle lens power and vertex distance are maximized, the magnification limit is only 1.8 to 2.0x. It is difficult to achieve a vertex distance greater than 20mm, and this is usually the limiting factor on the magnification achieved.
- Intraocular lens telescope is analogous to the contact lens telescope, but with the high-minus eyepiece in the form of an intraocular lens. This would typically be implanted when a cataract was removed, and a clear magnified retinal image would be achieved using a high-plus spectacle lens. As the separation between the two components is greater than in the contact lens telescope, higher (although still limited) magnification is possible.
- Implantable Miniature Telescope (VisionCare Ophthalmic Technologies Inc., Saratoga, CA, USA) is a small telescope sealed in a PMMA carrier, and designed to be implanted monocularly in a patient with age-related macular degeneration. The device provides magnified central vision for one eye while the non-operated eye gives peripheral vision for general navigation. It is available as a 2.2x or 3x telescope, focused for 50cm. Vision can be improved with spectacles for distance (≈ −2.00DS) and near (≈+2.00DS) as required.

Telescopes, near/intermediate

Telescopes in low vision work are often required to focus on objects closer than infinity, but all telescopes demonstrate an effect known as 'vergence amplification', in which the vergence of light from an intermediate or near object, which is slightly divergent when it reaches the telescope, becomes amplified by an amount proportional to the square of the magnification. This means that the accommodative demand, even for intermediate distances, is much greater than even a young subject can sustain. There are two practical ways in which a telescope can be modified to use for near or intermediate viewing:

- Focusing by increasing the telescope length. Increasing the separation of the objective and eyepiece is a practical method, the only limit being the physical restriction on practical tube lengths imposed by the particular device. In general, astronomical telescopes allow a greater range of focus than Galilean devices, some of which do not focus at all. The precise magnification provided for the task cannot be determined unless the powers of the component lenses of the telescope are known, but it will always be greater than the distance magnification given by that telescope.
- Adding a plus lens (reading cap) over the objective. This is the simplest practical solution, with the focal length of the plus lens being equal to the required working space. The task is therefore at the focal point of the added lens, so parallel light would now enter the telescope, which continues to act as an afocal system. This positive lens power can be incorporated into the objective lens, or can be clipped over the objective as a reading cap. The use of a reading cap is the more versatile option, since the cap can be removed or changed so that the telescope can be used for a variety of purposes. This modified system is often called a telemicroscope.

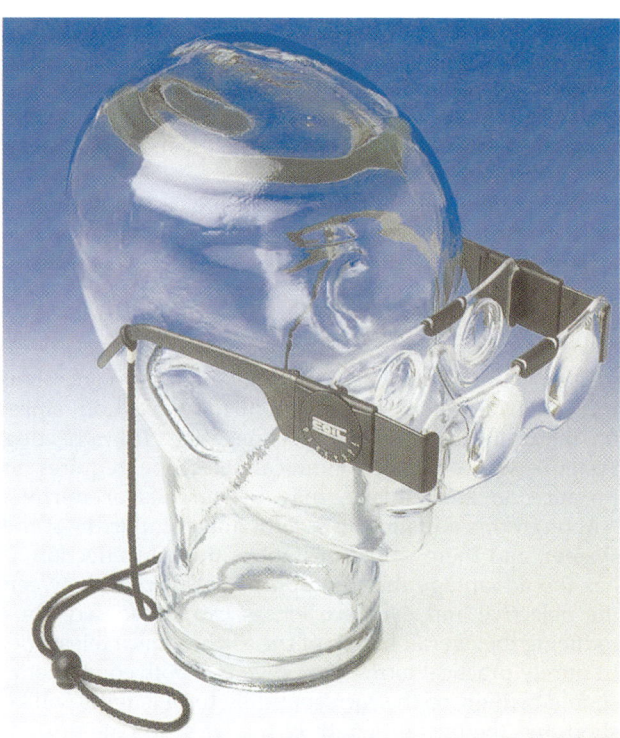

Figure T.4 • Spectacle-mounted Galilean telescope focusable for distance and intermediate tasks.

The magnification of the system is the product of that provided by its individual components, therefore:

Total magnification = afocal telescope magnification × plus-lens reading cap

As with all plus lens magnifiers, magnification of the reading cap = $F_{eq}/4$.

The advantage of using a near telescope rather than a plus lens magnifier is the increase in working space which it allows (for equivalent magnification). If a 2× distance telescope is used, working space is increased by 2×; that is, by a factor equal to the magnification of the telescope used. If a 3× telescope had been used to form the basis of the system, the working space would have been increased by 3×. This may allow manipulative tasks (such as writing and handicrafts) to be performed more easily, and higher degrees of binocular magnification are more practical (5× with telescopic, compared to 2.5× with a spectacle-mounted plus lens magnifier). The field of view of the system is extremely limited, however, which limits its usefulness for more active tasks such as performing music, or woodworking (Figure T.4).

Television reader

A television reader is an electronic magnifier with a mains-powered hand-held 'mouse' camera placed in contact with the material to be viewed, which produces a magnified image on a conveniently placed monitor. This monitor can be a standard domestic television, with a free channel being tuned to the signal. The television reader represented the first genuinely low cost closed circuit television system, now being comparable with optical aids. The magnification range is limited (and may be fixed at one value), but reverse polarity (see *Contrast*) can be selected. The camera itself is easily portable and can be plugged into any television. The patient could, for example, take it between work and home, or could use it on holiday. Versions are available with a small portable monitor, or with a stand to hold the camera so the patient can place a pen under the camera for writing.

Template method of measuring contact lens BOZR

- See *Profile matching, soft lens; Back optic zone radius*.

Tendency orientated perimetry

Tendency orientated perimetry (TOP) is incorporated in the Octopus range of perimeters (1-2-3 and 101). Rather than independently establishing the threshold at each test location with a series of presentations, TOP tests each location once and then combines the information from four locations to derive its threshold estimates. The version incorporated within the current Octopus range of instruments uses the standard 30/2 pattern of stimuli. The 76 test locations are divided into 19 groups of 4 and the results from the 19 groups are used to derive threshold estimates for all 76 test locations.

The TOP algorithm is much faster than both the full- and fast-threshold strategies. Its global indices, in patients with glaucoma, correlate well with those from the full-threshold strategy – a finding that owes much to the relatively infrequent occurrence of small scotomata.

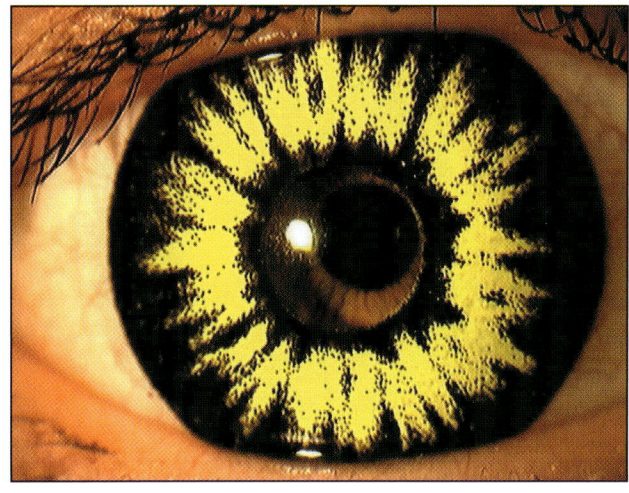

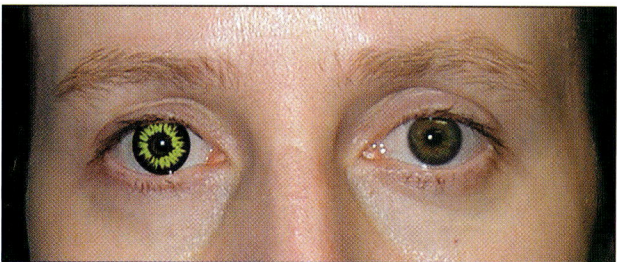

Figure T.5 • Theatric 'wolf eye' lens in the right eye.

Visual field defects investigated with TOP are found to have rounder edges and are shallower, giving a smoothed effect to the visual field.

Tetartanopia

'Tetartanopia' refers to a type of colour deficiency which might arise from inherited absence of a theoretical fourth type of middle wavelength ('yellow') sensitive cone photopigment. Abnormality of this photopigment would result in 'tetartanomalous trichromatism'. Since there are only three types of cone photopigment, 'tetartan' colour deficiency does not exist. Pseudoisochromatic designs intended to identify 'tetartan' defects are included in the HRR plates.

Theatric tinted contact lenses

Lenses can be designed and tinted – typically with opaque agents – to create dramatic or theatrical effects (Figure T.5). Such lenses are also known as 'costume' or 'party' lenses. Effects such as wolf eyes, national flags, hearts, stars, smiley faces etc. can be created, and some companies market afocal lenses specifically for this purpose.

Although these lenses are viewed as a fashion accessory, potential users must be advised to have a thorough initial eye examination to check that their eyes are suitable for wearing contact lenses, and that the fit is satisfactory. Regular aftercare examinations are also recommended. Users should also be warned that such lenses should never be 'shared' with anyone else because the contact lenses may not fit or may be contraindicated in another person, and because there is a danger of cross-contamination and infection. See *Tinted contact lenses*.

Theodore's superior limbic keratoconjunctivitis

- See *Filamentary keratitis, therapeutic lenses for*.

Therapeutic contact lenses

Contact lenses can be of therapeutic benefit in the following situations/conditions:
- distorted corneal shape
- relief of pain
- recurrent erosion syndrome
- dystrophies of the corneal epithelium
- filamentary keratitis
- dry eye
- degenerations of the corneal epithelium
- chemical injuries
- cicatricial conjunctivitis
- eyelid pathology
- post-trauma or post-surgery.

All types of contact lens have therapeutic uses, as follows:

1. Soft lenses. When considering the fitting of a 'bandage' lens, it is necessary to define or predict its probable pattern of use. The relevant considerations are:
- whether extended wear is necessary
- whether the patient (or, failing the patient, a relative or friend) can be taught to handle (or at least to remove) the lens
- the likely duration of therapeutic lens management
- whether the patient lives within practical travelling distance of the clinic or hospital
- whether the necessary topical medications are available unpreserved
- whether the risks of hypoxia, mechanical trauma and infection are outweighed by the perceived benefits of therapeutic lens wear.

Some hospital departments keep sets of 'bandage' lenses, custom made from high water content materials, in various radii and diameters. Others use commercially available lenses such as omafilcon A (Proclear, Biocompatibles-Hydron) or daily disposable lenses. Silicone hydrogel lenses have an important therapeutic role because of their very high gas permeability. In fitting, it is important to cover all anterior ocular areas requiring protection, and to aim for a little movement on blinking. There must be no compression of the limbus.

2. Silicone elastomer lenses. These lenses have an important range of therapeutic roles, especially in tear-deficient eyes. The material is tough and durable, and has good optical properties. The main practical problem is the frequent failure of the surface treatment, which confers wettability on a

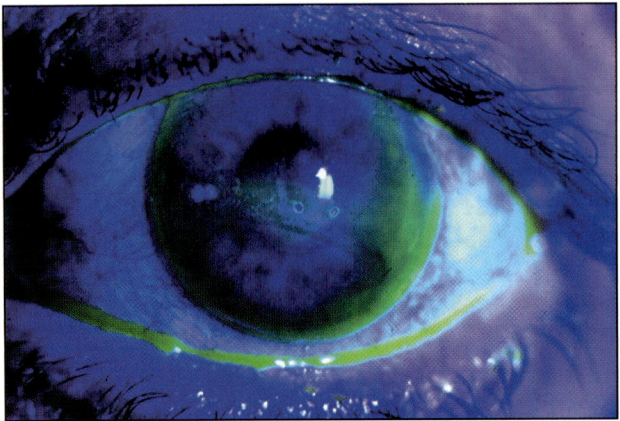

Figure T.6 • Large 'limbal diameter' rigid lens used to protect a neurotrophic corneal lesion in the early stages of the healing process.

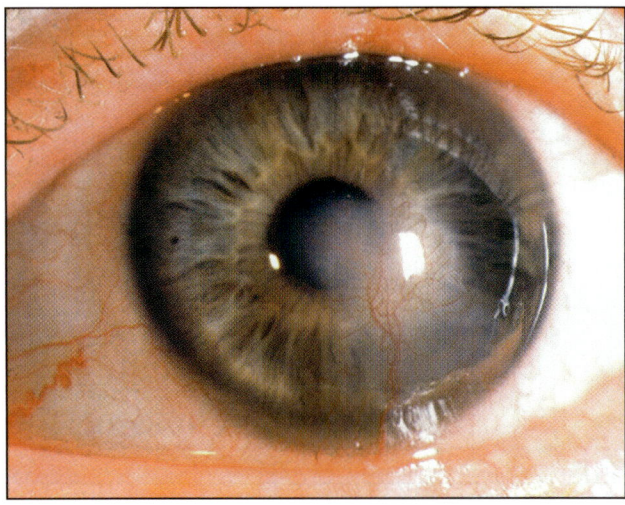

Figure T.7 • Neovascularization with lipid leakage following 40 years of PMMA scleral lens wear.

naturally non-wettable material. This results in lens binding and discomfort.

3. Rigid lenses. It is frequently necessary to use rigid lenses for a combination of optical and therapeutic indications. Although of less than corneal diameter, they may provide enough cover to protect the cornea from abnormal lashes, keratinized lid margins, and other hostile factors. Sometime lenses of large diameters are used (Figure T.6). In cases of ectatic conditions such as pellucid marginal degeneration, the cornea may become highly astigmatic, necessitating the fitting of a rigid bitoric lens.

4. Scleral lenses. These have a host of therapeutic roles. Their advantages include the following:

- corneal contact can be avoided
- any eye shape can be fitted
- complete protection of the cornea and bulbar conjunctiva is provided
- sealed fits are possible, using gas-permeable materials, which simplifies the fitting process and minimizes 'settling back'
- using gas-permeable materials, overnight wear is possible.

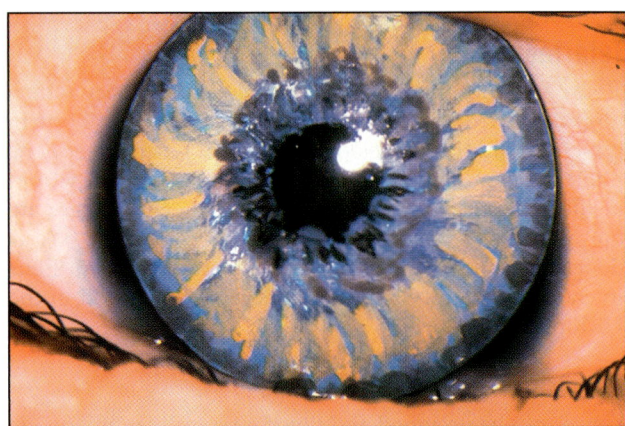

Figure T.8 • Large-diameter rigid lens with hand-painted artificial iris.

Therapeutic contact lenses, complications of

The adverse effects of contact lenses used therapeutically are similar to those used for general cosmetic wear, although the diseased or injured eye may be particularly at risk. Complications of particular concern in therapeutic contact lens prescribing include hypoxia (with or without neovascularization) (Figure T.7), sterile corneal infiltrates, and suppurative keratitis. Careful follow-up is vital after the fitting of a lens for a therapeutic indication, and there is as yet no reason to vary the convention of examining the eye on the day after fitting and not more than 1 week after that. If unplanned replacement lenses are used, spoilation may be observed to occur more quickly than with healthy eyes. Any change of the comfort or vision of the patient may be of great significance, and instruction should be given to the patient to remove the lens in such circumstances and to return to the clinic as an emergency if not rapidly relieved of the new symptoms.

Therapeutic contact lenses, tinted

A therapeutic tinted lens can be defined as a lens that is designed to treat an underlying defect or disease. Primary therapeutic applications of contact lenses include reducing excessive photophobia and glare due to aniridia (Figure T.8), eliminating monocular polyopia due to trauma, eliminating binocular diplopia in squint (in cases where surgical and optical intervention is not viable or is contraindicated), and variable nystagmus.

There are often secondary therapeutic benefits of tinted lenses designed for prosthetic use. These include the following examples:

- a lens with an opaque pupil masking a cataract but also eliminating disturbing light in a near-blind eye
- a rigid lens with an opaque iris pattern fitted to a distorted cornea in a sighted eye also having the effect of improving vision by neutralizing corneal optics, and

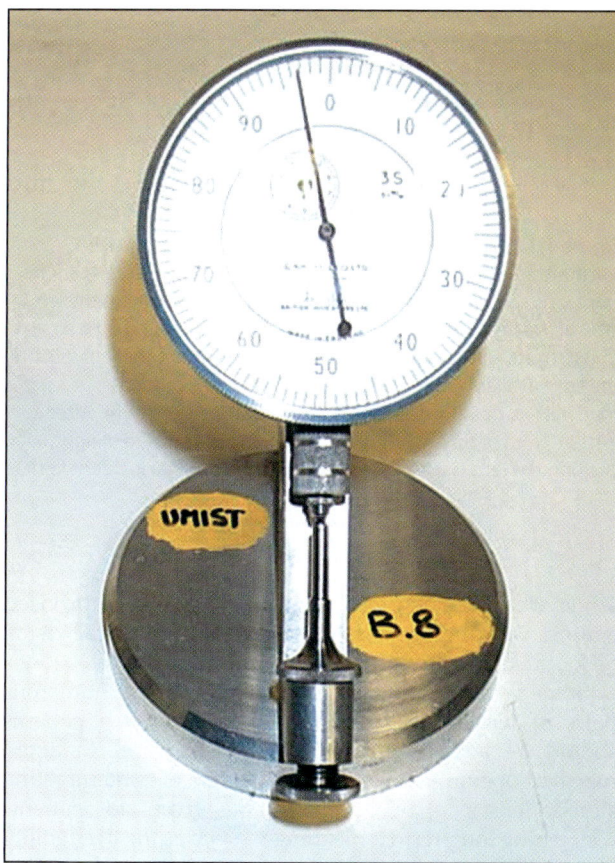

Figure T.9 • Rigid lens thickness caliper.

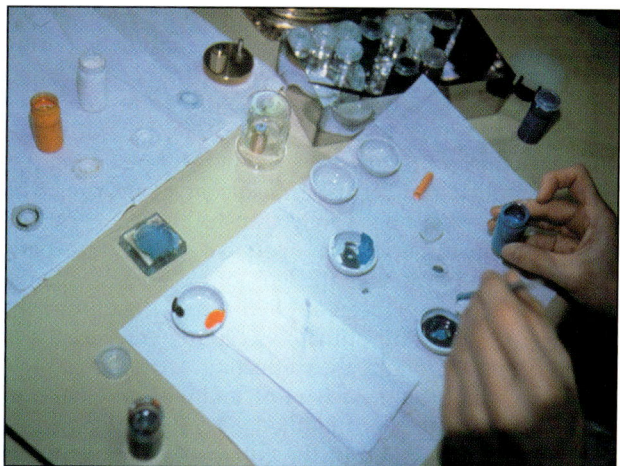

Figure T.10 • Hand-tinting rigid contact lenses.

the incorporation of appropriate lens power to correct vision
- a lens with an opaque iris pattern to mask aniridia in a sighted eye also reducing glare.

The prescription of tinted lenses to supposedly enhance colour vision in colour-defective patients, to cure dyslexia and to alleviate migraine can also technically be described as therapeutic applications, although in most cases improvements are attributed to a placebo effect rather than a true therapeutic effect. See *Tinted contact lenses; ChromaGen lenses.*

Thickness caliper, rigid contact lens

Knowledge of lens centre thickness is required for calculation of gas transmissibility and lens flexibility. The central and peripheral thickness can be measured using a contact lens thickness caliper; this may be a mechanical device where lens thickness is read off an analogue scale (Figure T.9), or it may be an electromechanical device where the thickness is displayed as a digital readout. Care must be exercised when touching the lens surfaces with the calipers, which depress the surface and give a lower reading than the true thickness.

Thickness measurement, soft contact lens

- See *Electrical contact thickness gauge, soft lens; Electromechanical thickness gauge, soft lens.*

Thimerosal disinfecting solution for contact lenses

- See *Chlorhexidine-thimerosal-preserved disinfecting systems.*

Thygeson's superficial punctate keratopathy

- See *Dystrophies of the corneal epithelium, therapeutic lenses for.*

Thyroid deficiency

- See *Systemic disease, contact lens wear in.*

Tight contact lens fit

A lens that moves or lags very little or not at all is deemed to be fitting tightly. Tight-fitting lenses induce greater levels of corneal staining than well-fitting lenses, and the prevalence of this staining increases with increasing tightness. Conjunctival staining corresponding to the lens edge may also be evident. Tight-fitting lenses tend to be comfortable, but patients occasionally complain of aching eyes later in the wearing period. Switching to a similar lens of flatter back optic zone radius or changing to a lens with a tendency towards flat fitting may solve the problem.

Tight contact lens syndrome

- See *Contact lens induced acute red eye (CLARE).*

Tinted contact lenses

A wide variety of manual (Figure T.10) and automated techniques can be used to apply translucent or opaque tints to soft and rigid lenses. An important initial consideration in deciding on the most appropriate tinted lens for a given patient is whether to use a soft or rigid lens. A particular lens type may be indicated for clinical reasons; for example, a rigid lens would be required in the case of a sighted eye with corneal distortion.

Soft lenses have the advantage of offering full corneal coverage and stability on the eye, and are thus particularly suited for cosmetic use. An advantage of rigid lenses is that it is possible to paint unique designs and so effect a more realistic iris appearance in terms of a more precise match of colour and iris features. However, full corneal coverage is not possible, and rigid lenses move on the eye. These effects can be minimized by fitting slightly tight, large-diameter lenses. In general, rigid lenses are best suited for prosthetic use. In certain cases of extensive ocular disfiguration, painted scleral lenses may give the best result.

The applied tint can be translucent or opaque. The resulting lens may be wholly translucent if translucent tints alone are applied, semi-opaque if opaque tints have been used on portions of the lens, or completely opaque if opaque tints have been applied across the entire lens surface. A translucent tint allows certain wavelengths of light to pass through, thus effecting a colour change. Light passing through such a tint, and reflecting back off the iris, will be further modified such that the cosmetic effect is a combination of the colour of the translucent tint and iris. Translucent tints can therefore be said to enhance or modify natural iris colours. This effect is only successful with relatively light coloured irides.

Opaque tints can substantially or completely block the passage of light. A coloured pattern can be applied over a totally opaque base to effect a complete change of eye colour while at the same time, for example, masking out underlying iris disfigurations. Thus, the primary cosmetic application of opaque tints is to change the colour of dark irides or have the prosthetic effect of restoring a normal appearance to a disfigured eye.

Tinted lenses are used for a variety of purposes, including lens handling, cosmetic, prosthetic, therapeutic, prophylactic and theatric applications.

Translucent tints can be created using four basic techniques; dye dispersion tinting, vat dye tinting, chemical bond tinting, and print tinting. Opaque tints can be applied using dot matrix printing, laminate tint constructions, or an opaque contact lens backing.

The procedures for fitting tinted lenses may differ from those employed for fitting non-tinted lenses. Tinted rigid lenses need to be of a large diameter so as to cover as much of the cornea as possible, and to minimize lens movement. Tinted soft lenses are also best fitted marginally more steep than non-tinted lenses to reduce lens movement. A full appreciation of the cosmetic effect of tinted lenses is gained by viewing the lenses in the eyes (using a mirror in the case of the patient) in environments that the patient anticipates being in – that is, both inside under artificial light and outside in natural light.

Chlorine-based disinfecting solutions can cause some lens fading. All other lens care products appear to be innocuous in this regard, including hydrogen peroxide disinfecting solutions and alcohol-based daily surfactant cleaning solutions. Intensive cleaners that employ acids, bases and oxidizing agents could cause tint fading, and so should not be used on tinted lenses.

Although tinting using laminate construction reduces oxygen transmissibility by increasing lens thickness, none of the other tint processes appear to affect lens oxygen performance.

Patients who wear opaque lenses with a clear pupil sometimes complain of haze or a veiling effect in their peripheral vision. This is due to a slight restriction of the visual field during the wear of such lenses. The phenomenon is more noticeable if the lens becomes decentred. In view of the measurable visual impairment

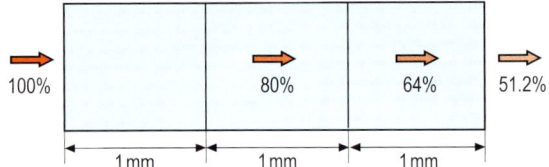

Figure T.11 • Transmission of light through a 3mm lens with transmittance of 80% per mm. 100% of the light is incident on the front lens surface. After travelling a further 1mm through the lens, 20% of the light has been absorbed and the remaining 80% is transmitted. After traveling a further 1mm through the lens, 80% of the light available at the beginning of the lens section is transmitted, or $0.8 \times 0.8 = 64\%$ of the initial incident light. After a further 1mm of travel through the lens, the proportion of light exciting the lens is $0.8 \times 0.64 = 51.2\%$ of the original incident light.

when wearing such lenses, patients should be advised against wearing them when undertaking critical visual tasks, such as driving.

Some fashion-conscious patients may possess numerous pairs of lenses of different tint designs. Such patients should be advised to mark their lens cases to avoid repeated opening, thus reducing the risk of contaminating stored lenses. Advice should be given to patients concerning long-term lens storage – such as the desirability of periodic lens cleaning even if lenses have not been worn.

Although disposable tinted lenses are available, some products, such as theatric lenses, are more expensive and are retained for long periods of time. Long-term lens maintenance therefore becomes an important issue. Some tinting processes can alter the lens surface charge. This could facilitate increased protein deposition, the consequences of which may be decreased vision and comfort, sensations of dryness, susceptibility to adverse eye reactions, lens distortion, and alterations to lens fitting characteristics.

Tinting processes can alter lens surface chemistry, which in turn can reduce surface wettability and lead to symptoms of dryness. Slight irregularities caused by surface tints may render tinted lenses slightly less comfortable than equivalent non-tinted lenses. Ocular lubricants can help alleviate these sensations.

Tinted ophthalmic lenses

Ophthalmic lenses may be tinted using a variety of techniques. Solid tints are produced by introducing tinting materials into the lens mixture at the time of manufacture. For example in glass, oxides of iron and manganese give green and pink colours, respectively. Only very small amounts are needed, and the mixture must be very carefully controlled in order to give consistent results. As the tinting material is distributed evenly throughout the lens material, this means that the tint density will depend on the lens thickness. In Figure T.11, the transmission through a 3mm sample lens is illustrated, where the material has a basic transmission of 80% per mm. Ignoring reflections, 80% is transmitted after 1mm; 80% of 80%, or 64%, is transmitted after 2mm; and 80% of 64%, or 51.2%, is transmitted after

Table T.3 • Examples of calculations using optical density.

Solid Tint Transmission		Example A	Example B	Example C
Transmission (%)	TR	25.00	64.00	80.00
Transmission (max 1.0)	T = TR/100	0.25	0.64	0.80
Thickness (mm)	d	2.00	2.00	1.00
Density	D = Log(1/T)	0.60	0.19	0.10
New thickness (mm)	n	3.00	1.00	3.00
New density	ND = D × n/d	0.90	0.10	0.29
New transmission (Max 1.0)	NT = $1/(10^{ND})$	0.1250	0.8000	0.5120
New transmission (%)	NTR = 100 × NT	12.50	80.00	51.20

3mm. Such calculations are quite straightforward; however in reality the situation is often more complex than in this simple example, and transmission is rather more difficult to calculate. It is therefore better to use optical density for the calculation of lens transmission, as densities can be arithmetically manipulated. For example, a lens 3mm in thickness will have an optical density three times that of one 1mm thick. The relationship of transmission to optical density is given by:

Density = 1/(Log T)

where T is the transmission and is given on a scale of zero to 1.0 (whereby 1.0 is equivalent to 100%). Examples of calculations using optical density are shown in Table T.3. Note that for simplicity these calculations assume that there is no loss of transmitted light from reflection. It can be seen from this table how a lens with the same optical density becomes less transmissive with increasing thickness (examples A and C). In practical terms, a solid tint will appear darker in thicker portions of the lens. For example, the edges of a highly negative lens, the centre of highly positive lens, or the higher powered lens of an anisometropic correction, will appear more deeply tinted.

Solid glass tints have been largely replaced by thin-film vacuum coated tints. A thin metallic film is deposited by evaporation on to the rear surface of a spectacle lens in a vacuum chamber. This gives an even tint that is independent of prescription and lens thickness. A very wide range of colour options is possible, but the precise tint is difficult to reproduce at a later date, making single lens replacement problematical. The lenses should be considered purely as cosmetic unless transmission spectra are available.

The standard method for producing tints on thermoset plastic materials (e.g. CR39) is to dip the lens into hot liquid dye – the 'dipped tint'. In the simplest form of manufacture, the density of tint is controlled by visual matching against standard samples. This is an inexpensive and effective way of tinting, but is not easily reproducible unless more sophisticated control methods are used. Lenses should be supplied as matched pairs, rather than individually, and should be regarded as being cosmetic in nature rather than providing specific protection unless transmission spectra are available. Gradient tints can be produced by slowly pulling the lens out of the tint bath, so that different parts of the lens are immersed for different periods of time.

Solid tints will vary in density depending on the lens prescription, so that a +6.00D lens will transmit less than a plano lens in the same diameter, particularly in the thicker central part of the lens. This can cause problems in anisometropia, where the lenses will cosmetically appear to be different colours. Also, when prescribing tints, the prescription must be considered along with the density of the material so that the required transmission will be achieved. In order to overcome these problems, laminated tints (also described as 'equi-tints') are sometimes used, where a plano layer of solid tinted material is bonded to a powered component, which may be of high refractive index material if the prescription is significant. Such laminations naturally increase the cost of manufacture, and are sometimes thicker than a standard lens. One special purpose lamination, which has been used both for glass and plastic lenses is where a polarizing tint is required. In this case, a sheet of plastic polarizing material is embedded between the front and back layers of a lens. Polarized lenses prevent plane-polarized light reflected from horizontal surfaces from entering the eye. As such they are found useful by drivers, fishermen and skiers. Another special form of lamination uses a wedge shaped cross section of tinted material in order to give a gradient tint.

Tints for low vision

Discomfort glare (see *Glare*) can often be removed by simply reducing the light level with a tint. The colour and percentage transmission are often selected on the basis of subjective reports and cosmetic acceptability. In order to be successful, particularly outdoors, a very dark tint (transmission 20 to 30%) is usually required. This can however significantly impair visual performance when the lenses need to be used in a variety of circumstances. It may be most appropriate therefore to consider plano tinted overspectacles with additional overhead and side shielding, which can be worn alone, or over prescription spectacles and quickly removed when necessary. Such a tint is also helpful in avoiding the delayed adaptation which would otherwise occur when moving from a very bright to a dimmer ambient illumination. Standard prescription photochromic lenses – which have a tint that darkens in response to high ambient levels of ultraviolet radiation (present in natural daylight, but not from artificial sources) but fades once the source is withdrawn – would appear to be an ideal alternative. Clinical experience, however, suggests that standard photochromic lenses are not particularly useful; patients find the tint ineffective in full sunlight, and too slow to react as they move, for example, from a bright street to indoor conditions.

The question of whether tinted lenses can reduce disability glare and actually improve visual performance is much more controversial. Reduction of the disability glare (and improvement of the image contrast) will require that the tint preferentially absorbs the light which is being scattered by the eye. The use of a non-selective neutral grey filter with equal absorption throughout the visible spectrum will not change the retinal image contrast, since both the light and dark areas within the image will be equally attenuated. Scatter of light by the medium through which it is travelling occurs when very small particles (a fraction of the wavelength of light) deflect a portion of the incident light beam approximately equally in all directions, and this scatter is wavelength dependent, being greater for shorter (blue) wavelengths. Theoretically, tints which absorb wavelengths below 500nm would minimize light scatter and improve retinal image contrast. Available transmissions range between 70% and 2%, and the lenses are typically yellow, amber, brown or even red in colour. Whether the situation is quite this simple within the eye is debatable, since the exact mechanisms for the scatter are unknown. Several groups of researchers have tested the potential of such tints to increase retinal image contrast, and hence improve vision, in patients with a variety of ocular pathologies. Such experiments have found it difficult to show objectively that tints are beneficial, and any positive effects are small.

There is no objective test to determine which particular tint from among those available may be best suited to a particular patient (with a particular pathology, or at a particular stage of the disease). Tinted lenses are obviously beneficial to some patients, but prescribing at present is by 'trial-and-error' with the eventual lens choice often based on the patient's subjective judgement, rather than objective measurement of visual performance. Examples of such tints are the Corning CPF glass photochromic lenses, which can be in plano clip-on, or prescription spectacle form (Corning Ophthalmic, Fontainebleau, France). It is often more effective to use overspectacles such as the NoIR range (NoIR Medical Technologies, South Lyon, MI) since the over-the-brow and side-shielding act to further reduce the amount of glare.

Tolerances for contact lenses

Contact lens manufacture is an inexact science, and manufacturers strive to supply lenses that have dimensions and optical characteristics in accordance with those specified. Manufacturing tolerances are the range of acceptable discrepancies between what is specified and what is supplied. Tolerances are agreed by consensus among a range of stakeholders in contact lens manufacture and clinical practice, with regard to known capabilities of currently available manufacturing techniques, and the likely clinical effects of discrepancies in lens dimensions from those specified. Currently agreed specifications for soft and rigid lenses are given in Appendix G.

Tonometry

Tonometry is the indirect measurement of intra-ocular pressure (IOP), and it is an important part of the full eye examination. As well as providing useful baseline data for the future examination of a patient's eye, tonometry has important implications in screening for eye disease. There is a well-established association between IOP and primary open-angle glaucoma. The insidious nature of the onset of this disease requires that an optometrist, with regular access to examine routinely a patient's apparently healthy eyes, employs a variety of clinical techniques to assess ocular health. A dramatic increase in IOP after pupil dilation requires monitoring and occasionally intervention as it may be evidence of an angle closure glaucoma attack. Raised IOP may also present a risk factor for developing a retinal vein occlusion. A drop in IOP may suggest an increased loss of aqueous through an alternative drainage route, as may occur with a retinal tear. As such, tonometry should be undertaken at least once at an initial examination, to establish a baseline reading; if there is any clinical sign warranting exclusion of IOP variation (such as possible retinal damage, pigment on the corneal endothelium and so on); as part of the dilation routine; and on everyone at risk of possible glaucoma (typically everyone over a certain age, 30 years being a sensible choice).

Most population studies among patients over 40 years of age indicate that IOPs measured with a Goldmann tonometer are distributed in a manner similar to a normal distribution with a mean pressure reading of approximately 16mmHg. However, the normal distribution curve is slightly distorted, since IOPs over two standard deviations above the mean (that is greater than 21mmHg) account for 5 to 6 per cent of the patients rather than the 2.5 per cent predicted by a normal distribution. A patient with an IOP greater than 21mmHg on a consistent basis is said to be an ocular hypertensive.

Tonometry relies upon the application of an external force to cause a deformation of the cornea (or the sclera in eyes where this is not possible, such as when anaesthesia cannot be used and the cornea is grossly scarred) and relating the deformation to the internal pressure of the eye. Tonometers may thus be classified according to the deformation produced.

Indentation tonometry (performed with the now rarely used Schiotz tonometer) relies upon a plunger of variable weight to indent the cornea; the level of indentation with differing weights is related to the IOP. All other tonometers, both contact and non-contact, rely upon a measurement of the force required to flatten an area of cornea (this being related to the IOP) and are hence known as applanation tonometers (Figure T.12). The basis of this is given by the Imbert-Fick law, which states that an external force against a sphere equals the pressure in the sphere times the area applanated or flattened by the external force. Contact tonometers, such as the Goldmann tonometer (with which the original population IOP studies were undertaken) and its portable variant, the Perkins tonometer (Figure T.12), use

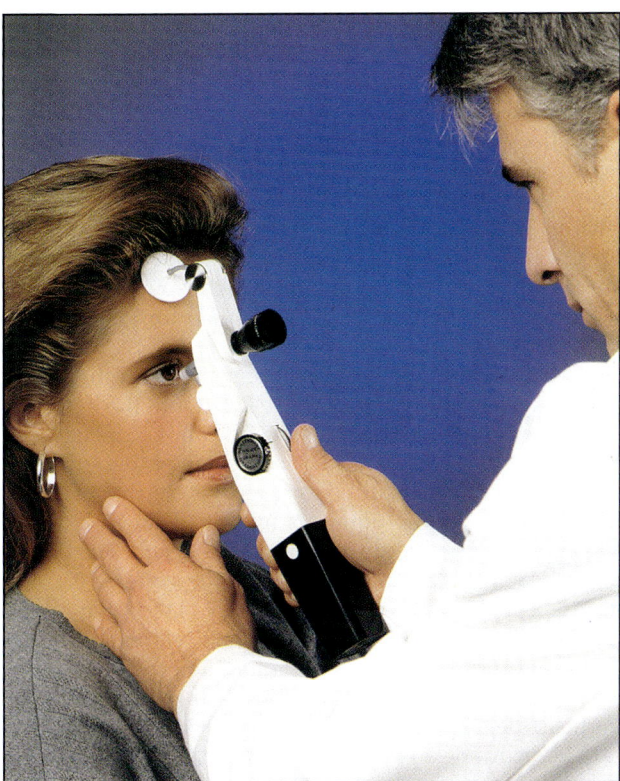

Figure T.12 • Perkins tonometer fitted with examination telescopes.

a flat ended probe incorporating a prism, which is pressed against the cornea. The circular meniscus around the flattened area of cornea is viewed through an optical doubling prism, and the amount of doubling is adjusted by altering the pressure of the cone to achieve a precise area of corneal flattening. A pre-determined flattening area is chosen so that errors due to surface tension from the tears and corneal elasticity are approximately cancelled out.

Non-contact tonometers, of which there are several, project a short-duration jet of air on to the central cornea and measurement is made of the time taken for the cornea to flatten and recover its normal profile. The extent of corneal deformation and recovery is monitored by the reflection of an infra-red beam off the central cornea into a detector. A slower rate of corneal deformation equates to a higher intra-ocular pressure. As non-contact methods are very rapid, taking a few milliseconds, several readings are taken and averaged out to overcome differences due to IOP fluctuation.

There are many physiological influences on IOP, such as ocular pulse, accommodation, pupil size, extraocular muscle action and so on, that make IOP a constantly changing measurement. The IOP is also found to change diurnally, so for accuracy, a series of readings should be taken at different times of day to arrive at a mid-level, peak and trough value. Central corneal thickness has a significant impact upon IOP measurements obtained by tonometry. A thicker cornea is likely to offer greater resistance to any force attempting to deform the corneal surface, thus giving a higher reading of IOP. Patients are found to have lower IOP – measured using conventional applanation tonometry – after refractive surgery than before, because the thinner cornea has less resistance to the tonometer force. Corneal rigidity and state of hydration are also thought to influence IOP measurements.

Toric contact lens design, rigid

Although spherical rigid lenses in general may be successfully fitted to astigmatic patients, with either apical clearance or apical contact, it is generally more satisfactory to fit such lenses with toroidal back optic zones in or near alignment. The physical fit, as denoted by the fluorescein pattern, will be similar to that seen with a well-fitted spherical lens in alignment with a cornea devoid of clinically significant astigmatism. Conversely, a toric lens aligning too closely with the cornea can lead to poor tear interchange. Consequently, it is advisable to use a toroidal back optic zone with the steeper radius fitted slightly flatter (longer radius) than the corresponding corneal radius so as to assist the interchange of tears. The flatter radius will generally be fitted 'on K' or else a little steeper than its corresponding corneal radius.

The peripheral radii are usually chosen to reflect the type of peripheral fit preferred by the practitioner concerned. Each meridian is considered separately, and the peripheral fittings in the two principal meridians are selected to provide the same difference between back optic and peripheral radii most commonly used by the practitioner in fitting spherical corneas. In addition, the peripheral curves will usually have the same degree of toricity as the BOZR.

For lenses with a spherical back optic zone and a toroidal peripheral zone, the peripheral curve region should be as large as possible to increase the likelihood of alignment with the toric cornea. These lenses are usually fitted fairly small to minimize meridional sag differences and slightly steeper centrally than the flatter corneal meridian to achieve a compromise fit. The meridional difference in the peripheral curves should be at least 0.6mm to help minimize lens rotation.

For spherical lenses, the power of the contact lens in air plus the power of the tear lens in air should add up to the ocular refraction. With toric lenses, the same rule applies, but here the two separate meridians must be considered. See *Compensated rigid bitoric lenses; Cylindrical power equivalent rigid toric lenses; Induced astigmatism with rigid toric lenses; Residual astigmatism with rigid toric lenses; Stabilization of rigid toric lenses; Toric lens, rigid.*

Toric contact lens fitting, soft

The fitting principles for soft toric lenses are very similar to those for spherical soft lenses. A well-fitting lens is comfortable in all directions of gaze, gives complete corneal coverage, and appears properly centred. On blinking, there should be about 0.3mm of vertical movement when the eye is in the primary position. On upwards gaze or lateral movements of the eye, the lens should lag by no more than 0.5mm. Generally, when specifying the lens diameter, the practitioner should err on the large side, as a larger diameter means that more area is available for the stabilization zones to take effect in the periphery of the lens. A well-fitting lens will reveal stable lens orientation with a quick return to axis if mislocated. A tight-fitting lens will show stable lens orientation but a slow return to axis if mislocated. A loose-fitting lens will demonstrate an unstable and inconsistent lens orientation.

Due to the absence of a tear lens, the back vertex power for a soft toric lens should be similar to the spectacle refraction (or ocular refraction if the vertex distance effect is significant). The back vertex power of the lens can be determined either empirically or by performing a spherocylindrical over-refraction (SCO) over a diagnostic lens. With empirical prescribing, the BVP ordered for the soft toric lens will be equal to the ocular refraction of the patient, based on the assumption of an afocal tear layer under the soft toric lens. For the latter method, a SCO may be performed over a spherical trial lens. The resultant toric lens power is simply calculated by adding the SCO to the BVP of the trial lens. With both methods, some arbitrary allowance for lens rotation may have to be incorporated into the final lens prescription.

Factors affecting the orientation of a soft toric lens in the eye include variations in lid tension (tightness), lid location, lid angle and lid symmetry; the type of fit (steep, alignment or flat); and the thickness profile of the lens. If it is expected that the soft toric lens to be ordered will rotate when placed on the eye of the patient, then an allowance must be made for this rotation, otherwise the cylinder axis of the lens in situ will not adopt the correct orientation for the ocular correction.

When allowing for nasal rotation in the right eye, the amount of rotation should be subtracted from the required cylinder axis, and vice versa for the left eye. When allowing for temporal rotation in the right eye, the amount of rotation should be added to the required cylinder axis, and vice versa for the left eye. Hence:

- if left eye and nasal rotation – add
- if left eye and temporal rotation – subtract
- if right eye and nasal rotation – subtract
- if right eye and temporal rotation – add.

The acronym 'LARS' (left add, right subtract), relating to nasal rotation of the inferior aspect of the lens, can be quite useful.

Many practitioners work on the principle that clockwise rotation necessitates adding the allowance for rotation to the required cylinder axis, and counter-clockwise rotation requires subtracting the allowance for rotation to determine the final cylinder axis. Hence:

- if clockwise rotation – add
- if counter-clockwise rotation – subtract.

If, at the dispensing or aftercare visit, the lens rotation is not what was expected (but the lens location is stable), the lens can simply be reordered with the revised allowance for lens rotation. Generally speaking, rotational stability is a more important factor than the degree of rotation. Lenses that give sub-optimal but stable acuity are likely to be more acceptable than lenses that give moments of clear vision followed by moments of poor vision as the lens rotates. See *Stabilization of soft toric lenses; Toric lens rotation, soft; Toric lens, soft.*

Toric contact lens manufacture

Either surface of a rigid lens will sometimes require a toric form for the correction of astigmatism and/or to achieve rotational stabilization. This can be achieved by directly lathing a toric surface on to a plastic button (or the xerogel in the case of soft lenses), or by a technique known as crimping. The process of directly lathing a toric back surface onto the lens button is achieved by using a 'fly-cutter', which is a diamond tool that has its cutting tip set at right angles to the axis of its support shank. The position of the fly-cutter and lens blank are reversed, so that the lathe manoeuvres the lens button in an arc around the fly-cutter, which spins in a fixed position. A similar principle is applied for generating a front toric surface.

To generate a toric back surface using the technique of crimping, a spherical back curve is cut into the button in the usual way, except that a stepped rim is also engraved into the base of the blank. The curvature of this surface is the average of the required toric radii of the finished lens. The thickness of the button is machined down to about 0.20mm thick so that the button can be flexed. The button is placed in a crimping tool with the concave surface facing upwards; this tool is a form of clamp that allows pressure to be incrementally applied to the rim of the button until it bends by a measured amount. The extent of bending is monitored optically using a conventional radiuscope.

The crimping assembly containing the flexed button is fixed to the spindle of a lathe and set spinning. A spherical surface is cut into the rotating flexed button. When the button is eventually released from the crimping tool, it reverts back to its natural shape and the lathed surface assumes a toric form. The lens is blocked and a spherical curve can be generated on the front surface. Crimping is used again to generate a toric front surface if required.

Toric soft lenses can be manufactured using moulding technology by designing the toric form into the moulds.

Toric contact lens orientation, soft

- See *Toric lens rotation, soft.*

Toric contact lens, rigid

The use of rigid toric lenses (in preference to rigid spherical lenses) is indicated under the following circumstances:

- to improve the vision in cases where a lens employing spherical front and back optic zone radii is unable to provide adequate refractive correction.
- to improve the physical fit in cases where a lens with a spherical back optic zone radius (BOZR) and spherical back peripheral zone radii fails to sit properly on the cornea.

These two applications are not always distinct, and occasionally a toric lens will be used for both physical and optical reasons.

There are many varieties of rigid toric lens available to the practitioner. Most commonly, such lenses will consist of a toroidal back optic zone and peripheral zone. These lenses are generally used in attempting to obtain a good physical fit on a cornea that is too toroidal to allow a good fit with a lens having a spherical BOZR and spherical peripheral radii. Lenses with toroidal back optic and peripheral zones can be produced with or without a toroidal front optic surface. A lens that has a toroidal back optic zone and a toroidal front surface is said to have a 'bitoric' construction. If the principal meridians are not parallel, then the lens is designated as having an 'oblique bitoric' construction.

Occasionally, a rigid toric lens may be prescribed that consists of a spherical back optic zone and a toroidal peripheral zone. This type of lens can also be produced with or without a toroidal front surface, the latter usually being the preferred option. Lenses with spherical back optic zones and toroidal peripheral zones are used as a means of attempting to improve the physical fit of a lens on an astigmatic cornea without the optical complications inherent in the use of lenses with toroidal back optic zones.

A rigid toric lens with a spherical back optic zone and spherical peripheral zone combined with a toroidal front optic surface is required in the situation where there is a significant amount of residual (non-corneal) astigmatism but minimal corneal astigmatism. In this case, the residual astigmatism needs to be corrected by means of a toroidal front surface, with a spherical optic zone indicated for the back surface due to the negligible corneal astigmatism.

Since rigid lenses with both spherical BOZR and peripheral radii are often used successfully on corneas with medium to high degrees of astigmatism, it is important to decide what degree of corneal astigmatism should indicate the use of toroidal back optic zones. In general, these lenses should only be used when a lens with a spherical BOZR cannot be made to fit successfully. It is rare to find that toroidal back optic zones are necessary unless the corneal astigmatism exceeds 2.50D (i.e. the difference in the corneal radii, as measured with a keratometer, exceeds approximately 0.5mm).

In cases of uncertainty (for example, where the corneal astigmatism is between 2.00 and 3.00D), a toroidal back optic zone would be used in preference to a spherical back surface curve when:

- a spherical lens exhibits poor centration or excessive movement
- excessive lens flexure is noted with a spherical lens
- fluorescein patterns with a spherical lens reveal excessive bearing along the flatter corneal meridian, regardless of the BOZR that is fitted
- Significant 3 and 9 o'clock staining occurs with a spherical lens
- there is marked corneal distortion and spectacle blur upon removal of the spherical lens from the eye; this occurs as a result of poor alignment between the spherical lens and the toric cornea, with the spherical lens subsequently having a moulding effect on the toric cornea
- there is significant residual astigmatism; in this case a spherical back surface may provide an adequate fit, but a toric back surface is utilized to stabilize the lens and prevent rotation, due to the presence of the correction for the residual astigmatism on the front surface of the lens.

A great deal depends on factors other than corneal astigmatism. Lid positions and tension are important. In a case of high with-the-rule corneal astigmatism and a drooping, loose lower lid, a toroidal back optic zone may

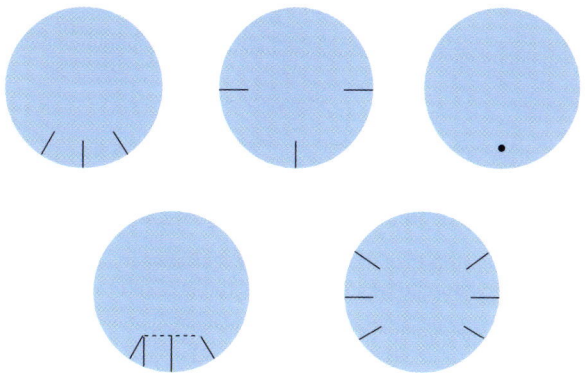

Figure T.13 • Various markings used by different manufacturers to assist practitioners in determining the angle of rotation of soft toric lenses in the eye.

be needed to obtain a good physical fit and centration. However, a similar eye with a firm, high lower lid may well be successfully fitted using a lens with spherical back surface curves.

The majority of cases of corneal astigmatism are found with the steeper corneal curve in the vertical meridian (with-the-rule). If an attempt is made to fit such an eye with a spherical BOZR, the lens often drops low on the cornea, causing physical discomfort and/or poor vision. The presence of against-the-rule corneal astigmatism usually necessitates the use of a toroidal back optic zone earlier than would be required with an equivalent amount of with-the-rule corneal astigmatism. This is due to the tendency for rigid spherical lenses to decentre laterally on corneas with even just moderate amounts (1.50–2.00D) of against-the-rule astigmatism. See *Compensated rigid bitoric lenses; Cylindrical power equivalent rigid toric lenses; Induced astigmatism with rigid toric lenses; Residual astigmatism with rigid toric lenses; Stabilization of rigid toric lenses; Toric lens design, rigid.*

Toric contact lens rotation, soft

Soft toric lenses contain markings at a specific reference point so the degree of rotation can be assessed when the lens is on the eye (Figure T.13). The markings may be in the form of laser traces, scribe lines, engraved dots or ink dots. These markings do not represent the cylinder axis; they are simply a point of reference with regard to which the rotation of the lens can be assessed. They may be either at the 6 o'clock position of the lens, or in the horizontal lens meridian at the 3 and 9 o'clock positions. The latter situation is preferable, as the markings can be then observed without having to retract the lower eyelid (which would interfere with the dynamic stabilizing forces that normally act to orient the lens). In addition, having two widely-spaced markings about 14mm apart at the 3 and 9 o'clock positions, as opposed to one mark or a set of marks at the 6 o'clock position, makes it easier to quantify the angle of rotation. Many laboratories that opt for the 6 o'clock indication provide three lines on their lenses, each separated by the same known angle, thus also facilitating a determination of lens rotation. Unfortunately, there is no standardization with respect to the angles used by different manufacturers (Figure T.14).

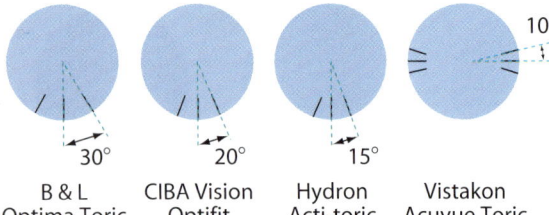

Figure T.14 • Examples of the different angles between axis location marks adopted by some manufacturers of soft toric lenses.

Estimation is a straightforward and reasonable technique for assessing the degree of lens rotation, made simpler if the practitioner remembers that the difference between each hour on a clock face is 308. Clinical experience has shown that this is a satisfactory method of assessing lens rotation, with errors more likely to occur when evaluating higher amounts of lens rotation. See *Stabilization of soft toric lenses; Toric lens fitting, soft; Toric lens, soft*.

Toric contact lens, soft

The use of soft toric lenses (in preference to soft spherical lenses) is indicated when there is ocular astigmatism present (whether corneal or non-corneal) that warrants correction. Unlike rigid lenses, soft lenses do not mask corneal astigmatism, but rather conform to the shape of the cornea. Consequently, correcting ocular astigmatism with soft lenses requires that cylinder be incorporated into the back vertex power (BVP) of the lens.

When deciding whether or not to prescribe a soft toric lens, the following factors need to be taken into account:

1. The degree of astigmatism. As a generalization, 1.00D or more of astigmatism should be corrected, although there will be significant variability between patients. About 45% of the population require a cylindrical correction of up to 0.75D, and 25% of the population require a correction of 1.00D or more.
2. The cylinder axis. An uncorrected cylinder with an oblique axis will cause greater degradation of the visual image compared with an equivalent amount of uncorrected with-the-rule or against-the-rule astigmatism.
3. Ocular dominance. Uncorrected astigmatism is far more likely to be accepted by the patient if it is in the non-dominant eye or in the eye with the poorer acuity.
4. Viability of other alternatives. The practitioner needs to consider whether soft toric lenses are the best option or if the patient would be better off with spectacles or rigid lenses. For example, a patient with high degrees (>5.00D) of both corneal and spectacle astigmatism would probably achieve better acuities with a rigid toric lens.
5. Visual needs of the patient. Usually, the less critical the visual task, the greater the amount of astigmatism that can be left uncorrected (and vice versa).

The two principal categories of surface optics of soft toric lenses are:

1. Toroidal back surface with a spherical front surface
2. Spherical back surface with toroidal front surface.

Regardless of which of these configurations is prescribed, the end result on the eye will be a bitoric lens form due to the wrapping of the front and back surface of the lens onto the cornea. The choice of design configuration is generally based more on considerations relating to manufacture. See *Stabilization of soft toric lenses; Toric lens fitting, soft; Toric lens rotation, soft*.

Toric lenses

A lens with a toroidal surface is known as a toric lens. Toric lenses may very occasionally have two toroidal surfaces, for example, in order to make a very high power cylindrical lens, but such items are rare.

Conventionally, a toric lens will have one spherical surface and one toroidal surface. The toroidal surface may be the front or back surface. The specification is commonly written as, for example:

$$\frac{+6.00DS}{-3.00DC \times 30/ -5.00DC \times 120}$$

The spherical front surface is written above the line, with the specification of the toroidal rear surface being written beneath. This lens could also have been specified as:

$$\frac{+5.00DS \times 120/ +7.00DC \times 30}{-4.00DS}$$

This second example is a front surface toroidal lens, the first being a back surface toroidal lens. Rear surface toroidal lenses are currently the most commonly used form, mainly for reasons of manufacturing convenience. If the lenses are considered to be 'thin', then both the above examples will have the same power. The first step is to add the first power of the toroidal surface to the spherical power, giving $+1.00 \times 120$. Next, the second power on the toroidal surface is added to the spherical power, giving $+3.00 \times 30$. This is equivalent to a sphero-cylindrical power of $+1.00/+2.00 \times 30$. Unlike a sphero-cylindrical form of lens, where there are only two alternative specifications, a toric lens can have a virtually infinite variety of forms, depending on the curvature of the spherical surface.

The traditional nomenclature for a toric lens is:

Sphere curve: power of the spherical surface

Base curve: lowest absolute power (longest radius) on the toroidal surface

Cross curve: highest absolute power (shortest radius) on the toroidal surface

The terms 'base curve' and 'cross curve' originate from the traditional method of manufacturing front surface toric glass single vision lenses. The term 'base curve' is now more likely to be used to describe the front spherical curve of a semi-finished lens which is designed to have a toroidal surface subsequently placed on the back.

Transposition between toric forms can be deduced from the discussion above. Below are examples of the steps required for the various transpositions.

- Transposition from toric to sphero-cylindrical form
    1. Add sphere curve of toric to first power of toroidal surface to give first power and axis of cross cylinder form

2. Add sphere curve of toric to second power of toroidal surface to give second power and axis of cross cylinder form.
3. Convert cross cylinder form to sphero cylindrical form.

Example:

$$\frac{+3.00DS}{-5.00DC \times 50 \, / -6.00DC \times 140}$$

1. +3.00DS +(−5.00DC) × 50 ⇒ −2.00DC × 50
2. +3.00DS +(−6.00DC) × 140 ⇒ −3.00DC × 140
3. −2.00DS /−1.00DC × 140

- Sphero-cylindrical to toric form with specific base curve on toroidal surface
  1. Transpose sphero-cylindrical form to the sphero-cylindrical form with the same sign of cylinder as the power of the base curve
  2. Write down base curve with axis 90° to cylinder axis
  3. Cross curve is base curve plus cylinder power with axis the same as cylinder axis
  4. Subtract base curve from sphere of sphero-cylindrical form to give sphere surface of toric.

Example: +8.00DS / −3.00DC × 180, on +9.00DC toroidal base curve

1. +8.00/− 3.00 × 180 ⇒ +5.00 / +3.00 × 90
2. +9.00 × 180
3. +9.00 + (+3.00) × 90 ⇒ +12.00 × 90
4. +5.00 − (+9.00) ⇒ −4.00

Finished form:

$$\frac{+9.00 \times 180 \, / +12.00 \times 120}{-4.00}$$

- Sphero-cylindrical to toric form with specific spherical surface
  1. Convert to cross-cylindrical form
  2. Subtract spherical surface from each power of the cross-cylinder form to give the new powers and associated axes for the toroidal surface.

Example: −1.00 / +2.00 × 165 on +4.00DS curve

1. −1.00 × 75 / +1.00 × 165
2. −1.00 − (+4.00) ⇒ −5.00 × 75
   and +1.00 − (+4.00) ⇒ −3.00 × 165

Finished form:

$$\frac{+4.00}{-3.00 \times 165 \, / -5.00 \times 75}$$

Toroidal back surface contact lenses
- See *Stabilization of rigid toric lenses; Stabilization of soft toric lenses*.

Total diameter (TD) of contact lenses
The total diameter (TD) of a lens is measured from the very edge of the lens through the lens centre (Figure T.15;

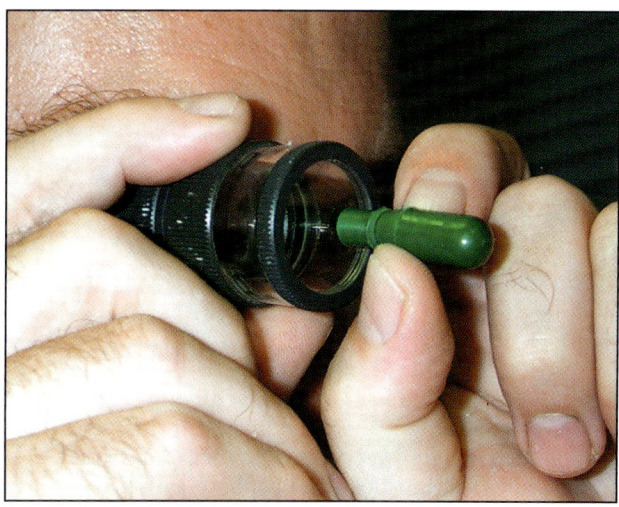

Figure T.15 • Measuring the overall diameter of a rigid lens using a loupe with calibrated scale on clear base plate.

see also Figure B.1). The fact that the water content and therefore the dimensions of some soft lens materials vary with temperature makes it difficult to compare the labelled diameter of one lens to another. Most non-ionic soft lenses, particularly those containing n-vinyl pyrrolidone, shrink by approximately 0.5mm when raised from room to eye temperature. Ionic lenses are also temperature sensitive, although they shrink much less than non-ionic lenses. Some lenses are made larger in diameter to compensate for this. A further complicating factor is that the on-eye diameter is affected by the sagittal depth of the lens. Lenses of similar nominal diameter can vary in sagittal depth by as much as 1mm and, since the periphery of a soft lens flattens to align with the bulbar conjunctiva, the sagittal depth can have a significant effect on lens diameter during lens wear.

Training patients about contact lenses
- See *Patient education*.

Training staff in optometric practice
- See *Staff training in optometric practice*.

Translating vision contact lenses
- See *Alternating vision lenses for presbyopia*.

Transposition of sphero-cylinder forms
Sphero-cylindrical lens combinations are common in ophthalmic optics. Such lenses can be made in alternative forms. Consider the example of a +3.00DS front surface combined with a +2.00DC axis 90 to give a thin lens. This is conventionally written as:

+3.00DS / +2.00DC × 90 or +3.00/ +2.00 × 90

For analytical purposes, it can be useful to write this in terms of purely cylindrical powers. Thus, the +3.00DS can be replaced by +3.00DC × 90 combined with +3.00DC × 180. If +2.00DC × 90 is now added in, the total effect is:

+5.00DC × 90/+3.00DC × 180

Note that the '/' symbol indicates 'combined with'. This notation is known as the 'cross-cylinder' form, and is useful for analytical purposes.

What would happen if the combination +5.00DS/−2.00DC × 180 were considered? Here the sphere would be represented by

+5.00DC × 90/+5.00DC × 180

Adding in the cylinder gives

+5.00DC × 90/+3.00DC × 180

which is the same result as achieved before. Thus there are two alternative sphero-cylindrical forms, and these can be exchanged by a process known as *transposition*.

The rules for transposition of sphero-cylindrical lenses are as follows:

1. Add sphere to cylinder to give new spherical power.
2. Change sign of cylinder to give new cylinder power.
3. Change axis by 90° e.g. if the original cylinder axis is = 90, then add 90; if the original cylinder axis is > 90, then subtract 90.

If a lens is considered to be 'thin' so that the thickness is neglected, then the two sphero-cylindrical forms can be considered as identical; however, in practise lenses of finite thickness would have some difference in optical properties.

Trial contact lens set disinfection

The vast majority of patients who wear soft lenses are fitted using disposable, single-use trial lenses, which are often supplied free by the manufacturer for this purpose. However, certain complex soft lenses (e.g. high-powered lenticular lenses, special tints, custom-made bifocal designs) are best fitted from trial lens sets. Although excellent success rates in fitting rigid lenses empirically (i.e. the lens is ordered based on measures of refraction and ocular dimensions) have been demonstrated, certain ocular conditions can only be corrected by fitting sophisticated designs from a trial lens set. An obvious case is keratoconus, and a practitioner who fits patients with this condition may have access to a number of trial fitting sets, each representing a different design concept. The issue arises as to how such trial fitting sets should be maintained so as to prevent cross-contamination of patients.

Proper application of the standard soft lens and rigid lens care protocols will be efficacious at killing most bacteria, viruses, fungi and protozoa, especially those known to cause infection in the eye. However, certain infectious agents that have more recently been identified are apparently resistant to current soft and rigid lens care regimes. Of particular concern at the present time is a proteinaceous vector known as a prion – a chameleon-like infectious agent that exists in different strains, has distinct biological properties, and can alter when the disease for which it is responsible crosses the species barrier. It has been suggested by health authorities in the UK that there is a remote theoretical risk of transmission of variant Creutzfeldt-Jacob disease (vCJD) between humans via transfer of bodily tissues and fluids such as tears. The prion is a vector for transmission of this disease.

An extension of the above argument leads to the conclusion that vCJD could theoretically be transmitted from an infected individual to another person via a trial contact lens contaminated with the offending prion. A solution containing 20000 ppm of available chlorine of sodium hypochlorite is effective in reducing transmissible spongiform encephalopathy (vCJD) infectivity; such a solution can be employed for disinfecting reusable rigid trial lenses.

Trial fitting, rigid contact lens
- See *Fitting rigid contact lenses.*

Trial fitting, soft contact lens
- See *Fitting soft contact lenses.*

Trichiasis
- See *Eyelid pathology, therapeutic lenses for.*

Trichromacy

Normal colour vision is trichromatic and mediated by three inherited cone photopigment types which have maximum sensitivity in the long, medium and short wavelength portions of the visible spectrum. The three photopigments have maximum sensitivity at about 560nm (L cones), 530nm (M cones) and 420nm (S cones) respectively (sometimes reported to have maximum sensitivity nearer to 565nm, 535nm and 440nm). The terms erythrolabe, chlorolabe and cyanolabe have been used to describe these photopigments. The three cone types are often referred to as 'red', 'green' and 'blue' sensitive to correspond with the three primary colours needed for additive colour mixing. This is convenient but is misleading because peak spectral sensitivity does not correspond with wavelengths normally associated with these colour names and all cone types are sensitive to a large range of wavelengths. The peak sensitivity of the L and M cones differs by only 30nm and there is a large overlap between the absorption spectra of these two pigments. This is due to the fairly recent evolution of the L and M cone photopigments from a common ancestor. The S cone photopigment appears to have evolved from rhodopsin (the rod photopigment) much earlier in genetic terms and although their spectral sensitivities overlap this is only significant in mesopic light levels when both types of receptor are stimulated. The spectral characteristics of visual photopigments can be measured using microspectrophotometry, cone electroretinograms and fundus (retinal) densitometry following selective colour adaptation.

The 'trichromatic colour vision' theory was advanced by Young and Helmholtz in the 18th century but was challenged by Hering who proposed the 'opponent pairs' theory based on colour appearance phenomena, such as afterimages, in which red is opponent to green, yellow opponent to blue and white opponent to black. It was originally considered that these two theories conflicted. However, it is now established that trichromacy occurs at the receptor level and that neural interactions within the retina result in three opponent pathways at the level of the retinal ganglion cells. Light is absorbed in the cones and converted into electrical signals by complex photochemical reactions. There are three channels transmitting colour information from the retina to the visual cortex. Electrical signals from the three classes of cones are processed in anatomically different retinal bipolar cells and ganglion cells to produce a luminance (light/dark) channel, derived from the sum of the L and M cone signals known as the magnocellular (phasic) pathway. The magnocellular channel adds L and M cone signals with a weighting of 2:1.

Recent analysis of the retinal cone mosaic has shown that there are large individual differences in the L:M cone ratio which appears to have no effect on colour perception. A post-receptoral gain mechanism must therefore exist in order to maintain the expected weighting. 'Unique yellow', a yellow which is neither reddish nor greenish, is the wavelength where the L:M cone input is 1:1. The contribution of S cones to the neurons of the magnocellular pathway is very small. The second red-green opponent channel is based on the difference in the L and M cone signals and is known as the parvocellular (tonic) pathway. The third channel, the koniocellular (K) pathway, is derived from the S cones and differenced with the sum of the L and M cone signals, hence often described as 'blue/yellow opponent'. Axons of the retinal ganglion cells serving the magnocellular and parvocellular pathways synapse in alternate layers in the lateral geniculate nucleus (LGN). Axons serving the K pathway synapse in thin (intercalated) layers adjacent to parvocellular layers in the LGN. Projections from these three pathways initially terminate in different layers of the primary visual cortex. Perception of colour is mediated by colour selective neurons in areas V1, V2 and in the extra-striate visual area V4 of the visual cortex.

Trifocal lenses

Trifocal lenses have three areas of discrete power, and are manufactured in a similar way to bifocal lenses (Figure T.16). The potential benefits of such lenses can best be illustrated by first considering an emmetrope with an amplitude of accommodation of 3.00D. Assuming that two thirds of this amplitude can be used for long periods of time, then the near addition required for near work at one third of a metre is +1.00D. If bifocals are used by this emmetrope, and ignoring any depth of field, then a range of clear vision from infinity to 0.33m is possible through the distance portion of the lens if maximum accommodation is used. Using the near segment, the furthest point of distinct vision will be 1m, and the nearest will be 0.25m, again assuming that maximum accommodation is used. Note that the two ranges overlap.

If an emmetrope who has 0.75D of accommodation is considered, then by making the same assumptions as before, 0.50D can be used for long periods, so that a +2.50D addition is (theoretically) required to see clearly at 0.33m. The clear ranges now become infinity to 1.33m in distance, and from 0.40m to 0.31m at near. These ranges clearly do not overlap, so there is a zone between the distance and near where no clear vision is possible.

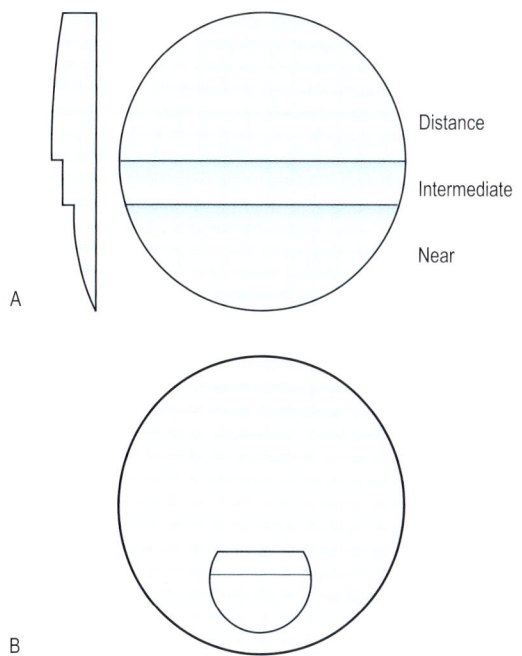

Figure T.16 • Two designs of tri-focal lens. (A) E style trifocal; (B) D segment trifocal, manufactured in solid plastic or fused glass.

The idea of a trifocal is to partially or wholly to fill in this intermediate range with a reduced addition. Thus, if a lens power for the intermediate of 50% of near was chosen, which is a commonly used ratio, then the intermediate power would be +1.25D, and an intermediate range of 0.80m down to 0.50m.

Thus, trifocals are required by the older presbyopes who require higher additions. Construction of these lenses follows the same principles as bifocal lenses, so that they can be manufactured in split, cement, fused glass or solid forms. Fused glass designs require a segment with two refractive indices of glass in order to give the intermediate and near powers. Although trifocal lenses have proved popular in the USA, they have largely been overtaken by the development of progressive addition lenses.

Trigeminal neuralgia
- See *Eyelid pathology, therapeutic lenses for.*

Truncation of contact lenses
- See *Stabilization of rigid toric lenses; Stabilization of soft toric lenses.*

Tungsten lamps
- See *Incandescent lamps.*

Two-step hydrogen peroxide disinfecting solution for contact lenses
- See *Hydrogen peroxide disinfecting solution.*

Typoscope

The typoscope was invented in 1897 by Charles Prentice, and is often known as the 'Prentice typoscope'. It consists of a rectangle of black card with a small central slit. The typoscope is designed to be placed over a page of text so that only about two to three lines of print can be seen within the slit area. The aim of the device is twofold:

- to help the patient to read along lines of text without straying up or down. When reaching the end of the line, the patient can first track back along the line which has just been read, and can then move the typoscope down to the next line. This is most valuable in cases of hemianopia (see hemianopia, aids for); patients with this condition may also value the edge of the slit aligned with the beginning (in left-sided hemianopia) or the end (in right-sided hemianopia) of the lines to help them read the whole of the lines.
- to increase retinal contrast by preventing intra-ocular scattering from the high luminance background. It is equivalent to the effect achieved with white-on-black print presented using reverse polarity on a closed circuit television system. The contrast of the object is identical to one which is black-on-white, but disability glare is greater with a white background since the overall luminance of the object is higher. (See *Glare.*)

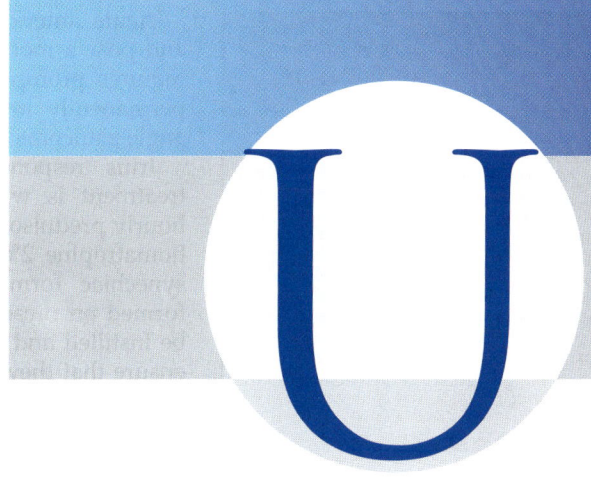

Ultrasound disinfection of soft contact lenses

This physical method of soft lens disinfection relies on sonic energy being imparted to micro-organisms to cause lethal cell changes. Such devices have a limited disinfection efficacy.

Ultraviolet radiation disinfection of soft contact lenses

Studies on the efficacy of ultraviolet radiation for contact lens disinfection have provided equivocal results. Using radiation of 253.7nm at an energy of 44.3µW/cm^2, Acanthamoeba cysts and trophozoites survive irradiation of 22 minutes in duration. Although the numbers of some micro-organisms are reduced by ultraviolet irradiation, the level of survivors is unacceptably high. However, adequate bacterial disinfection can be achieved at the same wavelength using an ultraviolet lamp with a higher energy output, 950µW/cm^2; lens parameter changes with this level of radiation are not clinically important.

Unit-dose saline for contact lenses

- See *Saline solutions*.

USAN classification of contact lens materials

- See *Water content, hydrogel*.

Uveitis, anterior

Uveitis is classified anatomically depending on the site of inflammation as being anterior (including iritis and iridocyclitis), intermediate (pars planitis), posterior and panuveitis. Iritis, or inflammation affecting the iris, is the most common type. Iritis is usually unilateral; if bilateral, it is more likely that there is an identifiable underlying cause. Iritis is also classified in terms of the severity and chronicity of inflammation: i.e. as acute, recurrent acute and chronic.

Causes of anterior uveitis include:

- External injury to the uvea, or other external agents
- Systemic diseases such as Sarcoidosis. In addition, 25% of iritis is associated with a histocompatibility antigen HLA-B27 positive systemic condition such as ankylosing spondylitis, Reiter's syndrome, psoriatic arthritis, juvenile rheumatoid arthritis, or inflammatory bowel disease (Crohn's disease, but not coeliac disease)
- Infections such as tuberculosis, candida, herpes zoster, toxoplasmosis
- Idiopathic specific uveitis, such as Fuch's uveitis syndrome
- Idiopathic non-specific (about 25%).

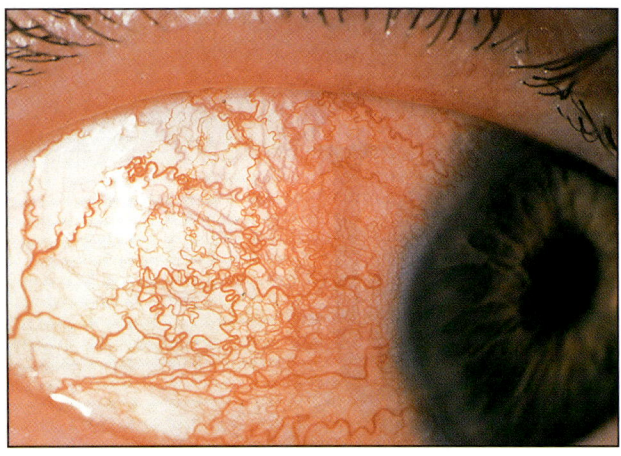

Figure U.1 • Characteristic circumlimbal 'ciliary flush' in acute anterior uveitis.

During an attack of anterior uveitis the affected eye is usually red, photophobic and has a dull ache. There is also often decreased vision and increased lacrimation. There may be a history of recurrent episodes. Chronic anterior uveitis is associated with exacerbations and remissions, but with much less of the acute symptoms. Some patients remain relatively asymptomatic despite significant inflammation. Symptoms of arthritis, back pain, skin rashes and urethritis should also be sought.

The classic findings of iritis are circumlimbal injection, anterior chamber cells and flare, keratic precipitates, anterior vitreous cells and posterior synechiae (Figure U.1). The pupil is often slightly miotic and slow to react and the intraocular pressure is often slightly low relative to the other eye. Intraocular pressure is occasionally high, especially with herpetic conditions. In granulomatous uveitis the keratic precipitates are typically large, termed 'mutton fat' precipitates, and there may be inflammatory nodules on the iris surface (Busacca nodules) or at the pupil margin (Koeppe nodules). Chronic recurrent iritis can lead to a band keratopathy or cataract formation.

Acute anterior uveitis can cause severe discomfort, and pose a moderate threat to sight if left untreated. It requires prompt investigation and treatment to avoid permanently impaired vision from pupil block, open angle glaucoma and cataract.

Iritis responds well to medical therapy. Initial treatment is with intensive topical steroids such as hourly prednisolone acetate 1% and a mydriatic such as homatropine 2% three times daily to prevent anterior synechiae formation. If there are already synechiae formed on presentation, a drop of homatropine should be instilled and the patient checked 30 minutes later to ensure that they have broken. If they are still present, a combination of mydriatics should be instilled, such as phenylephrine 10%, cyclopentolate 1% and tropicamide 1% in an attempt to break the synechiae. Following initial treatment, the drops are normally tapered, ceasing the dilating drop first. Mydriasis is not required once the anterior chamber reaction is under control as it will add to the photophobia as well as blurring vision. The corticosteroids are usually tapered over 4 to 6 weeks, unless there is a history of recurrent iritis where the tapering should be slower. Systemic steroids or periocular steroids may be required if the uveitis does not respond to hourly steroids.

No investigations are necessary for the first attack of iritis if it is unilateral. If recurrent, granulomatous, bilateral or posterior involvement is present, then appropriate blood tests could include: human leukocyte antigen B27, testing for e.g. HLA-B27 uveitis without systemic disease; erythrocyte sedimentation rate, testing for e.g. ankylosing spondylitis or Reiter's syndrome; chest X-ray, e.g. testing for tuberculosis or sarcoid; angiotensin-converting enzyme, testing for sarcoidosis; full blood examination, testing for any infection, e.g. testing for tuberculosis; Mantoux test, testing for tuberculosis; or antinuclear antibody, testing for juvenile arthritis. Other possible associations include inflammatory bowel disease, psoriatic arthritis, and Behçet's disease. As iritis is frequently recurrent patients should be advised to represent promptly if symptoms recur.

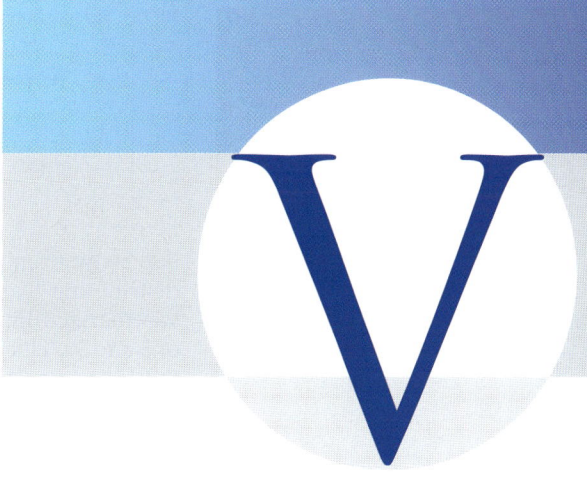

Vacuoles, contact lens associated

When the cornea is severely compromised, such as in the case of severe stromal oedema or an extensive microcyst response, the epithelium can also become oedematous; this manifests as the appearance of small fluid vacuoles in the epithelium. By observing the cornea using indirect retro-illumination on the slit-lamp biomicroscope, fluid vacuoles can be observed to display 'unreversed illumination'; that is, the distribution of light within the vacuole is the same as the light distribution of the background (Figure V.1). This indicates that the vacuole is acting as a diverging refractor, and therefore it must consist of material that is of a lower refractive index (fluid) than the surrounding epithelial tissue.

The aetiology of epithelial fluid vacuoles is two-fold. Epithelial oedema follows traumatic loss of surface epithelial cells. The fluid barrier (zonula occludens) that is normally found between surface epithelial cells is breached, resulting in the movement of fluid into the deeper layers of the epithelium. Since the cells are tightly fitted and attach snugly together, the oedema may not occur instantly, nor be widespread. Epithelial oedema can also form as a result of hypotonic ocular exposure, which can compromise the integrity of the fluid barrier. Epithelial oedema and the following thinning can co-exist during periods of rigid lens wear.

The flare observed with fluorescein in and around corneal abrasions is epithelial oedema. Histopathological evaluation of corneas following hypotonic exposure demonstrates that the oedema is extracellular and is present throughout the full thickness of the epithelium. Reflex tears are of

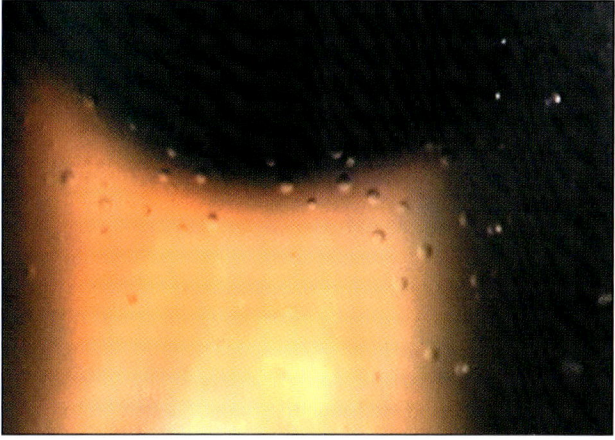

Figure V.1 • Fluid vacuoles at the epithelial surface displaying unreversed illumination.

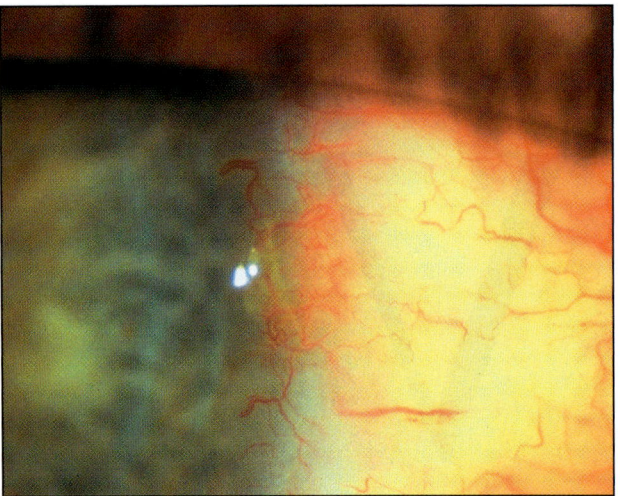

Figure V.2 • Vascularized limbal keratitis.

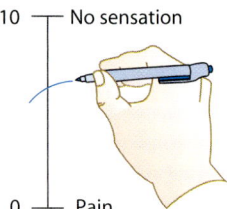

Figure V.3 • Vertical analogue scale used to quantify subjective comfort, whereby a higher number indicates greater comfort.

low tonicity and may also provoke epithelial oedema, such as during adaptation to rigid lenses.

Breakdown of the corneal fluid barrier, as indicated by the presence of fluid vacuoles, can lead to secondary problems. For example, contaminated low tonicity water – such as that which may be found in a jacuzzi or hot tub – has an association with contracting an Acanthamoeba keratitis. The amoeba may use the spaces created between cells by the oedematous state to gain entry to the cornea. This scenario is possible in both contact lens wearers and non-lens wearers. Fluid vacuoles can break through the anterior epithelial surface, leading to a very painful condition. Practitioners should therefore take action to eliminate fluid vacuoles from the epithelium by treating the underlying cause, which generally equates to the prescription of highly gas-permeable contact lenses that afford optimal corneal oxygenation.

Variant Creutzfeldt-Jakob disease
- See *Trial lens set disinfection*.

Varifocal lenses
- See *Progressive addition lenses*.

Vascularization, contact lens induced
- See *Neovascularization*.

Vascularized limbal keratitis, contact lens induced

This condition is observed in patients wearing rigid contact lenses on an extended wear basis. It manifests as a limbal inflammation, typically at either the 3 or 9 o'clock positions, and an encroachment of limbal vessels (Figure V.2). The adjacent conjunctiva may be oedematous and hyperemic, and the lesion may be surrounded by fine superficial punctate epithelial staining and mild corneal infiltration. The patient may only be mildly symptomatic, complaining of ocular dryness. The problem may be exacerbated if the lens surface is crazed or deposited.

This condition often occurs in regions of the limbus that have become desiccated due to poor wetting of the ocular surface. This problem is caused by bridging of the lids away from the globe, thus preventing the lids from distributing tears over the affected area. In this regard, vascularized limbal keratitis may be an advanced form of 3 and 9 o'clock staining. In late stages of this condition the lesion can become slightly raised, in the form of a thickened mass of epithelial tissue through which blood vessels traverse at various depths. This epithelial hypertrophy may be related to the fact that the limbus contains a high concentration of stem cells, creating a greater capacity for epithelial cell mitosis and movement. Also, the limbus hosts a vast array of immunologic mechanisms mediated via the mononuclear phagocyte system in limbal vessels.

Vascularized limbal keratitis is reversible, and cessation of lens wear for a few weeks will allow most of the pathology to resolve. Converting the patient from extended-wear to daily-wear lenses, and refitting with a smaller diameter rigid lens, may prevent the problem from recurring. Changing from rigid to soft lenses will certainly eliminate the problem.

Vascular pannus, contact lens induced
- See *Pannus*.

Vasoconstrictors
- See *Decongestants, ocular*.

Vat dye tinting of soft contact lenses

This process is used for creating translucent tints in soft lenses. The finished contact lens is soaked in a water-soluble dye for a fixed amount of time and at a specified temperature. The lens is then exposed to air, rendering the dye insoluble and trapped within the lens matrix. Because the dye only enters the lens surface to a depth of about 10μm, the lens will appear to have a uniform tint across its entirety, the intensity of which will be independent of optical power. The dye is held in position by strong absorptive forces, resulting in a stable, permanent tint that can only be extracted by the use of powerful solvents. See *Tinted lenses*.

VCJD
- See *trial lens set disinfection*.

Vertical analogue scale

This is a tool for quantifying subjective sensations (e.g. lens comfort). The patient is invited to mark the position on a vertical scale corresponding to the level of comfort (Figure V.3). The reason that the scale is oriented vertically is to avoid the potential bias, as a result of 'handedness', that may invalidate the use of a horizontal scale. The distance along the scale from the zero position is measured and taken as an index of the degree of sensation.

Vertometer
- See *Focimeter*.

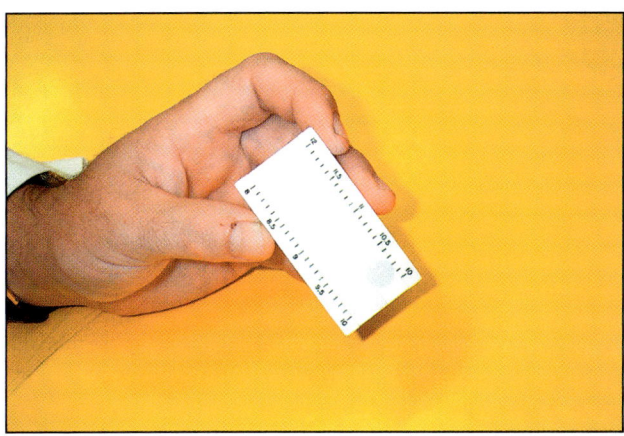

Figure V.4 • V-gauge with a double channel used to measure total lens diameter. In this case, the lens has a total diameter of 10.2mm.

Vessel ingrowth, contact lens associated
- See *Neovascularization*.

V-gauge, contact lens
The total diameter (TD) of a rigid lens can be measured using a V-gauge. This is a triangular channel cut into a plastic strip with markings and numerical diameter values arranged in descending order of magnitude towards the apex of the channel. The lens is placed at the wide end of the channel and pushed gently along towards the narrow end (or allowed to roll down within the channel as the V-gauge is tilted with the narrow end of the channel downwards) until it becomes lightly 'wedged' in the V-gauge channel (Figure V.4). Care must be taken to ensure that the V-gauge does not flex the lens, as this would underestimate lens diameter. The overall diameter is read off the pre-calibrated scale.

Videokeratoscope for corneal measurement
- See *Corneal topographic analysis*.

Videokeratoscope for lens measurement
Videokeratoscopes are ideal for checking aspheric front lens surfaces, with the lenses on or off the eye. Also, videokeratoscopes can be used to monitor lens front surface shape in cases of suspected lens flexure or dimensional instability. Videokeratoscopes are not generally suited for lens back surface analysis because the inherent software packages are designed for analysing convex surfaces only.

Visibility
The ability to perform a task safely, efficiently and comfortably depends upon its visibility, as well as on the visual capabilities of the employee. Naturally, the better the visibility, the easier it is to perform the task. Factors that influence the visibility of a task can be listed as follows:
- size of task
- distance of task
- illumination
- contrast
- colour
- time available to view task
- movement of the task
- glare
- atmospheric conditions.

How these factors affect visibility has been investigated by many researchers using different methods. One method is indirect: the influence of lighting, contrast, size of task, etc. upon job performance is assessed by measuring, for example, speed and accuracy. The simplest of the factors to adjust is the illumination; therefore, many studies have investigated the influence of illumination on job performance. The aim is to establish the range of lighting conditions that permits an improvement in performing a given task. With any study – either in a real environment or laboratory simulated conditions – certain factors must be taken into account and controlled if possible, e.g. motivation, methods of payment of employees, and type of work (and therefore level of visual difficulty of the task). There are other problems that are encountered in studies in the real environment:

- It is difficult to define the contrast in a task by reflectances from the detail and background because it is rare for the surfaces to be perfectly matt.
- The exposure time can be difficult to control. The viewing time allowed for many tasks is not externally controlled.
- The size of the task can be difficult to control. It can be altered by the employee by moving closer to the task and hence increasing the angular subtense at the eye (hence increasing the size of the task).

The principle effects of illumination, size and contrast upon visual performance are:

- Increasing the illumination produces an increase in performance, but this follows the law of diminishing returns.
- The point of the maximum performance is different for tasks of different sizes and contrast. The smaller the size and the lower the contrast, the higher the level of illumination at which maximum performance occurs.
- Larger improvements in performance can be achieved by changing the task size or contrast than by increasing the illumination.
- Increasing the illumination does not make a visually difficult task (i.e. small size and poor contrast) reach the same level of performance as a visually easy task (Figure V.5).

Although the findings above do, in principle, apply to all tasks, the relationship between illumination on the task and performance achieved will vary according to the type of task. In summary, the effect of illumination upon task performance will vary according to the visual difficulty of the task and the extent to which the visual part of the task determines the overall performance. The greater the visual difficulty, the greater the effect of the illuminance, whereas in a task such as audio typing, where there is only a small visual component, the effect of illuminance upon the overall task performance will be small.

Visibility meter
The principle of visibility meters is to reduce the visibility of a task to threshold and then relate the

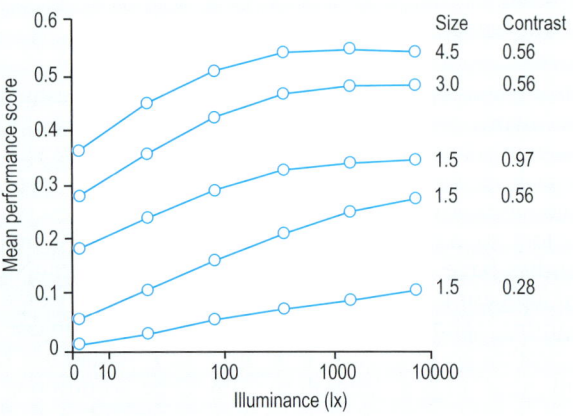

Figure V.5 • Mean performance scores for Landolt ring charts (after Weston H. C., Industrial Health Research Board Report No. 87, HMSO, London, 1945).

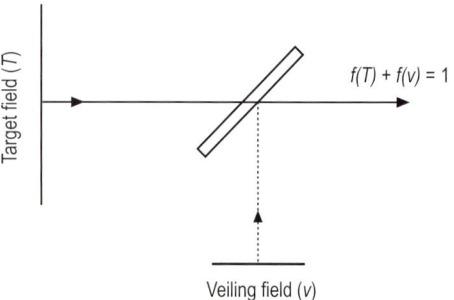

Figure V.6 • Visibility meter. f(T) fraction of total luminance from the target field reaching the observer's eye; f (υ) fraction of total luminance from the veiling field reaching the observer's eye (after A. A. Eastman (1968), J. Illum. Eng. Soc. 63: 36–40).

amount of reduction to a measure of visibility. Visibility meters can be used in several ways:

- To assess the relative visibility of a task and compare it to a standard condition.
- Once the level of visibility is established, it can be used to assess how much illumination is required to make the task as visible as the standard.
- The effects of illumination, contrast, colour, and polish of objects on the visibility can be assessed immediately.

Some meters reduce the visibility of the task to threshold by increasing the amount of veiling luminance and simultaneously decreasing the luminance from the task. This means that the overall luminance at the eye of the observer does not change, nor does the state of adaptation of the eye. A variable beam splitter can be used to achieve this effect, as shown in Figure V.6. The veiling luminance is provided by either the task background or a standard reflecting surface placed beside the task. Other meters use an internal light source to provide the veiling luminance.

If a light meter is not available to measure the illumination level, an approximate guide as to the level, which may be provided by a 60 and 100 watt bulb in a simple reflector such as an angle-poise, is given in Table V.1. If the visibility is poorer at work or at home, it may be that the illumination level is inadequate and that an additional light source will improve the visibility.

Visibility tints for contact lenses

- See Handling tints.

Vision impairment

- See Low vision.

Vision, measurement in contact lens practice

Vision should always be one of the first measurements in any contact lens examination. In this way, the vision measurement will be most indicative of the habitual vision of the patient and will be unaffected by the lights and ocular manipulations associated with later test procedures. It is equally important to establish a baseline measure of vision for medicolegal reasons.

The computer-presented visual acuity chart has advantages over other types of vision chart for contact lens practice (Figure V.7). Computer-generated optotypes can be randomized to prevent the contact lens patient from learning the letter sequences at successive visits. In addition, computerized vision charts can usually present letters down to 6/3 – a level of vision that can be achieved by many younger contact lens wearers.

Vision should be measured with and without the habitual distance spectacles of the patient at both distance and near. The level of vision can be related to the clinical history and to the results of the refraction and the binocular vision examinations. The unaided vision is of interest because patients who are commonly or intermittently uncorrected will compare that to the level of acuity they achieve with contact lenses.

Vision, poor

- See Poor vision, investigation of.

Vision screening

The general purpose of any vision screening programme is to detect those people who have defective vision but who do not present with symptoms that result in them

Table V.1 • Approximate levels of illumination (lux) that can be expected from 100-W and 60-W pearl bulbs (reproduced by kind permission of J.W. Grundy and Optometry Today, 1989).

	Distance (cm)							
	30	40	50	60	70	80	90	100
60-W bulb	900	500	320	225	165	125	100	80
100-W bulb	1800	1000	640	450	330	250	200	160

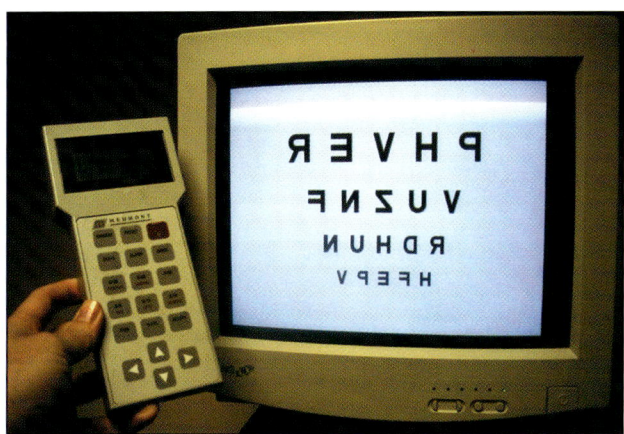

Figure V.7 • Computerized visual acuity chart. The letters on the screen are reversed for mirror display.

seeking optometric attention. Every occupation has specific visual requirements that must be met to perform tasks efficiently, safely, and with comfort. Therefore the main aim of vision screening is to detect those people whose visual ability is below the standard required. The advantages to industry of vision screening can be summarized as follows:

- Selection of personnel. Visual ability can be used in the selection of new employees or the transfer of an employee to a task they can perform efficiently.
- Identify employees with visual disabilities. These may be due to an uncorrected refractive error or ocular pathology. If the visual problems cannot be corrected then the employee can be transferred to a task they would be visually capable of performing efficiently.
- Improved employee–employer relationship.
- Improved visual efficiency can result in: increased productivity; fewer accidents and therefore reduced insurance costs; and reduced absenteeism as the task is less visually fatiguing.
- Compensation claims can be settled more easily.

Three techniques for screening vision may be used:
- Modified clinical technique
- Instrument screeners
- Computer programs.

The ideal screening programme should maximize screening success, i.e. correct referral and non-referral, and minimize screening errors, i.e. low over and under referral rate. In other words the test needs good sensitivity and specificity. Instrument screeners are widely used for vision screening of adults, and are often the method of choice used in industry and by government organizations. However, it must be remembered that whichever technique is used, it is only a screening test, and not a substitute for a full ophthalmic examination.

Vision screening, modified clinical technique of

This method of screening is carried out by qualified personnel, e.g. optometrists, who assess the visual functions considered to be particularly important to job performance. The screening examination may therefore consist of any of the following:

- History and symptoms. This is particularly useful as the history of a squint or amblyopic eye may be noted and this may reduce unnecessary referral. The presence of eyestrain when performing certain tasks can also be assessed.
- Visual acuity at any distance. The measurement can be taken at the exact distance required, with the appropriate size of letters or task.
- External eye examination and ophthalmoscopy. This allows detection of pathology of the eye that may otherwise go unnoticed. Ocular diseases do not always cause a reduction in vision that results in the person seeking medical attention.
- Retinoscopy. This permits the precise degree of hyperopia or myopia to be assessed objectively. It will also indicate whether or not poor vision is due to the fact that spectacles are required.
- Amplitude of accommodation. The result of this test will indicate whether the person can focus clearly and comfortably on a near task. Spectacles will generally be required by the older presbyopic person to see the task clearly.
- Binocular vision assessment. This can include a cover test at the viewing distance required, motility, near point of convergence, and stereopsis. To avoid eyestrain, binocular vision needs to be stable and these tests will indicate whether the binocular functions are under stress for a particular task. The presence of a squint or phoria will be detected by the cover test.
- Visual field. This can be assessed quite simply by a confrontation test, to determine whether there is any marked reduction, such as a homonymous hemianopia or quadrantic defects. The central visual field can be assessed using an Amsler chart. When held at 30cm, this chart covers the central 10° of the field either side of fixation.
- Colour vision. This can be assessed rapidly using the Ishihara pseudoisochromatic plates to identify red-green colour-deficiency. The Farnsworth D15 test or the City University test 2nd edition can be used as a second test to grade the severity of red-green deficiency and to identify significant congenital or acquired tritan defects. If an occupational task requires fine line discrimination, examination with the Farnsworth Munsell 100 hue test is helpful.

Advantages of the modified clinical technique for vision screening include:
- Flexibility – tests can be selected depending on the visual functions considered to be important for the task
- Tests can be performed at the appropriate distance
- The type and magnitude of refractive error can be assessed
- Ocular pathology may be detected
- Presence of a squint will be detected
- Very few false referrals.

The disadvantages of this technique are the high cost due to the use of professional personnel, such as optometrists, and that it is time-consuming.

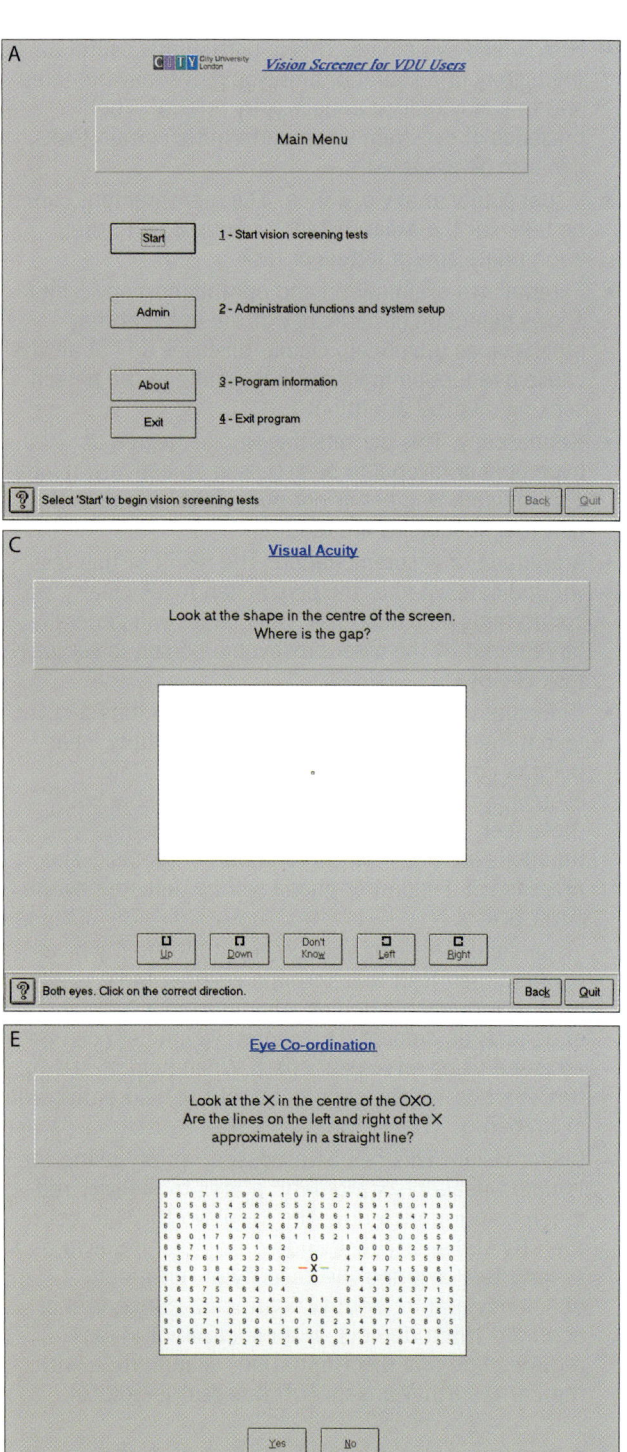
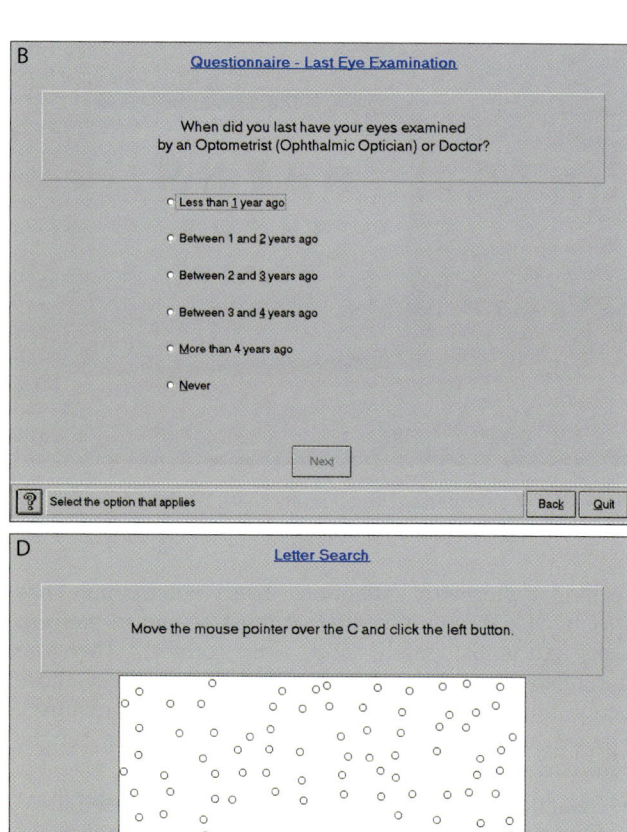

Figure V.8 (A)–(E) • City University Vision Screener for VDU users: examples of the questionnaire and vision tests, including visual acuity, letter search and fixation disparity tests (reproduced by kind permission of David Thomson and City Visual System Ltd.).

Vision screening, computer programs for

There are computer programs available that can be used to screen the vision of those who use visual display units (VDUs). The City University Vision Screening program can either be used in the consulting room or on-site. When used on-site, the system provides a direct assessment of the visual performance under the actual working conditions. It includes assessment of seven different tests of visual function including visual acuity, search tasks, oculomotor balance, fixation disparity and central visual fields. Visual acuity is measured using an illiterate E target monocularly and binocularly. Two search tasks have been included to assess if clear single vision can be sustained. The first task is to locate a single broken circle (C) that is hidden among a series of circles. The second task requires the observer to count the number of times that a certain digit/number occurs within an array of numbers. This task requires the observer to make a series of precise eye movements and maintain clear single vision. The oculomotor balance tests require the observer to wear red/green goggles to dissociate the eyes. One test displays a red line and a green scale and the observer reports the number that the line passes through. The fixation disparity test is based on the Mallett test and the observer views an OXO target through the red/green goggles. A red and green marker located on either side of the X is seen monocularly with each eye. The presence or absence of fixation disparity is recorded. The central visual fields are assessed using a multiple stimulus screening strategy. The programme also includes a questionnaire to determine any problems that VDU users may experience. The results of both the questionnaire and the visual function tests are analysed and a report is then provided giving advice and recommendations for each person (Figure V.8).

In addition, computerized vision screeners have been designed for use in schools, which include measurements of visual acuity and stereopsis, with colour vision being tested by selected Ishihara plates. Visual acuity is measured by a single line of letters surrounded by crowding bars being presented on the computer screen. The letter size is increased from LogMAR = 0.1(6/7.5) until all the letters are read correctly and the order of the letters are randomized in order to avoid learning effects. To assess stereopsis, the child views the computer screen through red/green goggles. Four pairs of red and green circles are displayed with one pair having a greater separation than the other three. The child is asked to indicate which one 'stands out' more than the others. The test can assess stereoacuity levels of 110, 220 and 330 seconds of arc.

The use of visual acuity measures alone as a method of screening children is not sensitive enough, especially when compared to the modified clinical technique (MCT) or use of instrument screeners. Compared to the use of instrument screeners or a battery of vision tests, the MCT is found to be the most sensitive, with the lowest under- and over-referral rate. The newer computerized screeners have been shown to have a high sensitivity and specificity.

Vision screeners, instrument

There are many different instrument vision screeners available, but most are basically modified stereoscopes. The eyepiece lenses are arranged so that their prismatic components simulate the viewing of a distant object and the near vision is simulated by either:

- moving the targets closer
- decreasing the separation between the half stereograms
- changing the lens power, i.e. introduce negative lenses.

The screeners usually have internal lighting and the targets are mounted either on a rotary drum or separately on cards, which are changed manually or by remote control. The types of tests commonly included in the instrument screeners are:

- visual acuity – distance and near (occasionally intermediate)
- heterophoria – horizontal and vertical at distance and near
- stereopsis
- fusion
- colour vision

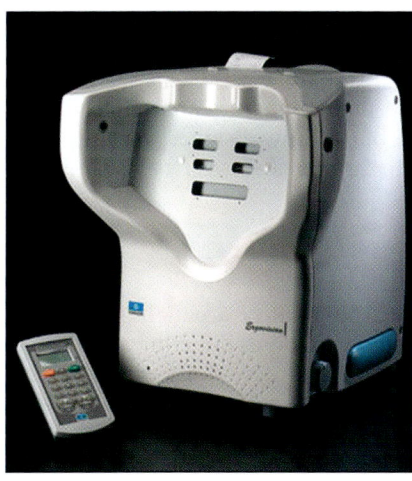

Figure V.9 • Ergovision screener (courtesy of Essilor Ltd).

- fogging test
- visual field
- astigmatism.

Advantages of instrument vision screeners include:

- operated by lay technicians
- rapid screening
- always available for use
- low maintenance costs
- cheap method of screening.

Disadvantages of instrument vision screeners include:

- lack of flexibility of tests and testing distance, especially for those screeners where the targets are on a rotary drum
- does not detect ocular pathology unless inferred by a reduction of visual acuity
- cannot detect squints
- awareness of the actual target distance may induce proximal accommodation and convergence, even when distance viewing conditions are simulated. This can effect the visual acuity measurement and induce a relative esophoria at distance
- there can be unnecessary referral by a lay operator of people with amblyopia or a squint
- reproductions of pseudoisochromatic plates or other designs but none of these are efficient for colour vision screening.

The Keystone and Rodenstock instruments offer a wide range of tests and are used by many organizations. The Ergovision screener incorporates some additional tests including dynamic visual acuity, variable contrast acuity, visual fatigue and dazzle recovery time (Figure V.9). The instrument uses a voice synthesizer to carry out the standard tests and the results are printed out at the end of the programme. All the tests can also be carried out at three different lighting levels: 15, 150, 300 cd/m^2. It is intended not only as a diagnostic test but also for studying vision in the working conditions. The wide range of tests should allow those visual examinations that are thought to be more closely matched to those of the task.

The Binoptometer is a vision screener that apparently overcomes the problem of proximal convergence. The tests are presented in free space, e.g. they are seen against a distant wall, thus eliminating proximal effects. Also tests can be carried out at any distance varying from infinity to 0.3m due to the optical design that is similar to a Badal Optometer.

Visual acuity

Visual acuity is a measurement of a patient's ability to resolve detail and usually involves directing a patient to identify targets – which are of ever decreasing size and typically of high contrast – at a set distance, until they can no longer be identified. The recognition of high contrast targets at the highest spatial frequency as described is useful for standardized assessment but is not representative of a normal visual environment and hence will not truly represent the patient's visual ability. The unaided visual acuity (usually called the 'vision') is useful in estimating refractive error before assessment and represents important baseline data where a patient does not use, or perhaps does not need to use, their correction all the time. The acuity with their current correction is known as the 'habitual visual acuity' and the resultant visual acuity after refraction and full correction of the current refractive error is known as the 'optimal visual acuity'. It is essential for an optometrist to note either the vision or habitual visual acuity prior to any clinical assessment in case of any legal action taken as a result of the examination. Both monocular and binocular acuity should be noted as there may be a discrepancy, such as when a nystagmus patient shows significant acuity improvement when in the binocular state.

Although there are several ways to specify target size on test charts, the most widely used system was introduced by Snellen in 1862. He assumed that the 'average' eye could just read a letter if the thickness of the limbs and the spaces between them subtended one minute of arc at the eye. Thus, the just-resolved letter 'E' would subtend five minutes of arc vertically. Snellen notation requires the acuity allowing the eye to resolve such a letter to be noted down as a fraction with the viewing distance (usually in metres and commonly 6 m) over the distance at which such a target would subtend 5 minutes of arc vertically. Thus, at 6m a 6/6 letter subtends five minutes of arc vertically, a 6/12 letter 10 minutes and a 6/60 letter 50 minutes. The Snellen fraction may also be written as a decimal, e.g. 6/6 = 1, 6/12 = 0.5 and 6/60 = 0.1.

An alternative is to record the minimum angle of resolution (MAR). The MAR relates to the resolution required to resolve the elements of a letter. Thus, 6/6 equates to an MAR of 1 minute of arc, 6/12 to an MAR of 2 and 6/60 to 10. The logMAR score is the $\log_{10}$ of the MAR, so it is 0 for 6/6 and 1 for 6/60. This means that targets smaller than the 6/6 letters, which would be expected to be resolved by a young healthy adult, would carry a negative score value. Some acuity values are shown in different notation in Table V.2.

Though Snellen notation is still in widespread use, there are criticisms of the standard Snellen chart (Figure V.10). There are fewer large letters so providing an unequal challenge to those with reduced vision, the letter spacing reduces leading to crowding on lower lines, the line separation is not regular so the challenge changes on reading down the chart which means that moving charts to different working distances alters the demand on acuity.

Table V.2 • The relationship between different acuity scales.

Snellen	Decimal	MAR	logMAR
6/60	0.10	10	1.000
6/24	0.25	4	0.602
6/12	0.50	2	0.301
6/6	1.00	1	0.000
6/4	1.50	0.667	–0.176

LogMAR charts, such as the Bailey-Lovie chart (Figure V.11), address some of these shortcomings by having spacing between letters on each line related to the width of the letters and between rows relating to the height of the letters, and an equal number of letters on each line. This provides a constant task as the patient reads down the chart, allowing it to be viewed at different working distances and the acuity to be more easily correlated. Such charts give greater repeatability of measurement and are more sensitive for detecting interocular acuity differences.

LogMAR scores may be noted on record cards either relating to the smallest target line size seen or using the Visual Acuity Rating where 0.02 is added for every letter missed on the line. So where a patient just manages the 6/6 line and no more they are scored as 0. If they miss two letters on this line they are scored as 0.04. Until this notation becomes universally accepted, Snellen notation is still appropriate for referrals and interprofessional communication. Most logMAR charts in use are calibrated for a working distance of 4m. When one has to reduce the distance, for example for a low vision patient, it is useful to remember to add 0.3 to the score every time the distance is halved. For example the ability to read the top line at 4 metres would be scored as an acuity of 1.0. At 2m, this would be scored as 1.3.

Where letter recognition is not possible, for example with small children or patients of different literacy, a range of picture and line targets is available. Some require identification and others matching of targets with a separate key card. The Landolt ring test requires the observer to identify where a gap appears (top, bottom, left or right) in a series of black circles of different size, all set against a white background. In the 'tumbling E' test, the letter E is presented in different orientations and sizes to the observer, who is asked to identify the orientation of the fingers of the E (i.e. up, down, left or right). For the very young, the use of gratings of different spatial frequency next to blank targets may be presented to see if the infant's attention is directed to the grating. Such preferential-looking tests have been found to show good repeatability in paediatric assessment. See *Contrast sensitivity testing; Ametropia and refractive error.*

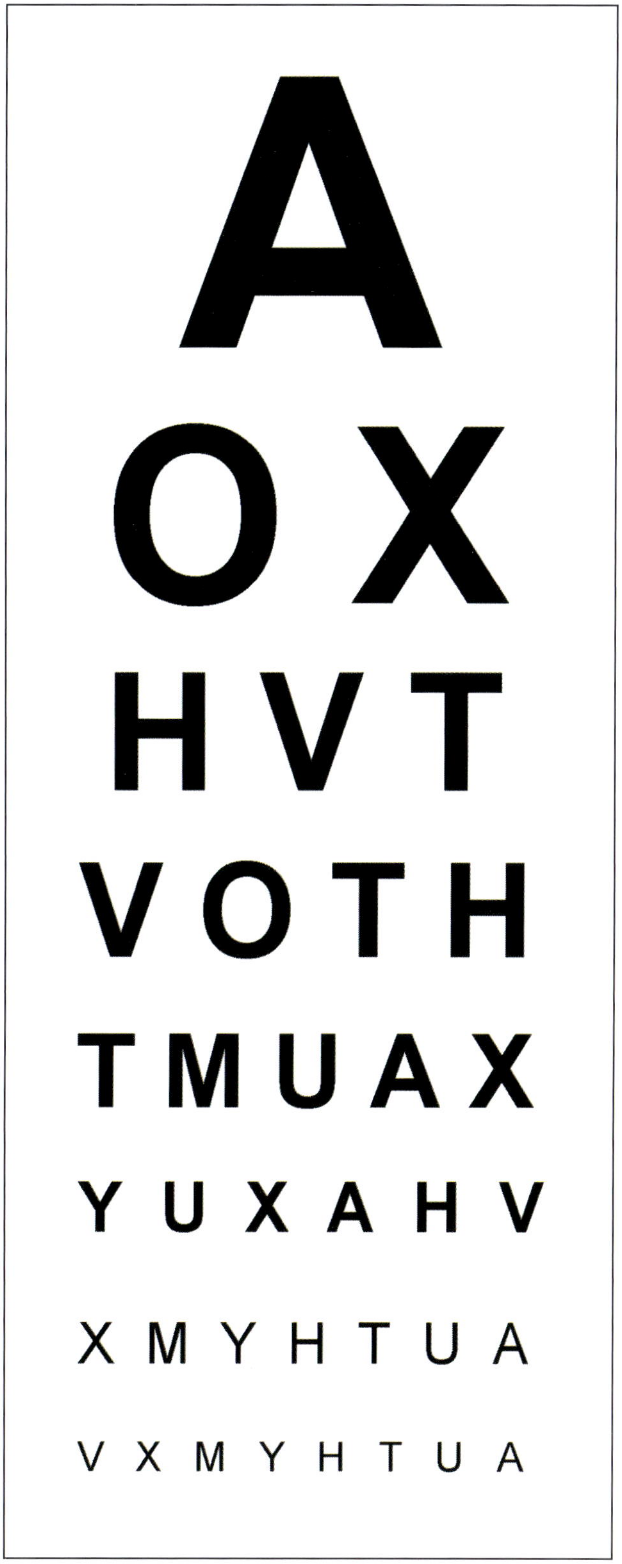

Figure V.10 • Snellen chart

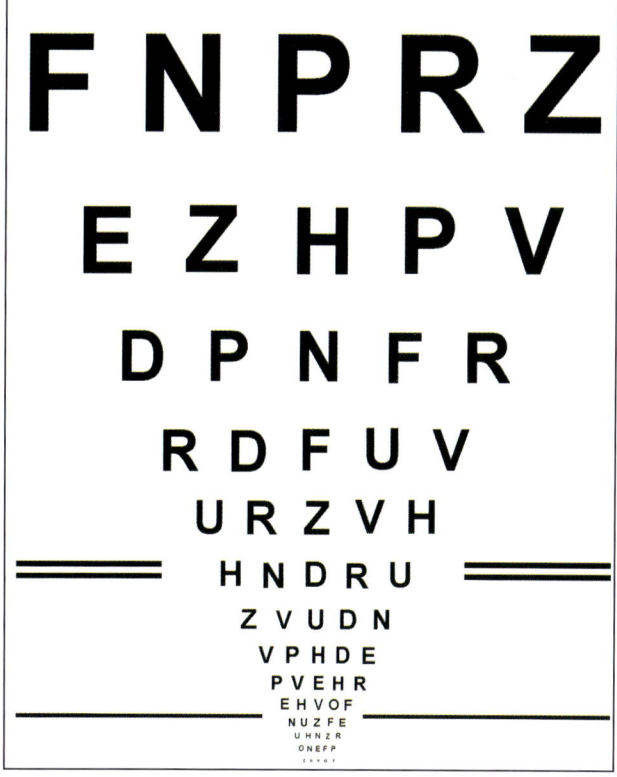

Figure V.11 • Bailey-Lovie chart.

Visual acuity measurement, low vision

The most commonly used technique for measuring visual acuity on a patient with low vision is the Snellen chart, although a logMAR chart (such as the Bailey-Lovie chart or the ETDRS chart) is preferable because of the larger number of letters available at larger sizes, which allows greater precision. It is preferable to have both internally and externally-illuminated charts, allowing assessment of the effect of different lighting conditions, and the option of different viewing distances to allow a wider range of acuities to be tested. It is usually inappropriate to use projector charts since the range of letter sizes is inadequate, and they are often of low contrast: computer generated displays avoid these shortcomings.

Testing should begin at a very close viewing distance (1m or less) to ensure that the patient can read across a line of at least 5 letters. If the letters are of mixed shape, greater difficulty in identifying circular letters may indicate significant uncorrected cylindrical error. It may also be possible to deduce the position of any (central) scotomas by noting where on the line the letters are missed. It is only necessary to revert to a 3 or 6m viewing distance if the smallest letters are obviously well within the capabilities of the patient when viewed from 1m. The aim should be to encourage patients, always giving them the impression that they are doing much better than expected. The patient should be given longer to make judgements, and encouraged to view eccentrically if this helps. The patient should be reassured that this is not 'cheating'. The acuity of each eye in turn should be recorded as accurately as possible; thus, '<6/60' is not adequate, and it should not be necessary to resort to 'counting fingers'. If patients can count the number of fingers held up, they will also be able to see letters at 1m or 0.5m. A patient report during history taking that one eye 'can't see anything' should be confirmed. The monocular acuity of each eye should be recorded, along with any comments on performance (for example, 'using

Table V.3 • Definitions and examples of functioning and disability according to the ICF.

	Functioning described at level of		
	Body part	Whole person	Individual interacting with society
Disability	Impairment	Activity limitation	Participation restriction
Examples	Crystalline lens opacity: visual acuity loss	Unable to read	Unable to vote in election
Possible interventions	Surgical treatment	Magnifier	Design for accessibility (all documents in large print)

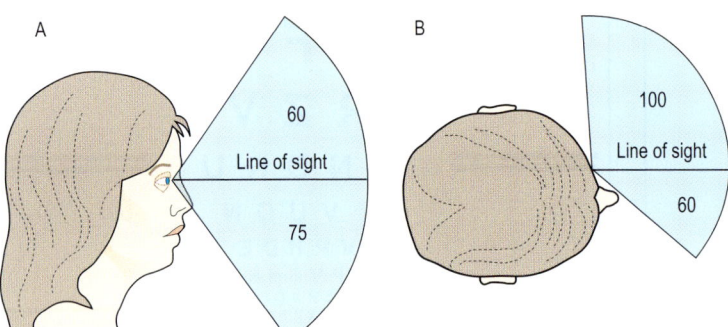

Figure V.12 • (A) Vertical and (B) horizontal extent of the normal visual field.

eccentric viewing to the right'; 'only reads first two letters on each line').

Visual disability

Low vision can be considered in terms of the part of the eye or visual pathway affected (e.g. the crystalline lens), the disease affecting it (e.g. cataract), and the impairment caused to physiological function (e.g. reduction in visual acuity or contrast sensitivity). As far as the affected individual is concerned, however, visual difficulties are more likely to be identified in functional terms, such as limitations of activities of daily living (e.g. reading, writing). This may affect interaction with the society in which a person with visual disability lives, creating restriction in participation in some areas of life (e.g. visiting an art gallery, or voting in an election).

The International Classification of Functioning, Disability and Health (ICF) published by the World Health Organization provides the language which can describe the body structures and functions, and the activities and events in which the individual would be expected to participate. Disability is a global term for any impairment, activity limitation or participation restriction, and the ICF creates a model of disability which recognizes the importance not just of considering the 'whole person' rather than the 'body part', but also of the crucial role played by the society in which a disabled person lives. This is summarized as 'contextual factors', which will be both 'environmental' (such as social attitudes, architectural characteristics, legal and social provisions) and 'personal' (such as gender, age, occupation, character, religious beliefs). Appropriate interventions may include medical treatment of the disorder such that the impairment is removed or reduced, assistive devices (such as magnifiers in the case of visual disability) to remove the activity limitation, and anti-discrimination legislation to bring about changes in how disabled individuals are provided for in society. A brief summary of the ICF model is given in Table V.3.

Visual field

The visual field can be defined as 'all the space that one eye can see at any given instant'. The term 'space' highlights the fact that the eye is looking at a 3 dimensional volume of space rather than a 2 dimensional area. The normal extent of the visual field, for a bright stimulus is:

- 60 degrees up
- 75 degrees down
- 100 degrees temporal
- 60 degrees nasal (Figure V.12).

The bridge of the nose influences the nasal extent, such that patients with prominent bridges will have a reduced nasal field. The superior extent is also affected by facial contours. Patients with deep-set eyes or prominent brows will have a restricted superior field. The effect of facial contours can, to some extent, be overcome during perimetry by getting the patient to turn his/her head. For example, in a patient with a prominent brow the full extent of the field can be measured lifting the chin slightly, turning the face upwards. With both eyes open the visual field has a horizontal extent of approximately 200° (100° temporal for each eye) while the vertical extent obviously remains the same. The binocular visual field – i.e. the region where both eyes can see the stimulus – extends for approximately 60° on either side of the vertical midline, 60° up and 75° down. The inferior extent of the binocular field is, however, often restricted by the nose.

Table V.4 • The size of stimuli used by Goldmann.

Goldmann size	Nominal size (mm²)	Angular subtence (min of arc)
0	0.0625	3.78
I	0.25	7.68
II	1.0	15.36
III	4.0	30.71
IV	16	61.3
V	64	122.56

By convention, the position of a stimulus within the visual field is described in terms of its eccentricity, how far it is away from the fixation point (measured in degrees), and the meridian along which the target lies. The horizontal corresponds to the 0 and 180° meridian and the vertical to the 90 and 270° meridian. It is also common for the eccentricity of the target to be described in general descriptive terms, such as peripheral, central, mid-periphery, centro-cecal etc. and for the radial position to be specified according to which quadrant it falls in, i.e. superior temporal, superior nasal, inferior nasal and inferior temporal.

The specification of stimulus size varies with the type of examination/perimeter. Most instruments now specify the size in terms of the angle subtended at the eye, e.g. a target subtends 30min of arc (0.5°). There are, however, 2 major exceptions to this. With bowl type perimeters it is common to refer to the stimulus size as being equivalent to one of those used in the Goldmann bowl perimeter. Goldmann's bowl perimeter has 6 different target sizes, labelled 0, I, II, III, IV and V. The nominal size and angle subtended by these stimuli is given below in Table V.4. The other exception is when a tangent screen is used. A tangent screen is a large flat cloth or screen often attached to a wall. It is common with this type of instrument to specify the target as a fraction, the numerator being the target diameter and the denominator the testing distance. For example, a target specification of 2/1000 means that the diameter of the target is 2mm and the testing distance is 1000mm (1m).

Most visual field instruments refer to the intensity of a stimulus in decibels. This value refers to the attenuation of the stimulus intensity from some preset value. In the case of projection instruments it is the depth of the filter placed in front of the bulb. The preset value is instrument specific, which means that decibel values often differ from one instrument to another.

Visual field artefacts

A variety of artefact can arise in the visual field due to extraneous factors. A common artefact is that caused by the rim of the lens in a pair of spectacles being worn by the patient during visual field measurement. It is important to use a correcting lens when examining the visual field. If the size or position of the correcting lens is incorrect then a correcting lens rim artefact is likely. This type of artefact normally occurs at the edge of the central field, at an eccentricity of 25 to 30°, and can mimic the appearance of a nerve fibre defect. Lens rim artefacts are more common in the elderly, especially those with deep-set eyes, and in patients with hyperopia, particularly those with lens powers over +6.00D.

Lens rim artefacts are more frequently encountered when using automated, as opposed to manual and semi-automated, strategies. The most likely explanation for this is that when using manual and semi-automated strategies, the perimetrist recognizes when the lens rim is causing problems and corrects for it by re-instructing the patient. In automated perimetry, the results are collected in a pre-programmed manner and then analysed at the end of the test. By the time the perimetrist recognizes that a problem may exist the data has already been collected and the test completed.

Various strategies can be adopted to reduce the incidence of lens rim artefacts:

- Use patient's own prescription. Whenever possible, use the patient's own spectacle correction as this usually gives a larger field of view then the equivalent prescription in trial lens form. It is also presumably more comfortable. Of course, when using the patient's own prescription, only single vision (not bifocal, multifocal or varifocal) spectacles can be used, and the prescription in the spectacles must be appropriate for the testing distance.
- Use ready-glazed spectacles. An alternative is to use sets of ready glazed spectacle frames. A large number of frames are required to cover the necessary range of corrections.
- Use a perimetric lens set and frame. Perimetric lens sets use large diameter lenses and can have fields of view that exceed 48° in all directions. Perimetric lens sets that use a trial frame, rather than simply attaching to the perimeter, are preferable; they are easier to align and move with the patient and thereby overcome artefacts due to the patient adjusting their head position during an examination.

Droopy eyelids or prominent eyelashes can result in an apparent loss of the superior peripheral field. This problem is more apparent in patients with prominent brows and deeply set eyes. It can also result from the patient being improperly positioned at the perimeter, i.e. the patient's face being tilted forward. Dermatochalasis is a common upper lid disorder in which there is redundancy of the upper eyelid skin. It is often associated with protrusion of orbital fat through weakened orbital septum and has been reported to cause apparent supero-temporal quadrant field defects.

The central retinal artery and vein pass out of the optic disc and then branch into a number of divisions that spread out over the internal surface of the retina. Because these vessels lie in front of the visual cells of the retina they can mask the receptors from a stimulus. With static techniques of investigation, 'angioscotoma' show up as the occasional missed stimuli, which, because of the size and location of these vessels, are more likely to occur near the blind spot and along the superior and inferior arcades. The effects are also more likely to show up with small rather than large stimuli.

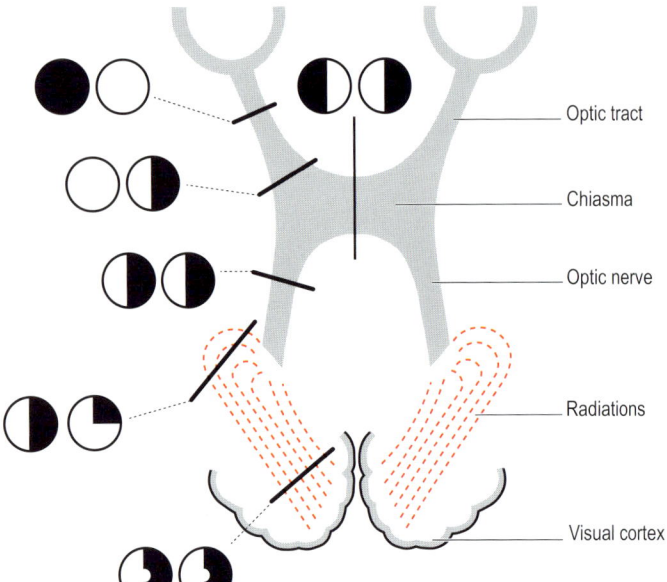

Figure V.13 • Visual field defects associated with lesions at various sites along the optic pathways.

Visual field catch trials

Most visual field tests incorporate a number of catch trials that are used to derive an estimate of patient reliability. In a false-positive catch trial, the perimeter goes through the motions of presenting a stimulus but does not actually present one. If the patient presses the button then this is classified as a false-positive. In a false-negative catch trial, the perimeter retests an already tested location at a supra-threshold test intensity. If the patient fails to respond positively to this presentation then this is classified as a false-negative.

The number of catch trials and errors are normally presented in the form of a fraction; the numerator represents the number of errors while the denominator represents the number of trials. Clearly, if the patient makes a high proportion of errors, then the results must be viewed with a certain amount of suspicion. There are, however, no published results giving the relationship between the number of errors and reliability. The precision of the catch trial estimates is dependent upon the number of catch trials. It has been estimated that for a true false positive rate of 33% (33% chance that the patient will press the button when no stimulus is presented) estimates derived from catch trials could lie anywhere between 7 and 57% (95% confidence limits). The poor precision of the catch trial estimate brings into question the current policy of using a single cut off value for accepting the visual field test as being 'reliable'.

A number of test programmes, e.g. SITA (see *Visual field tests, SITA*), use patient response times rather than catch trials to derive an estimate of the false positive rate. Analysing response times may prove to be a more precise measure of patient reliability than catch trials. The number of false-negative responses increases with the extent of glaucomatous field loss. This is likely to be an artefact of the algorithm used to test for false-negatives, which does not take into account the increased variability of responses at locations with reduced sensitivity.

Visual field defects associated with chasmal disorders

The type of visual field loss resulting from lesions to the chiasm is dependent upon the site of the lesion. Figure V.13 summarizes the many different types of field loss that can be expected from chiasmal lesions. While this figure gives a relatively clear and unambiguous description of the types of field loss associated with chiasmal lesions, it is not always possible to predict the site of the original lesion from the visual field defect. Other factors such as the nature of any tumour, be it hard or soft, its speed of growth, and the ability of the chiasma to distend can all have a significant effect upon the resultant field loss.

As the chiasma lies approximately 10mm above the roof of the pituitary fossa, it follows that a pituitary tumour must grow to a considerable size before it begins to compress the chiasma. For this reason, patients with endocrine secreting tumours, such as the chromophilic adenomas, usually seek medical advice for the hormonal changes that occur before the tumour has reached a sufficient size to put any pressure on the chiasma and cause any visual field loss. Patients with non-secreting chromophobe adenomas often have visual field loss when they first seek medical advice.

The classic visual field defect associated with a pituitary tumour is a bitemporal hemianopia, starting with early loss in the upper temporal quadrant, gradually extending inferiorly to form a bitemporal hemianopia. If left unchecked it continues around to involve the inferior nasal and finally the superior nasal fields. Visual field defects are often more apparent in the central isopters and relative rather than absolute. The exact nature of the visual field loss is dependent upon the position of the tumour in relation to the chiasma. Normally, the tumour puts slightly more pressure on the anterior part of the chiasma and produces the sequence of field defects described above. If, however, the chiasma is prefixed, then the tumour will press more on the posterior part of

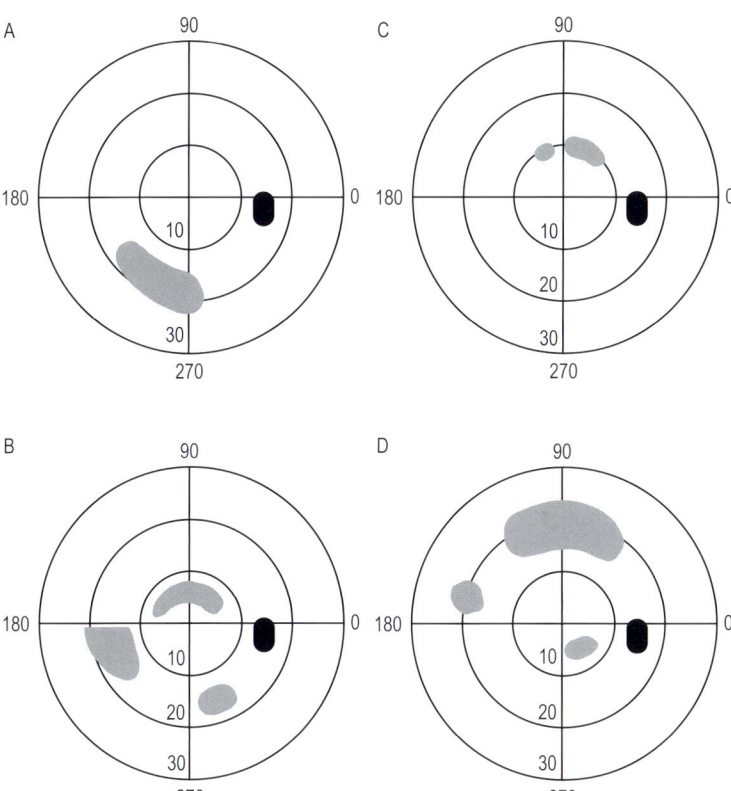

Figure V.14 • Paracentral defects, isopter diagrams.

the chiasma. A significant number of patients with pituitary tumours have atypical visual field defects such as unilateral central defects, unilaterally blind, and bitemporal paracentral scotoma. These atypical defects can easily lead to an incorrect diagnosis. Another factor to consider with pituitary tumours is the direction in which the tumour is enlarging. If it puts more pressure towards one side of the chiasma then the resultant defects will show a large degree of right/left asymmetry. With removal of the pituitary tumour there is a recovery of the visual field over a 1 to 2 month period although this is rarely complete. The extent of residual loss is dependent upon the degree of atrophy that has occurred.

Visual field defects associated with glaucoma

The types of visual field loss associated with glaucoma are as follows:
- paracentral,
- arcuate,
- nasal step,
- overall depression,
- baring of the blind spot,
- enlargement of the blind spot.

It is important to note that glaucomatous visual field defects are not confined to these categories; they can occur anywhere. Most of the defects, however, occur within the central 30° although the peripheral field is frequently involved. The visual field defects falling in the first 3 groups are collectively known as nerve fibre bundle defects. While the existence of one of these defects often indicates the presence of glaucoma, they can arise from a number of other pathological conditions such as anterior ischaemic optic neuropathy, optic nerve drusen, congenital pits and colobomas of the optic nerve head.

Paracentral defects – examples of which is shown in Figure V.14 – are frequently found in the early stages of glaucoma. These defects occur more frequently in the superior rather than the inferior field, are more common in the arcuate areas (between 10 and 20° of eccentricity) and are only rarely found at the macular or in the inferior temporal region. Paracentral defects respect the nerve fibre distribution within the retina in that they tend to follow the course of the nerve fibres and often show abrupt changes when they meet the horizontal midline. It is not unusual for there to be more than one paracentral defect although in the early stages they tend to be confined to either the superior or the inferior field. When plotted with kinetic techniques, these defects are often shown as having sharp edges and smooth contours. When plotted with static techniques, the defects are found to have irregular borders and to demonstrate a good deal of variability from one session to another.

Arcuate defect represents a more advanced stage of glaucomatous visual field loss. It is often viewed as a coalition of a group of paracentral defects (Figure V.15). As the name implies, these defects lie in the arcuate, or Bjerrum, regions, above and/or below the macula often extending from the horizontal midline to the disc. These defects, like the paracentral defects, are more often found in the superior rather than the inferior field. They respect the horizontal midline and again, when kinetically plotted, are often represented as smooth edged defects. Static instruments show a more irregular pattern and significant amounts of variability from one session to another.

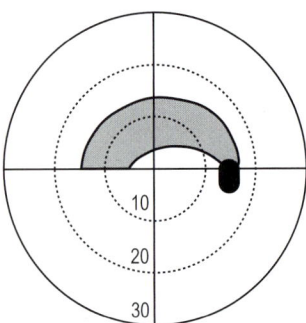

Figure V.15 • Superior arcuate defect, result from kinetic examination.

Nasal step is a characteristic defect associated with a difference in the sensitivity above and below the horizontal midline in the nasal field. This sensitivity difference, when investigated with a kinetic strategy, gives rise to a 'step' in the isopter (Figure V.16). The sensitivity loss associated with this type of defect is more frequent in the superior field. It is important to realize that small steps are not uncommon in normal patients. It is only when these steps exceed a certain value that they are considered significant. The critical value, differentiating normal from suspicious, has not been clearly defined although it varies with eccentricity being greater in the periphery than in the central field. Most published examples cite steps of around 5 to 10° as significant. The existence of a nasal step is a particularly valuable sign for several reasons. It occurs in a large percentage of patients with glaucomatous loss and it is highly specific to glaucoma, although there are other conditions that affect the optic nerve head that may also give rise to nasal steps. Its known location means that the perimetrist only needs a few moments to establish its presence. While nasal step occurs in a large percentage of cases with early field loss, it is rarely seen in isolation. The static correlate of nasal step would be a difference in the sensitivity above and below the horizontal midline.

An overall depression of the visual field, as the name implies, is a gradual sinking of the island of vision resulting in reduced sensitivity measures and a contraction of isopters. This type of defect is very different to the focal lesions described above which result from damage to specific nerve fibre bundles at the optic nerve head. Overall depression is believed to be the result of a diffuse loss of nerve fibres throughout the optic nerve. Its existence has been noted to occur in around 30% of patients with glaucomatous loss. Overall depression is, however, not specific to glaucoma. Changes to the crystalline lens (cataracts) cause a similar overall depression, as do the normally occurring age changes in the retina. While this defect can often be detected in retrospective studies, its existence contributes little to diagnosis.

Baring of the blind spot is often associated with glaucoma although its importance in both differential diagnosis and detection of glaucoma has been questioned. It results from a sensitivity difference above and below the disc, the area below the disc invariably being a little more sensitive than that above the disc. When the field is plotted kinetically with a stimulus whose intensity is set to be just above that of the retinal threshold below the disc, then it is not unusual to plot an isopter that curves around the disc. This type of defect is called baring of the blind spot because the isopter no longer includes the disc. While this type of defect is found in glaucoma patients, often as part of an arcuate defect, it is no longer considered to be specific to glaucoma. It is possible, provided the correct stimulus is chosen, to bare the blind spot in normal patients.

There are many different pathologies that can give rise to an enlarged blind spot. When enlargement is due to glaucoma it is usually in the form of an elongation along the course of the nerve fibres. While this type of defect has been reported in a relatively high proportion of glaucoma cases, it is no longer believed to have much value in the early diagnosis of the disease. It is only rarely found in isolation and is difficult to differentiate from the normal disc, which shows a wide range of different sizes and shapes.

Visual field defects associated with lesions to the visual cortex

There are 3 main causes of lesions to the visual cortex, vascular, tumours and trauma. The majority of lesions affecting the visual cortex are vascular in origin, caused by arteriosclerosis of the posterior cerebral artery. These lesions are invariably confined to one hemisphere, producing homonymous defects, which are perfectly congruent and often show macular sparing. Patients will typically report having had previous episodes of blurring or even blackouts, which are indicative of

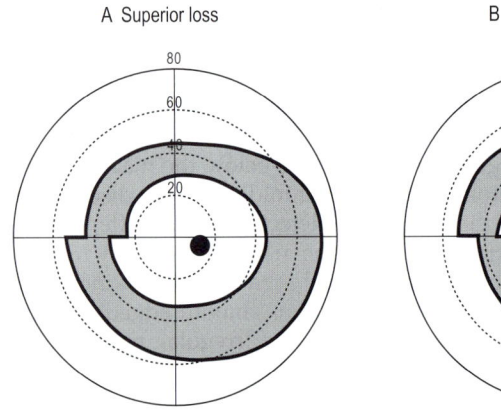

A Superior loss   B Inferior loss

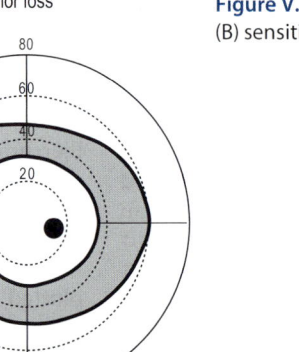

Figure V.16 • Nasal steps due to superior (A) and inferior (B) sensitivity loss.

vascular insufficiency. The edges to the visual field defects are usually steep and there is little if any recovery.

Visual field defects associated with tumours progress more slowly than those resulting from vascular lesions or trauma. They progress to give a homonymous hemianopia. Neighbouring tissue is often affected, giving rise to a large number of syndromes that together affect practically all the senses. A tumour may interfere with the vascular supply thereby mimicking a vascular lesion.

The diagnosis of trauma to the visual cortex is unambiguous. The resulting visual field defects are again homonymous, the extent being entirely dependent upon the amount and position of the damage. Traumatic lesions can affect both hemispheres, producing bilateral homonymous defects. Superior altitudinal defects are rare since damage to the corresponding region of the cortex invariably involves areas of the brain that are critical to survival. Loss of the field around the horizontal meridian is also rare, presumably because this region of the field is represented in the depths of the calcarine fissure, an area that is less likely to be involved in survivable trauma. Some recovery of function is common during the healing process. Macular sparing is far less common in trauma than in vascular lesions.

Visual field defects associated with lesions to the visual pathways

The position of the optic tracts, which are embedded in the cerebral hemispheres, makes the occurrence of an isolated tract lesion very rare. When other regions of the brain are involved, the non-visual effects are invariably more obvious than the visual ones. Those isolated lesions that do occur are most often caused by pituitary tumours affecting the chiasmal end of the tracts.

Damage to the lateral geniculate body cause homonymous defects (affecting either the right or left field of both eyes). However, the position of the lateral geniculate body makes it extremely rare for this structure to be involved in an isolated lesion. When neighbouring tissues are affected, the damage can often be so severe that it precludes any visual field examination.

Lesions to the optic radiations are normally vascular in origin and occur in patients who have generalized circulatory diseases such as arteriosclerosis. They normally have an abrupt appearance, which differentiates them from the slowly progressing defects associated with tumours. Visual field defects that involve the optic radiations are normally confined to one hemisphere and produce visual field defects which are confined to one hemifield. Lesions to the radiations also tend to be more congruous (alike in both eyes) than those of the optic tracts but less congruous than those from the visual cortex.

Temporal lobe lesions, which affect the radiations shortly after they have left the lateral geniculate can produce what is known as a 'pie in the sky' field defect. This is caused by the lesion selectively involving the fibres in Meyer's loop. Another characteristic of temporal lobe lesions is their tendency to split the macula. Lesions involving both the temporal and occipital lobes usually give rise to macular sparing.

Lesions further back, towards the visual cortex, can often result in quadrantanopsias (loss of a quadrant). This is due to the continuing process of sorting and alignment that occurs along the visual pathways. Within the radiations there is a clear separation of the fibres emanating from the different regions of the visual field. Additionally, there is a separate blood supply to the dorsal and ventral fibres. The dorsal fibres are supplied by the middle cerebral artery, which if occluded would produce an inferior quadrantanopsia, while the lateral fibres are supplied by the posterior cerebral artery. As the posterior cerebral artery goes onto supply the visual cortex, occlusion of this vessel produces a complete homonymous hemianopia rather than a superior quadrantanopsia as would be predicted from a consideration of the radiations in isolation.

Visual field defects associated with optic nerve disorders

A tilted optic disc is a congenital anomaly in which the optic disc appears tilted to the nasal rather than temporal side. It is also known as Fuchs' coloboma, congenital crescents, conus, dysversion of the optic nerve head and situs inversus. The last name refers to the course of the emerging vessels, which tend to leave on the nasal rather than temporal side of the disc. It is bilateral in approximately 80% of cases. Tilted optic disc is due to an abnormality at the optic nerve head that results in hypoplasia of the retina and choroid and ectasia of the fundus. It is associated with myopia and has a reported incidence of around 3%. The main type of visual field defect associated with tilted discs is a temporal depression which could easily be confused with chiasmal disorders, especially when the condition is bilateral. The depression does, however, often cross the vertical midline, a characteristic not found in chiasmal lesions. The defects are believed to be the result of diffuse hypoplasia of the optic nerve, the inferior nasal sector of which is more affected. The defects are also more evident in the central field although they are not confined to it.

Optic disc drusen are formed by the accumulation of deposits (chiefly calcified mitochondria) in the optic nerve head. It is a congenital defect that is thought to be related to the size of the lamina cribosa. The drusen tend to remain buried during the early years of life becoming visible during the second and third decade when they appear as white swellings often extending beyond the disc margin. The incidence of optic disc drusen has been put at approximately 1 to 2% of the population. The condition is invariably bilateral and progressive, although it rarely affects visual acuity. The best technique for identifying disc drusen is B-mode ultrasonography. Visual field defects have been reported to occur in over 80% of cases of optic nerve head drusen, and are generally relative and arcuate in nature. The extent of visual field loss is dependent upon the size of the drusen which also cause a thinning of the nerve fibre layer. The visual field defects are believed to result from the drusen pressing on the optic nerve bundles.

Anterior ischaemic optic neuropathy (AION) results from acute ischaemia of the anterior part of the optic nerve (the part supplied by the posterior ciliary artery). It is caused by circulatory occlusive disorders and is often associated with temporal arteritis and diabetes mellitus. It most often involves a segment of the nerve and only rarely involves the whole nerve. Visual acuity is affected in the majority of cases – more so in those with temporal arteritis than those without. While some patients show a slight improvement with time to both their acuity and extent of visual field loss, the majority are left with a severe disability. There is also a high incidence of the fellow eye becoming involved. The type of field loss associated with AION is dependent upon whether the temporal artery is involved, in which case the visual field loss is often severe. Because the lesion in ischaemic optic neuropathy is sited at the optic nerve head, the visual field defects usually relate to the course of the retinal nerve fibres, often ending at the horizontal rafé. This means the defects can often resemble those seen in glaucoma. Differences between the defects seen in AION and glaucoma are:

- In AION the defects occur suddenly with the result that the patient is often aware of the visual field loss. Patients with primary open angle glaucoma are rarely aware of any field loss until is has reached a significant portion of their visual field.
- It is not uncommon for defects in AION to involve the inferior field and the macula. The macula, by comparison, is rarely involved in the early stages of glaucoma.

Papilloedema, a non-inflammatory swelling of the disc, is caused by raised intra-cranial pressure. In the early stages of the disease, papilloedema is difficult to differentiate from papillitis, which is an inflammatory condition involving the optic nerve head. Papilloedema causes recognizable swelling at the nerve head. Patients have symptoms that relate to the raised intra-cranial pressure, such as headaches, diplopia and vomiting. The condition is bilateral and does not affect the visual acuity until it has reached an advanced stage. The classic visual field defect found in papilloedema is bilaterally enlarged blind spots, although this may not be present in the early stages. In later stages, papilloedema can result in both peripheral and central loss. While release of the raised intra-cranial pressure can often result in a substantial recovery of the visual field, the amount of recovery is dependent upon the length of time and extent of the raised intra-cranial pressure. If the pressure has been raised for a significant amount of time then some optic atrophy will have occurred, resulting in permanent visual field loss.

Optic neuritis is a term used to describe a series of conditions that can affect both the optic nerve and nerve head. It includes both inflammations and demyelinating degenerations of the optic nerve. When it involves the nerve head, giving the ophthalmoscopic sign of a swollen disc, it is called papillitis. When it is confined to an area behind the disc, thereby giving no visible signs, it is called retrobulbar neuritis. Generally speaking, papillitis is more common in children while retrobulbar neuritis is more common in adults. The retrobulbar form of optic neuritis is often associated with multiple sclerosis. Exact statistics on the subject vary enormously from one report to another. A recent review paper found that anywhere from 13 to 85% of patients who have an attack of optic neuritis have been reported to eventually develop multiple sclerosis and that 50% of patients with multiple sclerosis have electrophysiological and neuropathological evidence of previous optic neuritis. The high incidence of electrophysiological and neuropathological evidence of optic neuritis may signify that in certain instances the attacks do not give rise to any symptoms. These patients may well have subtle visual field defects which do not involve the macula. Visual field loss in optic neuritis is invariably monocular, although it is feasible for both optic nerves to be involved. A wide variety of defects can occur, including diffuse loss, nerve fibre bundle defects and centrocecal loss. The pattern of field loss reflects the region of nerve affected. If the central section is involved (axial neuritis) then there will be central field loss. If, on the other hand, only the peripheral section of the nerve is involved (periaxial neuritis) then the central field will be preserved. The field defects associated with optic neuritis show a great deal of fluctuation and can change in both their size and extent from one day to the next. The existence of visual field loss during the symptomatic acute phase of optic neuritis is almost universal and common in asymptomatic eyes.

Optic atrophy, which is a general term used to describe a degeneration of the optic nerve fibres and not a specific disease, can be evaluated and/or substantiated with visual field measures. Optic atrophy is characterized by a pallor of the optic nerve head that may appear greyish, yellowish or white. The wide range of normal disc appearances can make it difficult to establish whether the 'pallor' of a disc is physiological or pathological. If a visual field defect can be found, then this indicates that a pale disc is a true optic atrophy rather than physiological pallor. The nature of the field defect in optic atrophy is dependent upon its cause. See *Visual field loss associated with glaucoma*.

Visual field defects associated with retinal disorders

Occlusions of the central retinal artery cause an abrupt painless loss of vision and rapid death of the ganglion cells. In such cases the presence of a cilioretinal artery may lead to a residual island of vision, usually in the central and centrocecal area. Branch occlusions of the central retinal artery produce sector and arcuate defects, the exact location of the defect being dependent upon the affected branch. Visual field defects associated with arterial occlusions are characterized by their permanence and sharp edges.

Occlusions of the central retinal vein also cause an abrupt, painless loss of vision. In the majority of cases the acuity is reduced to less than 6/60 and there is little if any recovery even when followed for a number of years. Branch retinal vein occlusions give more variable results and while acuity is often affected, the loss is not as severe and the prognosis for recovery is better than with central vein occlusion. This is especially true in the younger patients where the extent of recovery is often surprising.

The haemorrhaging and oedema that follow a branch vein occlusion would be expected to produce irregular shaped relative defects, which regress with the re-absorption of the blood. In some cases the defect is not only absolute and permanent, but also follows the nerve fibre distribution. Investigation of these patients has demonstrated that, in addition to the vein occlusion,

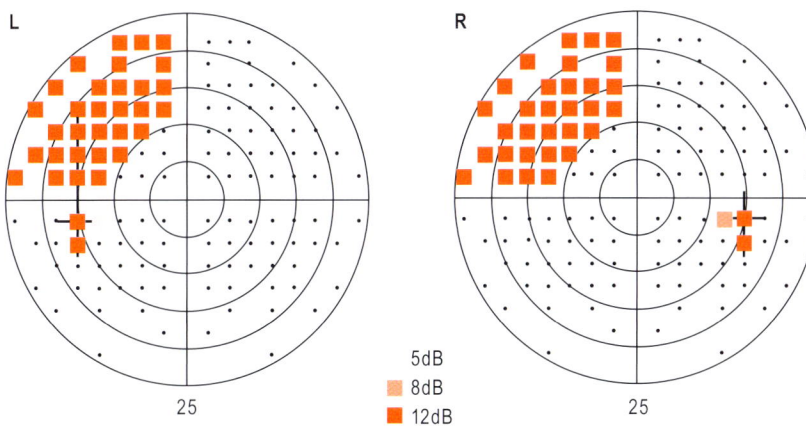

Figure V.17 • Centrocecal scotoma due to nutritional deficiency.

there is often some arterial disease and it is the arterial disease that has led to the more severe field loss. Two important points to remember about venous occlusions are: a) they are common in patients with primary glaucoma, and b) they give rise to secondary glaucoma.

Various nutritional deficiencies and certain drugs are known to produce retinal neuropathies. The effects are varied but primarily involve the central part of the visual field. This makes them particularly easy to detect with Amsler charts. The neuropathies related to nutritional deficiency and the abuse of tobacco and alcohol are normally grouped together because they present with identical clinical signs. Many clinicians believe that all three conditions are related, with dietary deficiency being the common denominator. Prognosis for recovery is good although this can take a considerable time (from 3 to 9 months). Treatment consists of a well balanced diet with B-complex vitamin supplement. Bilateral, relatively symmetrical, centrocecal scotoma (Figure V.17), are the most commonly reported type of field defect. The defects are most prominent with red or green targets, which is a manifestation of the acquired red/green dyschromatopsia that is often present in these patients. While field loss is often associated with reduced visual acuity, there have been reports of patients retaining normal acuity while having significant visual field loss and deficits in colour discrimination. It is not known why these conditions have a predilection for the fibres supplying the centrocecal area or in fact why other types of toxic optic nerve neuropathies produce different types of field loss.

The antimalarial drugs, chloroquine phosphate and hydroxychloroquine sulphate, which are also used in the treatment of rheumatoid arthritis and other immunological diseases of connective tissue, are known to produce ocular damage in a cumulative dose-related fashion. In the case of hydroxychloroquine, it is not so much the cumulative dose that is associated with retinopathy but the size of the daily dose. A particularly worrying aspect of this type of retinopathy is that once detected it often progresses even when the drug therapy is discontinued. The types of ocular damage seen with chloroquine include corneal deposits, loss of accommodation and retinopathy, the latter being the most serious. Visual field defects are central (within the central 30°) and may or may not involve the macula. They can also be present when there are no observable ophthalmoscopic changes. The defects are more noticeable with red targets, although they can often be detected with white stimuli, especially when sensitive techniques, such as full-threshold perimetry, are used. One type of central field defect found in chloroquine retinopathy is a perifoveal ring depression. This defect has been reported in a wide variety of macular pathologies, leading to the conclusion that it might be a stereotyped response of the retina to macular insults. It is the superior part of the central field that is often the most susceptible to damage.

Retinitis pigmentosa is a generic term used to describe a group of retinal degenerations. While it has for a long time been viewed as an inherited condition, with several different inheritance patterns, a significant number of cases appear to have no family history of the disorder. The diagnosis of retinitis pigmentosa is based upon a number of factors including: night blindness, progressive peripheral visual field loss, 'bone-spicule' pigmentation in the mid-peripheral retina, arterial attenuation, and attenuated or non-existent electro-retinograms. There is no known treatment for retinitis pigmentosa and patients gradually, over a period of many years, lose more and more of their peripheral field until they become totally blind or are left with only a small central island of vision. While loss of the central field does occur, either from the progressive nature of the degeneration or as a result of separate macular lesions, it is important to note that 25% of patients retain good central acuity throughout life. Retinitis pigmentosa is associated with a variety of field defects which, in the early stages, are more pronounced when the background illumination is reduced. Loss of the peripheral field is an early sign, along with a ring scotoma, the outer edge of which is beyond the central 30°. The defects are bilaterally symmetrical and progress slowly until there is either a complete loss of vision or a small central island at the fovea.

Field defects associated with retinal detachments correspond to the position and size of the detachment. In the case of simple detachments, the defects normally break through (extend out) to the periphery. In solid detachments, caused by neoplasms, the edge of the defect tends to be less severe and may not break through to the periphery.

Visual field indices

Three global indices have been developed to quantify glaucomatous visual field results obtained with threshold perimetry. Patients with glaucoma often show an overall depression of their visual field. The mean defect/deviation value is designed to give a measure of this overall loss in sensitivity. Each tested location is compared with that from a population of age matched normal values. The results are then averaged to give a mean value. The mean defect/deviation is affected by all types of visual field loss although it is more sensitive to generalized depression than to small local defects. On its own, mean defect is neither very sensitive nor specific to glaucomatous loss. Its greatest value is not in the detection of abnormality but in the long term monitoring of patients with established loss.

Mean defect is used in the Octopus range of instruments while mean deviation is used in the Humphrey Zeiss range of instruments. The Humphrey calculation of mean deviation differs from the Octopus calculation of mean defect by the addition of a measure of variance. The effect of this addition is to weight each measure of deviation according to the normal degree of variance found at that location.

It is known that patients with early glaucoma show an increase in the variability of their responses. The fluctuation index was designed to help clinicians recognize this. If the fluctuation was high then the clinician would become suspicious. The fluctuation estimate is also used when assessing change in the visual field. Fluctuation is estimated from repeat threshold estimates at certain test locations (normally 10 locations). This measure of fluctuation is more correctly termed 'short-term fluctuation', the prefix 'short-term' being used to specify the type of variability that occurs within a single examination session. When looking at the results from different examinations of the same patient, the variability between sessions is found to be greater than that within a session. There is an additional component of variability, which is called 'long-term' fluctuation. Short-term fluctuation is a global index, i.e. it gives a single measure of variability that applies to the whole visual field. Variability is dependent upon sensitivity and it cannot be accurately represented by a global value. For example, if a patient had an early arcuate defect where the sensitivity is reduced, then the variability, or fluctuation, in this region of the visual field would be much greater than in the other areas of the visual field. The concept of a global index of fluctuation is no longer considered to be correct.

Patients with glaucoma often have localized areas of sensitivity loss. Loss variation (LV) and pattern standard deviation (PSD) are designed to give a measure of this localized loss. These indices give a measure of the dispersion of defect values (the difference between the measured threshold and the expected threshold). Where there is localized loss, the defect values will be higher and there will be an increase in the dispersion of defect values. The dispersion of defect values can be represented by the statistical measures 'variance' or 'standard deviation'. The Octopus range of instruments use 'variance' and call this index LV while the Humphrey range of perimeters use standard deviation and call this index PSD. The LV and PSD indices include a component which is due to variability and are, therefore, unlikely to ever be zero even in a normal eye. To overcome this it has been proposed that LV and PSD should be corrected by a value that represented the patient's normal variability in threshold estimates. A measure of variability already exists in the index fluctuation. The fluctuation index is, therefore, used to reduce the values of LV and PSD to produce two new indices – corrected LV and corrected PSD – the values of which are centred around zero in normal eyes.

Global measures for kinetic perimetry include the area falling within a given isopter and those for supra-threshold perimetry include the percentage of missed stimuli, e.g. Estermann score.

Visual field learning and fatigue effects

It has been known for some time that performance in a visual field examination improves as the patient gains experience with the test. This effect, which results in an apparent increase in the patient's sensitivity and a reduction in the amount of variability, is known as a learning effect. The rate of the learning is not the same for all patients: some show no obvious improvement in sensitivity with repeat testing; some demonstrate a gradual increase in their sensitivity across several sessions; and some exhibit a large increase in sensitivity from the first to the second session which then levels off on subsequent sessions. The improvement in sensitivity is not consistent across the whole visual field; it often being greater in the superior compared to the inferior field and in the periphery as compared to the central field. Because of learning effect the first or first two sessions should be ignored.

Patient fatigue manifests itself as either an increase in the threshold or an increase in variability. These effects are not due to an actual fatiguing of the visual system but rather to difficulties in the maintenance of attention. In patients exerting accommodative effort during a visual field examination, fatigue may manifest itself as an inability to sustain this effort thereby producing effects similar to defocus.

In normal patients the effects are minimal, being in the order of 1 to 1.5dB, when the threshold is measured continuously over a period of 30min.

Glaucoma patients show an enhanced fatigue-like effect, the overall magnitude of which is dependent upon whether the test location is in:

- A relatively normal region of the field, in which case the effect is minimal and similar to that seen in normal patients.
- A defective region of the field, in which case the fatigue effects are much larger having an average extent of nearly 6dB.
- An area adjacent to a defective region of the field, in which case there is an increased fatigue effect similar in magnitude to that found in defective regions.

Fatigue effects are dependent upon the examination strategy. Fully automated techniques place considerable demands upon the patient with respect to maintaining their attention. Semi-automated techniques, in which the patient is given verbal feedback during the examination, help to maintain attention and reduce the effects of fatigue. Threshold strategies are also found to be more demanding, and therefore fatiguing, than suprathreshold strategies. Verbal encouragement helps to reduce fatigue effects as will interruption of the test sequence with rest periods.

Visual field loss due to malingering and hysteria

Patients with functional loss vary from the deliberate malingerer, who feigns visual loss, to the highly suggestive hysteric. Visual field defects associated with the malingering patient are typically a contraction of the field with steep gradients at the edge. The malingerer can often be exposed by altering the testing distance and checking that the diameter of the defects adjusts itself according to the laws of physics, i.e. as the patient moves away from the screen his defect should cover a larger area.

The same type of defect is often found in the hysteric patient and again altering the testing distance can often expose the problem. A second type of defect associated with hysteria is the spiral field. This occurs in kinetic perimetry when the patient's hysteria produces a smaller and smaller field as the examination progresses. It is, of course, dependent upon the perimetrist plotting the field in a regular clockwise or anticlockwise manner. When the second eye is tested, or the first eye repeated, the patient normally exhibits a severely constricted tubular field. An important aspect of the hysteric field is the susceptibility of the patient to suggestions. The extent and nature of field loss is thus dependent upon the perimetrist.

When functional disorders are investigated with automated static perimetry, where there is no regular sequence of presentations, it is very difficult to differentiate them from genuine loss. Reliability indices are not helpful; for example, false positives are uncommon and false negatives are often elevated but not out of proportion to that seen in cases of severe loss. Fixation losses, as measured by blind spot presentations, are again often within normal limits.

Visual field probability plots

Total deviation and pattern deviation probability maps take the threshold data from a visual field examination and calculate, for each test location, whether or not the threshold values are significantly different from those of a normal eye of the same age. They rely upon the perimeter having a database of threshold values from normal eyes which not only gives the average sensitivity for each test location (from which defect information is be derived) but also the distribution of threshold values. Data is normally presented as being beyond the 5, 2, 1 or 0.5% level. This simply means that there is a less than 5, 2, 1, or 0.5% chance that the measured sensitivity value comes from a normal eye.

Pattern deviation probability values differ from total deviation probability values in that they have been adjusted for overall shifts in sensitivity. For example, a patient might have an overall sensitivity that is below that of a normal patient of the same age. The pattern deviation probability map takes the overall shift in intensity into account by looking at some of the most

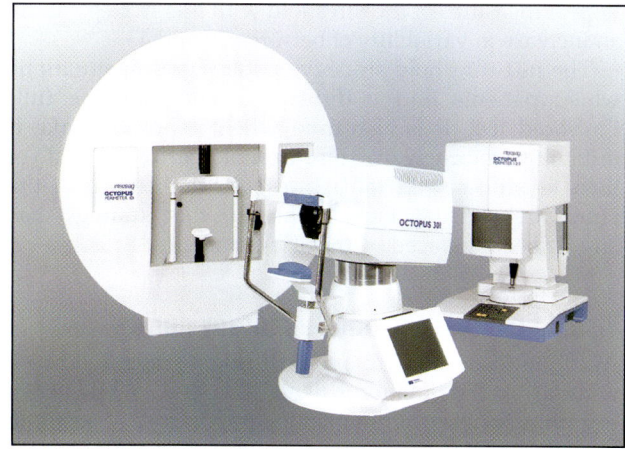

Figure V.18 • Octopus range of perimeters.

sensitive results and compares these to the most sensitive results from normal eyes. Any difference is compensated for by shifting all the values either up or down. Pattern deviation probability maps mask diffuse loss.

Visual field tests, dynamic

The variability of a patients responses increases as the sensitivity of the tested location decreases. This has important implications for the calculation of the optimal (speed and accuracy) threshold algorithms. Simulations show that as the variability increases so should the step size of the optimal staircase algorithm. The logical conclusion is that step sizes should increase as the estimated sensitivity reduces. This is exactly what the dynamic strategy does. The step size increases from 2 to 10dB and because the dynamic strategy remains optimal in regions of reduced sensitivity, the total number of presentations and overall test times are reduced in comparison to the full-threshold strategy. This algorithm is available in the Octopus range of perimeters (Figure V.18) and can be also be added to the Humphrey test battery.

In the current generation of Octopus perimeters, the dynamic strategy is used with a one-reversal staircase. By using a one-reversal staircase, Octopus have further reduced the examination times (approximately 40% of the full-threshold strategy). One-reversal techniques are, however, less accurate and hence the overall precision of this application of the dynamic strategy is reduced. The Octopus programmes do, however, allow retesting of all locations to improve repeatability.

Visual field tests, fast-threshold

The fast-threshold strategy was designed to overcome one of the main drawbacks of the full threshold strategy – that is, long test times. Rather than use a two-reversal staircase it uses just one reversal and rather than have two step sizes (4 and 2dB) it uses a single step size of 3dB. Stimuli which are not seen are gradually increased (3dB steps) until seen and those initially seen are gradually decreased in intensity until not seen.

While this strategy achieves its objective of being faster than the full-threshold strategy (it saves approx. 5.5min/eye) it does so at the cost of reduced accuracy.

Repeat measures of the threshold with this strategy show an increase in variability of between 20 and 43%.

The fast-threshold strategy is often used in situations where patients find it difficult to complete the full-threshold test. It is also used when resources make it difficult to routinely use full-threshold perimetry and yet there is still a need for a threshold test result. In the Humphrey Visual Field Analyzer, this strategy has largely been replaced by the SITA strategies.

Visual field tests, fixation accuracy during

Accurate fixation is important during a visual field test; without it, repeatability is likely to be low. While at the beginning of the examination the importance of accurate fixation can be emphasized to the patient, it is also important to have a means of monitoring fixation throughout the examination. If fixation is not being maintained then appropriate action can be taken e.g. telling the patient to keep their eye still.

The simplest technique for monitoring fixation is observation by the perimetrist. The observation can be direct, as is the case in most tangent screen instruments, or with the aid of a telescope or camera, as is the case in most bowl perimeters. Such techniques are dependent upon the judgement and continued vigilance of the perimetrist. The fact that the perimetrist needs to be present in order to make this judgement is an obvious disadvantage, as is the lack of any formal way for the perimetrist to comment on the accuracy of fixation. Despite this obvious limitation, the technique has been shown to have a good correlation with precise measures of fixation.

The perimeter can incorporate a fixation monitor that either indicates to the perimetrist when fixation is inaccurate or, in the more sophisticated instruments, automatically repeats any measurements made while fixation was inaccurate. While this is a very attractive option – as it does not require the perimetrist to be continually vigilant – most fixation monitors cannot differentiate between rotations of the eye, which occur when the patient looks away from the fixation target, and translations of the eye, which occur when the patient fidgets (a common event). A translation of the eye, such as will occur with a slight sideways movement of the head, does not necessarily mean that fixation has been lost or that the angular subtence of the perimetric stimuli has been changed by a large amount. A 10mm lateral displacement of the eye will only change the angular subtence of a stimulus at 30° by 1.7°.

Automatic fixation monitors are generally insensitive to small fixation errors (e.g. 1°). Some of the early-computerized perimeters had automatic fixation monitors that allowed sensitivity to be varied. It soon became evident that if the fixation monitor was set to be sensitive to small fixation inaccuracies (≤ 3°) then the incidence of fixation errors became so great that it was almost impossible to record any data. The solution was to either turn the fixation monitor off or to lower its sensitivity. While the later approach may have given the perimetrist a sense of well being, believing that fixation was being monitored, in reality it was too crude to be of any real benefit.

Fixation can be monitored by occasionally presenting targets in the region of the patient's blind spot (the Heijl-Krakau technique). If fixation is accurate during these presentations the stimulus will not be seen. If, on the other hand, fixation is inaccurate then the stimulus is likely to fall outside of the blind spot and elicit a response. The results of this technique are usually presented in the form of a fraction, in which the numerator represents the number of times the patient reported seeing the blind spot stimulus and the denominator gives the number of times it was presented. A frequently quoted fixation criteria for accepting the results of a visual field test is if the number of fixation errors is < 33%. There is no evidence on which to base this threshold value and the relatively small number of fixation tests (on average there are only 10 to 12 fixation tests in a perimetric test) mean that the precision of the estimated percentage is very low. As the position of the blind spot varies from one individual to another it is necessary, at the onset of the examination, to establish the location of the blind spot. Inaccurate location of the blind spot may result in numerous fixation errors in a patient who has maintained good fixation. The major advantages of this technique are its simplicity and ease of implementation. Its disadvantages are:

- It only samples fixation; ideally, fixation should be monitored every time a stimulus is presented.
- It increases the examination time.
- It is unlikely to detect small fixation errors.

At present, the best fixation monitor is the perimetrist looking at an image of the eye displayed on a monitor. This technique is not only sensitive but, via verbal feedback, can result in an improvement in the fixation accuracy for subsequent presentations. It is helpful if the judgement of the perimetrist is supported by an objective estimate derived from a procedure such the Heijl-Krakau technique. Perimetrists should, however, be encouraged to write on the record chart when they believe that the 'automatic' system has given an erroneous impression of the fixation accuracy of the patient.

Visual field tests, full-threshold

The full-threshold strategy was developed for the first computerized perimeter, the Octopus 201. It has since been adopted by almost all computerized static perimeters although recently it has been largely superseded by the SITA algorithm in the Humphrey Visual Field Analyzer.

The full threshold strategy was based upon a theoretical evaluation (simulation) that considered various staircase procedures and concluded that the optimal one (time and precision) was a two-reversal staircase in which the step size reduced from 4dB to 2dB after the first reversal. Figure V.19 gives four examples of how this algorithm would derive its threshold estimate.

The full-threshold strategy became the standard technique for monitoring glaucomatous visual field loss and as such has been used in a large number of research projects. It is not, however, ideal. It suffers from four major drawbacks:

- Long test time – Total test time for the 24/2 pattern of stimuli, including setting the patient up, giving instruction and demonstrating the programme, is approximately 20min/eye.

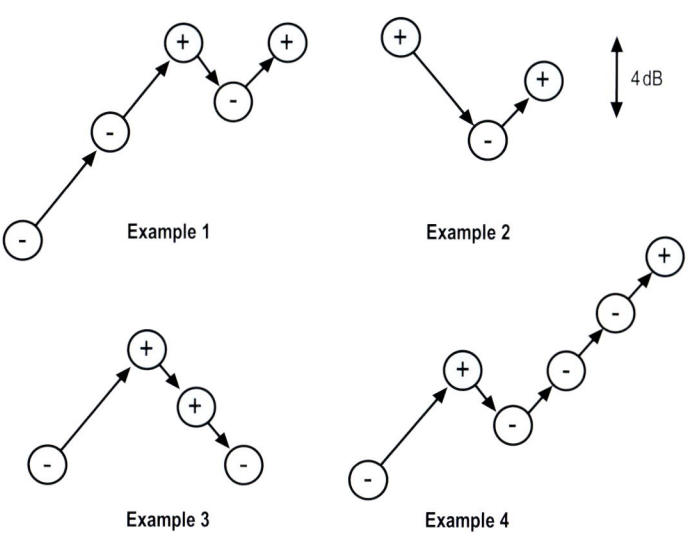

Figure V.19 • Examples of how the threshold is established in the full threshold strategy. Plus indicates the stimulus was seen, minus that it was missed.

- Demanding task – This strategy is very demanding for the patient. Patients are continuously being asked whether or not they can see a stimulus that is very close to their threshold and, by definition, difficult to see.
- Poor repeatability – Threshold estimates, especially at locations where there is some loss in sensitivity, show large amounts of variability. This makes it very difficult to differentiate between progressive loss and random noise.
- There is a significant learning effect (see *Visual field learning effects*).

Visual field tests, kinetic

Kinetic examination strategies rely upon the fact that the centre of the visual field is normally more sensitive than the periphery. A stimulus that is a little too weak to be seen at the edge of the visual field becomes visible as it is brought towards the centre. With kinetic examination strategies the perimetrist selects a stimulus of a given size and intensity and moves it from outside the visual field towards its centre noting the position at which it first becomes visible. This is repeated along a series of different meridians and the points at which the stimulus first became visible are then joined together by a line which is called an isopter (Figure V.20). Scotomata within the area of an isopter are detected by continuing to move the stimulus towards the centre of the visual field after it has first been detected. The patient is asked to report if, at any time, it disappears. Once a scotoma has been detected its extent is plotted by moving the stimulus along a series of radial directions from within the scotoma until it is detected.

The perimetrist can repeat the whole process with stimuli of differing size and/or intensity, in order to build up a map of the patient's visual field. The similarity between isopter diagrams and relief maps is frequently brought out in the terminology used by perimetrists. It is common for perimetrists to talk about the 'island of vision', the 'height' of the sensitivity profile and the 'depth' of a defect.

Kinetic examination strategies were very popular in the early days of perimetry. They have, however, been

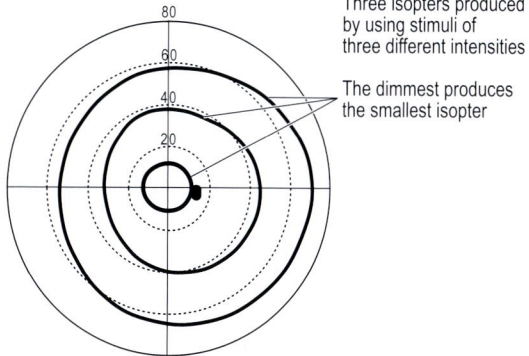

Figure V.20 • Three isopters produced by kinetic strategy.

largely replaced by static techniques. One of the major advantages of kinetic examination strategies is that the perimetrist has almost total control over the examination. The perimetrist can examine as much or as little as required; the field can be examined in any order; it is possible to pay particular attention to specific regions of the field or completely ignore whole regions; and the stimulus can be moved in any direction and at any speed. This flexibility allows the perimetrist to tailor the examination technique to the specific problems presented by the patient. The examination can be slowed down when the patient appears flustered. A patient making errors can be re-instructed and it is possible to reduce any variability in the results by repeating measurements that appear unusual. This degree of flexibility can be extremely valuable. When re-examining a patient who has an established defect the previous field chart can be used as a template to quickly check if the extent of field loss has changed. The major disadvantage of kinetic examination strategies is that they are relatively time consuming and do not lend themselves well to a quick screening of the visual field.

Kinetic tests are less sensitive when it comes to the detection of scotoma. It has been suggested (somewhat facetiously) that if one did not know where the blind spot was one would be unlikely to find it in a routine kinetic examination. One explanation for this lowered sensitivity is that when moving a stimulus within the boundary of an isopter, the perimetrist is relying upon the patient to report if it disappears or dims. The majority of patients want to be helpful and want to be able to see the stimulus. As a consequence of this they often fail to report or notice the momentary disappearance that occurs when the stimulus passes through a scotoma. Lapses of attention by the patient, which are not uncommon during the fairly tedious procedure of a visual field examination, may also result in the patient failing to recognize that the stimulus has disappeared. The ideal examination strategy would be one where any lapses of attention resulted in the assumption that a defect exists, rather than – as in the case of kinetic perimetry – that the field is normal.

The flexibility of kinetic examination strategies, which was cited as one of its advantages, can, ironically, also be seen as a disadvantage. When several different perimetrists are employed to collect visual field data, there is a danger that they will not examine the visual field in exactly the same way. In these situations, it can be difficult to decide whether changes in the visual field are the product of changes in the technique of examination or real changes in the patient's visual field.

Kinetic examination strategies are ideal in an environment where a great deal of flexibility is of value, e.g. in a neurological clinic, where in one patient a clinician may be looking for a hemianopia, the next a central loss and the next an enlarged blind spot. If, on the other hand, perimetry is going to be practised in an environment where a large number of patients have similar defects and the ideal form of examination can be more precisely defined, e.g. in a glaucoma clinic, then this flexibility becomes redundant and could even be considered a disadvantage.

Kinetic perimetry is often used to map the residual field of patients who are known to have severe visual field loss. An example would be a patient who has only a small central island of vision that does not extend beyond the central 5 degrees. The kinetic strategy is also found to be useful in patients who, for a variety of reasons, cannot cope with static techniques. This would include young children and those with attention problems.

Visual field tests, SITA

The SITA (Swedish Interactive Thresholding Algorithm) is one of the latest developments in automated perimetry. It is only available on the Humphrey 700 series of instruments. The aim of its developers was to create a faster threshold algorithm with a level of repeatability that is the same as that of the full-threshold strategy. This is achieved by:

- taking more account of prior knowledge
- doing away with the need for false-positive catch trials
- speeding up the rate of stimulus presentation in patients who respond quickly.

The full- and fast-threshold strategies were developed at a time when our understanding of the nature of visual field loss in glaucoma was far less advanced than it is today. While these strategies used some prior knowledge, the starting level is set according to the thresholds of neighbouring locations when these are available, SITA uses prior knowledge more extensively. This has made it possible to reduce the number of presentations at certain locations.

The SITA algorithm uses an analysis of patient response times (the time between stimulus presentation and the patient pressing the response key) to estimate what the false-positive response rate would be. An analysis of response times has shown a relationship between the false-positive rate and the number of response times that fall outside the normal response time window (either much faster or longer than normal). This relationship is used to get an estimate of the false-positive response rate.

The stimulus presentation rate is set to a constant value in the full- and fast-threshold strategies (it can be changed by the operator but in reality is rarely altered). The standard rate has to take into account slow responders and is, therefore, slower than it need be for many patients. The SITA algorithm monitors the patient's response times and adjusts the presentation rate accordingly. In this way those patients that respond quickly will be presented with stimuli at a faster rate and thereby complete the test in less time.

There are currently 2 versions of the SITA test: SITA standard and SITA fast. The SITA standard test saves approximately 7min/eye in comparison to the full-threshold strategy and its repeatability is as good, if not a little better, than the full-threshold test. Its threshold estimates are, on average, approximately 1dB higher than the full-threshold value – a factor which needs to be taken into account when comparing the results from the full-threshold strategy to those from SITA. The SITA fast test, as the name implies, was designed to be even faster at the expense of poorer repeatability (similar to the fast-threshold strategy). This test is almost 10min faster per eye than the full-threshold test and 4min faster than the fast-threshold test.

Visual field tests, static

A number of different visual field techniques employ static examination strategies. While some may have been developed to quickly screen the visual field, others have been designed to give detailed information concerning the depth and extent of any visual field loss. They are grouped together under the term 'static' because the stimuli in these strategies do not move.

Static examination strategies have become increasingly popular and in many clinics have almost entirely replaced kinetic ones. This change has resulted from a variety of factors, among which are the following:

- Operator independence – Static examination strategies are, on the whole, less sensitive to operator variability. Some are almost entirely independent of the operator whose task is simply to explain the test, align the patient and start the programme.
- Speed – Static strategies can be used to rapidly screen the visual field.
- Numerical analysis – The results from static measures of the threshold lend themselves well to a wide variety of analytical techniques. These techniques are used to reduce the relatively large amount of numerical data obtained from a static examination to one or more

numbers that summaries the extent of defect. They can also be used to analyse any differences that have occurred between visits and establish whether or not these are significant.
- Computer control – The advent of low cost computers which can collect, store and graphically present and print the results from static investigations has made static examination strategies more viable.

Some static strategies derive an estimate of the threshold of the eye at a series of different test locations. These are known as threshold visual field tests (see *Visual field tests, threshold*). Others present their stimuli at an intensity that is calculated to be slightly above the patient's threshold and simply record whether or not the stimuli are seen. These are known as suprathreshold tests (see *Visual field tests, suprathreshold*).

Visual field tests, suprathreshold

In a suprathreshold examination strategy the stimuli are initially presented at an intensity that is calculated to be above the patient's threshold. If the stimuli are seen, then it is assumed that no significant defect exists. This strategy has largely been developed as a screening procedure for conditions such as glaucoma. In comparison to other examination strategies, e.g. threshold strategies, they can test a far greater number of locations in the same amount of time or the same number of locations in far less time.

Selection of the test intensity is an important part of a suprathreshold test. If the intensity is set too high, then there is a danger that shallow defects will be missed. The test becomes insensitive to shallow defects, and produces too many false-negatives. On the other hand, if the test intensity is set too low, close to the threshold of the patient, then a large number of patients with normal visual fields will miss stimuli. In this case, the test has a low specificity and produces too many false-positives. Most suprathreshold tests present stimuli at an intensity calculated to be between 4 and 6dB above the patients' threshold.

Threshold sensitivity declines with age and hence what might be a suprathreshold intensity for a young person could be close to the threshold of an older patient. Some strategies use the relationship between threshold and age to set the test intensity; these are known as age-related suprathreshold tests. Other strategies derive an estimate of the patient's threshold at the beginning of the test and use this estimate to derive the suprathreshold test value; these are known as threshold-related suprathreshold tests.

At the adaptation levels used in perimetry (lower photopic), the foveal region of the visual field is more sensitive than the periphery. To retain a constant relationship between the intensity of the stimuli and the threshold, it is necessary for the stimulus intensity to vary with test location. Most modern instruments incorporate a map of expected thresholds and use this to keep the increment constant.

In a single stimulus, suprathreshold strategy stimuli are presented one at a time and the patient is usually asked to press a response button each time a stimulus is seen. The test is fully automated in that once started there is no need for the perimetrist to do anything other than to give the odd encouraging comment to the patient and to ensure that the test is progressing smoothly. Single stimulus tests incorporate false-positive catch trials (see *Visual field catch trials*) that break up long sequences of positive responses. Without these catch trials there is the danger that patients will simply get into a rhythm of pressing the button after each presentation, even when they do not see a stimulus.

Several machines, such as the Dicon LD400 and the Henson range of instruments, are also capable of presenting patterns of 2, 3, or 4 stimuli at a time. The task of the patient is to verbally report to the perimetrist the number of stimuli seen. If the number reported is correct, the perimetrist progresses to the next pattern. The number of stimuli varies from pattern to pattern in a manner that the patient cannot predict. If the number reported is incorrect then the perimetrist asks the patient to report the locations at which the stimuli were seen. It is then the task of the perimetrist to establish and enter the location/s of any missed stimuli. One of the major advantages of multiple stimulus strategies is that they are faster than single stimulus ones, taking approximately half the amount of time for the same number of stimuli. Multiple stimulus tests also promote a dialogue between the patient and the perimetrist. This has certain psychological advantages and has been shown to reduce variability in comparison to single stimulus tests.

A disadvantage of the multiple stimulus strategy arises when a patient has a large area of defect affecting many of the stimuli. In these situations the perimetrist has to ask the patient to identify the stimulus locations in a high proportion of the patterns. This process slows down the test and can lead to a certain amount of frustration and anxiety in the patient who is continually being reminded of all the stimuli that cannot be seen.

Suprathreshold strategies vary on the basis of what happens when a stimulus is missed. In the most basic strategy, suprathreshold test stimuli are either seen or missed and marked accordingly on the printout. A slightly more sophisticated form of suprathreshold test will retest any missed stimuli at the same intensity. If stimuli are seen on the second presentation, then it is assumed that the initial miss was a false-positive. (It should be remembered that in a non-selected population, a missed stimulus is more likely to be a false-positive than a true positive). It is generally accepted that a test with repeats is significantly better (much higher specificity) and well worth the extra examination time.

An even more sophisticated type of suprathreshold test will present missed stimuli at higher intensities to obtain some measure of defect depth. There are two widely used versions of this more sophisticated test:

- those that retest defect areas at higher suprathreshold increments. In these instances defects are normally graded into 3 or 4 categories and the field charts marked accordingly.
- those that retest defect areas with a threshold strategy in order to get an estimate of defect depth at damaged test locations.

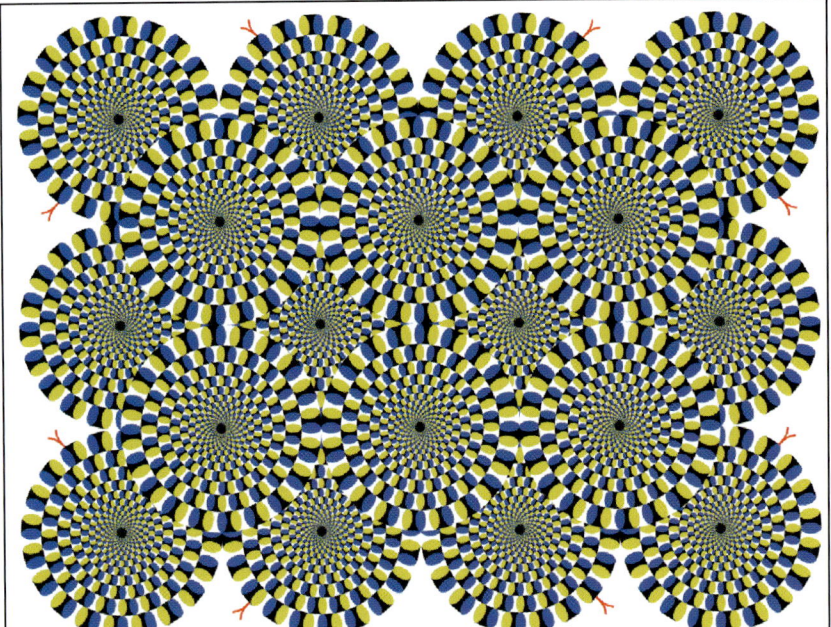

Figure V.21 • The rotating snake illusion. (Reprinted with permission from Akiyoshi Kitaoka, www.ritsumei.ac.jp/~akitaoka/index-e.html)

Visual field tests, threshold

A threshold strategy is one in which the threshold is estimated at a series of different test locations. There are many different ways of deriving a threshold estimate and, therefore, many different types of threshold test.

The results obtained from any threshold technique will be prone to a certain amount of error, i.e. difference between the true threshold at any given location and the measured threshold. The smaller this error, the better is the technique. In general, the more elaborate, and hence time consuming, a technique is the more accurate is its threshold estimate. The problem for perimetry (and indeed for many other clinical measures) is that time is not unlimited. Patients cannot be expected (even if the other facilities exist) to spend long periods of time undergoing the demanding task of a visual field investigation. If a limit is set on examination time, then the longer it takes to derive a threshold measure at each test location the fewer locations can be tested.

The 5 most widely used threshold strategies are the full-threshold strategy, the fast-threshold strategy, the dynamic strategy, Tendency Orientated Perimetry (TOP) and the recently developed Swedish Interactive Thresholding Algorithm (SITA). All threshold strategies, with the exception of TOP, require several stimulus presentations at each test location. These do not occur one after another but are mixed up with the presentations at the other test locations. This mixing up makes it impossible for the patient to predict the location of the next stimulus and thus discourages eye movements made in response to the expected stimulus location.

Threshold strategies are widely used for the monitoring of glaucomatous visual field loss. When used for this purpose the most widely used pattern of test locations is known as the 24/2. This pattern presents stimuli on a 6 degree square matrix across the central 24 degrees of the visual field. The matrix is displaced 3° from the vertical and horizontal midlines. Another commonly used pattern is the 30/2 which extends out to 30°. The 24/1 and 30/1 patterns are similar square matrix distributions that are not displaced from the midlines. They are not so widely used as the '/2' distributions which are better for visual field defects that are likely to have scotomata that respect the vertical or horizontal midlines, e.g. neurological and glaucomatous defects.

Visual function assessment, low vision
- See *Outcome measures*, *low vision*.

Visual illusion

A visual illusion (also known as an optical illusion) refers to the perception of a two- or three-dimensional geometric drawing or object that does not correspond with the physical construct of that drawing or object. The illusions may relate to apparent distortions or false impressions of space, texture, colour or movement. Figure V.21 is the 'rotating snake' illusion, which creates a false impression of movement. When any one circle is fixated, many of the other circles appear to be rotating. Aside from their entertainment and curiosity value, visual illusions are used extensively in visual psychophysics experimentation as a vehicle for gaining a more complete understanding of human visual perception.

Visual impairment
- See *Low vision*.

Visual loss, adjustment to

Most patients with low vision have acquired their visual loss (rather than having the condition from birth), and it will obviously have been a traumatic event in their lives and that of their families and friends. The reaction of the patient to their loss of vision, and the attitudes of those around them, may have a considerable influence on how rehabilitation is planned, and will certainly affect its outcome. Family support may be psychological or practical (arranging the lighting at home, or moving a chair closer to the television), but can also be negative if the carer takes over all daily tasks from the patient and they can no longer be independent.

The loss of vision has been likened to bereavement in the effect it has on patients, and the way in which they cope follows a similar pattern. This model describes a series of emotional stages which patients must go through as they come to terms with their loss – shock, depression and anxiety, anger, disbelief and denial – all being superseded in time by realistic acceptance. This is the optimum stage for patients to reach; they understand and accept the eye condition and its prognosis, and try not to worry unduly about what may happen in the future. They can strike the right balance between accepting help from others, and making the most effective use they can of their remaining vision, using whatever aids and strategies are necessary. They are not embarrassed to acknowledge their visual status, and do not mind being seen using an aid in public.

The loss model of adjustment to visual impairment leads to useful descriptions of patient behaviour but has been criticized because it does not suggest how the patient can be helped to reach this final stage. Models which do this tend to concentrate on concepts of locus of control, self-efficacy and self-esteem. When patients first lose their vision, they find it difficult to carry out simple daily tasks, making them fear that they will no longer be able to live alone. Early intervention using aids to give the patient back the ability to perform these tasks can prevent depression and over-dependence on external help.

It can be seen that the rehabilitation process and the adaptation of the patient are inextricably linked. Whilst successful rehabilitation can aid adaptation, it is important that the patient has a positive attitude, strong motivation and realistic expectations of what rehabilitation can achieve in order to benefit from it. Whether it occurs as a natural progression, or is assisted and speeded by the rehabilitation process, it is assumed that when the patient is well adapted to their visual loss, its negative effects will be minimized and their quality of life will be greater. Therefore questions about adaptation, and thoughts and feelings concerning the vision loss, are often the basis of questionnaires, or are included as a domain in a more general instrument. See *Outcome measures, low vision*.

Visual standards

There are two methods of determining the appropriate visual standard for a particular occupation, namely by the use of predetermined visual standards or by the establishment of the relationship between visual ability and job performance/competence.

Lists of standards of vision for various occupations may be found in the Association of Optometrists handbook and other optical diaries. They include such occupations as visual display unit operators, private motorists and pilots. The standards listed can also be applied to occupations that are considered to have comparable visual requirements.

While it is quite simple to establish an employee's visual ability, relating this to their job competence is more complicated. There is no satisfactory method of grading job competence due to non-visual factors influencing the assessment. For example, job competence may be influenced by age, intelligence, attitude, motivation, manual dexterity, and motor reaction times.

A five-step programme for establishing a vision standard is as follows:

- Choose a method for grading job competence.
- Analyse the visual factors required for the task (see *Visual task analysis*).
- Decide on criteria for visual competence, e.g. visual acuity of 6/9 or better, and stereopsis.
- Screen the vision of two groups of employees who are judged to be 'job competent' and 'job incompetent'. These two groups should be age-and sex-matched if possible.
- Compare their grading of visual competence to job competence. If the appropriate vision standard has been chosen, then the majority of the visually incompetent should fall into the job incompetent group.

Grading job competence can be done in a number of ways and may include:

- supervisor rating
- quality and quantity of production
- accident frequency
- absenteeism
- employee turnover
- wages (if on piece-rate).

Visual standards for visual display units (VDUs)

In the past the UK Association of Optometric Practitioners (AOP) has recommended a visual standard for VDU users. However, it is now felt that setting a standard is of little value as many VDU users who do not meet the criteria often have no visual problems. Therefore the AOP now provides general guidance about the visual problems that may lead to discomfort or symptoms whilst using VDUs. Consideration should be given to the working distances, screen height, binocular vision and visual fields. The VDU user should be able to see the range of visual tasks, e.g. screen and keyboards; the top of the VDU should be positioned just below eye level; decompensated phorias should be corrected; poor convergence may require correction of treatment; and visual field loss is not normally a problem unless there are binocular central defects.

It is not uncommon for VDU operators to complain of asthenopia. The symptoms may be due to an uncorrected visual defect but they may also be due to other factors. The main causes of asthenopia include:

- ocular status
- personal factors – physiological and psychological
- work station factors – glare, luminance, flicker, colour, contrast, alphanumeric design, and postural factors
- environmental factors – room temperature, relative humidity, and air movement.

Table V.5 • Occupational analysis (reproduced with kind permission of J.W. Grundy and Optometry Today, 1987).	
Name and general description of the task	
Working distances	a. Far (beyond 200cm) b. Intermediate (200–55cm) c. Near (55–30 cm) d. Very near (Less than 30cm)
Size of detail	a. Large (Angular size of critical detail over 10') b. Medium (5'–10') c. Small (3'–5') d. Very small (2'–3') e. Extremely small (1'–2') f. Minute (less than 1')
Main working position	a. Sitting b. Standing c. Moving d. Mixture
Size of working areas (in which critical vision is required)	a. Large b. Medium c. Small
Head movements	a. Side to side b. Up and down c. Mixture
Direction of gaze	a. Ahead b. Up. c. Down d. Side e. Mixture
Changes in direction of gaze	a. Frequent b. Occasional c. Seldom
Movement of the task	a. Stationary b. Slow movement c. Fast
Potential danger	a. High risk b. Medium risk c. Low risk
Special accuracy or care	a. Required b. Limited requirements c. Not required
Binocular vision and stereoscopic requirements	a. Required b. Not important c. Monocular vision adequate
Colour vision requirement	a. Good colour discrimination required b. Limited requirements acceptable c. Not required
Visual fields	a. Good field required b. Fair field acceptable c. Not important
Visibility (i.e. the relationship between the size of detail, working distances, contrast, and time available for viewing the task)	a. Good b. Fair c. Poor
Type of lighting in use, its adequacy and suitability	
Eye protection requirements	a. Required b. Not required
Hazard(s)	a. Basic b. Impact 2 c. Impact 1 d. Molten metal e. Dust f. Gas g. Chemicals h. Radiation i. Laser j. Other

Visual task analysis

In order to determine the visual standard for a task, a visual task analysis must be carried out. Factors such as distance and size of the critical detail of the task should be assessed, along with need for colour discrimination, depth perception, body, head and eye posture, field of vision, eye movements required, and the contrast and illumination of the task. From the subsequent analysis the important visual factors can be identified.

The visual task analysis should be carried out on-site; however, this is not always possible. A logical method for determining the visual factors required for a particular task has been designed to act as a simple reference guide for use by optometrists in a consulting room (Table V.5).

From the knowledge of the distance and size of the critical detail of the task, the visual acuity necessary to discriminate the smallest detail can be determined. This can be calculated easily from a simple graphical method using a nomogram (Figure V.22). For example, a task has a critical detail of 0.6mm and it is viewed at 70cm. When a straight line is drawn through these values it will intercept the right-hand scale to indicate that the corresponding visual angle is 3.0min of arc and the minimum visual acuity required is 6/18. It is important to remember that the values given are a measure of the resolving power of the eye and higher standards are required for the task to be carried out for prolonged periods of time.

It has been suggested that the visual acuity necessary for a demanding task should be approximately twice the minimum value. Therefore, in the above case a visual acuity of 6/9 is advised. The employee can often move closer to the task, increasing the angular subtense at the eye, but this depends on the amount of accommodation and convergence available. The older presbyopic employee, who has a reduced amount of accommodation, may need an intermediate and/or a near prescription, depending on the distance of the task.

After analysis of the visual task and thus allowing the important visual factors to be determined, a standard can be set by either:

- choosing a standard believed to be necessary to work efficiently and safely, e.g. visual acuity 6/12, distinguish principal colours. This can be tested by relating visual competence to job competence as described previously; or
- insisting on the normal level of visual capabilities for each factor chosen, e.g. visual acuity 6/6, normal colour vision. This approach would exclude some who were capable of performing the task comfortably.

Vitreous humour

The vitreous humour is a transparent viscoelastic gel that fills the posterior chamber of the eye. The vitreous

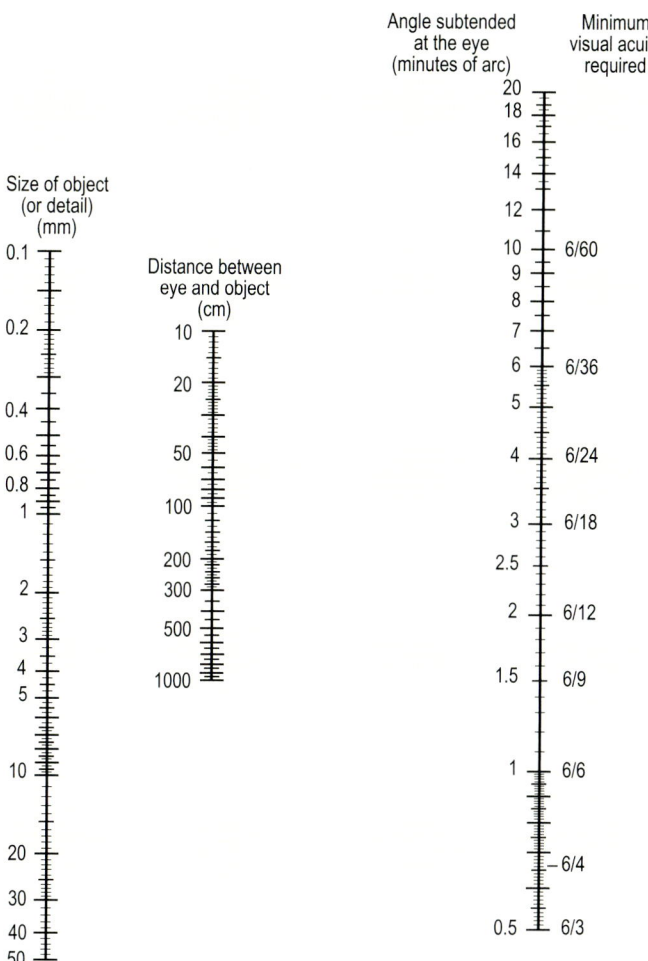

Figure V.22 • Nomogram for finding the visual angle subtended by objects of which the size and distance are known (after H.C Weston (1962) Sight, Light and Work, 2nd Edition. H.K. Lewis & Co Ltd, London).

contacts the ciliary body laterally and retina posteriorly, and shows an anterior depression (the hyaloid fossa) to accommodate the lens. Traditionally, the vitreous is regarded as consisting of two portions: a 'cortex' of densely arranged collagen fibrils and a central zone of more liquid vitreous with diffuse fine collagen fibrils. The cortical vitreous forms firm attachments to adjacent tissues such as the margins of the optic disc, the vitreous base (a 3–4mm wide band that spans the ora serrata) and the posterior lens capsule. Glycosaminoglycans (principally hyaluronon) fill the space between collagen fibrils. The vitreous gel liquefies with age and commonly, the posterior vitreous separates from the retina (a process referred to as a posterior vitreous detachment).

Waggoner (Hardy, Rand and Rittler) pseudoisochromatic plates
- See *Pseudoisochromatic plates*.

Warpage of contact lenses
- See *Corneal warpage; Dimensional instability, rigid lens*.

Water content, soft contact lens

The function of the chemical groups in hydrogels is primarily to attract and bind water within the structure. The extent of this water-binding ability controls the equilibrium water content (EWC), which is the single most important property of a hydrogel. It is defined as:

$$\text{EWC (\%)} = \frac{\text{Weight of water}}{\text{weight of hydrated gel}} \times 100\%$$

It is important to define the temperature at which the measurement was made and the nature of the hydrating medium (e.g. pure water or saline solution). The apparent equilibrium water content of a gel measured in water at 20°C in isotonic saline can be quite different from its value when maintained at 35°C in isotonic saline in a laboratory, or in the eye (at a presumed temperature of 35°C) (Figure W.1).

Poly-HEMA hydrogel has an equilibrium water content of approximately 38% (depending upon the degree of cross-linking and conditions of measurement). This can be reduced by co-polymerizing with a hydrophobic monomer such as methyl methacrylate, or increased by co-polymerizing with more hydrophilic monomers such as N-vinyl pyrrolidone (NVP) or methacrylic acid. By using a range of monomers in various combinations it is possible to purpose-design or tailor-make polymers for contact lens use. In order to achieve a particular water content, a mixture of monomers is chosen such that the balance of more hydrophilic and less hydrophilic monomers gives the required water content. A cross-linking agent (usually at around 1% of the total monomer mix) is added to produce a network that will give elastic stability.

A particular combination of monomers and cross-linking agent is classified in the USA in two ways. It is given a USAN (United States Adopted Name) identity (e.g. etafilcon-A), which is unique to that specific composition. It will also fall into one of the four groups of the FDA classification scheme, which offers a simple but effective subdivision of lens materials, on the basis of water content and ionic character, into four groups:

1. Group I – low water content non-ionic
2. Group II – high water content non-ionic
3. Group III – low water content ionic
4. Group IV – high water content ionic.

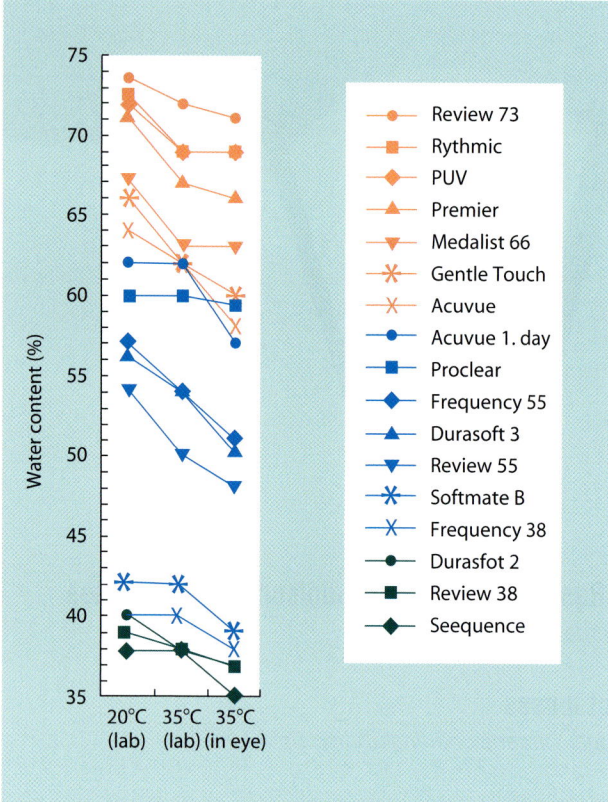

Figure W.1 • Change in the water content of a wide range of hydrogel lenses when the environment is changed from (left) laboratory room temperature (20°C) to (centre) 35°C maintained in a temperature-controlled laboratory water bath to (right) lens wear (35°C).

Table W.1. • Measurement of chromatic mechanisms using intense selective colour adaptation.

Background colour	Colour mechanism measured
Yellow (red + green)	Blue (short wavelength sensitive)
Magenta (red + blue)	Green (medium wavelength sensitive)
Blue-Green (blue + green)	Red (long wavelength sensitive)

The division between low and high water content is set at 50%, and an ionic hydrogel is defined as one containing more that 0.2% ionic material. Although the classification was designed many years ago to deal with differences in solution sensitivity, it remains a useful method for the broad segregation of materials, particularly those in Groups II and IV.

One or two types of classification anomaly do exist, however. The first arises in high water content polymers with levels of methacrylic acid only marginally above 0.2%, such as perfilcon. Although placed in Group IV, they do not behave like typical Group IV materials such as etafilcon and vifilcon. The principal difference is found in the way that they interact with tear components. The second type of anomaly lies in the fact that, some years ago, the same USAN name appears to have been given to two or more different ratios of the same ingredients, and as a result the same USAN name is given to materials of different water content that appear in more than one FDA Group (e.g. bufilcon and phemfilcon). See *Refractometer, soft lens*.

Wavelength detection thresholds

Wavelength detection thresholds are measured in the presence of high intensity background adaptation fields. This measurement technique is particularly useful for demonstrating tritan colour deficiency. Detection thresholds for a 1° field measured on a high intensity 10° white background produce a curve with 3 maxima, at approximately 520nm, 600nm and 440nm, which are associated with three opponent colour vision mechanisms. The maxima occur in spectral regions where 2 photopigments are stimulated differentially. The short wavelength component of the curve is absent in tritanopia.

High intensity adapting fields consisting of broad wavelength bands are used to adapt two cone photopigment response mechanisms so that the third mechanism can be isolated and studied. Chromatic mechanisms can be measured using intense selective colour adaptation, with background colour and colour mechanisms measured. See Table W.1.

The technique was introduced by Wald to study normal colour vision and adapted for the study of acquired colour deficiency by Marré. This so-called 'Wald-Marré technique' shows that in the early stages of Type 3 (tritan) colour deficiency there is an isolated disturbance of the short wavelength mechanism. At a later stage both the short wavelength and the middle wavelength mechanism are affected and finally all three mechanisms are abnormal.

Short wavelength detection thresholds, measured on an intense yellow background-adapting field, as in the TNO test, provide the 'gold standard' for identifying tritanopia. The TNO test examines the short wavelength detection threshold centrally and is therefore mainly concerned with identifying congenital colour deficiency. The adapting field subtends 10° to 15° and consists of wavelengths greater than 560nm. The 1° test field is 460nm. Short wavelength automatic perimetry (SWAP) is used to assess peripheral areas of reduced short wavelength sensitivity associated with acquired (Type 3) colour deficiency in patients with glaucoma and diabetes. The examination conditions vary in different perimeters.

The use of monochromatic adapting fields was pioneered by Stiles in 1949. A total of 7 spectral responses were determined and are derived from complex interactions in the visual pathway. Pi 1, Pi 2 and Pi 3 are derived from short wavelength (blue) sensitivity and have peaks at about 435nm. Pi 4 and Pi 4' are middle wavelength (green) sensitive and peak at about 535nm. Pi 5 and Pi 5' are long wavelength (red) sensitive and peak at about 570nm.

Wavelength discrimination

Wavelength discrimination ability is defined by measuring the smallest change in wavelength (or dominant wavelength hue) that can be detected at each wavelength value when lightness differences have been eliminated. Normal wavelength discrimination has 3 minima located in spectral regions where 2 cone photopigments are being stimulated differentially. The characteristics of different types of colour deficiency can be demonstrated in terms of wavelength discrimination deficits. These data clearly show that protanopes and deuteranopes cannot distinguish wavelengths greater than 540nm when only one cone photopigment is stimulated. This feature of red-green dichromacy provides the basis for identifying protanopes and deuteranopes with a spectral anomaloscope. Hue discrimination usually refers to the ability to discriminate non-spectral desaturated, pigment colours that can be identified according to dominant wavelength. The F-M 100 hue test is the equivalent clinical test.

Wearing schedule for contact lens wearers

In the past, all patients fitted with lenses for the first time were advised to adopt a wearing schedule, which means progressively increasing lens wearing time over the first few days or weeks of wear. Such advice was also given when lenses were worn following a period of prolonged cessation of lens wear. The said purpose of advising adherence to a wearing schedule was to allow patients to 'adapt' to lenses. Failure to adapt to early generation, low oxygen performance, PMMA and thick soft lenses (by exceeding the adaptation wearing schedule) resulted in worsening discomfort and red and watery eyes towards the end of the wearing period. The physiological basis of this adaptation process remains unclear, but appears to be related to the effects of prolonged hypoxia. Guidelines relating to wearing schedules for soft and rigid lenses are as follows:

1. Soft lenses. Soft contact lens wearers used to be advised to wear their lenses for no more than 4 hours on the first day, and to increase the wearing time by no more than 2 hours each day over subsequent wearing days up to a maximum of 12 hours wear per day. New modalities and improvements in soft lens materials and design have now largely rendered this approach redundant. Some gradual adaptation may be advised if the patient is being prescribed lenses of relatively low oxygen performance (e.g. very high-powered lenses). Inevitably, the more frequently lenses are worn, the greater the level of adaptation. Patients should be warned not to over-wear daily-wear soft contact lenses in spite of how comfortable they may feel. The introduction of 1-day disposable soft lenses in the mid-1990s has meant that a number of patients wear their lenses on a part-time basis; however, adaptation is not required when wearing such lenses.

2. Rigid lenses. These lenses generally require some adaptation. Some practitioners, to alleviate discomfort during the fitting appointment and the dispensing visit, have advocated topical anaesthetics. Nominally, patients are instructed to wear lenses on the first day for about 2 hours, building up by an extra 2 hours per day. Some practitioners accelerate this process by advising patients to wear lenses in the morning, followed by a break during the afternoon, and then to recommence wear in the evening. The adaptation process is patient-dependent, and the level of comfort can act as a guide. For a variety of reasons, it sometimes takes a few days for the surface of rigid lenses to attain an optimal level of wettability and comfort. First, some hydrophobic polishing compounds may not have been completely removed from the lens surface prior to delivery (although thorough lens cleaning prior to dispensing the lens to the patient can alleviate such problems). Secondly, until becoming coated with the natural constituents of the tears, rigid lenses may remain slightly hydrophobic on the first day of wear, especially if they have been delivered in a dry state. Storing 'dry-supplied' rigid lenses in solution for about 24 hours prior to dispensing will minimize this effect.

Wetting solutions, rigid contact lens

In addition to their role in lens disinfection, most rigid lens 'storage' solutions also act to 'wet' or 'condition' the lens. This role is principally to act as a lubricant, affording a degree of protection to the cornea and lid margins when the lens is inserted. The cushioning effect minimizes discomfort at insertion. The secondary effects of successful lens wetting are that the lens surface is rendered hydrophilic to aid a stable pre-lens tear film, and is made more 'biocompatible', which might reduce protein deposition.

Various agents are incorporated into rigid lens solutions to aid surface conditioning. Polyvinyl alcohol is a positively charged polymer that is attracted to the negatively charged surface of lenses containing methacrylic acid to provide more wettable lenses. Another agent used to increase wettability is the viscosity agent hydroxyethylcellulose. In addition to preservatives and conditioning/wetting agents, rigid lens care solutions also contain buffering agents to maintain a stable pH, and chelating agents to increase antimicrobial action and assist in lens cleaning.

Wilhelmy plate measurement

This method of measuring contact lens surface wettability is also known as dynamic contact angle analysis (see Figure C.1). During the Wilhelmy plate technique, the sample is held in a microbalance and immersed into a liquid by means of a moveable platform. The angle that the meniscus of the immersion fluid makes with the test sample as it is lowered into the immersion fluid (the 'advancing angle'), and the angle that the meniscus of the immersion fluid makes with the test sample as it is removed from the immersion fluid (the 'receding angle'), is calculated from force measurements obtained during sequential immersion cycles. The difference between the advancing and receding angles is known as hysteresis, and this provides a measure of surface characterization.

Wing cells of the epithelium
- See *Corneal epithelium*.

Wrinkling, contact lens induced

Corneal wrinkling is a rare but severe ocular complication of contact lens wear, characterized by the appearance of a series of deep parallel grooves, giving the impression of a 'wrinkled' cornea. In white light, the ridges of the wrinkles can be seen as bright reflexes (Figure W.2). These take the form of linear wave patterns of fluorescein

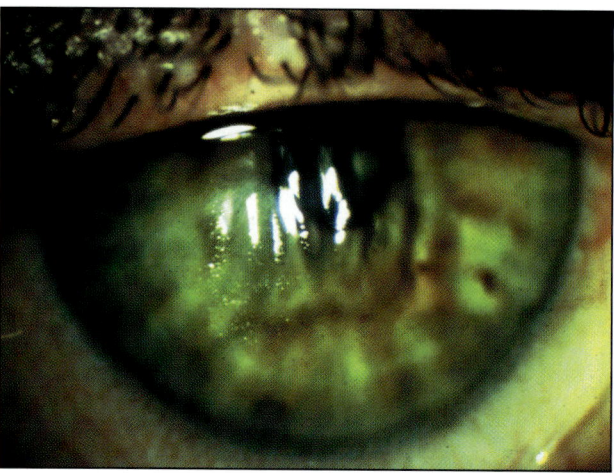

Figure W.2 • Wrinkling of the corneal epithelium caused by an experimental soft lens of high elasticity (the lens is in the eye).

pooling across the cornea and intersecting at different angles. Several discrete spots of fluorescence may be observed at the points of intersection of the two wave patterns.

This condition is observed in patients wearing steeply fitted, highly elastic, ultra-thin, middle water content lenses; such lenses are typically custom made and are not standard commercial products. Excessive elastic forces are thought to draw corneal tissue inwards from the limbus, causing the cornea essentially to 'collapse' in a concertina-like fashion, creating a wrinkled appearance. These forces could be derived from intrinsic elastic energy created when a relatively steep lens is compressed against the eye and then attempts to return to its original shape. Corneal wrinkling may also have an osmotic aetiology in view of the observation that complete evaporation of the tear film in normal humans can cause an almost identical corneal wrinkling and vision loss to lens-induced wrinkling.

As would be expected with such a dramatic distortion of the corneal surface, vision drops to less than 6/60 within 5 minutes of lens insertion. The condition is also extremely painful. Clinical evaluation of corneal wrinkling is best achieved by slit-lamp examination under white light, and with fluorescein under cobalt blue light. Computerized videokeratoscopy can provide useful supplementary information by viewing both the unprocessed image of the reflected mires and the processed, colour-coded surface map.

Corneal wrinkling probably involves the epithelium and anterior stroma. This view is based upon observations of the extreme variance in intensity of fluorescence across the ridges of a wrinkled cornea, implying deep furrows, and the extreme distortion of photokeratometric mires. The intensity of the wrinkling pattern increases with time following a blink, indicating fluorescein pooling within deep troughs.

The treatment protocol for a patient experiencing corneal wrinkling is to cease lens wear immediately. Although the appearance of wrinkling will indeed have disappeared within 24 hours, the patient should not wear any lenses for 1 week as a precaution so as to allow possible sub-clinical compromise to resolve. The patient should then be refitted with a soft lens that is devoid of inherently high elastic forces. Alternatively, rigid lenses can be fitted because corneal wrinkling does not occur with such lenses. The time course of recovery of corneal wrinkling is directly related to the period of lens wear that induced the changes, whereby more intense wrinkling takes longer to recover.

Wolfring gland

- See *Accessory lacrimal glands*.

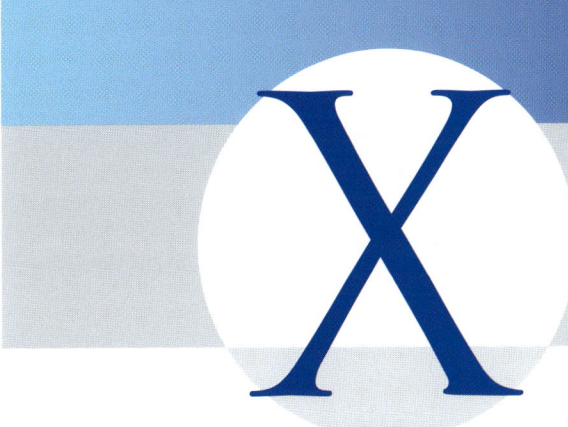

X-Chrom contact lens
A rigid lens with a red tint, designed to be worn in the non-dominant eye, with a clear lens in the contralateral eye. It has been claimed that wearing this lens combination improves colour perception in red-green colour-deficient patients. The lens transmits light above 570nm. Any improvement in colour discrimination is obtained by comparing learned lightness contrast differences when objects are viewed monocularly. See *ChromaGen lenses*.

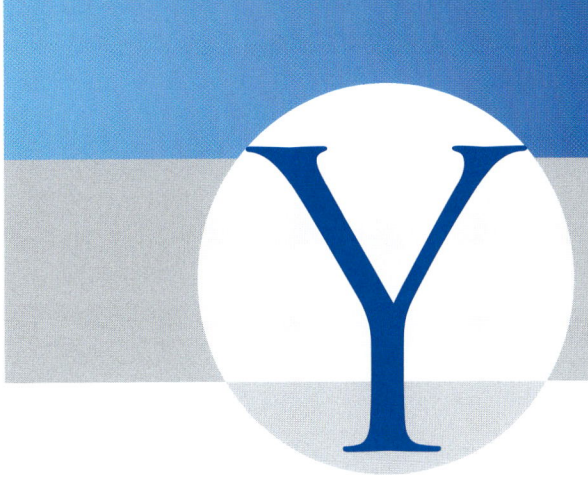

Young contact lens patients
- See *Paediatric contact lens fitting*.

Young's modulus

In solid mechanics, Young's modulus (also known as the Young modulus, modulus of elasticity, elastic modulus or tensile modulus) is a measure of the stiffness of a given material. It is defined as the limit, for small strains, of the rate of change of stress with strain. This can be experimentally determined from the slope of a stress–strain curve created during tensile tests conducted on a sample of the material. Young's modulus is named after Thomas Young, the English physicist, physician and Egyptologist.

Young's modulus is often used to describe the stiffness of soft and rigid contact lenses. Values of Young's modulus are around 1500 to 2000 MPa for rigid lenses, 0.4 to 1.5 MPa for silicone hydrogel lenses, and 0.3 to 0.5 MPa for hydrogel lenses.

The stiffness of a material will influence patient comfort and visual performance, and will affect the durability of the lens. A lens made from a material that is less stiff (lower Young's modulus) will generally offer improved comfort compared with a lens made from a stiffer material; however, a stiffer material has the advantage of masking greater amounts of astigmatism. Thus, a rigid lens will mask astigmatism, whereas a soft lens will mask very little, if any, astigmatism, because in the latter case the lens will flex to assume the shape of the astigmatic cornea. It is also worth remembering that modulus is a material parameter and so the effective stiffness of a particular contact lens will be influenced by its specific geometry. Thus, a lens with a low modulus may still be relatively stiff if it has a thick design.

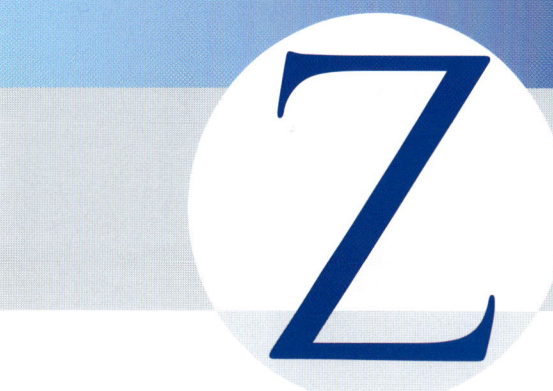

Zeis glands
- See *Glands of Zeis*.

Appendices

APPENDIX

Appendix A

Reported ocular side effects of selected systemically administered drugs

Ocular effect	Non-proprietary name	Principal use
Extraocular muscle paresis	Atenolol	Antihypertensive
	Fluoxetine	Antidepressant
	Indomethacin	Rheumatic disease
	Phenelzine	Antidepressant
	Propranolol	Antihypertensive
External ophthalmoplegia	Phenytoin	Anticonvulsant
Periorbital oedema	Diltiazem	Antianginal/antihypertensive
	Nifedipine	Antianginal/antihypertensive
	Verapamil	Antianginal/antihypertensive
Eyelid – retraction or lag	Thyroxine sodium	Hypothyroidism
Eyelid – allergic oedema	Enalpril	Antihypertensive
Eyelid – ptosis	Atenolol	Antihypertensive
	Fluoxetine	Antidepressant
	Levodopa	Parkinsonism
	Phenelzine	Antidepressant
	Propranolol	Antihypertensive
Tears – increased	Thyroxine sodium	Hypothyroidism
	Warfarin sodium	Anticoagulant
Tears – decreased	Amiodarone	Antiarrhythmic
	Amitriptyline	Antidepressant
	Atorvasstatin	Lipid regulation
	Chloropromazine	Antipsychotic
	Fluoxetine	Antidepressant
	Hydrochlorothiazide	Antihypertensive
	Imipramine	Anti-emetic
	Isotretinoin	Acne
	Loratadine	Anti-allergic
	Paroxetine	Antidepressant
	Simvastatin	Lipid regulation
	Thioridazine	Antipsychotic
	Triamterene	Diuretic
Keratoconjunctivitis sicca	Cyclophosphamide	Neoplastic disorders
	Methyldopa	Antihypertensive
	Propranolol	Antihypertensive
Conjunctiva – injection	Thyroxine sodium	Hypothyroidism
Conjunctiva – conjunctivitis	Amiodipine	Antianginal/antihypertensive
	Fluoxetine	Antidepressant
	Paroxetine	Antidepressant
	Ranitidine	Ulcer-healing drug
	Terazosin	Antihypertension
	Warfarin sodium	Anticoagulant
Blepharoconjunctivitis	Amoxicillin	Antibacterial
	Cyclophosphamide	Neoplastic disorders
	Isotretinoin	Acne
Cornea – sub-epithelial opacities	Isotretinoin	Acne
Cornea – keratopathy	Tamoxifen	Breast cancer
Cornea – deposits	Flecainide	Antiarrhythmic
	Indomethacin	Rheumatic disease
Cornea – vortex keratopathy	Amiodarone	Antiarrhythmic
	Chloroquine	Antimalarial
	Procainamide	Antiarrhythmic
Mydriasis	Amitriptyline	Antidepressant
	Digoxin	Cardiac failure
	Fluoxetine	Antidepressant
	Levodopa	Parkinsonism
	Loratadine	Anti-allergic
	Nitrazepam	Hypnotic for insommnia

Reported ocular side effects of selected systemically administered drugs (continued)

Ocular effect	Non-proprietary name	Principal use
	Orphenadrine	Parkinsonism
	Paroxetine	Antidepressant
	Phenoxymethylpenicillin	Antibacterial
Mydriasis & cycloplegia	Amitriptyline	Antidepressant
	Dicyclomine	Gastro-intestinal disorders
	Hyoscine	Gastro-intestinal disorders
	Imipramine	Anti-emetic
Accommodation – reduced	Loratadine	Anti-allergic
	Phenoxymethylpenicillin	Antibacterial
Accommodation – paralysed	Amitriptyline	Antidepressant
	Warfarin sodium	Anticoagulant
Intra-ocular pressure – increased	Amitriptyline	Antidepressant
	Beclomethasone	Asthma
Intra-ocular pressure – decreased	Capotril	Antihypertensive
	Donepezil	Alzheimer's dementia
	Methyldopa	Antihypertensive
	Propranol	Antihypertensive
	Rivastigmine	Alzheimer's dementia
Lens – posterior subcapsular cataract	Beclomethasone	Anti-allergic
Lens – opacities	Amiodarone	Antiarrhythmic
	Phenytoin	Anticonvulsant
Myopia – transient	Chlorthalidone	Antihypertensive
	Isosorbide dinitrate	Antianginal
Retinopathy	Tamoxifen	Breast cancer
Transient retinal ischaemia	Nifedipine	Antianginal/antihypertensive
	Verapamil	Antianginal/antihypertensive
Retinal haemorrhage	Diltiazem	Antianginal/antihypertensive
Central retinal artery occlusion	Propranol	Antihypertensive
Cystoid macular oedema/toxic maculopathy	Amiodarone	Antiarrhythmic
	Chlorpropamide	Diabetes mellitus
	Ethambutol	Antituberculous
	Isoniazid	Antituberculous
	Nictonic acid	Lipid regulation
	Streptomycin	Antituberculous
	Vigabatrin	Antiepileptic
Papilloedema	Cyclosporin	Immunosuppressant
Optic neuritis/neuropathy	Amiodarone	Antiarrhythmic
	Chlorpropamide	Diabetes mellitus
	Ethambutol	Antituberculous
	Isoniazid	Antituberculous
	Minoxidil	Antihypertensive
	Naproxen	Rheumatic disease
	Streptomycin	Antituberculous
	Vigabatrin	Antiepileptic
Nystagmus	Amitriptyline	Antidepressant
	Ethacrynic acid	Diuretic
	Fluoxetine	Antidepressant
	Frusemide	Diuretic
	Phenelzine	Antidepressant
	Phenytoin	Anticonvulsant
Blurred vision	Amitriptyline	Antidepressant
	Carbamazepine	Antiepileptic
	Ciprofloxacin	Antibacterial
	Digoxin	Cardiac failure
	Diltiazem	Antianginal/antihypertensive
	Disopyramide	Antiarrhythmic
	Frusemide	Diuretic

Reported ocular side effects of selected systemically administered drugs (*continued*)

Ocular effect	Non-proprietary name	Principal use
	Indomethacin	Rheumatic disease
	Lisinopril	Antiarrhythmic/antihypertensive
	Loratidine	Anti-allergic
	Nabumetone	Rheumatic disease
	Nifedipine	Antianginal/antihypertensive
	Phenytoin	Anticonvulsant
	Ranitidine	Ulcer-healing drug
	Sertraline	Antidepressant
	Simvastatin	Lipid regulation
	Terazosin	Antihypertension
	Triamterene	Diuretic
Increased light sensitivity/photophobia	Ciprofloxacin	Antibacterial
	Fluoxetine	Antidepressant
	Nabumetone	Rheumatic disease
	Nalidixic acid	Antibacterial
	Paroxetine	Antidepressant
	Thyroxine sodium	Hypothyroidism
	Triamterene	Diuretic
Coloured haloes around lights	Digoxin	Cardiac failure
Ocular irritation	Diltiazem	Antianginal/antihypertensive
	Lisinopril	Antiarrhythmic/antihypertensive
	Nifedipine	Antianginal/antihypertensive
Ocular pain	Amiodipine	Antianginal/antihypertensive
	Amitriptyline	Antidepressant
	Cyclosporin	Immunosuppressant
	Fluoxetine	Antidepressant
	Paroxetine	Antidepressant
Peri-orbital/orbital pain	Phenytoin	Anticonvulsant
Colour vision defects	Carbamazepine	Antiepileptic
	Digoxin	Cardiac failure
	Ethambutol	Antituberculous
	Indomethacin	Rheumatic disease
	Phenytoin	Anticonvulsant
	Ranitidine	Ulcer-healing drug
	Valproic acid	Anticonvulsant/antidepressant
Convergence insufficiency	Methyldopa	Antihypertensive
Diplopia	Amiodipine	Antianginal/antihypertensive
	Amoxicillin	Antibacterial
	Carbamazepine	Antiepileptic
	Digoxin	Cardiac failure
	Enalapril	Antihypertensive
	Fluoxetine	Antidepressant
	Guanethidine	Antihypertension
	Loratadine	Anti-allergic
	Oxprenolol	Antianginal/antihypertensive
	Phenelzine	Antidepressant
	Phenoxymethylpenicillin	Antibacterial
	Phenytoin	Anticonvulsant
Visual field defects – general	Indomethacin	Rheumatic disease
	Nifedipine	Antianginal/antihypertensive
	Vigabatrin	Antiepileptic
Visual field defects – scintillating or pericentral scotoma	Digoxin	Cardiac failure
Visual field defects – centrocaecal scotoma	Ciprofloxacin	Antibacterial

Reported ocular side effects of selected systemically administered drugs (*continued*)		
Ocular effect	**Non-proprietary name**	**Principal use**
Visual field defects – central or centrocaecal scotoma	Chloropropamide	Diabetes mellitus
Visual hallucinations	Amitriptyline	Antidepressant
	Atenolol	Antihypertensive
	Cyclosporin	Immunosuppressant
	Digoxin	Cardiac failure
	Diltiazem	Antianginal/antihypertensive
	Isosorbide dinitrate & mononitrate	Antianginal
	Levodopa	Parkinsonism
	Loratadine	Anti-allergic
	Mexiletine	Antiarrhythmic
	Orphenadrine	Parkinsonism
	Phenytoin	Anticonvulsant
	Propranolol	Antihypertensive
Xanthopsia	Frusemide	Diuretic
	Triamterene	Diuretic

Appendix B
Optometric grading scales (with permission from Richard M. Pearson)

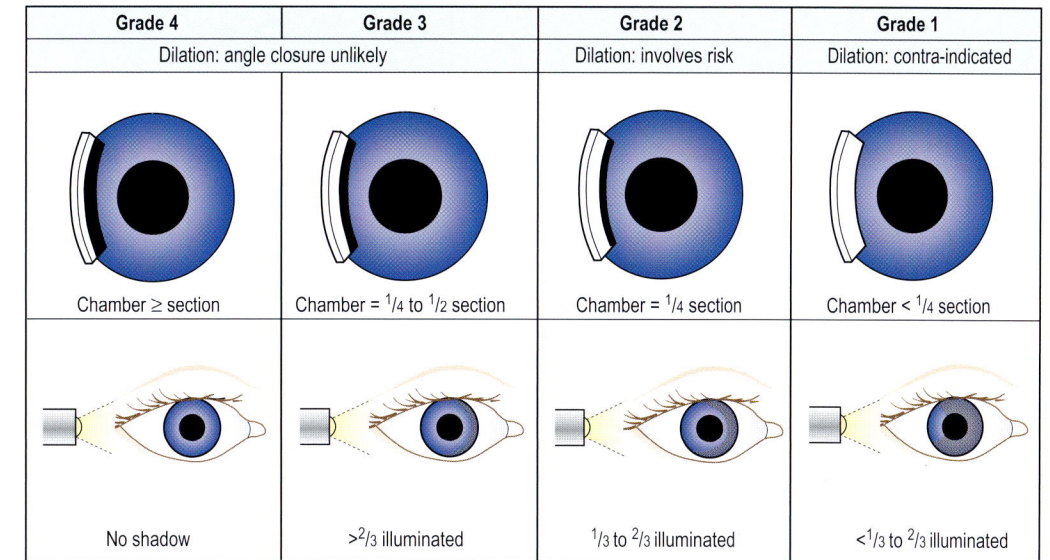

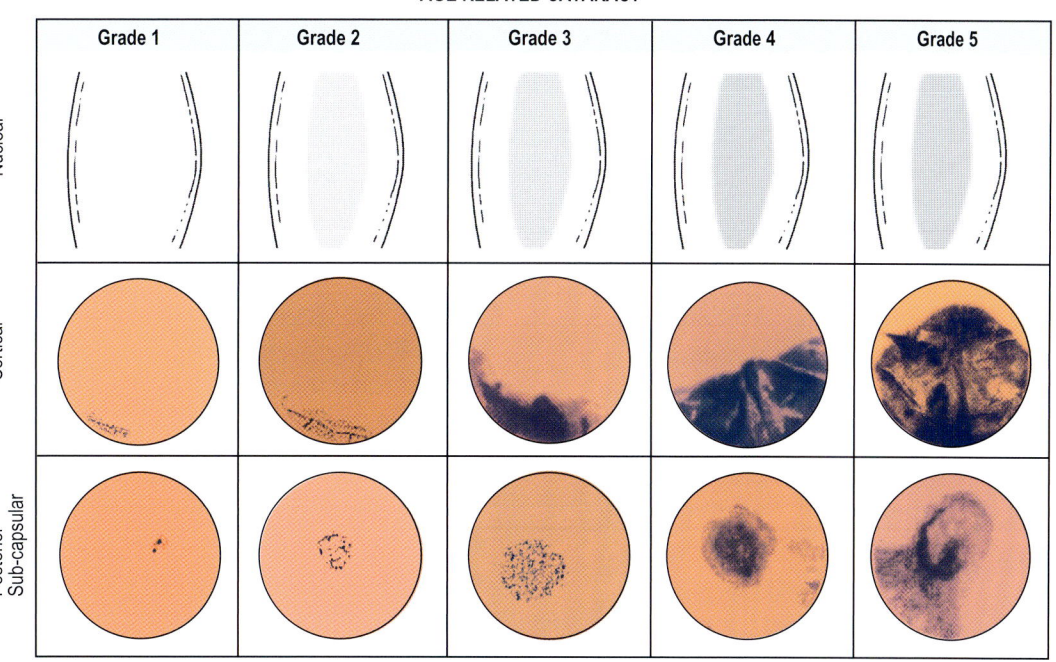

Optometric grading scales (*continued*)

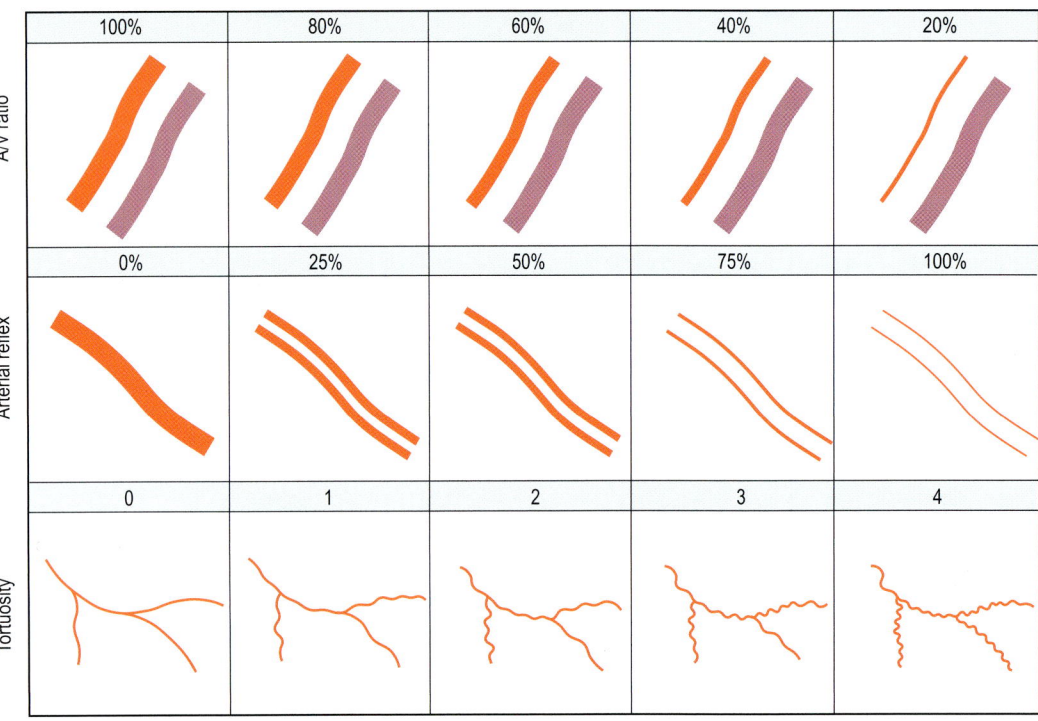

Appendix C
Efron grading scales for contact lens complications

The grading scales presented on the following pages were devised by Professor Nathan Efron and painted by the ophthalmic artist, Terry R. Tarrant.

These grading scales are presented in two panels and are designed to assist practitioners quantify the level of severity of a variety of contact lens complications. The eight complications on the first panel are those that are more likely to be encountered in contact lens practice. Many of these complications are graded routinely by some practitioners. The eight complications on the second panel are less commonly encountered in contact lens practice, or represent pathology that is rare or unusual. The order of presentation of the complications on each panel, from top to bottom, reflect the likely order in which these complications would be encountered in the course of a systematic examination using the slit lamp biomicroscope.

Opposite each of the two grading scale panels is a table – set out in the same format as the corresponding panel of complications – that briefly explains the salient features of each image.

The development of these grading scales was kindly sponsored by CooperVision. A handy plastic-coated A4-sized version of these grading scales, which comes in a protective slip case with comprehensive instructions for use, is available free from CooperVision. Simply send a request, with your full postal address, to: gradingscales@coopervision.co.uk

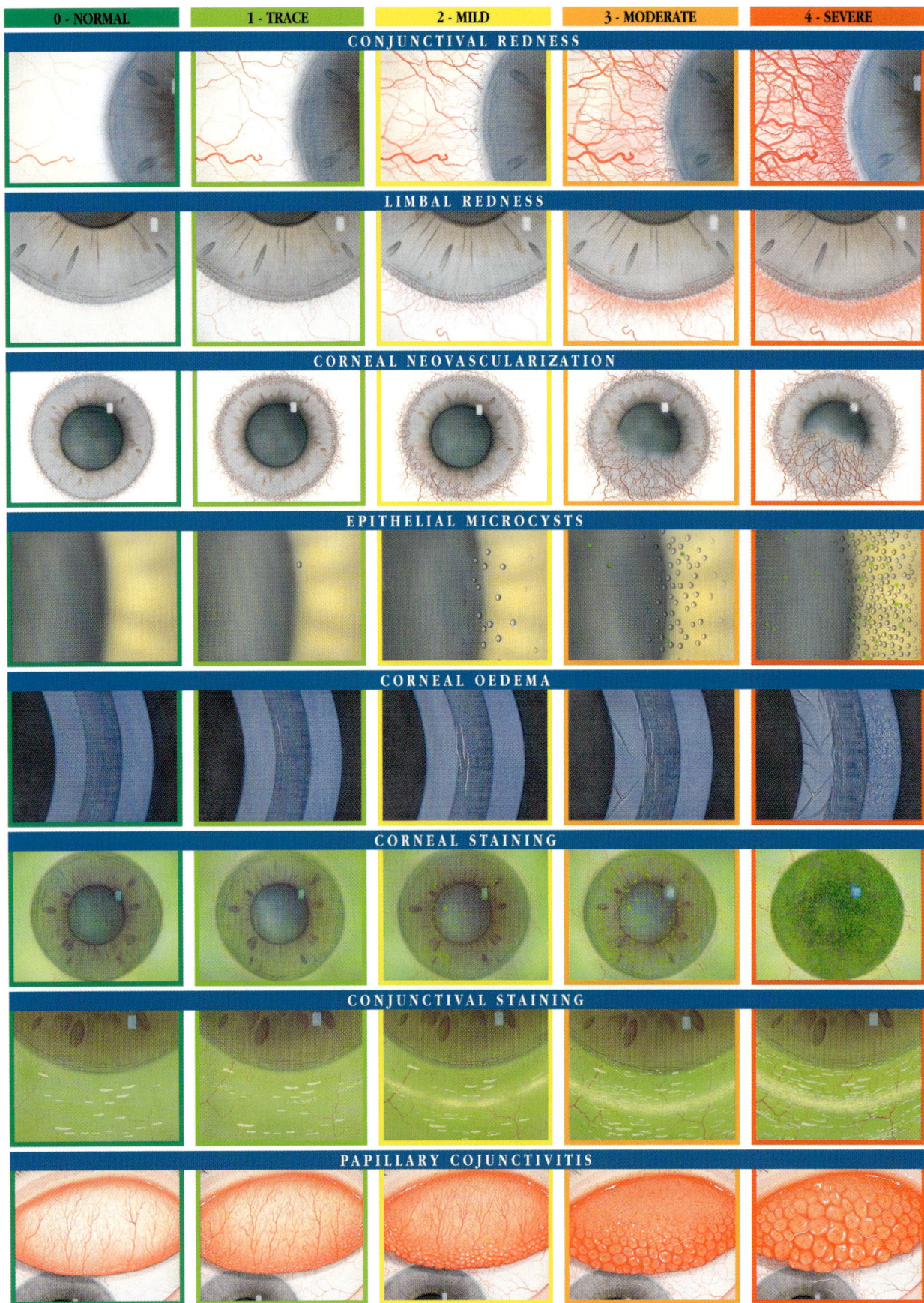

0 - NORMAL	1 - TRACE	2 - MILD	3 - MODERATE	4 - SEVERE
CONJUNCTIVAL REDNESS				
'White' bulbar conjunctiva One major vessel Clear cornea	Small increase in conjunctival redness Major vessel more engorged	Further increase in conjunctival redness Limbal redness Slight ciliary flush	Conjunctiva very red Increased limbal redness Ciliary flush	Conjunctiva extremely red Limbus very red Intense ciliary flush Reflex on major vessel
LIMBAL REDNESS				
'White' limbus White corneal reflex	Slightly increased limbal redness White corneal reflex	Increased limbal redness Increased conjunctival redness White corneal reflex	Limbus very red Increased conjunctival redness Speckled corneal reflex	Limbus extremely red Conjunctival redness Hazy corneal reflex
CORNEAL NEOVASCULARIZATION				
Clear cornea White reflex	Vessels encroach <1 mm from lower left quadrant (LLQ)	Vessels encroach 2–3 mm from LLQ Limbal redness Reflex less crisp Central corneal haze	Vessels encroach 4–5 mm from LLQ Corneal haze around vessels Speckled reflex	Vessels encroach 6mm from LLQ Lipid at leading edge of vessels Very diffuse reflex
EPITHELIAL MICROCYSTS				
High magnification view of pupil margin Clear cornea	Single microcysts at pupillary margin Microcyst displays reversed illumination	16 microcysts Some appear faint (newly formed)	About 70 microcysts Some microcysts at the surface stain with fluorescein	About 180 microcysts Many at the surface stain with fluorescein
CORNEAL OEDEMA				
Clear cornea and 3 mm wide parallelepiped Left: endothelium Centre: stroma Right: epithelium	Single vertical stria in posterior cornea	Three vertical striae in posterior cornea	Many vertical striae in posterior cornea Folds in endothelium	Many vertical striae in posterior cornea Many folds in endothelium Epithelial bullae
CORNEAL STAINING				
Clear cornea No staining Fluorescein in eye Cobalt blue reflex	Light punctate staining Slight conjunctival redness	More punctate staining Increased redness	Light pan-corneal punctate staining Diffuse reflex	Heavy pan-corneal punctate staining Very diffuse reflex
CONJUNCTIVAL STAINING				
Clear cornea Fluorescein pooling in some folds Cobalt blue reflex	Increased fluorescein pooling in folds Slight staining at position of lens edge	More fluorescein pooling in folds Interrupted lens edge staining Increased conjunctival redness	Widespread fluorescein pooling in folds Continuous lens edge staining Conjunctival redness	Widespread fluorescein pooling in folds Heavy lens edge staining Conjunctival redness Limbal staining
PAPILLARY CONJUNCTIVITIS				
Pale conjunctiva Vessels clearly visible Slight roughness at tarsal fold	Pink conjunctiva Vessels visible Increased roughness at tarsal fold	Red conjunctiva Vessels less visible Papillae at tarsal fold Reflexes on some papillae	Very red conjunctiva Vessels barely visible Large papillae Bright papillary reflexes Single mucus strand	Extremely red conjunctiva Vessels not visible Very large papillae Bright papillary reflexes More mucus strands

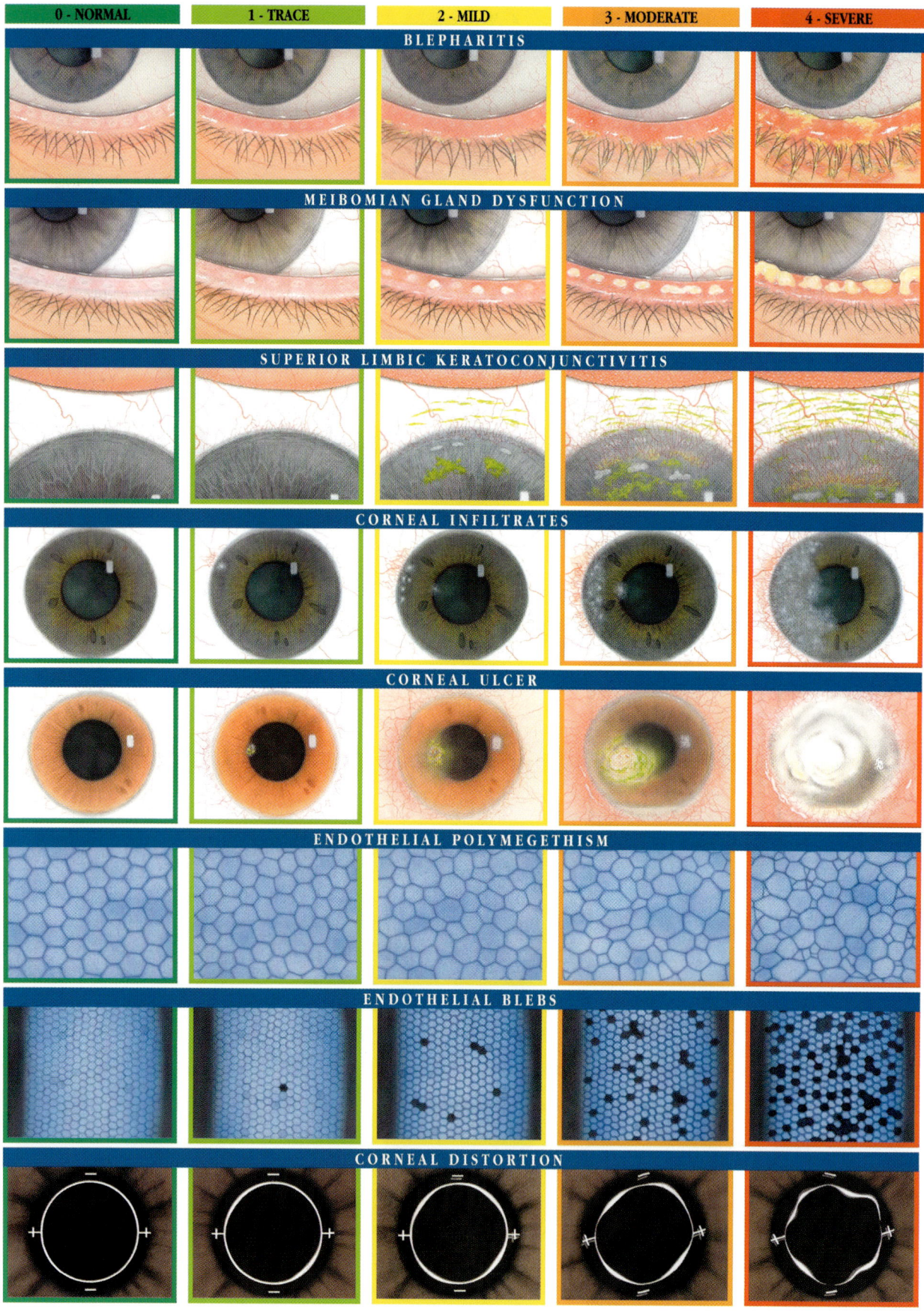

0 - NORMAL	1 - TRACE	2 - MILD	3 - MODERATE	4 - SEVERE
BLEPHARITIS				
Pale lid margin Openings of meibomian glands visible Clean lashes	Pink lid margin Openings of meibomian glands less visible Clean lashes	Red lid margin Openings of meibomian glands barely visible Yellow crust at base of lashes Some lashes stuck together	Telangiectasis of lid margin Increased crusting More lashes stuck together Bulbar conjunctival redness	Severe telangiectasis of lid margin Excess yellow crusting Lashes stuck together Increased bulbar conjunctival redness Skin irritation
MEIBOMIAN GLAND DYSFUNCTION				
Pale lid margin Openings of meibomian glands visible Clean lashes	Pink lid margin Cloudy expression at some gland orifices	Red lid margin Milky expression at most gland orifices Increased tearing	Red lid margin Yellow expression at all gland orifices Expressions becoming continuous	Thick creamy yellow expression at all gland orifices Expressions continuous Bulbar conjunctival redness
SUPERIOR LIMBIC KERATOCONJUNCTIVITIS				
Clear conjunctiva Clear superior limbus Clear cornea Clear reflex	Increased conjunctival redness Slight limbal redness Clear cornea	Conjunctival redness and staining Increased limbal redness Corneal staining and infiltrates	Greater conjunctival redness and staining Increased limbal redness 2–3 mm fibrovascular pannus Greater corneal staining and infiltrates	Severe conjunctival redness and staining Severe limbal redness 5 mm fibrovascular pannus Severe corneal staining and infiltrates
CORNEAL INFILTRATES				
Clear cornea Clear conjunctiva and limbus Clear reflex	Single small grey infiltrate at 10 o'clock near limbus Adjacent limbal redness	Five small grey infiltrates at 9–10 o'clock near limbus Adjacent limbus more red	Numerous small hazy gray infiltrates at 8–10 o'clock in peripheral cornea Adjacent limbus very red	Hazy grey confluent infiltrates that cover left half of cornea Adjacent limbal redness from 5 to 11 o'clock Mild conjunctival redness
CORNEAL ULCER				
Clear cornea Clear conjunctiva and limbus Clear reflex	<1 mm corneal ulcer at left pupil margin Stains with fluorescein Mild limbal redness at 7–11 o'clock	2–3mm corneal ulcer Haze around ulcer Intense limbal redness at 7–11 o'clock Ciliary flush	6 mm corneal ulcer Haze around ulcer General corneal haze Intense circumlimbal redness Conjunctival redness Increased ciliary flush	White pan-corneal ulcer Cornea opaque Intense circumlimbal and conjunctival redness Intense ciliary flush
ENDOTHELIAL POLYMEGETHISM				
Cells same size Hexagonal shape Coefficient of variation (COV) = 0.15	Small variance in cell size COV = 0.25	Increased variance in cell size COV = 0.35 Some five-, six- and seven-sided cells	Considerable variance in cell size COV = 0.45 Some three-, four-, five-, six- and seven-sided cells	Substantial variance in cell size COV = 0.55 Some three-, four-, five-, six-, seven-, eight- and nine-sided cells
ENDOTHELIAL BLEBS				
Cells same size Hexagonal shape No blebs	One bleb	Three single blebs Two double-cell blebs	Large number of blebs 'Thickened' cell borders	Very large number of blebs Increased spacing between cells
CORNEAL DISTORTION				
Bright, sharp, circular keratometer mire	Slightly distorted keratometer mire Variation in thickness of circle	Distorted keratometer mire Variation in thickness of circle Loss of focus of right and top ± signs	Very distorted keratometer mire Greater variation in thickness of circle Loss of focus and distortion of all ± signs	Extremely distorted keratometer mire Greater variation in thickness of circle with some gaps Loss of focus and distortion of all ± signs

Appendix C

Appendix D
Vertex distance correction
Effective power (D) of plus- and minus-prescription spectacle lenses at the corneal plane for various vertex distances (mm)*. Courtesy of Adrian S. Bruce

Spec Rx (D)	Power (D) at Corneal Plane for Different Vertex Distances (mm)									
	8 mm		10 mm		12 mm		14 mm		16 mm	
	plus	minus	plus	minus	plus	minus	plus	minus	plus	minus
4.00	4.13	3.88	4.17	3.85	4.20	3.82	4.24	3.79	4.27	3.76
4.25	4.40	4.11	4.44	4.08	4.48	4.04	4.52	4.01	4.56	3.98
4.50	4.67	4.34	4.71	4.31	4.76	4.27	4.80	4.23	4.85	4.20
4.75	4.94	4.58	4.99	4.53	5.04	4.49	5.09	4.45	5.14	4.41
5.00	5.21	4.81	5.26	4.76	5.32	4.72	5.38	4.67	5.43	4.63
5.25	5.48	5.04	5.54	4.99	5.60	4.94	5.67	4.89	5.73	4.84
5.50	5.75	5.27	5.82	5.21	5.89	5.16	5.96	5.11	6.03	5.06
5.75	6.03	5.50	6.10	5.44	6.18	5.38	6.25	5.32	6.33	5.27
6.00	6.30	5.73	6.38	5.66	6.47	5.60	6.55	5.54	6.64	5.47
6.25	6.58	5.95	6.67	5.88	6.76	5.81	6.85	5.75	6.94	5.68
6.50	6.86	6.18	6.95	6.10	7.05	6.03	7.15	5.96	7.25	5.89
6.75	7.14	6.40	7.24	6.32	7.34	6.24	7.45	6.17	7.57	6.09
7.00	7.42	6.63	7.53	6.54	7.64	6.46	7.76	6.38	7.88	6.29
7.25	7.70	6.85	7.82	6.76	7.94	6.67	8.07	6.58	8.20	6.50
7.50	7.98	7.08	8.11	6.98	8.24	6.88	8.38	6.79	8.52	6.70
7.75	8.26	7.30	8.40	7.19	8.54	7.09	8.69	6.99	8.85	6.90
8.00	8.55	7.52	8.70	7.41	8.85	7.30	9.01	7.19	9.17	7.09
8.25	8.83	7.74	8.99	7.62	9.16	7.51	9.33	7.40	9.50	7.29
8.50	9.12	7.96	9.29	7.83	9.47	7.71	9.65	7.60	9.84	7.48
8.75	9.41	8.18	9.59	8.05	9.78	7.92	9.97	7.80	10.17	7.68
9.00	9.70	8.40	9.89	8.26	10.09	8.12	10.30	7.99	10.51	7.87
9.25	9.99	8.61	10.19	8.47	10.40	8.33	10.63	8.19	10.86	8.06
9.50	10.28	8.83	10.50	8.68	10.72	8.53	10.96	8.38	11.20	8.25
9.75	10.57	9.04	10.80	8.88	11.04	8.73	11.29	8.58	11.55	8.43
10.00	10.87	9.26	11.11	9.09	11.36	8.93	11.63	8.77	11.90	8.62
10.25	11.17	9.47	11.42	9.30	11.69	9.13	11.97	8.96	12.26	8.81
10.50	11.46	9.69	11.73	9.50	12.01	9.33	12.31	9.15	12.62	8.99
10.75	11.76	9.90	12.04	9.71	12.34	9.52	12.65	9.34	12.98	9.17
11.00	12.06	10.11	12.36	9.91	12.67	9.72	13.00	9.53	13.35	9.35
11.25	12.36	10.32	12.68	10.11	13.01	9.91	13.35	9.72	13.72	9.53
11.50	12.67	10.53	12.99	10.31	13.34	10.11	13.71	9.91	14.09	9.71
11.75	12.97	10.74	13.31	10.51	13.68	10.30	14.06	10.09	14.47	9.89
12.00	13.27	10.95	13.64	10.71	14.02	10.49	14.42	10.27	14.85	10.07

Effective power (D) of plus- and minus-prescription spectacle lenses at the corneal plane for various vertex distances (mm)*. Courtesy of Adrian S. Bruce (continued)

Spec Rx (D)	Power (D) at Corneal Plane for Different Vertex Distances (mm)									
	8 mm		10 mm		12 mm		14 mm		16 mm	
	plus	minus	plus	minus	plus	minus	plus	minus	plus	minus
12.25	13.58	11.16	13.96	10.91	14.36	10.68	14.79	10.46	15.24	10.24
12.50	13.89	11.36	14.29	11.11	14.71	10.87	15.15	10.64	15.63	10.42
12.75	14.20	11.57	14.61	11.31	15.05	11.06	15.52	10.82	16.02	10.59
13.00	14.51	11.78	14.94	11.50	15.40	11.25	15.89	11.00	16.41	10.76
13.25	14.82	11.98	15.27	11.70	15.76	11.43	16.27	11.18	16.81	10.93
13.50	15.13	12.18	15.61	11.89	16.11	11.62	16.65	11.35	17.22	11.10
13.75	15.45	12.39	15.94	12.09	16.47	11.80	17.03	11.53	17.63	11.27
14.00	15.77	12.59	16.28	12.28	16.83	11.99	17.41	11.71	18.04	11.44
14.25	16.08	12.79	16.62	12.47	17.19	12.17	17.80	11.88	18.46	11.60
14.50	16.40	12.99	16.96	12.66	17.55	12.35	18.19	12.05	18.88	11.77
14.75	16.72	13.19	17.30	12.85	17.92	12.53	18.59	12.23	19.31	11.93
15.00	17.05	13.39	17.65	13.04	18.29	12.71	18.99	12.40	19.74	12.10
15.25	17.37	13.59	17.99	13.23	18.67	12.89	19.39	12.57	20.17	12.26
15.50	17.69	13.79	18.34	13.42	19.04	13.07	19.80	12.74	20.61	12.42
15.75	18.02	13.99	18.69	13.61	19.42	13.25	20.21	12.90	21.06	12.58
16.00	18.35	14.18	19.05	13.79	19.80	13.42	20.62	13.07	21.51	12.74
16.25	18.68	14.38	19.40	13.98	20.19	13.60	21.04	13.24	21.96	12.90
16.50	19.01	14.58	19.76	14.16	20.57	13.77	21.46	13.40	22.42	13.05
16.75	19.34	14.77	20.12	14.35	20.96	13.95	21.88	13.57	22.88	13.21
17.00	19.68	14.96	20.48	14.53	21.36	14.12	22.31	13.73	23.35	13.36
17.25	20.01	15.16	20.85	14.71	21.75	14.29	22.74	13.89	23.83	13.52
17.50	20.35	15.35	21.21	14.89	22.15	14.46	23.18	14.06	24.31	13.67
17.75	20.69	15.54	21.58	15.07	22.55	14.63	23.62	14.22	24.79	13.82
18.00	21.03	15.73	21.95	15.25	22.96	14.80	24.06	14.38	25.28	13.98
18.25	21.37	15.92	22.32	15.43	23.37	14.97	24.51	14.54	25.78	14.13
18.50	21.71	16.11	22.70	15.61	23.78	15.14	24.97	14.69	26.28	14.27
18.75	22.06	16.30	23.08	15.79	24.19	15.31	25.42	14.85	26.79	14.42
19.00	22.41	16.49	23.46	15.97	24.61	15.47	25.89	15.01	27.30	14.57
19.25	22.75	16.68	23.84	16.14	25.03	15.64	26.35	15.16	27.82	14.72
19.50	23.10	16.87	24.22	16.32	25.46	15.80	26.82	15.32	28.34	14.86
19.75	23.46	17.06	24.61	16.49	25.88	15.97	27.30	15.47	28.87	15.01
20.00	23.81	17.24	25.00	16.67	26.32	16.13	27.78	15.63	29.41	15.15

* Based on the equation: OR = SR/(1−[d × SR]), where
OR = ocular refraction
SR = spectacle refraction
d = vertex distance (m)
* The lens powers enclosed within the heavy border relate to the standard vertex distance of 12mm that will apply in most cases.

Appendix D

Appendix E
Extended keratometer range conversion
Conversion of keratometer reading (D) to its extended value (D) when a +1.25D lens (for steep corneas) or a −1.00D lens (for flat corneas) is held in front of the keratometer*. Courtesy of Adrian S. Bruce

Steep Corneas (using a +1.25D lens)[a]

Keratometer Reading (D)	Extended Value (D)	Keratometer Reading (D)	Extended Value (D)	Keratometer Reading (D)	Extended Value (D)
43.00	50.13	46.13	53.78	49.25	57.42
43.13	50.28	46.25	53.92	49.38	57.57
43.25	50.42	46.38	54.07	49.50	57.71
43.38	50.57	46.50	54.21	49.63	57.86
43.50	50.72	46.63	54.36	49.75	58.00
43.63	50.86	46.75	54.51	49.88	58.15
43.75	51.01	46.88	54.65	50.00	58.30
43.88	51.15	47.00	54.80	50.13	58.44
44.00	51.30	47.13	54.94	50.25	58.59
44.13	51.44	47.25	55.09	50.38	58.73
44.25	51.59	47.38	55.23	50.50	58.88
44.38	51.74	47.50	55.38	50.63	59.02
44.50	51.88	47.63	55.53	50.75	59.17
44.63	52.03	47.75	55.67	50.88	59.32
44.75	52.17	47.88	55.82	51.00	59.46
44.88	52.32	48.00	55.96	51.13	59.61
45.00	52.47	48.13	56.11	51.25	59.75
45.13	52.61	48.25	56.25	51.38	59.90
45.25	52.76	48.38	56.40	51.50	60.04
45.38	52.90	48.50	56.55	51.63	60.19
45.50	53.05	48.63	56.69	51.75	60.34
45.63	53.19	48.75	56.84	51.88	60.48
45.75	53.34	48.88	56.98	52.00	60.63
45.88	53.49	49.00	57.13		
46.00	53.63	49.13	57.27		

[a] Based on the equation: Extended = (1.166 × Keratometer) − 0.005

Conversion of keratometer reading (D) to its extended value (D) when a +1.25D lens (for steep corneas) or a −1.00D lens (for flat corneas) is held in front of the keratometer*. Courtesy of Adrian S. Bruce (continued)

Flat Corneas (using a −1.00D lens)[b]

Keratometer Reading (D)	Extended Value (D)	Keratometer Reading (D)	Extended Value (D)	Keratometer Reading (D)	Extended Value (D)
36.00	30.87	38.12	32.70	40.25	34.52
36.12	30.98	38.25	32.80	40.37	34.63
36.25	31.09	38.37	32.91	40.50	34.73
36.37	31.19	38.50	33.02	40.62	34.84
36.50	31.30	38.62	33.12	40.75	34.95
36.62	31.41	38.75	33.23	40.87	35.06
36.75	31.52	38.87	33.34	41.00	35.16
36.87	31.62	39.00	33.45	41.12	35.27
37.00	31.73	39.12	33.55	41.25	35.38
37.12	31.84	39.25	33.66	41.37	35.48
37.25	31.94	39.37	33.77	41.50	35.59
37.37	32.05	39.50	33.88	41.62	35.70
37.50	32.16	39.62	33.98	41.75	35.81
37.62	32.27	39.75	34.09	41.87	35.91
37.75	32.37	39.87	34.20	42.00	36.02
37.87	32.48	40.00	34.30		
38.00	32.59	40.12	34.41		

[b] Based on the equation: Extended = (1.858 × Keratometer) −0.014

* Derived from data in: Mandell, R.B. (1988) Dioptral and mm curves for extended keratometer range. Appendix 7. In Contact Lens Practice 4th ed. pp. 998–999. Charles C. Thomas.

Appendix F
Corneal curvature – corneal power conversion
Conversion between corneal front surface radius of curvature (r; mm) and corneal power (K; D)*. Courtesy of Adrian S. Bruce

r (mm)	K (D)	r (mm)	K (D)	r (mm)	K (D)	r (mm)	K (D)	r (mm)	K (D)
6.30	53.57	6.99	48.28	7.63	44.23	8.27	40.81	8.91	37.88
6.36	53.07	7.00	48.21	7.64	44.18	8.28	40.76	8.92	37.84
6.37	52.98	7.01	48.15	7.65	44.12	8.29	40.71	8.93	37.79
6.38	52.90	7.02	48.08	7.66	44.06	8.30	40.66	8.94	37.75
6.39	52.82	7.03	48.01	7.67	44.00	8.31	40.61	8.95	37.71
6.40	52.73	7.04	47.94	7.68	43.95	8.32	40.56	8.96	37.67
6.41	52.65	7.05	47.87	7.69	43.89	8.33	40.52	8.97	37.63
6.42	52.57	7.06	47.80	7.70	43.83	8.34	40.47	8.98	37.58
6.43	52.49	7.07	47.74	7.71	43.77	8.35	40.42	8.99	37.54
6.44	52.41	7.08	47.67	7.72	43.72	8.36	40.37	9.00	37.50
6.45	52.33	7.09	47.60	7.73	43.66	8.37	40.32	9.01	37.46
6.46	52.24	7.10	47.54	7.74	43.60	8.38	40.27	9.02	37.42
6.47	52.16	7.11	47.47	7.75	43.55	8.39	40.23	9.03	37.38
6.48	52.08	7.12	47.40	7.76	43.49	8.40	40.18	9.04	37.33
6.49	52.00	7.13	47.34	7.77	43.44	8.41	40.13	9.05	37.29
6.50	51.92	7.14	47.27	7.78	43.38	8.42	40.08	9.06	37.25
6.51	51.84	7.15	47.20	7.79	43.32	8.43	40.04	9.07	37.21
6.52	51.76	7.16	47.14	7.80	43.27	8.44	39.99	9.08	37.17
6.53	51.68	7.17	47.07	7.81	43.21	8.45	39.94	9.09	37.13
6.54	51.61	7.18	47.01	7.82	43.16	8.46	39.89	9.10	37.09
6.55	51.53	7.19	46.94	7.83	43.10	8.47	39.85	9.11	37.05
6.56	51.45	7.20	46.88	7.84	43.05	8.48	39.80	9.12	37.01
6.57	51.37	7.21	46.81	7.85	42.99	8.49	39.75	9.13	36.97
6.58	51.29	7.22	46.75	7.86	42.94	8.50	39.71	9.14	36.93
6.59	51.21	7.23	46.68	7.87	42.88	8.51	39.66	9.15	36.89
6.60	51.14	7.24	46.62	7.88	42.83	8.52	39.61	9.16	36.84
6.61	51.06	7.25	46.55	7.89	42.78	8.53	39.57	9.17	36.80
6.62	50.98	7.26	46.49	7.90	42.72	8.54	39.52	9.18	36.76
6.63	50.90	7.27	46.42	7.91	42.67	8.55	39.47	9.19	36.72
6.64	50.83	7.28	46.36	7.92	42.61	8.56	39.43	9.20	36.68
6.65	50.75	7.29	46.30	7.93	42.56	8.57	39.38	9.21	36.64
6.66	50.68	7.30	46.23	7.94	42.51	8.58	39.34	9.22	36.61
6.67	50.60	7.31	46.17	7.95	42.45	8.59	39.29	9.23	36.57
6.68	50.52	7.32	46.11	7.96	42.40	8.60	39.24	9.24	36.53
6.69	50.45	7.33	46.04	7.97	42.35	8.61	39.20	9.25	36.49
6.70	50.37	7.34	45.98	7.98	42.29	8.62	39.15	9.26	36.45
6.71	50.30	7.35	45.92	7.99	42.24	8.63	39.11	9.27	36.41
6.72	50.22	7.36	45.86	8.00	42.19	8.64	39.06	9.28	36.37
6.73	50.15	7.37	45.79	8.01	42.13	8.65	39.02	9.29	36.33
6.74	50.07	7.38	45.73	8.02	42.08	8.66	38.97	9.30	36.29
6.75	50.00	7.39	45.67	8.03	42.03	8.67	38.93	9.31	36.25
6.76	49.93	7.40	45.61	8.04	41.98	8.68	38.88	9.32	36.21
6.77	49.85	7.41	45.55	8.05	41.93	8.69	38.84	9.33	36.17
6.78	49.78	7.42	45.49	8.06	41.87	8.70	38.79	9.34	36.13
6.79	49.71	7.43	45.42	8.07	41.82	8.71	38.75	9.35	36.10
6.80	49.63	7.44	45.36	8.08	41.77	8.72	38.70	9.36	36.06
6.81	49.56	7.45	45.30	8.09	41.72	8.73	38.66	9.37	36.02

Conversion between corneal front surface radius of curvature (r; mm) and corneal power (K; D)*. Courtesy of Adrian S. Bruce (continued)

r (mm)	K (D)	r (mm)	K (D)	r (mm)	K (D)	r (mm)	K (D)	r (mm)	K (D)
6.82	49.49	7.46	45.24	8.10	41.67	8.74	38.62	9.38	35.98
6.83	49.41	7.47	45.18	8.11	41.62	8.75	38.57	9.39	35.94
6.84	49.34	7.48	45.12	8.12	41.56	8.76	38.53	9.40	35.90
6.85	49.27	7.49	45.06	8.13	41.51	8.77	38.48	9.41	35.87
6.86	49.20	7.50	45.00	8.14	41.46	8.78	38.44	9.42	35.83
6.87	49.13	7.51	44.94	8.15	41.41	8.79	38.40	9.43	35.79
6.88	49.06	7.52	44.88	8.16	41.36	8.80	38.35	9.44	35.75
6.89	48.98	7.53	44.82	8.17	41.31	8.81	38.31	9.45	35.71
6.90	48.91	7.54	44.76	8.18	41.26	8.82	38.27	9.46	35.68
6.91	48.84	7.55	44.70	8.19	41.21	8.83	38.22	9.47	35.64
6.92	48.77	7.56	44.64	8.20	41.16	8.84	38.18	9.48	35.60
6.93	48.70	7.57	44.58	8.21	41.11	8.85	38.14	9.49	35.56
6.94	48.63	7.58	44.53	8.22	41.06	8.86	38.09	9.50	35.53
6.95	48.56	7.59	44.47	8.23	41.01	8.87	38.05	9.51	35.49
6.96	48.49	7.60	44.41	8.24	40.96	8.88	38.01	9.52	35.45
6.97	48.42	7.61	44.35	8.25	40.91	8.89	37.96	9.53	35.41
6.98	48.35	7.62	44.29	8.26	40.86	8.90	37.92	9.54	35.38

* Based on the equation: Surface power (D) = (1.3375 − 1.0)/radius (m)

Appendix G
Contact lens manufacturing tolerances
Dimensional tolerances for soft, PMMA and rigid lenses (all units in mm)

Dimension	Soft Lenses	PMMA Lenses	Rigid Lenses
Back optic zone radius	±0.20	±0.025	±0.05
Back optic zone radii of toroidal surfaces where the difference in radii is:			
<0.20		±0.25	±0.05
0.2–0.4		±0.35	±0.06
0.4–0.6		±0.55	±0.07
>0.6		±0.75	±0.09
Sagitta at specified diameter	±0.05		
Back optic zone diameter	±0.20	±0.025	±0.05
Back peripheral radius		±0.10	±0.10
Front peripheral radius		±0.10	±0.10
Back peripheral diameter		±0.20	±0.20
Total diameter	±0.20	±0.10	±0.10
Front optic zone diameter	±0.20	±0.20	±0.20
Bifocal segment height		−0.10 to +0.20	−0.10 to +0.20
Centre thickness		±0.02	±0.02
Centre thickness, where the nominal value is:			
≤0.10	±0.010 + 10%		
>0.10	±0.015 + 5%		

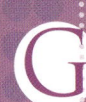

Optical tolerances for soft, PMMA and rigid lenses

Dimension	Soft Lenses	PMMA Lenses	Rigid Lenses
Back vertex power			
≤5D		±0.12D	±0.12D
≤10D	±0.25D	±0.18D	±0.18D
≤15D		±0.25D	±0.25D
≤20D	±0.50D	±0.37D	±0.37D
>20D	±1.00D	±0.50D	±0.50D
Cylinder power			
≤2D	±0.25D	±0.25D	±0.25D
2–4D	±0.37D	±0.37D	±0.37D
>4D	±0.50D	±0.50D	±0.50D
Cylinder axis	±5°	±5°	±5°
Prismatic error			
(measured at the geometric			
centre of the optic zone)			
Back vertex power <6D		±0.25cm/m	±0.25cm/m
Back vertex power >6D		±0.50cm/m	±0.50cm/m
Prescribed prism		±0.25cm/m	±0.25cm/m

Material property tolerances for soft lenses

Material Property	Tolerance
Refractive index	±0.005
Water content	±2%
Oxygen permeability	±20%

- The tolerances outlined in this appendix were obtained from the following standards:
  ISO 8321–1: 1991 Optics and optical instruments – Contact Lenses – Part 1: Specification for rigid corneal and scleral contact lenses.
  BS ENISO 8321–2: 2000 (BS 7208–24:2000) Ophthalmic optics – Specifications for material, optical and dimensional properties of contact lenses – Part 2: Single-vision hydrogel contact lenses.
- PMMA tolerances are given here because trial lens fitting sets are often fabricated from this material due to its resilience.
- See also: Hough, T. (2000) A Guide to Contact Lens Standards. British Contact Lens Association.

Appendix H
Terms, symbols and abbreviations
Terms, symbols and abbreviations used to describe contact lenses

Term	Symbol	Abbreviation
Back optic zone radius	r_0	BOZR
Back peripheral radius	$r_1, r_2, ...$	BPR1, BPR2, ...
Front optic zone radius	r_{a0}	FOZR
Front peripheral radius	$r_{a1}, r_{a2}, ...$	FPR1, FPR2, ...
Back optic zone diameter	$\varnothing_0$	BOZD
Back peripheral zone diameters	$\varnothing_1, \varnothing_2, ...$	BPZD1, BPZD2, ...
Total diameter	$\varnothing_T$	TD
Front optic zone diameter	$\varnothing_{a0}$	FOZD
Front peripheral zone diameters	$\varnothing_{a1}, \varnothing_{a2}, ...$	FPZD1, FPZD2, ...
Geometric centre thickness	t_c	tc
Carrier junction thickness	t_{a0}	tj
Peripheral junction thickness	$t_{a1}, t_{a2}, ...$	ta1, ta2, ...
Radial edge thickness	t_e	RET
Axial edge thickness	t_{ak}	AET
Radial edge lift	l_r	REL
Axial edge lift	l_a	AEL
Front vertex power	F_v	FVP
Back vertex power	F_v'	BVP
Oxygen flux	j	j
Oxygen permeability	Dk	Dk
Oxygen transmissibility	Dk/t	Dk/t

- The terms and symbols outlined above were obtained from the following standard:
  ISO8320–1986 Optics and optical instruments – Contact Lenses – Vocabulary and symbols.
- The abbreviations given above were modified from those suggested by:
  Hough, T. (2000) A Guide to Contact Lens Standards. British Contact Lens Association.